Yamada's Handbook of Gastroenterology

Yamada's Handbook of Gastroenterology

John M. Inadomi
University of Washington
Seattle
WA, USA

Renuka Bhattacharya
University of Washington
Seattle
WA, USA

Joo Ha Hwang
Stanford University
Stanford
CA, USA

Cynthia Ko
University of Washington
Seattle
WA, USA

FOURTH EDITION

WILEY Blackwell

Edition History [3e, 2013]

Registered Office(s)
John Wiley & Sons, Inc., 111 River Street, Hoboken, NJ 07030, USA
John Wiley & Sons Ltd, The Atrium, Southern Gate, Chichester, West Sussex, PO19 8SQ, UK

Editorial Office
9600 Garsington Road, Oxford, OX4 2DQ, UK

For details of our global editorial offices, customer services, and more information about Wiley products visit us at www.wiley.com.

Wiley also publishes its books in a variety of electronic formats and by print-on-demand. Some content that appears in standard print versions of this book may not be available in other formats.

Library of Congress Cataloging-in-Publication Data

Names: Inadomi, John M., author. | Bhattacharya, Renuka, author. | Hwang, Joo Ha, author. | Ko, Cynthia W., author.
Title: Yamada's handbook of gastroenterology / John M Inadomi, Renuka Bhattacharya, Joo Ha Hwang, Cynthia Ko.
Other titles: Handbook of gastroenterology | Yamada's textbook of gastroenterology.
Description: Fourth edition. | Hoboken, NJ : Wiley-Blackwell, 2020. | Includes bibliographical references and index.
Identifiers: LCCN 2019030447 (print) | LCCN 2019030448 (ebook) | ISBN 9781119515692 (paperback) | ISBN 9781119515760 (epub) | ISBN 9781119515746 (adobe pdf)
Subjects: MESH: Gastrointestinal Diseases | Handbook
Classification: LCC RC801 (print) | LCC RC801 (ebook) | NLM WI 39 | DDC 616.3/3–dc23
LC record available at https://lccn.loc.gov/2019030447
LC ebook record available at https://lccn.loc.gov/2019030448

Cover Design: Wiley
Cover Images: 4th and 7th image from left courtesy of John Inadomi, © SEBASTIAN KAULITZKI/Getty Images, © u3d/Shutterstock, © Explode/Shutterstock, © Magic mine/Shutterstock, © Victor Josan/Shutterstock, © Adao/Shutterstock

Set in 9.5/13pt Meridien by SPi Global, Pondicherry, India

SKY876D37D7-E149-4B42-A495-275E8A731907_032122

Contents

Color Plates List

Preface

On behalf of my co-authors, Drs. Bhattacharya, Hwang, and Ko, I am pleased to introduce the fourth edition of *Yamada's Handbook of Gastroenterology*. *Yamada's Handbook* is based on the *Textbook of Gastroenterology* and *Principles of Clinical Gastroenterology* by Dr. Tadataka Yamada and is divided into two major sections: symptom-based evaluation chapters and disease-based management chapters. In addition to updating the content for this version of *Yamada's Handbook*, in most chapters we have incorporated Key Practice Points, Essentials of Diagnosis, and Potential Pitfalls, easily identified in "call-out boxes," that highlight the most important factors that guide clinical care. We have written case scenarios accompanied by discussions for many of the chapters that we hope will provide the context necessary to translate medical knowledge to clinical practice. In addition, we have included a series of questions, with detailed answers located in the back of *Yamada's Handbook*, that provide a means to test and solidify the reader's knowledge base. New to this edition are references to recent national society clinical practice guidelines that have improved the timeliness of our recommendations. Finally, we have added endoscopic and radiographic images that illustrate the breadth and depth of our specialty (see the color plates section).

We hope *Yamada's Handbook of Gastroenterology* is a useful companion to the Yamada *Textbook of Gastroenterology* and *Principles of Clinical Gastroenterology*, especially for readers interested in a condensed reference guiding the care of patients with gastrointestinal and liver diseases. In addition, we expect that trainees of all levels will benefit from *Yamada's Handbook* by providing a solid foundation upon which they may build a comprehensive understanding of this exciting and rapidly evolving field of medicine.

John M. Inadomi
2019

List of Abbreviations

5-ASA 5-aminosalicylate
6-MMP 6-methylmercaptopurine
6-MP 6-mercaptopurine
6-TG 6-thioguanine
ACCR amylase-to-creatinine clearance ratio
ACE angiotensin-converting enzyme
ADH alcohol dehydrogenase
AFP α-fetoprotein (AFP
AIDS acquired immunodeficiency syndrome
AIH autoimmune hepatitis
ALD alcoholic liver disease
ALDH acetaldehyde dehydrogenase
ALT alanine aminotransferase
AMA antimitochondrial antibody
ANA antinuclear antibody
APC adenomatous polyposis coli; argon plasma coagulation
ASCA anti-*Saccharomyces cerevisiae* antibody
ASMA anti-smooth muscle antibody
AST aspartate aminotransferase
BRIC benign recurrent intrahepatic cholestasis
BUN blood urea nitrogen
CBC complete blood count
CC chronic constipation
CCK cholecystokinin
CDC Centers for Disease Control and Prevention
CEA carcinoembryonic antigen
CHRPE congenital hypertrophy of the retinal pigment epithelium
CREST calcinosis, Raynaud phenomenon, esophageal dysmotility, sclerodactyly, and telangiectasia
CRP C-reactive protein
CT computed tomography
CTC computed tomography colonography
DES diffuse esophageal spasm
DS double strength
EAC esophageal adenocarcinoma
ECG electrocardiogram
EGD esophagogastroduodenoscopy
EGG electrogastrography
EHEC enterohemorrhagic *Escherichia coli*
EIEC enteroinvasive *Escherichia coli*

ELISA enzyme-linked immunosorbent assay
EMR endoscopic mucosal resection
EPEC enteropathogenic *Escherichia coli*
ERCP endoscopic retrograde cholangiopancreatography
ERP endoscopic retrograde pancreatography
ESD endoscopic submucosal dissection
ESR erythrocyte sedimentation rate
ETEC enterotoxigenic *Escherichia coli*
EUS endoscopic ultrasound
FAP familial adenomatous polyposis
FIT fecal immunochemical test
FNA fine needle aspiration
FOBT fecal occult blood test
GABA γ-aminobutyric acid
GAVE gastric arteriovenous ectasia, gastric antral vascular ectasia
GERD gastroesophageal reflux disease
GGT γ-glutamyl-transferase
GI gastrointestinal
GIST gastrointestinal stromal tumor
HAART highly active antiretroviral therapy
HAV hepatitis A virus
HBIG hepatitis B immune globulin
HBV hepatitis B virus
HCC hepatocellular carcinoma
HCT hematocrit
HCV hepatitis C virus
HDV hepatitis D virus
HE hepatic encephalopathy
HEV hepatitis E virus
HGD high-grade dysplasia
HHC hereditary hemochromatosis
HIAA hydroxyindoleacetic acid
HII hepatic iron index
HIV human immunodeficiency virus
HNPCC hereditary nonpolyposis colorectal cancer
HPF high-power field
HVPG hepatic venous pressure gradient
IBD inflammatory bowel disease
IBS irritable bowel syndrome
IBS-C irritable bowel syndrome – constipation predominant
ICU intensive care unit
Ig immunoglobulin
IGF insulin-like growth factor
IHC immunohistochemistry
IL interleukin
IM intramuscular
I-MIBG I-labeled metaiodobenzylguanidine
INR international normalized ratio
IPMN intraductal papillary mucinous neoplasm
IPSID immunoproliferative small intestinal disease

IU international unit
IV intravenous
LAP leucine aminopeptidase
LDH lactate dehydrogenase
LES lower esophageal sphincter
MALT mucosa-associated lymphoid tissue
MCV mean corpuscular volume
MELD Model for End-Stage Liver Disease
MEN multiple endocrine neoplasia
MRCP magnetic resonance cholangiopancreatography
MRI magnetic resonance imaging
NADH nicotinamide adenine dinucleotide
NAFLD nonalcoholic fatty liver disease
NASH nonalcoholic steatohepatitis
NCCN National Comprehensive Cancer Network
NG nasogastric
NSAID nonsteroidal anti-inflammatory drug
OLT orthotopic liver transplantation
pANCA perinuclear antineutrophil cytoplasmic antibody
PAS periodic acid-Schiff
PBC primary biliary cirrhosis
PCNA proliferating cell nuclear antigen
PCR polymerase chain reaction
PDGFR platelet-derived growth factor receptor
PEG polyethylene glycol
PEI percutaneous ethanol injection
PET positron emission tomography
PFIC progressive familial intrahepatic cholestasis
PICC peripherally inserted central catheter
PJS Peutz–Jeghers syndrome
po *per os*
PPI proton pump inhibitor
PPN peripheral parenteral nutrition
PSBL primary small bowel lymphoma
PSC primary sclerosing cholangitis
PTC percutaneous transhepatic cholangiography
PUD peptic ulcer disease
qid *quater in die*
RFA radiofrequency ablation
RUQ right upper quadrant
SAAG serum-ascites albumin gradient
SBP spontaneous bacterial peritonitis
SCC squamous cell carcinoma
SGOT serum glutamic oxaloacetic transaminase
SGPT serum glutamic pyruvic transaminase
SLA soluble liver antigen
SO sphincter of Oddi
SOD sphincter of Oddi dysfunction
SVR sustained virological response
TACE transarterial chemoembolization

TARE transaterial radioembolization
TCA tricyclic antidepressant
TGF transforming growth factor
TIBC total iron-binding capacity
TIPS transjugular intrahepatic portosystemic shunt
TLESR transient lower esophageal sphincter relaxation
TNF tumor necrosis factor
TPMT thiopurine methyltransferase
TPN total parenteral nutrition
TSH thyroid-stimulating hormone
tTG tissue transglutaminase
TTS through-the-scope
UES upper esophageal sphincter
UGT uridine diphosphate glucuronosyltransferase
VCE video capsule endoscopy
VEGF vascular endothelial growth factor
VIP vasoactive intestinal peptide
WBC white blood count
WDHA watery diarrhea, hypokalemia, and achlorhydria
ZES Zollinger–Ellison syndrome

PART 1

Approach to Patients with Gastrointestinal Symptoms or Signs

CHAPTER 1
The Patient with Dysphagia or Odynophagia

Dysphagia is the sensation of food hindered in its passage from the mouth to the stomach. Dysphagia is differentiated from odynophagia (pain on swallowing) and from globus sensation (perception of a lump, tightness, or fullness in the throat that is temporarily relieved by swallowing). The act of swallowing has four phases: the oral preparation phase, the oral transfer phase, the pharyngeal phase, and the esophageal phase. An abnormality of any of the phases can produce dysphagia. Dysphagia is usually divided into two categories: (i) oropharyngeal: disorders of the oral preparation, oral transfer, or pharyngeal phases of swallowing; and (ii) esophageal: dysfunction of the esophageal phase of swallowing (Table 1.1). The etiology and evaluation of oropharyngeal and esophageal dysphagia differ, whereas odynophagia also has a distinct underlying differential diagnosis (Figure 1.1).

Clinical presentation

History

The patient's history helps define whether symptoms are oropharyngeal or esophageal in location and structural or neuromuscular in origin. If dysphagia occurs within one second of swallowing or is associated with drooling, choking, coughing, aspiration, or nasal regurgitation, an oropharyngeal process is likely. Conversely, an esophageal cause is more likely if dysphagia occurs more than one second after swallowing, if there is retrosternal pain, or if there is regurgitation of unchanged food. Dysphagia perceived in the cervical area may result from either oropharyngeal or esophageal disease. Dysphagia perceived below the suprasternal notch is nearly always diagnostic of an esophageal source. Structural esophageal disorders generally produce solid food dysphagia with progression to liquid dysphagia only if luminal narrowing becomes severe. Patients with neuromuscular disorders of the esophagus usually report both

Yamada's Handbook of Gastroenterology, Fourth Edition. John M. Inadomi, Renuka Bhattacharya, Joo Ha Hwang, and Cynthia Ko.

Table 1.1 Differential diagnosis of dysphagia and odynophagia

Oropharyngeal dysphagia
Neurologic disorders
Cerebrovascular accident
Parkinson disease
Amyotrophic lateral sclerosis
Brainstem tumors
Multiple sclerosis
Bulbar poliomyelitis
Myogenic disorders
Myasthenia gravis
Muscular dystrophies
Polymyositis
Local mechanical lesions
Inflammation (pharyngitis, abscess, tuberculosis, radiation, syphilis)
Neoplasm
Congenital webs
Extrinsic compression (thyromegaly, cervical spine hyperostosis, adenopathy)
Radiation or caustic damage
Foreign body
Upper esophageal sphincter(UES) disorders
Primary cricopharyngeal dysfunction
Cricopharyngeal bar
Zenker diverticulum
Esophageal dysphagia
Motor disorders
Achalasia
Scleroderma or other rheumatologic conditions
Spastic motor disorders, such as jackhammer esophagus or diffuse esophageal spasm
Esophagogastric junction outflow obstruction
Chagas disease
Ineffective esophageal motility
Fragmented esophageal peristalsis
Intrinsic mechanical lesions
Benign stricture (peptic, caustic, radiation)
Schatzki ring
Carcinoma
Eosinophilic esophagitis
Esophageal webs
Esophageal diverticula
Benign tumors
Foreign bodies
Extrinsic mechanical lesions
Vascular compression – aberrant subclavian artery or thoracic aortic aneurysm
Mediastinal abnormalities
Cervical osteoarthritis
Foreign body
Functional dysphagia

Table 1.1 *(cont'd)*

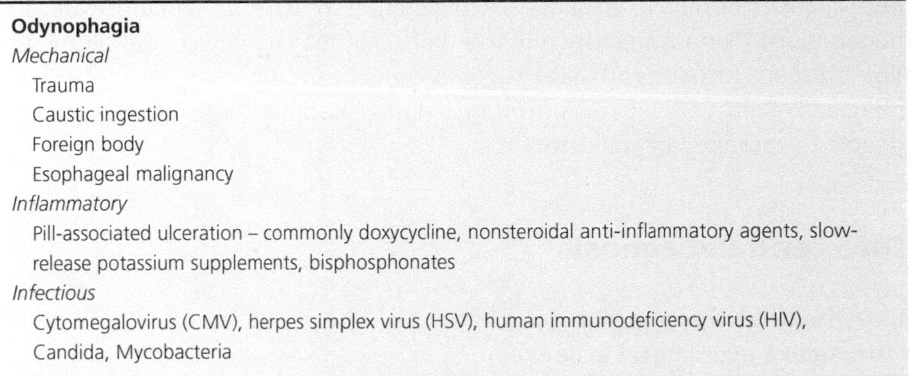

Odynophagia
Mechanical
Trauma
Caustic ingestion
Foreign body
Esophageal malignancy
Inflammatory
Pill-associated ulceration – commonly doxycycline, nonsteroidal anti-inflammatory agents, slow-release potassium supplements, bisphosphonates
Infectious
Cytomegalovirus (CMV), herpes simplex virus (HSV), human immunodeficiency virus (HIV), Candida, Mycobacteria

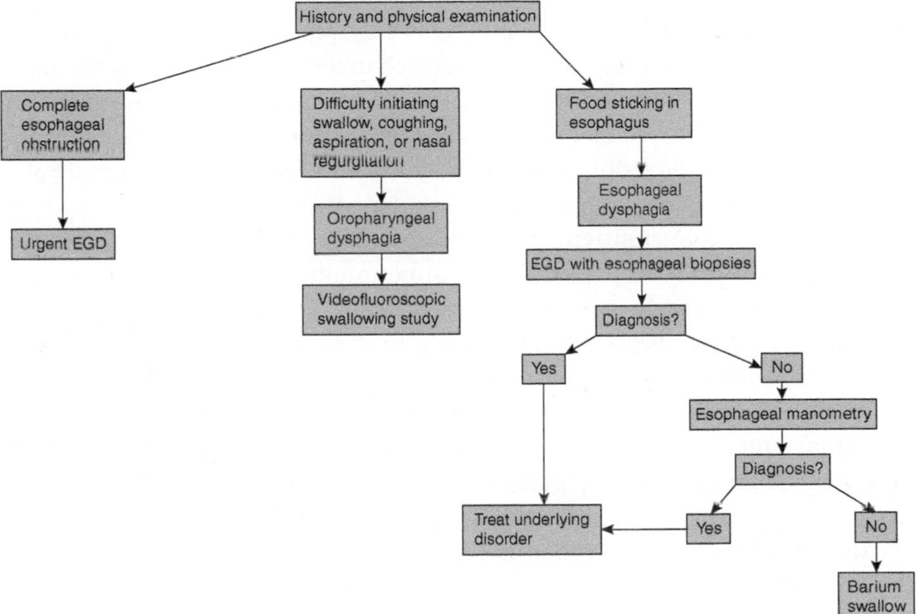

Figure 1.1 Evaluation of dysphagia or odynophagia. EGD, esophagogastroduodenoscopy.

liquid and solid dysphagia from symptom onset. Both structural and neuromuscular oropharyngeal disorders produce early liquid dysphagia. Patients with oropharyngeal dysphagia are commonly evaluated and co-managed with otolaryngologists or neurologists.

In patients with odynophagia, risk factors for opportunistic infection should be assessed and a careful medication history taken.

Physical examination

The head and neck must be examined for sensory and motor function of the cranial nerves, masses, adenopathy, or spinal deformity. Evidence of systemic disease, including sclerodactyly, telangiectasias, and calcinosis in scleroderma; neuropathies or muscle weakness from generalized neuromuscular disease; and hepatomegaly or adenopathy due to esophageal malignancy should be sought. The presence of oral candidiasis suggests fungal infection as a cause of odynophagia. Weight and general nutritional status should be assessed in case dysphagia has resulted in malnutrition.

Differential diagnosis

Esophageal dysphagia

Obstructive esophageal lesions

Esophageal dysphagia is most commonly caused by structural lesions that physically impede bolus transit. Patients with esophageal strictures secondary to acid peptic damage may present with progressive dysphagia after a long history of heartburn. These strictures usually are located in the distal esophagus, but more proximal strictures may develop at the transition point to columnar mucosa in patients with Barrett esophagus. A Schatzki ring, a thin, circumferential mucosal structure at the gastroesophageal junction, causes episodic and nonprogressive dysphagia. Eosinophilic esophagitis should be considered in younger patients who present with intermittent solid food dysphagia or food impaction, particularly in those with a history of allergic or eosinophilic disorders. Patients with esophageal malignancies report progressive symptoms, often starting primarily with solid food dysphagia but progressing to dysphagia for liquids. Relatively recent onset of symptoms and presence of alarm symptoms should prompt rapid evaluation to rule out a malignant etiology. Other mechanical lesions (e.g. abnormal great vessel anatomy, mediastinal lymphadenopathy, and cervical vertebral spurs) can cause dysphagia.

Motor disorders of the esophagus

Primary and secondary disorders of esophageal motor activity represent the other main etiology of esophageal dysphagia. Primary achalasia is an idiopathic disorder characterized by dysmotility of the esophageal body and failure of lower esophageal sphincter (LES) relaxation on swallowing with or without associated LES hypertension. Primary achalasia can be categorized into three types using esophageal manometry. Type 1 achalasia is characterized by poor or absent esophageal peristalsis along with incomplete relaxation of the LES. Type 2 is characterized by pan-esophageal pressurization, and type 3 by spastic esophageal contractions.

Conditions that mimic primary achalasia include secondary achalasia, a disorder with identical radiographic and manometric characteristics caused by malignancy at the gastroesophageal junction or by paraneoplastic effects of a distant tumor, and Chagas disease, which results from infection with

Trypanosoma cruzi. Some patients have esophagogastric junction outflow obstruction, which can be defined by esophageal manometry and may be due to incompletely expressed achalasia or mechanical obstruction. Other spastic esophageal disorders, such as jackhammer esophagus or diffuse esophageal spasm, have also been associated with dysphagia. Many patients with esophageal dysphagia have ineffective motility or fragmented esophageal peristalsis, which are best diagnosed with esophageal manometry. Systemic diseases (e.g. scleroderma and other rheumatic diseases) also cause dysphagia because of reduced rather than spastic esophageal motor function.

Odynophagia

Oropharyngeal odynophagia most commonly results from malignancy, foreign body ingestion, or mucosal ulceration. Esophageal odynophagia usually is a consequence of caustic ingestion, infection (e.g. *Candida albicans*, herpes simplex virus, cytomegalovirus), radiation damage, pill esophagitis, or ulcer disease induced by acid reflux (see Table 1.1).

Diagnostic investigation

Patients who present with complete obstruction with inability to handle oral secretions should undergo urgent upper endoscopy. Contrast radiography is not only associated with an aspiration risk; lesions found on radiography may be obscured by the contrast media. Airway protection is mandatory, so there should be a low threshold for endotracheal intubation or use of an esophageal or gastric overtube.

In the absence of complete obstruction, the history further dictates the next step in investigation. For dysphagia of presumed esophageal origin, upper endoscopy is the test of choice for evaluation and possibly treatment of anatomic abnormalities. Strictures or Schatzki rings can be dilated at the time of endoscopy. If no structural lesion is found, biopsies from the proximal-to-mid and distal esophagus should be taken to exclude eosinophilic esophagitis. If no etiology is identified on upper endoscopy, esophageal manometry should be performed to determine if an esophageal motility disorder is present. Barium swallow radiography can also be helpful to evaluate esophageal transit or to reveal subtle anatomic abnormalities.

Oropharyngeal dysphagia is best evaluated by a video-fluoroscopic swallowing study. Videofluoroscopy of mastication and swallowing of thin liquids, thick liquids, and solids is helpful in examining the coordination of the swallowing process in patients with suspected neuromuscular disease and potentially directing therapy. In some instances, specialized manometry can reveal abnormal upper esophageal sphincter (UES) relaxations. Transnasal or peroral endoscopy also may reveal vocal cord dysfunction but is rarely diagnostic in this setting.

Because mucosal lesions are common, endoscopy is the procedure of choice for odynophagia. If endoscopy is nondiagnostic, esophageal manometry can be useful to identify motility disorders than can cause odynophagia, such as achalasia or diffuse esophageal spasm.

Management

Dysphagia

Selected causes of oropharyngeal dysphagia, including Parkinson disease, hypothyroidism, polymyositis, and myasthenia gravis, may have specific therapies. Surgical myotomy may benefit patients with Zenker diverticulum or cricopharyngeal achalasia. A few limited studies suggest that myotomy also may be useful in treating selected cases of neuromuscular disease. For untreatable neuromuscular conditions, consultation with a speech pathologist may afford development of a rehabilitation program to improve swallowing. Techniques include altering food consistency, motor retraining, controlled breathing, coughing, and head positioning. When adequate nutrition cannot be maintained, alternative routes for enteral feedings such as a gastrostomy may be indicated.

Management of esophageal dysphagia depends on its cause. Benign strictures, webs, and rings can be dilated at the time of upper endoscopy. Rigid bougie dilators or controlled radial expansion (CRE) balloon dilators have equivalent efficacy in treating strictures. Patients with underlying gastroesophageal reflux disease should be treated with intensive acid suppression. Eosinophilic esophagitis may improve with dietary modifications such as the six-food elimination diet or topical steroids. Early malignancies may be surgically resected, whereas palliation via endoscopic stenting or chemoradiotherapy may be used for unresectable lesions. Achalasia can be treated with surgical myotomy or large-caliber endoscopic balloon dilation. Botulinum toxin injection into the LES is used rarely for palliation of symptoms in patients with achalasia who are not candidates for more definitive therapy. The newest endoscopic option for treatment of achalasia is per-oral endoscopic myotomy (POEM). Other primary esophageal motility disorders may respond to nitrates, calcium channel antagonists, and, in rare instances, botulinum toxin or surgical myotomy.

Odynophagia

Therapy for odynophagia secondary to opportunistic infection relies on anti-infective treatments, whereas pill esophagitis and caustic ingestion may be managed with medications such as proton pump inhibitors to reduce acid reflux or slurries to coat the irritated esophagus.

Complications

The most serious complication of oropharyngeal dysphagia is tracheal aspiration, with development of cough, asthma, or pneumonia. Esophageal dysphagia may also result in aspiration, especially in the case of complete obstruction, and with more chronic symptoms in malnutrition and failure to thrive because of reduced oral intake.

Complications from odynophagia are related to the underlying etiology. Bleeding or perforation from esophageal ulceration may occur.

Key practice points

Dysphagia

- Complete esophageal obstruction requires emergency endoscopy with attention to airway protection. Radiographic contrast studies should be avoided due to risk of aspiration and potential interference with subsequent endoscopy.
- Distinguish oropharyngeal from esophageal source with a thorough patient history. Patients with oropharyngeal dysphagia are often co-managed with otolaryngologists or neurologists, depending on the underlying disorder.
- Oropharyngeal symptoms are best evaluated by fluoroscopic imaging, whereas esophageal symptoms are best evaluated initially by endoscopy, followed by manometry to evaluate motility disorders and potentially barium swallow.

Odynophagia

- If a fungal etiology is likely, empirical antifungal treatment is reasonable.
- Endoscopy is the optimal test to evaluate odynophagia.

Case studies

Case 1

A 32-year-old man with a history of asthma presents to the emergency department with six hours of difficulty swallowing. The symptoms began after eating a steak and have progressed to the point where he can no longer swallow his own secretions. He states a prior history of similar symptoms two and six months earlier; both episodes resolved without medical intervention.

Physical examination reveals a healthy-appearing man who is sitting upright with a bucket into which he spits his saliva. No other abnormalities are noted. Laboratory tests are normal.

The patient is intubated. An upper endoscopy is performed, and a large piece of steak is removed from the distal esophagus. Multiple esophageal rings and longitudinal furrows are noted in the esophagus.

The patient is discharged. At follow-up endoscopy one month later, the patient has had no recurrence of symptoms, although he has been careful to cut his food into small pieces and chew his food thoroughly before swallowing. Biopsies show increased intraepithelial eosinophils in the proximal and distal esophagus.

Discussion and potential pitfalls

Esophageal food impaction requires urgent medical intervention. The inability to swallow one's own secretions is a red flag indicating complete esophageal obstruction. In these cases, it is important to avoid contrast radiography, which not only interferes with the endoscopic visualization but is also potentially hazardous due to the risk of pulmonary aspiration. Endoscopic removal of the food bolus should be conducted after ensuring airway protection with an esophageal overtube or by endotracheal intubation.

Eosinophilic esophagitis is commonly diagnosed in young men with a history of atopic disorders and recurrent food impactions. Suggestive features on endoscopy include multiple esophageal rings and longitudinal furrows. The condition can be diagnosed by taking multiple biopsies in the distal and mid-to-proximal esophagus. Patients with possible eosinophilic esophagitis may respond to proton pump inhibitor therapy, and consideration should be given to evaluation for food allergies and treatment with topical steroids.

Case 2

A 67-year-old man is referred to your office for symptoms of dysphagia that have been present for four years, which have not previously been evaluated. He describes progressive dysphagia to solids and liquids, intermittent chest discomfort, and a 15-pound weight loss over the past year. He is otherwise healthy and has no symptoms of heartburn or odynophagia.

Physical examination reveals a thin man whose examination is otherwise normal. Upper endoscopy reveals a dilated, tortuous esophagus. No mass or stricture is noted, and the endoscope passes through the esophagogastric junction with only mild resistance. Esophageal manometry illustrates aperistalsis of the esophageal body with nonrelaxation of the LES, consistent with type 1 achalasia. He is referred for consideration of surgical myotomy.

Discussion and potential pitfalls

Achalasia is classically diagnosed on esophageal manometry by nonrelaxation of the LES with dysmotility of the esophageal body. High-resolution manometry with esophageal pressure topography provides greater diagnostic accuracy and differentiation between the three subtypes of achalasia. The manometric findings of idiopathic achalasia are not specific and can also be seen with pseudo-achalasia or Chagas disease. Barium radiography classically shows a tortuous or dilated esophagus with a "bird's beak" appearance to the LES. The ganglion cell degeneration found in achalasia is presumed to be immune mediated, as opposed to pseudo-achalasia where infiltration of the esophageal wall by tumor causes obstruction with proximal dilation. In patients who are older and who have relatively rapid progression of symptoms, the diagnosis of pseudo-achalasia as a result of a paraneoplastic process without direct tumor stenosis of the esophagogastric junction must also be considered.

Case 3

A 26-year-old man known to be HIV-positive presents with odynophagia. He has no prior acquired immunodeficiency syndrome (AIDS)-defining diagnosis and has not been taking highly active antiretroviral therapy (HAART). Odynophagia with both liquids and solids has been noted for two weeks leading to a 12-pound weight loss. Physical examination is notable for the absence of oral candidiasis and no abdominal tenderness or masses. Laboratory tests include a CD4 count of 28.

The patient is prescribed oral antifungal medication but has no relief of symptoms after seven days. On upper endoscopy, multiple small discrete ulcers are seen in the mid-to-distal esophagus. Biopsies and viral cultures do not show evidence of herpes simplex virus (HSV) or cytomegalovirus (CMV) infection. HAART is initiated, and the patient improves within five days.

Discussion and potential pitfalls

Immunocompromised patients are at risk of opportunistic infections. Odynophagia in this group of patients is commonly due to fungal infections (*C. albicans*), CMV, and HSV. Empiric therapy with an oral antifungal agent is a reasonable first step. If symptoms do not improve, investigation with upper endoscopy is indicated to evaluate for the presence of the viral infections. Idiopathic ulcerations associated with HIV are also a cause of odynophagia and are diagnosed by the exclusion of evidence of other opportunistic infection on biopsies of the ulcer. Patients may improve with initiation of HAART, but in some cases oral corticosteroids are also necessary for treatment.

Further reading

ASGE Standards of Practice Committee (2014). The role of endoscopy in the evaluation and management of dysphagia. *Gastrointest. Endosc.* 79: 191–201.

Liu, L.W.C., Andrews, C.N., Armstrong, D. et al. (2018). Clinical practice guidelines for the assessment of uninvestigated esophageal dysphagia. *J. Can. Assoc. Gastroenterol.* 1: 5–19.

Vaezi, M.F., Pandolfino, J.E., and Vela, M.F. (2013). ACG clinical guideline: diagnosis and management of achalasia. *Am. J. Gastroenterol.* 108: 1238–1249.

CHAPTER 2
The Patient with Heartburn or Chest Pain

Clinical presentation

History

Gastroesophageal reflux disease (GERD) is a frequent cause of visits to primary care providers and gastroenterologists. GERD most commonly presents as heartburn, a burning sensation in the chest that is often accompanied by symptoms of regurgitation of fluid or solid foods. It is frequently postprandial or nocturnal but can be experienced at any time of day. Patients often note trigger foods, which frequently are spicy, acidic, or fatty. It is important to ask patients about symptoms that many indicate extraesophageal symptoms of GERD, such as asthma, hoarseness, or cough. The history should also ask about symptoms of complicated GERD, such as dysphagia, pulmonary aspiration, and unintentional weight loss.

Patients with GERD and other esophageal disorders including esophageal dysmotility may present with chest pain instead of classic heartburn. When evaluating patients for chest pain, it is important to rule out cardiac etiologies of chest pain, such as coronary artery disease, prior to attributing the pain to a non-cardiac etiology. However, 20–30% of patients who undergo cardiac catheterization for chest pain do not have significant coronary artery disease. If coronary artery disease has been excluded, symptoms may arise from diseases of the cardiopulmonary system, musculoskeletal structures, gastrointestinal tract, and central nervous system (Table 2.1). Less common causes include biliary tract disease, pleural and mediastinal inflammation, dissecting aortic aneurysm, and varicella zoster infection of the chest wall.

Chest pain of esophageal origin commonly is described as substernal and squeezing or burning in character. It may last from minutes to hours and radiate in a pattern similar to angina. Although it is often not associated with swallowing, it can be exacerbated by ingesting hot or cold liquids. In contrast to cardiac chest pain, exertion only rarely triggers esophageal chest pain. Relief may be

---

Yamada's Handbook of Gastroenterology, Fourth Edition. John M. Inadomi, Renuka Bhattacharya, Joo Ha Hwang, and Cynthia Ko.

Table 2.1 Causes of chest pain

Cardiopulmonary causes of chest pain
Coronary artery disease
Coronary artery spasm
Microvascular angina
Mitral valve prolapse
Aortic valve disease
Pericarditis
Dissecting thoracic aortic aneurysm
Mediastinitis
Pneumonia
Pulmonary embolus
Musculoskeletal causes of chest pain
Costochondritis
Fibromyalgia
Arthritis
Nerve entrapment or compression
Esophageal causes of chest pain
Gastroesophageal reflux
Achalasia
Diffuse esophageal spasm
Other spastic motor disorders
Infectious or pill-induced esophagitis
Food impaction
Neuropsychiatric causes of chest pain
Panic disorder
Anxiety disorder
Depression
Somatization
Miscellaneous causes of chest pain
Varicella zoster virus reactivation

provided by ingestion of antacids or nitroglycerin. Pain that lasts for hours, that is related to meals, that does not radiate laterally, and that is relieved by acid suppression suggests an esophageal origin.

Physical examination

Patients with uncomplicated GERD frequently have a normal physical examination, although the clinician should be alert to possible physical findings associated with GERD complications, such as symptoms of malnutrition if the patient has dysphagia related to an esophageal stricture. Physical examination occasionally helps to delineate the cause of chest pain. Reproduction of symptoms by chest wall palpation suggests a musculoskeletal source. Auscultation of pleural friction rubs or decreased breath sounds implies pleuropulmonary disease.

Cutaneous eruptions in a dermatomal pattern suggest varicella zoster. An abnormal cardiac exam may suggest a cardiac etiology, and abdominal tenderness raises concern for peptic or biliary tract disease.

Additional testing

Most patients with symptoms consistent with uncomplicated GERD can first be treated empirically by acid suppression with either histamine-2 (H2) receptor antagonists or proton pump inhibitors. Patients should also be counseled regarding lifestyle modifications, such as elevation of the head of the bed, avoidance of trigger foods, and weight loss if needed. If patients do not exhibit any alarm features and have an adequate response to lifestyle modification and acid suppression, further evaluation is not always needed. If symptoms do not respond well to acid suppression, there are symptoms of complicated GERD such as dysphagia or recurrent aspiration, or there is diagnostic uncertainty, upper endoscopy, esophageal manometry, or esophageal pH testing may be needed.

Endoscopy is superior for detecting esophagitis and affords the capability to perform a biopsy of abnormal mucosa, whereas radiographic techniques may detect subtle strictures or dysmotility. However, endoscopy often will not demonstrate esophagitis even in the presence of GERD, whether treated or untreated. Nevertheless, upper endoscopy is useful to exclude other esophageal disorders that may mimic heartburn and to look for anatomic abnormalities often associated with GERD such as a hiatal hernia or lax gastroesophageal flap valve.

Ambulatory esophageal manometry or pH testing (with or without impedance testing) allows better evaluation of esophageal physiology than upper endoscopy and can be helpful to define the underlying disorder in patients with GERD symptoms unresponsive to standard therapy or in patients with noncardiac chest pain. Esophageal manometry may define an underlying esophageal motility disorder. Esophageal motility disorders can be classified according to the Chicago classification (Table 2.2) and can generally be divided into spastic

Table 2.2 Chicago classification of esophageal motility disorders

Disorders with esophagogastric junction outflow obstruction
Achalasia
Esophagogastric junction outflow obstruction
Major disorders of peristalsis
Diffuse esophageal spasm
Jackhammer esophagus
Absent contractility
Minor disorders of peristalsis
Ineffective motility
Fragmented peristalsis

disorders, disorders of the esophagogastric junction, and hypomotile disorders. However, manometry detects potentially pathogenic motor abnormalities in only a minority of patients with noncardiac chest pain.

The best test for quantifying acid reflux and its relationship to symptoms is ambulatory pH monitoring of the esophagus. This can be accomplished with placement of a transnasal catheter or a wireless probe into the esophagus with measurement of pH over 24–48 hours. Esophageal pH monitoring allows quantification of the frequency and severity of reflux events as well as correlation of reflux episodes with such symptoms as heartburn or chest pain. Esophageal impedance testing can also be performed, which allows detection of non-acid reflux events. An esophageal pH less than 4 for longer than 5% of total exposure time suggests a diagnosis of GERD with a sensitivity of 85% and a specificity of 95%. Ambulatory pH monitoring is also helpful to define patients with reflux hypersensitivity, who have normal esophageal acid exposure but heartburn symptoms that correlate with reflux episodes, or functional heartburn, who have normal acid exposure and heartburn symptoms that do not correlate with reflux episodes.

The evaluation of a patient with chest pain is outlined in Figure 2.1. Initial diagnostic tests involve exclusion of cardiac disease, potentially with electrocardiography, exercise stress testing, echocardiography, or coronary arteriography, depending on the patient's age and risk factors. Once cardiac disease is excluded, noncardiac sources for chest pain may be evaluated.

In many patients with noncardiac chest pain, an empiric trial of high-dose proton pump inhibitor therapy is tried and can be expected to relieve symptoms in 80% if chest pain is due to underlying GERD. If this fails, or if more definitive evaluation is desired, upper endoscopy, esophageal manometry and pH monitoring, or barium swallow radiography can be used to exclude esophageal sources of chest pain.

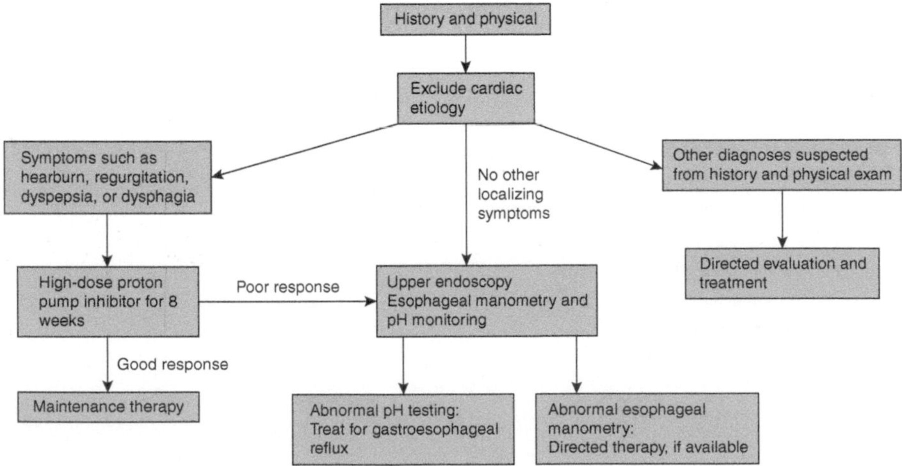

Figure 2.1 Evaluation of the patient with chest pain.

Differential diagnosis

Heartburn

Although heartburn is most frequently related to abnormal acid reflux, it can also be caused by such functional disorders as reflux hypersensitivity, where the patient reports symptoms of acid reflux with physiologic levels of reflux. Some patients with esophageal dysmotility can also present with symptoms of heartburn.

Chest pain

Cardiac disorders

Cardiac etiologies must be considered in a patient with unexplained chest pain, even in the absence of coronary atherosclerosis. Coronary artery spasm is reported in some individuals with chest pain. Exertional chest pain may be a consequence of abnormalities of the smaller endocardial vasculature without evidence of fixed lesions or spasm of the epicardial vessels, a condition termed *microvascular angina*. Diagnosis of this disorder may require measurement of coronary flow reserve with or without provocative testing. The relationship of chest pain to mitral valve prolapse is controversial. Furthermore, esophageal motor abnormalities may coexist with both microvascular angina and mitral valve prolapse that make the cause of chest pain uncertain in affected individuals.

Esophageal disorders

Esophageal disorders account for 20–60% of cases of noncardiac chest pain. Although heartburn is more typical, chest pain is a common atypical symptom of GERD. Primary spastic esophageal motor disorders are found in fewer than 50% of patients with noncardiac chest pain. One such condition, diffuse esophageal spasm, accounts for 5% of cases and is characterized by the presence of high-amplitude, nonperistaltic esophageal contractions on manometry. Functional disorders of the esophagus such as reflux hypersensitivity or functional heartburn may be the underlying etiology of noncardiac chest pain in many patients. Miscellaneous gastroesophageal sources of chest pain include infectious or pill-induced esophagitis, food impaction, and proximal gastric ulcers.

Musculoskeletal causes

Musculoskeletal conditions account for 10–30% of cases of noncardiac chest pain. Chest pain from musculoskeletal sources (e.g. costochondritis [Tietze syndrome], fibromyalgia, inflammatory arthritis, osteoarthritis, thoracic spinal disease) is characterized by localized chest wall tenderness and definable trigger points and may be reported at rest, with movement, or during sleep.

Neuropsychiatric causes

Panic disorder presents with at least three attacks in as many weeks of intense fear or discomfort accompanied by at least four of the following symptoms: chest pain, restlessness, choking, palpitations, sweating, dizziness, nausea or abdominal distress, paresthesia, flushing, trembling, and a sense of impending doom. Of all cases of noncardiac chest pain, 34–59% result from panic disorder. In addition to increased anxiety, these patients also exhibit an increased prevalence of depression and somatization.

Management

The cornerstone of managing typical GERD is therapy with acid suppressive medications such as proton pump inhibitors or H2-receptor antagonists. Lifestyle modifications such as avoidance of trigger foods, weight loss (if applicable), and elevating the head of the bed at night are also helpful. A subset of patients with documented abnormal reflux and incomplete response to conservative therapies may be candidates for endoscopic or surgical antireflux procedures. Patients with reflux hypersensitivity or functional heartburn may benefit more from such neuromodulators as tricyclic antidepressants than from acid suppression.

Treatment of esophageal chest pain may be unsatisfactory because of diagnostic uncertainties, the intermittent nature of symptoms, the side-effect profiles of available pharmaceutical agents, and the awareness that many of these conditions improve spontaneously without treatment. After a careful diagnostic examination, many patients respond to physician reassurance that no dangerous condition exists. Underlying gastroesophageal reflux can be treated in a similar manner as for those patients with typical symptoms. For painful esophageal motility disorders, nitrates and calcium channel blockers may be considered, although response rates for these agents are low. Some patients respond instead to tricyclic antidepressant agents (e.g. amitriptyline, imipramine) at doses lower than those used to treat depression. Limited data also suggests an improvement in chest pain with the selective serotonin reuptake inhibitors, which may be useful if there are concomitant anxiety disorders.

For panic disorders, anxiolytics may be effective, but their use may be limited by concerns about long-term dependence or tolerance. Cognitive behavioral therapy may produce significant improvements in chest pain, functional disability, and psychological distress in selected patient populations with psychogenic etiologies of chest pain.

Complications

GERD can lead to such complications as esophagitis, esophageal stricture formation, and Barrett esophagus predisposing to esophageal adenocarcinoma. Screening and surveillance for Barrett esophagus remain somewhat controversial, although it may be reasonable to screen high-risk populations for Barrett esophagus. These include older white men with chronic GERD, a history of smoking, central obesity, and a family history of Barrett esophagus or esophageal malignancy. Chest pain of esophageal origin may lead to potential complications of the underlying disorder. The major risk in evaluating a patient with unexplained chest pain is the premature exclusion of coronary ischemia, which may have life-threatening consequences.

Key practice points

Heartburn

- Heartburn is the most common symptom of typical GERD.
- Patients with typical GERD usually respond well to lifestyle modifications and acid suppression with H2-receptor antagonists or proton pump inhibitors.
- Patients with suspected gastroesophageal reflux with either typical or atypical symptoms but incomplete response to first-line therapies should undergo further evaluation, which may include upper endoscopy, esophageal manometry, and/or ambulatory esophageal pH monitoring.

Chest pain

- Cardiac etiologies must be considered in a patient with unexplained chest pain, even in the absence of known coronary atherosclerosis.
- Esophageal disorders are the most common causes of noncardiac chest pain. An empirical trial of high-dose proton pump inhibitor therapy for suspected GERD can be undertaken if cardiac causes of chest pain have been ruled out.
- Although heartburn is more prevalent, chest pain is a common atypical symptom of GERD.
- Chest pain from musculoskeletal sources is characterized by localized chest wall tenderness and definable trigger points and may be reported at rest, with movement, or during sleep.
- Upper endoscopy can exclude an esophageal mucosal source of pain.
- Esophageal manometry may define an underlying esophageal motility disorder.
- The best test for correlating symptoms with gastroesophageal reflux is ambulatory pH monitoring, ideally with impedance testing and symptom correlation.

Case studies

Case 1

A 56-year-old woman with a history of hypertension and diabetes controlled by oral agents presents to her primary care physician reporting intermittent substernal squeezing chest pain, radiating to the neck and lasting approximately 30–90 minutes. Her symptoms generally occur at rest and are not clearly related to meals. She has taken over-the-counter antacids with intermittent improvement in her symptoms. Physical examination reveals an obese woman in no distress and with no significant abnormalities noted. Laboratory tests are normal other than a mildly elevated fasting blood glucose. An electrocardiogram (ECG) is normal.

The patient is referred for a stress echocardiogram, which is normal. She starts a twice-daily proton pump inhibitor with improvement in her symptoms. The patient is referred to a gastroenterologist who performs upper endoscopy. The esophagus, stomach, and duodenum are normal. Esophageal manometry shows normal esophageal motility, and 24-hour esophageal pH monitoring off proton pump inhibitors shows abnormal distal esophageal acid exposure with a strong symptom association profile for chest pain.

Discussion

In patients with chest pain, coronary ischemia should be excluded. Nonerosive reflux disease is a common cause of noncardiac chest pain and cannot always be differentiated from coronary artery disease by history or physical examination. Most patients with esophageal chest pain will respond to high-dose proton pump inhibitor therapy, but esophageal manometry and 24-hour ambulatory pH monitoring off medications may be necessary to confirm the diagnosis of GERD and to correlate abnormal reflux episodes with symptoms of chest pain.

Case 2

A 25-year-old man with a history of depression is referred to the gastroenterology clinic for evaluation of recurrent heartburn occurring after meals and at night. Prior evaluation was unremarkable, including cardiac stress testing and upper endoscopy. A trial of high-dose proton pump inhibitors had no effect on his symptoms. The patient underwent esophageal manometry and 24-hour pH monitoring off proton pump inhibitors that revealed normal esophageal acid exposure but correlation of heartburn symptoms with physiologic reflux episodes. The patient was started on low-dose amitriptyline with modest improvement in his symptoms.

Discussion

This case highlights some of the challenges of treating heartburn that does not respond adequately to acid suppression. Performing upper endoscopy is useful to evaluate for signs of acid reflux disease, such as esophagitis. Esophageal manometry can help to rule out motility disorders. Ambulatory pH monitoring is useful to quantify the amount of acid reflux and to correlate with reported symptoms. This patient reported heartburn symptoms associated with physiologic reflux episodes, suggesting reflux hypersensitivity. This may be successfully treated with neuromodulators such as tricyclic antidepressants.

Further reading

ASGE Standards of Practice Committee (2015). The role of endoscopy in the management of GERD. *Gastrointest. Endosc.* 81: 1305–1310.

Katz, P.O., Gerson, L.B., and Vela, M.F. (2013). Guidelines for the diagnosis and management of gastroesophageal reflux disease. *Am. J. Gastroenterol.* 108: 308–328.

Shaheen, N.J., Galk, G.W., Iyer, P.G., and Gerson, L. (2016). ACG clinical guideline: diagnosis and management of Barrett's esophagus. *Am. J. Gastroenterol.* 111: 30–50.

CHAPTER 3

The Patient with Gastrointestinal Bleeding

Gastrointestinal (GI) bleeding is a common problem, ranging in severity from occult blood loss to life-threatening hemorrhage. In approaching the patient with GI bleeding, it is important to assess the acuity, severity, and site of blood loss by symptoms, hemodynamic status, and laboratory assessment. Hematemesis indicates an upper GI source proximal to the ligament of Treitz. Melena usually results from acute upper GI bleeding but can also indicate bleeding from the small intestine or the proximal colon. Hematochezia usually indicates a colonic source but may also be caused by brisk upper GI bleeding. Patients may also have occult GI bleeding without clinically visible hemorrhage.

Approach to Acute Gastrointestinal Bleeding

Initial assessment

Initial assessment of patients with acute GI bleeding should include a directed history. Prior peptic disease or dyspeptic symptoms suggest ulcer bleeding. Recent ingestion of aspirin, nonsteroidal anti-inflammatory drugs (NSAIDs), alcohol, or caustic substances should be ascertained. Known or suspected liver disease raises the possibility of varices or portal gastropathy. In patients with suspected lower GI bleeding, a history of hemorrhoids or inflammatory bowel disease is important to note. Abdominal pain or diarrhea suggests colitis or neoplasm. Malignancy also may be indicated by weight loss, anorexia, lymphadenopathy, or palpable masses.

Evaluation of hemodynamic status by vital signs is critical in patients with acute GI bleeding. Physical examination findings of cirrhosis such as ascites, spider angiomas, or splenomegaly may suggest portal hypertension. Rectal examination should be performed to identify stool color. Based on the history and physical examination, an initial assessment of the site of GI blood loss can frequently be made, directing subsequent management.

Yamada's Handbook of Gastroenterology, Fourth Edition. John M. Inadomi, Renuka Bhattacharya, Joo Ha Hwang, and Cynthia Ko.

Laboratory studies

A complete blood count and coagulation studies should be part of the initial laboratory evaluation. The first hematocrit may not reflect the degree of blood loss because acute hemorrhage produces loss of both erythrocytes and volume. Microcytic anemia suggests chronic blood loss. With massive upper GI bleeding, azotemia reflects intestinal absorption of nitrogenous breakdown products of blood, although azotemia with creatinine elevation suggests renal insufficiency. Abnormal liver tests raise concern about possible cirrhosis with portal hypertension.

Resuscitation and blood transfusion

The first step in managing a patient with GI bleeding from any source is to assess clinical severity (Figure 3.1). Hematemesis, melena, or hematochezia suggest major hemorrhage, whereas pallor, hypotension, and tachycardia indicate substantial blood volume loss and mandate immediate volume replacement. Two large-bore intravenous catheters should be placed, and crystalloid administered to replenish intravascular volume while awaiting blood products. Unstable patients should be admitted to an intensive care unit. A nasogastric tube can be placed to assess for ongoing active hemorrhage. However, clear aspirates can be found in some patients with duodenal bleeding, and assessment of hemodynamic stability should include all clinical parameters.

The need for blood transfusion is influenced by patient age, coexistent cardiovascular disease, and persistent hemorrhage. A limited transfusion approach targeting a hemoglobin of 7 g/dl is appropriate in patients without significant cardiovascular disease or ongoing hemorrhage. Packed erythrocytes are preferred for blood transfusion to avoid fluid load. If coagulation studies are abnormal, fresh-frozen plasma or platelets may also be needed, but studies in this area are limited.

Potential pitfalls

Hematochezia may be seen in patients with brisk upper GI bleeding. Placement of a nasogastric tube or upper endoscopy may be needed to exclude an upper GI source in unstable patients with hematochezia. A "clear" lavage indicates the absence of duodenal sampling, so only bilious lavage fluid rules out active duodenal hemorrhage.

Acute Upper Gastrointestinal Bleeding

Differential diagnosis

The most common causes of upper GI hemorrhage are peptic ulcer disease (35–40%), esophagitis or esophageal ulcers, and sequelae of portal hypertension. Other disorders comprise a small minority of cases (Table 3.1). Most cases of

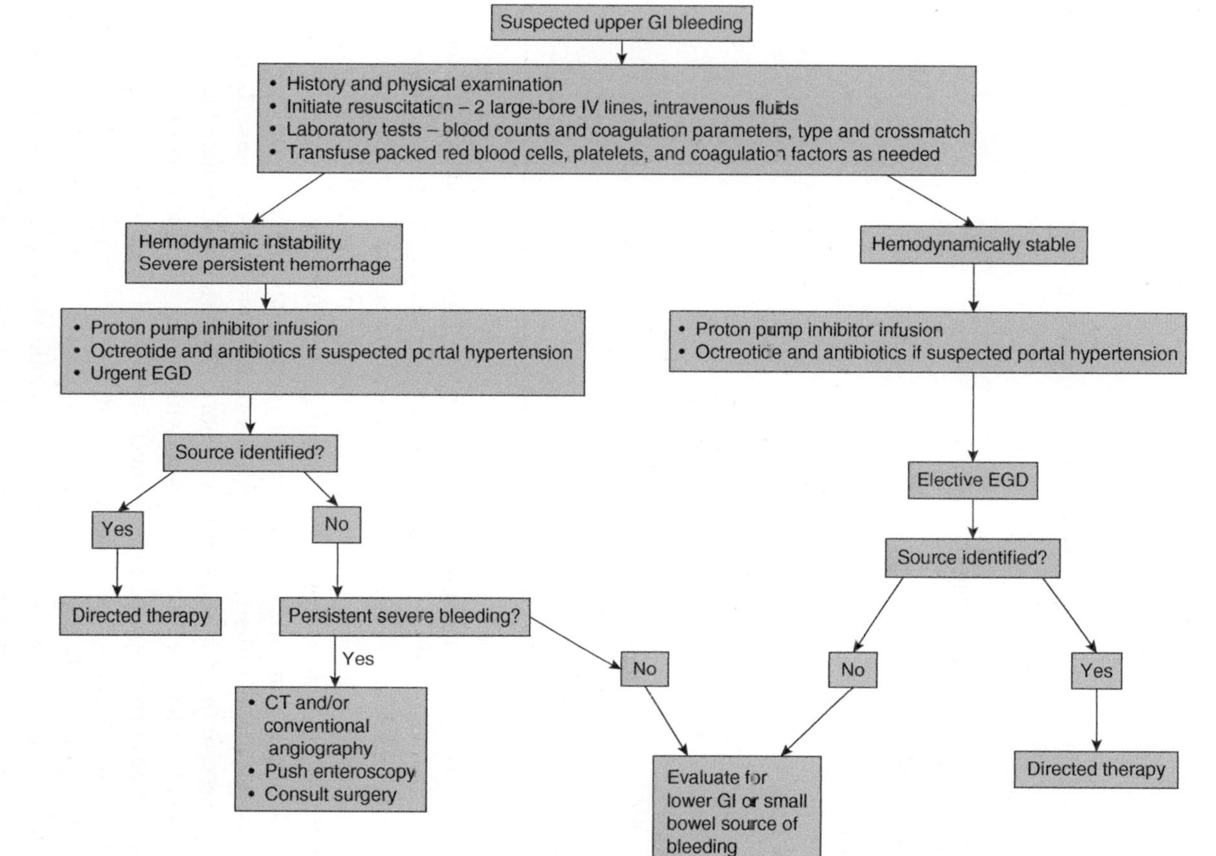

Figure 3.1 Suggested approach to acute upper gastrointestinal bleeding. CT, computed tomography; EGD, esophagogastroduodenoscopy; GI, gastrointestinal; IV, intravenous. Patients who have recurrent bleeding after identification and treatment of an upper GI source should undergo repeat upper endoscopy.

Table 3.1 Causes of overt gastrointestinal hemorrhage

Causes
Common upper gastrointestinal sources
Peptic ulcer disease (duodenal, gastric, stomal)
Esophagitis and esophageal ulcers (acid reflux, infection, pill induced, sclerotherapy, radiation induced)
Varices (esophageal, gastric, duodenal)
Portal hypertensive gastropathy
Mallory–Weiss tear
Neoplasms
Vascular ectasias and angiodysplasias, including hereditary hemorrhagic telangiectasia and gastric antral vascular ectasia
Dieulafoy lesion
Common lower gastrointestinal sources
Diverticulosis
Angiodysplasia
Hemorrhoids
Anal fissures
Neoplasms
Inflammatory bowel disease
Ischemic colitis
Infectious colitis
Radiation-induced colitis
Meckel diverticulum
Intussusception
Aortoenteric fistula
Solitary rectal ulcers
Nonsteroidal anti-inflammatory drug (NSAID)-induced cecal ulcers

peptic ulcer disease result from *Helicobacter pylori* infection or from chronic aspirin or NSAID use. Esophagitis most commonly results from gastroesophageal reflux disease. Esophageal ulcers may be caused by severe gastroesophageal reflux disease, viral infection, certain medications, and prior radiation therapy.

Esophagogastric varices and portal hypertensive gastropathy are frequent causes of GI bleeding in patients with portal hypertension. However, up to 50% of upper GI bleeds in patients with cirrhosis result from other causes. Gastric varices are present in 20% of patients with portal hypertension. Isolated gastric varices suggest splenic vein thrombosis, which may be a consequence of pancreatic disease and is treated by splenectomy. Portal hypertensive gastropathy appears endoscopically as a mosaic, snakeskin-like mucosa resulting from engorged mucosal vessels.

Miscellaneous causes of upper GI bleeding include Mallory–Weiss tears at the gastroesophageal junction induced by retching or vomiting. Hemorrhage from Mallory–Weiss tears usually resolves spontaneously without intervention. Neoplasms most commonly bleed slowly, but occasionally exhibit massive hemorrhage. Bleeding in a Dieulafoy lesion results from pressure erosion of the overlying epithelium by an ectopic artery without surrounding ulceration or inflammation.

Vascular ectasias in the stomach and duodenum can cause recurrent acute GI hemorrhage or chronic slow blood loss. They are associated with advanced age, chronic kidney disease, aortic valve disease, and prior radiation therapy. Hereditary hemorrhagic telangiectasia is an autosomal dominant disorder with telangiectasias of the tongue, lips, conjunctiva, skin, and mucosa of the gut, bladder, and nasopharynx. Gastric arteriovenous ectasia (GAVE), or watermelon stomach, has the appearance of columns of vessels along the tops of the antral folds.

Management

Medical therapy

Empiric medical treatment can be given for patients with suspected upper GI bleeding (Figure 3.1). For presumed peptic disease, intravenous proton pump inhibitor therapy can decrease the need for endoscopic therapy and reduce rates of rebleeding. For presumed portal hypertensive bleeding, intravenous octreotide can be initiated. Antibiotics (e.g. quinolones or ceftriaxone) should be administered to patients with cirrhosis and acute GI bleeding whether or not bleeding is variceal in origin.

Therapeutic endoscopy

Endoscopy in patients with upper GI bleeding allows identification of the bleeding site and possibly therapy. Ideally, patients should be hemodynamically resuscitated prior to endoscopy. Urgent upper endoscopy is indicated in patients with ongoing hemorrhage, suspected cirrhosis, or aorto-enteric fistulae. Patients who are hemodynamically stable without evidence of ongoing bleeding can undergo more elective endoscopy. Barium radiography may obscure endoscopic or angiographic visualization of the bleeding site and should not be used in the acute setting.

In patients with peptic ulcer bleeding, the presence of a nonbleeding visible vessel or an adherent clot within the ulcer increases the risk of rebleeding. Thus, endoscopic therapy for peptic ulcer disease should be performed for active bleeding, visible vessels, or adherent clots if (after removal) they are associated with visible vessels. Local injection with vasoconstrictors (epinephrine) or normal saline, thermal therapy with electrocautery or argon plasma coagulation, and mechanical therapy with hemostatic or over-the-scope clips are all widely used. Other sources amenable to thermal or mechanical therapy include refractory Mallory–Weiss tears, neoplasms, angiodysplasia, or Dieulafoy lesions.

Bleeding esophageal varices may be managed by endoscopic band ligation or sclerotherapy, with initial hemostasis rates of 85–95%. The role of endoscopy in managing gastric varices is less well established, although sclerotherapy, thrombin injection, cyanoacrylate injection, and snare ligation may be effective.

Scintigraphy and angiography

Scintigraphic and/or angiographic studies may be indicated if a bleeding site cannot be identified at endoscopy or if bleeding severity precludes endoscopy. Technetium-labeled erythrocyte scans can localize bleeding if the rate of blood loss exceeds 0.04 ml/minute. Scintigraphy is becoming less common because of evolving imaging techniques such as computed tomography (CT) angiography, which may provide more accurate localization. Conventional angiography can localize the bleeding site if the rate of blood loss is greater than 0.5 ml/minute and can offer therapeutic capability. Angiography with embolization or vasoconstrictor infusion may be effective when endoscopic therapy fails or is not indicated. Angiographic placement of a transjugular intrahepatic portosystemic shunt (TIPS) can effectively control bleeding secondary to portal hypertensive etiologies. A newer option for management of gastric varices is balloon-occluded retrograde or antegrade transvenous occlusion (BRTO or BATO).

Mechanical compression

When endoscopic therapy of variceal hemorrhage fails, balloon tamponade achieves initial hemostasis in 70–90% of cases. However, more definitive therapy such as variceal banding is still required after patient stabilization.

Surgery

Patients with recurrent peptic ulcer bleeding usually benefit from repeat endoscopy prior to proceeding to angiography or surgery. When endoscopy or angiography fail, emergency surgery may be required.

Complications

The most serious complication of upper GI bleeding is exsanguination and death. Mortality from acute upper GI hemorrhage increases from 8–10% to 30–40% in patients with persistent or recurrent bleeding.

Because of the high mortality of hemorrhage secondary to portal hypertension, prevention of rebleeding is crucial. Variceal obliteration with endoscopic band ligation or sclerotherapy reduces rebleeding rates. Nonselective beta-blocker therapy to reduce portal pressures also reduces recurrent hemorrhage from esophageal varices. In selected patients with esophageal or gastric varices, TIPS or BRTO/BATO may be useful to prevent recurrent bleeding.

Acute Lower Gastrointestinal Bleeding

Differential diagnosis

Bleeding colonic diverticula, angiodysplasia, and ischemic colitis are the major causes of acute lower GI bleeding (Table 3.1). Diverticular bleeding usually is painless with red or maroon stools. Colonic angiodysplasias are responsible for 10–40%

of acute lower GI bleeding episodes and usually are multiple, small (<5 mm in diameter), and localized to the right colon and cecum. They are associated with advanced age, renal insufficiency, prior irradiation, and aortic valve disease. Patients with ischemic colitis frequently present initially with abdominal pain followed by bleeding. Most cases occur in the setting of reduced visceral blood flow and do not require underlying fixed mesenteric vascular stenosis. Nevertheless, patients with ischemic colitis are frequently elderly with significant comorbid disease.

Chronic or recurrent lower GI hemorrhage is most often due to angiodysplasia, vascular ectasias, hemorrhoids, and colonic neoplasia. Hemorrhoids and anal fissures usually result in small volumes of bright red blood on toilet paper or on the stool. Benign and malignant colonic neoplasms can be associated with small-volume hematochezia or occult blood loss.

Colitis secondary to inflammatory bowel disease, bacterial infection, and radiation therapy rarely leads to bleeding that is more than small to moderate in volume. Patients who have recently undergone colonoscopic polypectomy may present with postpolypectomy bleeding. Portal hypertension may predispose to development of ileocolonic and anorectal varices, which may cause brisk blood loss.

Management

Principles of resuscitation in acute lower GI bleeding are similar to those for upper GI hemorrhage (Figure 3.2). Because brisk upper GI hemorrhage also may present with hematochezia, a potential upper GI source may need to be excluded by nasogastric tube placement or upper endoscopy.

Medical therapy

Certain lower GI sources are amenable to specific medical therapy. Hemorrhoids, anal fissures, and solitary rectal ulcers benefit from bulk-forming agents, sitz baths, and avoidance of straining. Inflammatory bowel disease usually responds to specific anti-inflammatory drug therapy.

Therapeutic endoscopy

Colonoscopy is recommended within 24 hours of presentation after rapid bowel preparation in patients with significant bleeding. Patients with less severe bleeding can undergo more elective evaluation. Diverticular and postpolypectomy bleeding can be treated with injection therapy, electrocautery, or endoscopic clip placement. Thermal therapy with electrocautery or argon plasma coagulation can successfully treat angiodysplasia and radiation proctopathy. Colonoscopy also may be used to ablate or resect bleeding polyps.

Therapeutic angiography

When colonoscopy fails or cannot be performed in patients with ongoing hemorrhage, angiography with selective arterial embolization or infusion of vasoconstrictors may be offered but carries a 13–18% risk of bowel ischemia.

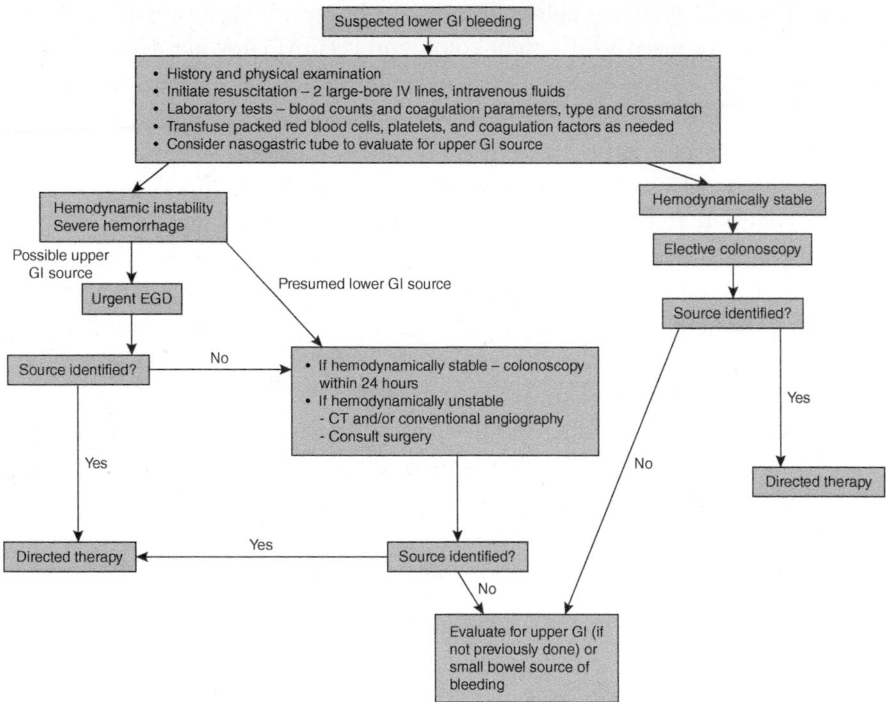

Figure 3.2 Suggested approach to a patient with acute lower GI bleeding. CT, computed tomography; EGD, esophagogastroduodenoscopy; GI, gastrointestinal; IV, intravenous.

Surgery

For certain diagnoses (e.g. Meckel diverticulum or some malignancies), surgery is the appropriate primary therapy. It may rarely be required for patients with recurrent diverticular bleeding. Emergency surgery carries high morbidity and mortality that increase with bleeding severity and comorbidity.

Complications

The most severe complications of lower GI bleeding include the potential need for surgery, exsanguination, and death. Chronic or recurrent lower GI bleeding is associated with significant morbidity and subjects the patient to the risks of frequent transfusions.

Obscure Gastrointestinal Bleeding

Obscure GI bleeding is defined as persistent or recurrent bleeding of unknown origin after an appropriate endoscopic evaluation. Obscure GI bleeding may be overt (i.e. visible) or occult (i.e. iron deficiency or fecal occult blood without visible bleeding). A suggested algorithm for the evaluation of obscure GI bleeding is shown in Figure 3.3.

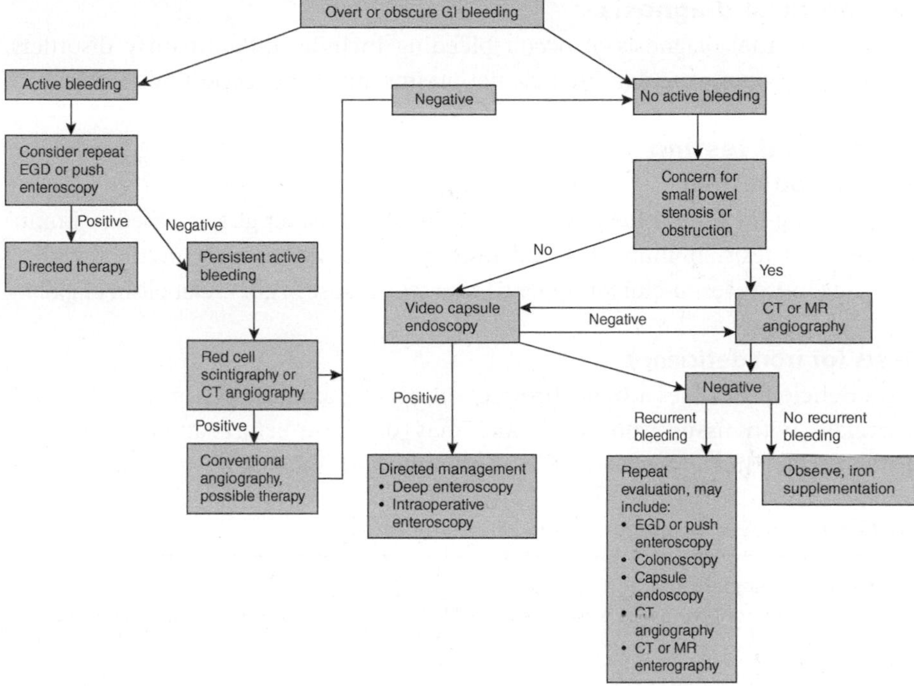

Figure 3.3 Suggested approach to obscure GI bleeding. CT, computed tomography; EGD, esophagogastroduodenoscopy; GI, gastrointestinal; MR, magnetic resonance.

Occult Gastrointestinal Bleeding

Clinical presentation

Most occult GI bleeding is chronic and, if significant, can produce marked iron deficiency anemia.

History

Patients with chronic occult blood loss most often are asymptomatic or report symptoms secondary to anemia. Dyspepsia, heartburn, or regurgitation suggest possible peptic causes, whereas weight loss and anorexia raise concern for malignancy. Recurrent episodes of occult blood loss in elderly patients without other symptoms are consistent with vascular ectasias.

Physical examination

Profound iron deficiency may present with fatigue, pallor, or hyperdynamic circulation with high cardiac output. Splenomegaly, jaundice, or spider angiomata raise the possibility of blood loss secondary to portal hypertensive gastropathy.

Differential diagnosis

The differential diagnosis of occult bleeding includes inflammatory disorders, infectious causes, vascular diseases, neoplasms, and other conditions (Table 3.2).

Additional testing

Fecal blood testing

Fecal testing for occult blood can be performed with either guaiac-based or immunochemical tests. Immunochemical tests are very sensitive for occult lower GI bleeding but are less useful for upper GI sources because of gut metabolism of globin.

Tests for iron deficiency

Iron deficiency causes a hypochromic, microcytic anemia. Serum ferritin levels correlate with tissue iron stores and may decrease before anemia develops. However, ferritin is an acute-phase reactant, and inflammatory conditions can

Table 3.2 Causes of occult gastrointestinal hemorrhage

Tumors and neoplasms
Primary adenocarcinoma – most commonly colorectal but also gastric, esophageal, and ampullary malignancies
Metastases
Large polyps
Lymphoma
Leiomyoma
Leiomyosarcoma
Lipoma
Infectious causes
Hookworm
Strongyloidiasis
Ascariasis
Tuberculous enterocolitis
Amebiasis
Vascular causes
Vascular ectasia, including gastric antral vascular ectasia (GAVE)
Portal hypertensive gastropathy
Hemangiomas
Blue rubber bleb nevus syndrome
Other disorders
Acid peptic disease
Hiatal hernia (Cameron erosions)
Inflammatory bowel disease
Radiation enteritis
Meckel diverticulum
Solitary rectal ulcer
Small bowel or colonic ulcer
Medications – nonsteroidal anti-inflammatory drugs (NSAIDs), potassium supplements, chemotherapeutic agents

cause false elevations. With iron deficiency, a reduced transferrin saturation is typically seen. Measurement of bone marrow iron stores remains the gold standard for diagnosing iron deficiency anemia.

Endoscopy and radiography

For the patient with occult blood-positive stools without anemia or iron deficiency, colonoscopy is the appropriate diagnostic procedure because risk of upper GI malignancy is low. Patients with unexplained iron deficiency anemia should undergo both upper endoscopy and colonoscopy. Small intestinal biopsies may be performed to exclude celiac disease. In patients with specific GI symptoms, the sequence of diagnostic testing should be directed to the anatomical site from which symptoms appear to arise. If no lesion is found, further evaluation of the small bowel by capsule endoscopy or by CT or magnetic resonance (MR) enterography should be considered (Figure 3.3). Abnormalities detected on any of these studies may need further evaluation by deep enteroscopy.

Management

Treatment of occult GI bleeding is dictated by the diagnostic evaluation. Chronic blood loss may require long-term oral or intravenous iron supplementation. Repletion of iron stores may take three to six months.

Complications

Chronic occult GI blood loss usually is well tolerated in young individuals; however, older patients or those with underlying cardiorespiratory disease may develop fatigue or other symptoms related to anemia.

Key practice points

- Initial evaluation and management of a patient with acute gastrointestinal bleeding should focus on assessment of hemodynamic status and fluid resuscitation. In most patients, endoscopy should be performed after patient stabilization. Endoscopy may be needed more urgently if in patients with ongoing large-volume bleeding.
- In patients with severe or ongoing hematochezia, an upper GI source should be ruled out by nasogastric lavage or upper endoscopy.
- Urgent colonoscopy within 24 hours of presentation after rapid bowel preparation is recommended in patients with severe lower GI bleeding.
- Occult GI hemorrhage without iron deficiency anemia warrants a colonoscopy only. An upper endoscopy is also indicated if iron deficiency is present.

Case studies

Case 1

A 63-year-old man with hepatitis C-related cirrhosis presents to the emergency department with several hours of light-headedness and dark stool. His pulse is 120bpm with a blood pressure of 90/50mmHg. Skin exam reveals scleral icterus, few spider angiomata, and melena on rectal exam. Initial laboratory studies are notable for a hemoglobin of 11g/dl, platelets of 85,000, blood urea nitrogen (BUN) 18mg/dl, creatinine 0.8mg/dl, international normalized ratio (INR) 1.5, albumin 2.8g/dl, bilirubin 1.7mg/dl. Nasogastric aspirate reveals clear fluid without blood or bile.

The patient is stabilized and admitted to the intensive care unit. Proton pump inhibitors, octreotide, and antibiotics are initiated. A repeat hemoglobin is 8.0g/dl. Urgent endoscopy reveals no varices and a 2cm duodenal bulb ulcer with a visible vessel that is successfully treated with epinephrine injection and bipolar electrocautery. The octreotide drip is subsequently discontinued. A stool antigen for *H. pylori* is positive and treated with antibiotics for two weeks and omeprazole for eight weeks. Repeat stool antigen testing for *H. pylori* is negative at three months.

Discussion

This case highlights important points in the management of acute upper GI bleeding. First, although this patient has evidence of cirrhosis, GI bleeding in this setting may not be due to sequelae of portal hypertension. Nevertheless, initiating octreotide therapy is reasonable while awaiting further evaluation. Second, empiric proton pump inhibitor therapy is reasonable in the setting of melena and suspected upper GI bleeding. This can be discontinued if an acid-related upper GI source of bleeding is not found. Third, antibiotics are indicated because they reduce morbidity and mortality for cirrhotics with GI bleeding. Fourth, despite the lack of anemia or blood on gastric aspirate, the hemodynamic alterations suggest significant blood loss, indicating a need for ICU admission and urgent endoscopy. Next, transfusion of packed red blood cells was not indicated as the patient's hemoglobin remained above 7g/dl without evidence of ongoing hemorrhage. Finally, testing for *H. pylori* is indicated for patients with peptic ulcer disease. In the setting of complicated peptic ulcer disease (i.e. with bleeding, perforation, or obstruction), documentation of eradication is recommended.

Case 2

A 76-year-old woman presents with sudden onset of painless hematochezia two hours earlier. She is otherwise healthy and not taking any NSAIDs or aspirin. On physical examination, her pulse is 115bpm and blood pressure 102/56mmHg. There are dark red clots on rectal exam. Laboratory studies are notable for a hemoglobin of 11.8g/dl, platelets of 315,000, BUN 7mg/dl, creatinine 1.0mg/dl, and INR 1.0. Nasogastric tube aspirate reveals clear bilious fluid.

The patient is admitted to the ICU and stabilized. A repeat hemoglobin is 9.6 g/dl. After bowel preparation, urgent colonoscopy reveals sigmoid diverticulosis. One diverticulum contains a clot with an underlying visible vessel. An endoscopic clip is successfully applied to the vessel.

Discussion

Diverticular hemorrhage is a common cause of acute lower GI bleeding and usually presents without abdominal pain. The absence of abdominal pain makes diagnoses such as ischemic or infectious colitis less likely. Despite a negative nasogastric lavage, studies have shown that up to 15% of hemodynamically significant hematochezia cases are due to an upper GI source. Therefore, it is appropriate to consider doing an upper endoscopy prior to colonoscopy in patients with hemodynamic instability in whom an upper GI bleed should be ruled out.

Case 3

A 60-year-old woman with adult-onset diabetes and chronic renal insufficiency is found to have iron deficiency anemia (hemoglobin 8.3 g/dl, ferritin 28 ng/ml, transferrin saturation 10%). She has no history of gross bleeding, takes no NSAIDs, and has an unremarkable physical exam. Colonoscopy with terminal ileal intubation and EGD with duodenal biopsies are normal. Small bowel capsule endoscopy is performed, revealing scattered vascular ectasias in the proximal-to-mid small bowel. Balloon enteroscopy is performed with cautery of multiple vascular ectasias. Oral iron therapy is continued with improvement of anemia at three-month follow-up.

Discussion

When the initial evaluation of iron deficiency anemia with colonoscopy and EGD is negative, the patient is said to have occult, obscure GI bleeding. Some practitioners will elect to proceed directly to small bowel evaluation with capsule endoscopy, while others will elect for a trial of iron replacement. Some patients may also need more extensive small bowel evaluation by CT or MR enterography. Deep enteroscopy may be needed for endoscopic therapy of small bowel lesions.

Further reading

ASGE Standards of Practice Committee (2017). The role of endoscopy in management of suspected small-bowel bleeding. *Gastrointest. Endosc.* 85: 22–31.

Garcia-Tsao, G., Albrades, J.G., Berzigotti, A., and Bosch, J. (2017). Portal hypertensive bleeding in cirrhosis: risk stratification, diagnosis, and management: 2016 practice guidance by the American Association for the Study of Liver Diseases. *Hepatology* 65: 310–335.

Gerson, L.B., Fidler, J.L., Cave, D.R., and Leighton, J.A. (2015). Diagnosis and management of small bowel bleeding. *Am. J. Gastroenterol.* 110: 1265–1287.

Laine, L. and Jensen, D.M. (2012). Management of patients with ulcer bleeding. *Am. J. Gastroenterol.* 107: 345–360.

Strate, L.L. and Gralnek, I.M. (2016). ACG clinical guideline: management of patients with acute lower gastrointestinal bleeding. *Am. J. Gastroenterol.* 111: 459–474.

CHAPTER 4

The Patient with Unexplained Weight Loss

Unexplained weight loss may result from combinations of biological and behavioral factors. Hunger is a consequence of physiological processes, whereas appetite is more heavily influenced by environmental and psychological input, including the aroma and appearance of food and a person's mood. Unintentional weight loss can be related to insufficient nutrient intake, poor absorption of nutrients, or catabolic states. Clinically important weight loss is generally defined as unintentional weight loss of more than 5% over 6–12 months. Malignancy causes up to 40% of cases of unintentional weight loss, and a substantial proportion of these malignancies arise in the gastrointestinal tract. Up to 20–25% have a psychiatric cause of weight loss.

Clinical presentation

History

The first step in evaluation is objective documentation of the reported weight loss. The pattern, quality, and quantity of dietary intake should be assessed. Medications (e.g. procainamide, theophylline, thyroxine, and nitrofurantoin) may be factors in older patients. Fever or chills may suggest infectious causes, and appropriate risk factors raise the possibility of acquired immunodeficiency syndrome (AIDS). Nausea, early satiety, dysphagia, abdominal pain, jaundice, or a palpable abdominal mass may suggest underlying gastrointestinal malignancy. Diarrhea or bulky, foul-smelling, oily stools indicate possible malabsorption. Other systemic diseases are suggested by specific symptom profiles.

The history should also include a search for psychiatric causes, including alcoholism and depression. Psychomotor retardation or loss of interest or pleasure in daily activities is characteristic of depression. A denial of significant weight loss is common in anorexia nervosa, whereas secretive purging is classic in bulimia.

Yamada's Handbook of Gastroenterology, Fourth Edition. John M. Inadomi, Renuka Bhattacharya, Joo Ha Hwang, and Cynthia Ko.

Anorexia nervosa may also be associated with symptoms of altered gut function (e.g. early satiety, bloating, vomiting, constipation) and endocrine activity (e.g. amenorrhea, loss of libido, symptoms of hypothyroidism).

Physical examination

Physical findings of weight loss relate to its cause and the degree of malnutrition. Attention should be paid to overall appearance as well as to mood and affect. Cutaneous examination may suggest endocrine disease or AIDS (e.g. Kaposi sarcoma). Jaundice reflects hepatobiliary disease. Malignancy is suggested by lymphadenopathy, occult or overt gastrointestinal bleeding, or masses, whereas obstruction produces abdominal distension and high-pitched bowel sounds. Demonstrably impaired mental function may be an underlying factor in older patients.

Manifestations of severe malnutrition include hypothermia, bradycardia and other arrhythmias, hypotension, hypothermia, and dehydration, especially in patients with anorexia nervosa. Some may show temporal wasting or loss of skeletal muscle mass. Brittle hair or nails, decreased fat stores, acrocyanosis, downy hair, yellow cutaneous discoloration (from hypercarotenemia), and loss of secondary sexual characteristics may be seen, especially in young patients with anorexia nervosa. Self-induced vomiting or regurgitation produces halitosis, pharyngitis, and gingival or dental erosions from reflux of gastric acid and also may lead to parotid swelling and abrasion or scarring of the knuckles from inserting the fingers into the mouth.

Additional testing

Laboratory, radiological, and endoscopic evaluations are guided by the history and physical examination, including associated symptoms, patient age, symptom duration, prior medical conditions, degree of malnutrition, and emotional factors (Figure 4.1). Laboratory studies should include a complete blood count, sedimentation rate, C-reactive protein, electrolytes, blood urea nitrogen (BUN), creatinine, total protein, albumin, urinalysis, thyroid function, and liver chemistries. Radiography of the chest and abdomen can detect malignancy or obstruction. In the absence of specific findings, routine age-appropriate screening for malignancy is indicated.

Other tests for organic disease may be indicated in some patients. Testing for tuberculosis or human immunodeficiency virus can be performed in at-risk patients. If malabsorption is suspected, screening tests such as celiac serologies, qualitative or quantitative fecal fat, fecal elastase, serum carotene, and prothrombin time may be obtained. Specific tests for small intestinal or pancreatic causes of malabsorption are ordered if results of screening tests are positive or if suspicion of malabsorption is high. Hydrogen breath tests may help in the diagnosis of small intestinal bacterial overgrowth, and fecal and serum alpha-1-antitrypsin levels can help in diagnosing a protein-losing

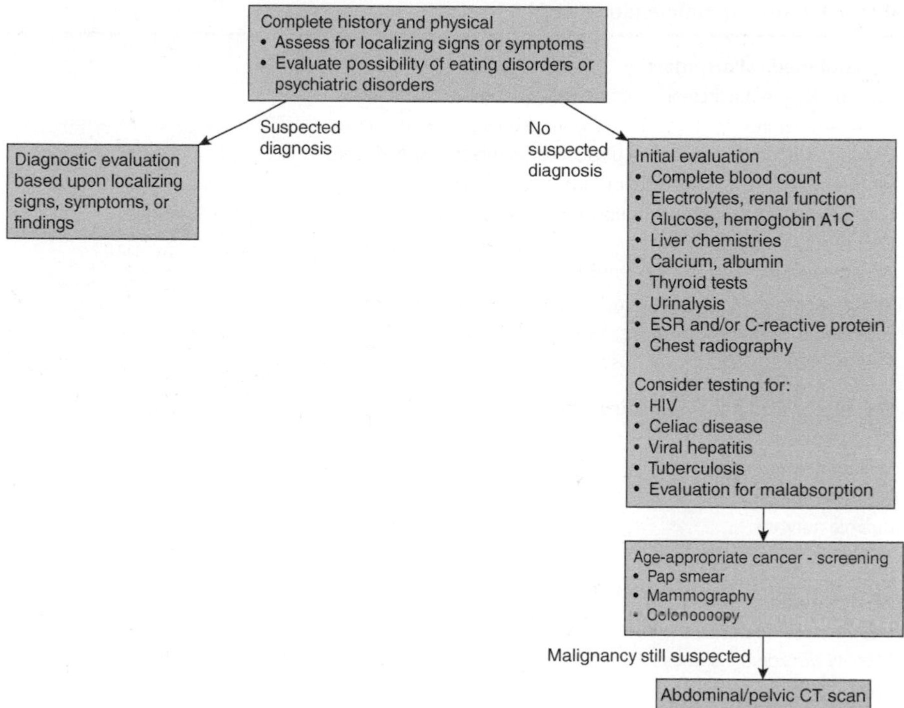

Figure 4.1 Evaluation of a patient with unexplained weight loss. CT, computed tomography; ESR, erythrocyte sedimentation rate; HIV, human immunodeficiency virus.

enteropathy. If structural disease is suspected, abdominal computed tomography or ultrasonography may detect underlying malignancies, and endoscopy may diagnose underlying ulcer disease, malignancy, or celiac disease. Mesenteric angiography or duplex ultrasonography can be considered if chronic mesenteric ischemia is suspected. When biological disease has been excluded, referral to a mental health specialist may help to exclude psychiatric causes of weight loss.

Differential diagnosis

In general, a person's weight fluctuates by as much as 1.5% per day. A sustained unintentional weight loss greater than 5% warrants concern and possible investigation. A variety of general medical, psychiatric, and gastrointestinal syndromes can produce unexplained weight loss (Table 4.1). About half of all cases of unexplained weight loss are attributable to organic disease, whereas psychiatric conditions, especially in the elderly, comprise the majority of the remaining cases.

Table 4.1 Causes of unintentional weight loss

General medical disorders
Malignancy – e.g. carcinoma, lymphoma, leukemia
Endocrinopathies – e.g. hyperthyroidism, diabetes mellitus, adrenal insufficiency, hypopituitarism
Chronic infections – e.g. tuberculosis, fungal infections, endocarditis, acquired immunodeficiency syndrome (AIDS), chronic helminth infection
Medications – e.g. metformin, nonsteroidal anti-inflammatory agents, antiviral medications
Chronic obstructive pulmonary disease
Congestive heart failure – e.g. cardiac cachexia
Renal disease – e.g. chronic kidney disease, nephrotic syndrome
Neurologic disease – e.g. stroke, Parkinson disease, dementia
Rheumatologic disease – e.g. systemic sclerosis
Psychiatric and behavioral disorders
Depression
Schizophrenia
Anorexia nervosa
Bulimia nervosa
Adult rumination syndrome
Gastrointestinal disorders
Gastrointestinal obstruction
Motility disorders – e.g. esophageal motility disorders, gastroparesis, chronic intestinal pseudo-obstruction
Pancreatic disease – e.g. pancreatic exocrine insufficiency
Protein-losing enteropathy
Malabsorption in the small intestine – e.g. celiac disease, inflammatory bowel disease
Small intestinal bacterial overgrowth
Chronic mesenteric ischemia
Gastrointestinal malignancy

General medical disorders

Malignancy should be considered early in evaluating weight loss, although neoplasm is not prevalent in patients without specific signs or symptoms. Endocrinopathies such as hyperthyroidism, diabetes mellitus, and adrenal insufficiency produce weight loss by varying mechanisms. Chronic infections (e.g. tuberculosis, fungal diseases, subacute bacterial endocarditis, AIDS) can cause weight loss, as can chronic kidney disease. In elderly patients, weight loss results from reduced taste or smell, physiological changes, comorbidities including neuropsychiatric syndromes, effects of medications, poor dentition, and lack of available food. Chronic obstructive lung disease and congestive heart failure produce weight loss by increasing caloric demands, causing anorexia, or increasing the work of eating.

Gastrointestinal disorders

Gastrointestinal diseases cause weight loss in several ways. Dysphagia from esophageal lesions or motility disorders can decrease nutritional intake. Luminal obstruction usually is associated with exacerbation of symptoms on meal ingestion, either immediately (esophageal stricture or cancer, achalasia), one to three hours postprandially (gastric or proximal intestinal obstruction), or several hours later (distal obstruction). Motor disorders such as gastroparesis or chronic intestinal pseudo-obstruction have similar effects. Likewise, pain from pancreaticobiliary sources may worsen after food ingestion, thus reducing intake. Malabsorption may result from disorders of the small intestine or pancreas or from small intestinal bacterial overgrowth. Weight loss occurs in ulcer disease because of meal-evoked pain. Constipation may cause anorexia. Postprandial abdominal pain is common with chronic mesenteric ischemia, leading to fear of eating and decreased oral intake.

Behavioral disorders

Depression is the most common behavioral disorder that decreases food intake and also is characterized by mood changes, sleep disruption, anhedonia, and low self-esteem. Alcoholism produces weight loss by mechanisms independent of its common association with depression. Weight loss may also occur with thought disorders (e.g. schizophrenia) because of distorted perceptions about food or eating.

Eating disorders

Eating disorders such as anorexia nervosa and bulimia nervosa, both of which may affect up to 5–10% of young women, are distinguished by the patient's altered body image and desire to maintain thinness. Eating disorders are much less common in older individuals. Adult rumination syndrome also produces weight loss and is often unrecognized.

Anorexia nervosa

Anorexia nervosa affects predominantly young women of all ethnic groups and socio-economic levels. Anorexia nervosa is characterized by distortion of body image and an inability to interpret hunger and satiety, with a preoccupation with eating and a sense of ineffectiveness. Patients are not truly anorectic but struggle against hunger to achieve an unrealistic degree of weight loss through dietary restriction, exercise, self-induced vomiting, or laxative abuse. Other psychosocial factors, including low self-esteem, obsessive–compulsive and avoidant personality traits, and perfectionistic tendencies, are common.

Bulimia nervosa

Bulimia nervosa is characterized by repetitive binges of overeating followed by acts to avert weight gain (e.g. self-induced emesis, laxative or diuretic abuse, excessive exercise). It occurs almost exclusively in women younger than 30 years, with a prevalence of 1–10%. There is a strong association of bulimia with affective disorders, low self-esteem, and family histories of mood disturbances, alcoholism, and drug addiction. Syndromes with occasional binge eating followed by purging may be present in up to 19% of college-age women.

Adult rumination syndrome

Rumination syndrome, or merycism, is an eating disorder in which the patient repetitively regurgitates food from the stomach, rechews it, and then reswallows it. The episodes are initiated by belching or swallowing and creating a common esophageal and gastric channel by reducing lower esophageal sphincter pressure. Diaphragmatic and rectus abdominis muscle contraction produces regurgitation, expelling gastric contents into the mouth, where they are rechewed and ingested. Adult patients generally report weight loss, regurgitation, and vomiting and are concerned about medical rather than psychiatric causes. The differential diagnosis includes esophageal strictures, gastroesophageal reflux disease, gastrointestinal (GI) dysmotility syndromes, and luminal obstruction. Characteristic manometric patterns may be seen in some patients with rumination syndrome.

Management

Therapy should be directed toward a specific etiology of weight loss, if identified. Nutritional assessment and support can promote weight gain in many patients with nonmalignant etiologies of weight loss. If no specific etiology is identified after appropriate investigations, a period of observation is indicated because more than 65% of these individuals do well on follow-up. For individuals with minor degrees of weight loss, nutritional supplementation may be sufficient. With severe malnutrition, hospitalization is necessary. Enteral refeeding may be attempted. If enteral feedings are poorly tolerated or refused, parenteral nutrition may be required. If the patient is severely malnourished, his or her fluid status and electrolytes need to be monitored closely for refeeding syndrome. Pharmacological therapy with progesterones and anabolic steroids has limited efficacy.

Antidepressant medications may produce striking weight gain in depressed patients. Medical and psychological management of behavioral disease should be initiated immediately along with any refeeding program. Potassium supplements may be needed for patients with anorexia or bulimia nervosa. Prokinetic medications and laxatives may reduce GI symptoms in anorexia nervosa, thus aiding the overall treatment plan. Antidepressants may reduce binge episodes and impulsive behavior in some patients with bulimia but play little role in anorexia nervosa. For anorexia nervosa, feedings are re-established at 200–250 cal above the intake at time of presentation and are increased by 250–300 cal every five days to ensure a weekly weight gain of 1.5 kg as an inpatient and 0.75–1.0 kg as an outpatient. The goal for refeeding is to achieve 90–100% of ideal body weight.

Psychological therapy for eating disorders addresses distorted beliefs about weight and eating, body image, fear of weight gain, self-criticism, and poor self-regulation. Therapies that have been efficacious for carefully selected patients with eating disorders include individual psychotherapy, interpersonal therapy, family therapy, and cognitive behavioral therapy. For patients with adult rumination syndrome, behavior modification and biofeedback appear to be the most effective approaches.

Complications

Profound weight loss has significant complications regardless of its cause. Cardiac complications include arrhythmias and sudden death, caused by either the primary disorder or metabolic consequences secondary to purging, such as hypokalemia. Electrocardiographic changes include bradycardia, decreased QRS amplitude, QT prolongation, ST segment changes, and U waves secondary to hypokalemia. Liver chemistry abnormalities result from hepatic steatosis. Fecal impaction can result from many of the causes of weight loss as well as from decreased oral intake and dehydration. Clinical features of hypothyroidism may develop, although free thyroxine levels usually are normal. Bulimia patients may develop pseudo-Bartter syndrome with fluid retention and peripheral edema after abruptly discontinuing diet pills and laxatives.

The prognosis of a patient with unexplained weight loss depends on the underlying etiology. Many organic conditions, especially malignancies, are fatal. For patients with anorexia nervosa, the recovery rate ranges from 32 to 71% at 20 years, although up to 5% die from complications of malnutrition. Nearly 75% of adolescents with anorexia nervosa continue to suffer from psychiatric diseases. Recovery rates for bulimia are 50–60%, although the condition is fatal in 1–5%.

Key practice points

- Sustained unexplained weight loss of 5% or more warrants investigation.
- The history and physical examination will often elucidate the cause of weight loss.
- Investigation for malignancy as directed by symptoms and patient age is recommended. Further evaluation should focus on adequacy of nutrition intake, looking for catabolic conditions, and ruling out malabsorption or calorie loss.
- Mental health disorders are a common cause of weight loss and often require a multidisciplinary approach to management.

Case studies

Case 1

A 30-year-old man with no significant past medical history presents with a 20-pound weight loss over the past three months. Review of systems is notable for mild diarrhea and generalized abdominal discomfort. Laboratory evaluation is notable for a normal complete blood count (CBC), comprehensive metabolic panel, and an elevated anti-tissue-transglutaminase IgA antibody. Esophagogastroduodenoscopy (EGD) reveals a normal esophagus and stomach and mild villous blunting in the duodenum. Histopathology from the duodenal biopsies confirms a diagnosis of celiac disease. The patient is placed on a gluten-free diet with gradual resolution of weight loss and improvement in symptoms.

Discussion

The initial evaluation of weight loss should be directed toward any symptoms. In this case, the patient's age makes malignancy less likely. The history of diarrhea suggests possible malabsorption, prompting investigation for celiac disease. Therapy directed at the underlying disorder results in resolution of weight loss.

Case 2

A 58-year-old woman with a past history of alcohol use disorder and smoking presents with a 32 lb. weight loss over the past four months. Her review of systems is unremarkable except for diarrhea without abdominal pain. Laboratory evaluation is notable for a normal CBC, serum electrolytes and renal function, liver transaminases, alkaline phosphatase, bilirubin, and thyroid function tests. Mammography and pelvic examination are normal. Colonoscopy and EGD with random biopsies are normal. Given ongoing weight loss, computed tomography (CT) of the abdomen and pelvis is performed, revealing an atrophic pancreas with calcifications. There are no pancreatic masses. Further laboratory evaluation reveals an elevated 24-hour fecal fat level with low fecal elastase levels. The patient begins pancreatic enzyme supplementation with improvement in diarrhea and resolution of weight loss.

Discussion

In the absence of historical features or symptoms to direct the diagnostic evaluation, most practitioners will begin by attempting to exclude malignancy. For women, this includes performing mammography; in both men and women of appropriate age, colonoscopy is also recommended. If colonoscopy is negative, many practitioners will perform EGD at the same setting. If structural disease is suspected, abdominal CT or ultrasonography may suggest malignancy or other underlying etiologies. In this case, the elevated fecal fat and low fecal elastase suggest pancreatic exocrine insufficiency, and there is no evidence of malignancy on CT. Pancreatic enzyme replacement results in resolution of weight loss.

Further reading

Alibhai, S.M., Greenwood, C., and Payette, H. (2005). An approach to the management of unintentional weight loss in elderly people. *Can. Med. Assoc. J.* 172: 773.

McMinn, J., Steel, C., and Bowman, A. (2011). Investigation and management of unintentional weight loss in older adults. *BMJ* 342: d1732.

CHAPTER 5

The Patient with Nausea and Vomiting

Nausea is the subjective sensation of an impending urge to vomit, and vomiting (emesis) is the forceful ejection of gastric contents from the mouth. Other symptoms may be misinterpreted by the patient as nausea or vomiting. Regurgitation is the effortless return of gastric or esophageal contents in the absence of nausea or involuntary spasmodic muscular contractions. Rumination is characterized by regurgitation of food into the mouth, where it is rechewed and reswallowed. Anorexia refers to loss of appetite. Early satiety is the sensation of gastric fullness before a meal is completed. Nausea may be part of a general complaint of indigestion that includes abdominal discomfort, heartburn, anorexia, and bloating.

Clinical presentation

History

Acute vomiting (for one to two days) most often results from infection, a medication or toxin, or accumulation of endogenous toxins, as in uremia or diabetic ketoacidosis. Chronic vomiting (longer than one week) usually results from a chronic medical or psychiatric condition. Vomiting soon after eating suggests gastric outlet obstruction or inflammatory conditions (e.g. cholecystitis and pancreatitis), whereas delayed vomiting is characteristic of gastroparesis or more distal obstruction. Psychogenic vomiting may occur soon after eating, but most patients control their emesis until the gastric contents can be expelled into a toilet or other receptacle. Early morning nausea characterizes endocrine conditions, such as pregnancy. Meals may relieve nausea associated with peptic ulcer or esophagitis. Patients with cannabinoid hyperemesis almost universally report relief of symptoms with hot showers or baths.

The character of the vomitus can provide diagnostic clues. Vomiting of undigested food is seen with Zenker diverticulum and achalasia. Partial digestion is observed with gastric outlet obstruction and gastroparesis. Bilious vomiting

Yamada's Handbook of Gastroenterology, Fourth Edition. John M. Inadomi, Renuka Bhattacharya, Joo Ha Hwang, and Cynthia Ko.

excludes gastric outlet obstruction, whereas vomiting of blood suggests mucosal damage. Voluminous acidic emesis is observed with gastrinomas, whereas feculent emesis occurs with distal obstruction, bacterial overgrowth, and gastrocolic fistulae.

Associated symptoms should be assessed. Pain is reported with ulcer disease, obstruction, or inflammatory disorders. Diarrhea, fever, or myalgias suggest possible infection. Weight loss occurs in many patients with chronic nausea. However, patients with psychogenic vomiting usually maintain stable weight. Headaches, visual changes, altered mentation, and neck stiffness raise the possibility of central nervous system etiologies, whereas tinnitus or vertigo indicate labyrinthine causes.

Physical examination

A physical examination assists in diagnosing and managing nausea and vomiting. Fever suggests inflammation or infection. Tachycardia, orthostatic hypotension, loss of skin turgor, and dry mucous membranes indicate dehydration. Oral examination may reveal loss of dental enamel, a common finding in bulimia. A succussion splash on side-to-side movement is found in gastric outlet obstruction and gastroparesis. An absence of bowel sounds signifies ileus, whereas high-pitched hyperactive bowel sounds with a distended abdomen are consistent with intestinal obstruction. Abdominal tenderness is noted with inflammation, infection, and luminal distension, whereas gross or occult fecal blood should prompt evaluation for ulcer, inflammation, or malignancy. Adenopathy and masses suggest malignancy; hepatomegaly is also found in malignancy and in benign hepatic disease. On neurological examination, focal signs, papilledema, and impaired mentation suggest central nervous system disease. Asterixis is present in metabolic conditions, such as uremia and hepatic failure. Gut motility disorders may be associated with peripheral and autonomic neuropathy.

Additional testing

A thorough history and physical examination will provide sufficient information to diagnose and treat most patients with nausea and vomiting. If there is a clear temporal association of the onset of vomiting with myalgias, cramps, and diarrhea or with initiation of a new medication, no further workup is needed. However, some patients with more chronic symptoms require further evaluation.

Laboratory studies

Several blood tests assist in evaluating the patient with nausea and vomiting (Figure 5.1). With long-standing symptoms or dehydration, serum electrolytes may show hypokalemia, metabolic alkalosis, or an elevated blood urea nitrogen (BUN) relative to creatinine. Other useful tests may include complete blood counts, amylase, lipase, liver chemistries, albumin, thyroid function, and plasma cortisol. Pregnancy should be excluded in appropriate patients. Specific serological

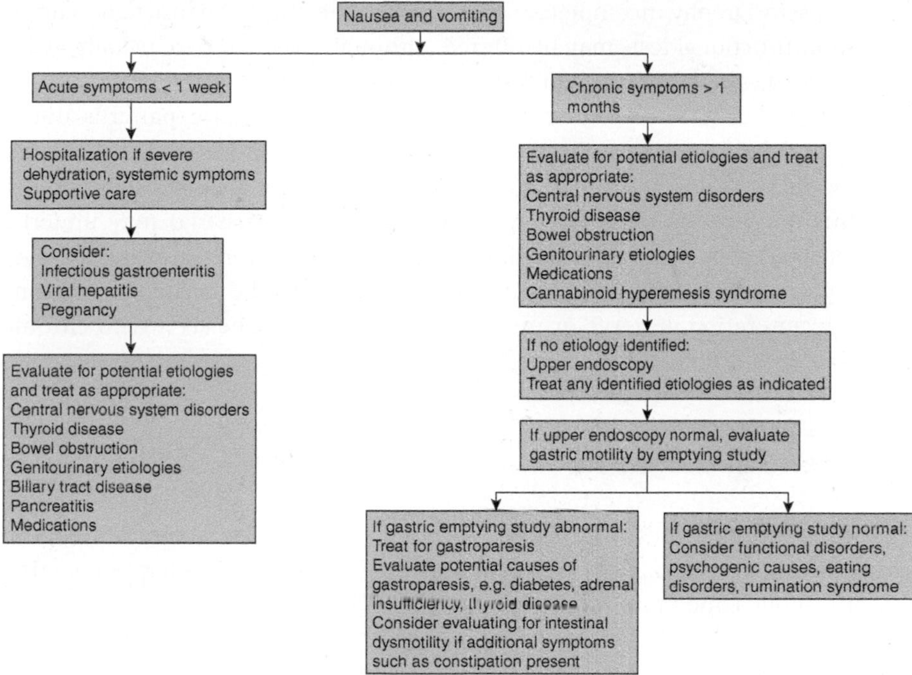

Figure 5.1 Workup of a patient with nausea and vomiting.

markers can screen for presumed collagen vascular diseases, and antineuronal antibodies may be positive with malignancy-associated motility disorders.

Structural studies

Structural investigation may be needed to exclude organic illness as a cause of vomiting. Flat and upright abdominal radiographs can screen for possible obstruction or ileus. Contrast radiography of the small intestine may confirm partial obstruction and can help evaluate intestinal transit time. If symptoms are intermittent, computed tomography (CT) or magnetic resonance (MR) enterography may provide more detailed assessment of the small bowel. Upper endoscopy can assess possible gastric outlet obstruction and allows biopsies if indicated. Retained food in the absence of obstruction is seen in gastroparesis. For suspected pancreaticobiliary disease, transabdominal or endoscopic ultrasound, abdominal CT, hepatobiliary scintigraphy, or MR cholangiopancreatography may be useful. CT or MR imaging of the head may be indicated for suspected central nervous system sources.

Functional studies

If luminal obstruction is excluded, motility disorders such as gastroparesis and chronic intestinal pseudo-obstruction should be considered. Gastroparesis is diagnosed by demonstrating delayed emptying of an ingested meal using scintigraphy.

When scintigraphy incompletely characterizes the cause of nausea and vomiting, other functional tests may be offered, although these tests are usually available only in specialized gastrointestinal physiology laboratories. Tests such as antral-duodenal or intestinal manometry can evaluate motor patterns under fasting and fed conditions. Electrogastrography measures electrical pacemaker activity of the stomach through electrodes affixed to the abdomen. Pacemaker rhythms that are too rapid (tachygastria) or slow (bradygastria) may underlie development of nausea and vomiting. In rare cases of severe unexplained dysmotility, a surgical full-thickness intestinal biopsy may be needed to demonstrate degeneration of nerve or muscle layers, which can be seen with chronic intestinal pseudo-obstruction.

Differential diagnosis

The differential diagnosis of nausea and vomiting includes medication effects, gastrointestinal and intraperitoneal disease, neurological disorders, endocrine and metabolic conditions, and infections (Table 5.1).

Medications

Drug effects are among the most common causes of nausea and vomiting and usually occur shortly after initiating therapy. Chemotherapeutic agents such as cisplatin and cyclophosphamide are potent emetic stimuli that act on central and peripheral neural pathways. Emesis from chemotherapy may be acute, delayed, or anticipatory. Analgesics such as aspirin or nonsteroidal anti-inflammatory drugs (NSAIDs) induce nausea by direct gastrointestinal mucosal irritation. Other classes of medications that produce nausea include cardiovascular drugs (e.g. digoxin, antiarrhythmics, antihypertensives), diuretics, hormonal agents (e.g. oral hypoglycemics, contraceptives), antibiotics (e.g. erythromycin), and gastrointestinal medications (e.g. sulfasalazine).

Disorders of the gastrointestinal tract and peritoneum

Gut and peritoneal disorders represent prevalent causes of nausea and vomiting. Gastric outlet obstruction often produces intermittent symptoms, whereas small intestinal obstruction is usually acute and associated with abdominal pain. Disorders of gut motor activity (e.g. gastroparesis and chronic intestinal pseudo-obstruction) evoke nausea because of an inability to clear retained food and secretions. Gastroparesis may be idiopathic or secondary to several systemic diseases (e.g. diabetes, scleroderma, lupus, amyloidosis, pancreatic adenocarcinoma, ischemia). Nausea is frequently a functional symptom without clearly defined etiology. Chronic intestinal pseudo-obstruction may be hereditary, result from systemic disease, or occur as a paraneoplastic syndrome (most commonly, small cell lung carcinoma). Superior mesenteric artery

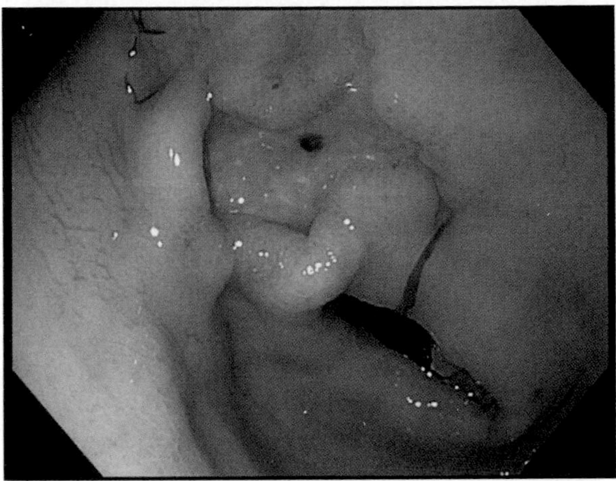

Chapter 20 Gastric ulcer: ulcer with a "flat pigmented spot" that is at low risk for recurrent hemorrhage.

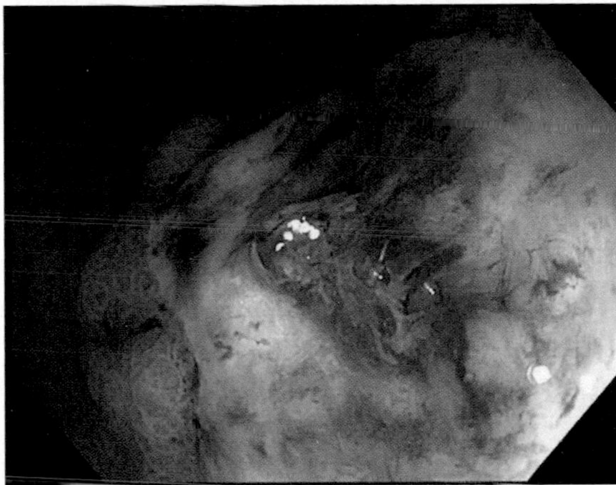

Chapter 20 Gastric ulcer: ulcer with a "pigmented protuberance (visible vessel)" that is at high risk for recurrent hemorrhage.

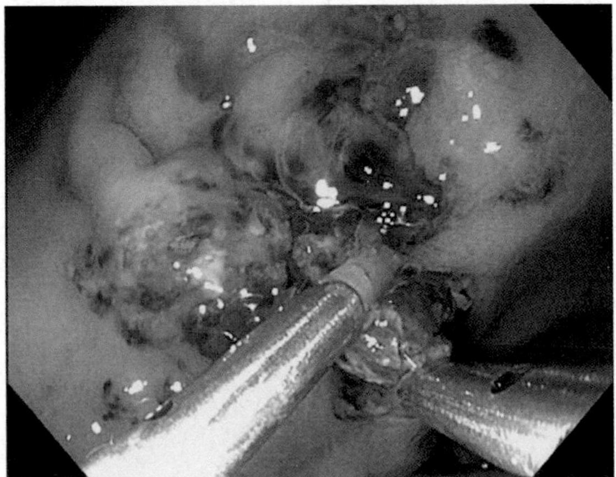

Chapter 20 Gastric ulcer: ulcer after endoscopic treatment with hemoclips placed at site of visible vessel.

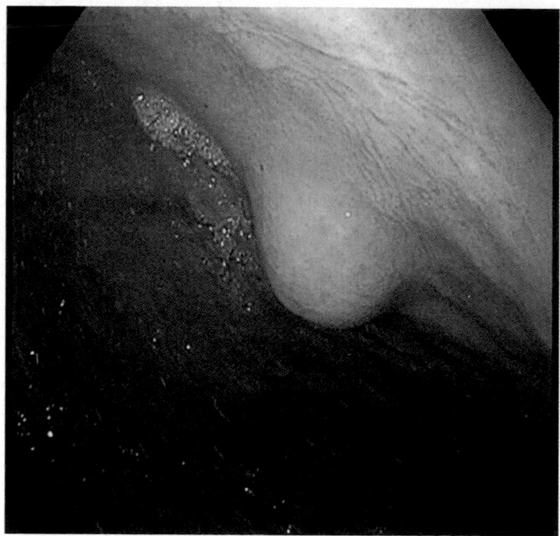

Chapter 22 Subepithelial mass: endoscopic image of tumor deep to the epithelial layer of the gastric mucosa.

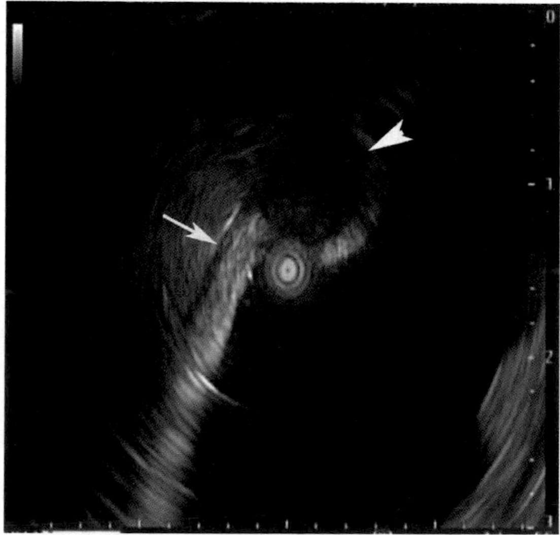

Chapter 22 Subepithelial mass: endoscopic ultrasound image of subepithelial mass (white arrow) and cytology aspiration needle (yellow arrow).

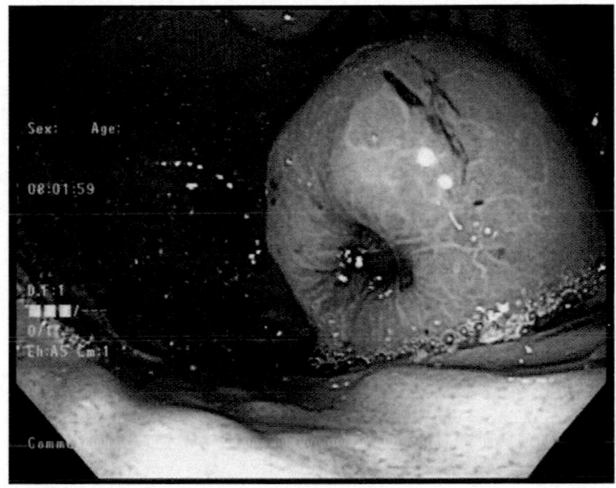

Chapter 22 Gastrointestinal stromal tumor (GIST).

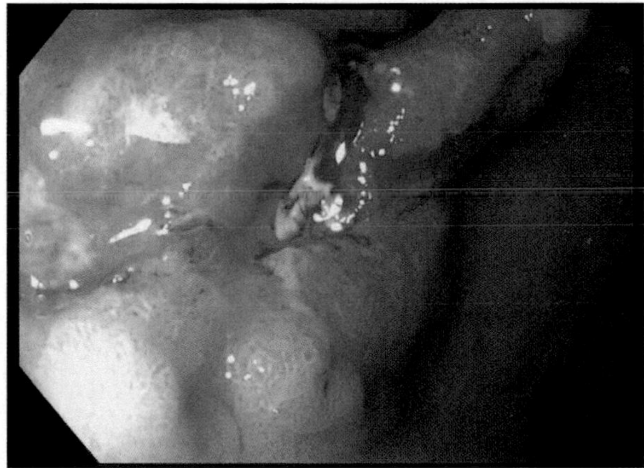

Chapter 22 Gastric cancer: ulcerated malignancy of gastric body.

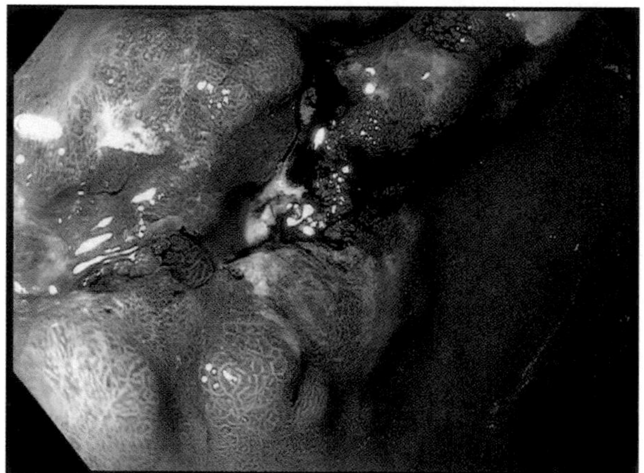

Chapter 22 Gastric cancer: narrow band imaging via endoscopy of gastric malignancy.

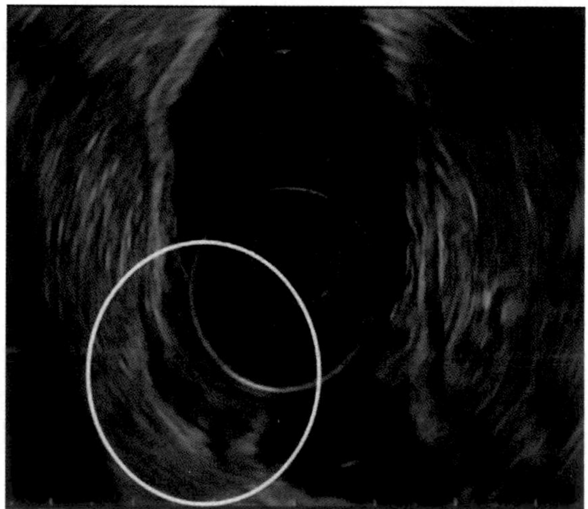

Chapter 22 Gastric cancer: endoscopic ultrasound image of gastric cancer.

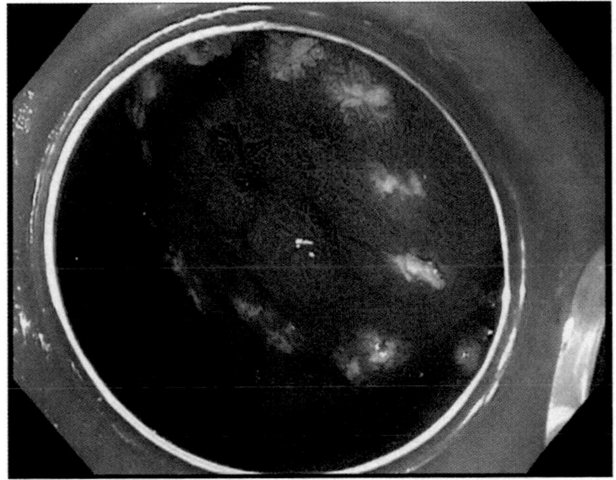

Chapter 22 Gastric cancer: early stage gastric cancer being prepared for removal by endoscopic submucosal dissection (ESD).

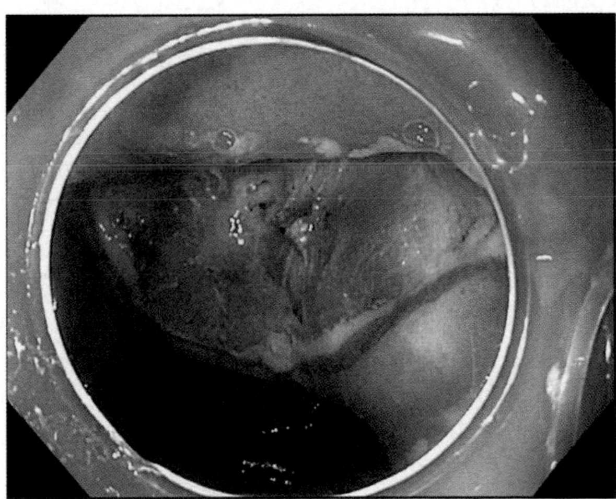

Chapter 22 Gastric cancer: after removal by ESD.

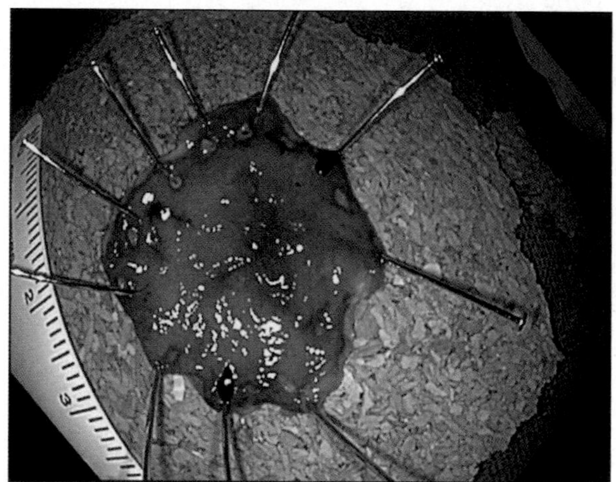

Chapter 22 Gastric cancer: ESD specimen.

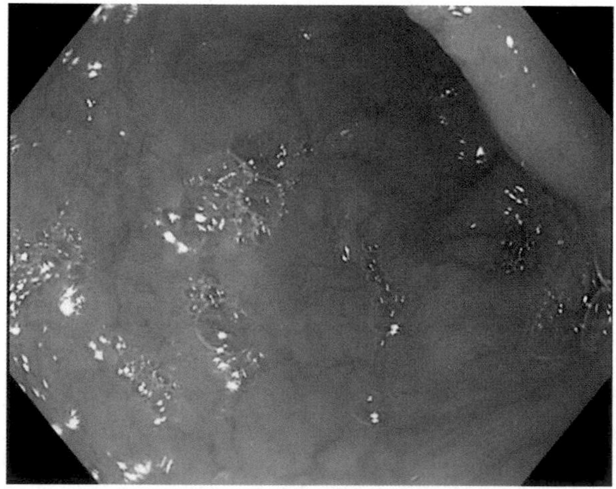

Chapter 23 Celiac disease: "scalloped mucosa" in duodenum.

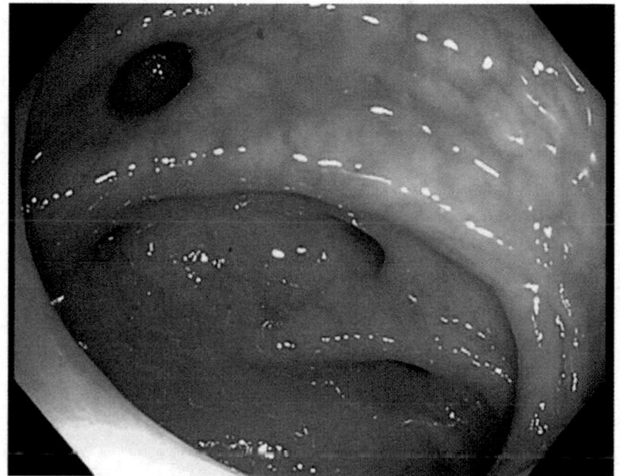

Chapter 26 Diverticulosis.

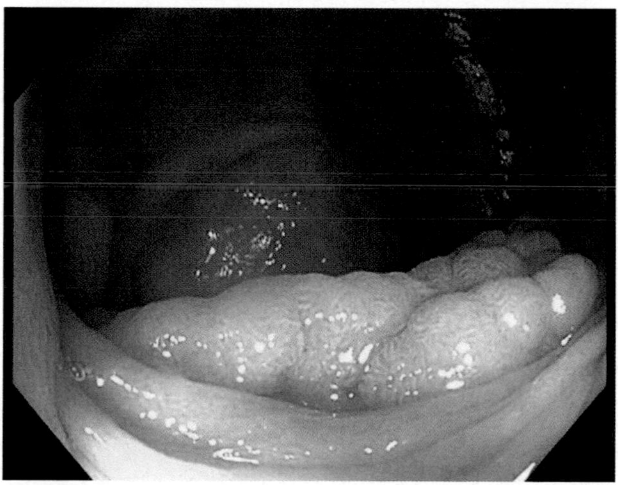

Chapter 29 Adenomatous polyp.

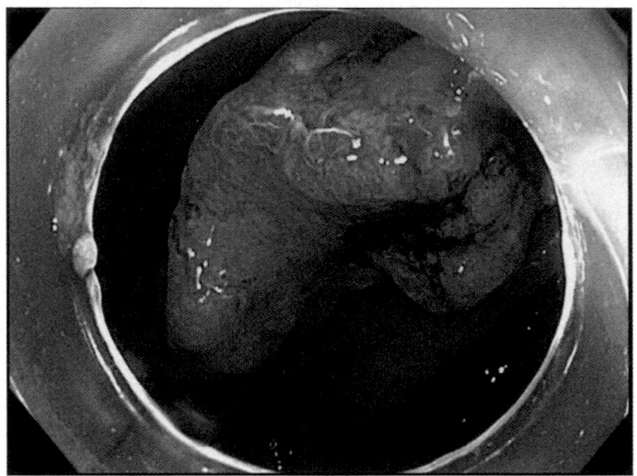

Chapter 29 Colon cancer: endoscopic image prior to submucosal dissection removal.

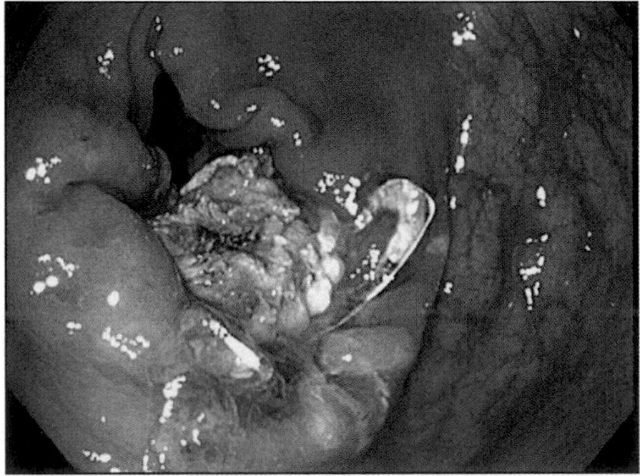

Chapter 29 Colon cancer: colon cancer after removal via ESD.

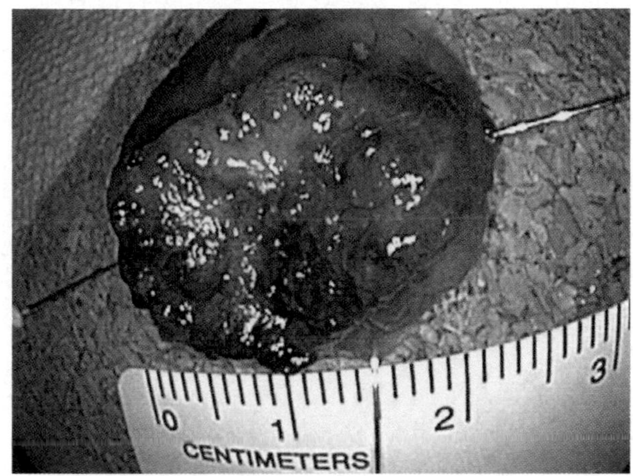

Chapter 29 Colon cancer: ESD specimen.

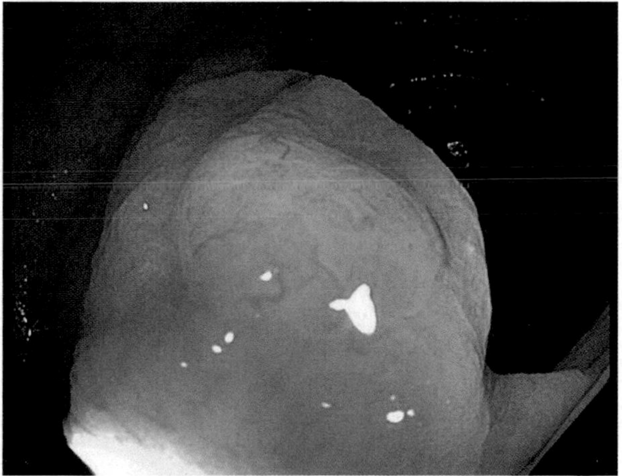

Chapter 29 Colon polyp: sessile serrated polyp.

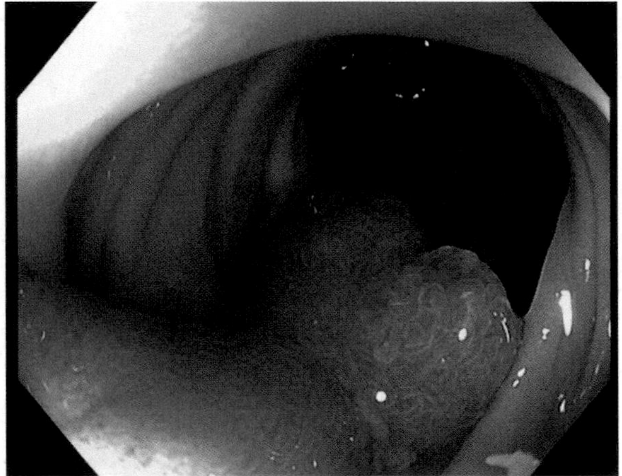

Chapter 29 Colon polyp: pedunculated adenomatous polyp.

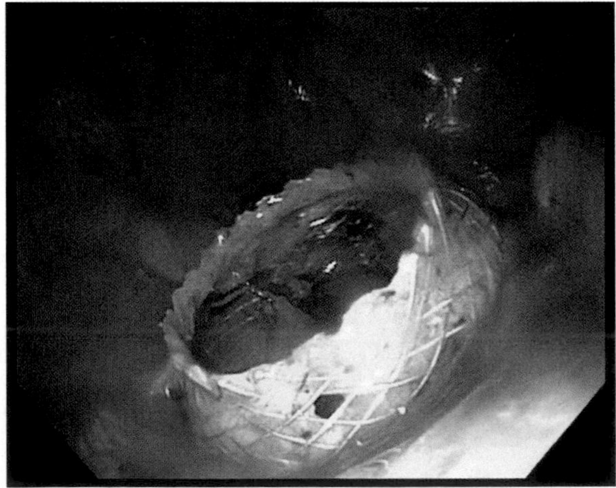

Chapter 31 Lumen-opposing metal stent: endoscopic image of the gastric aspect of stent connected to pancreatic pseudo-cyst.

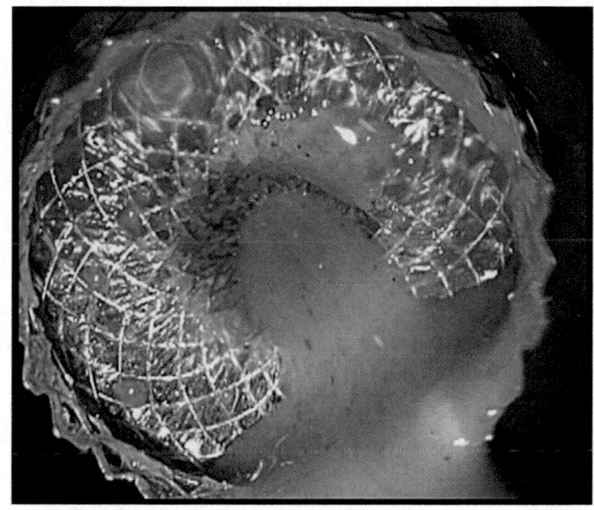

Chapter 31 Lumen-opposing metal stent: endoscopic image of pseudo-cyst drainage.

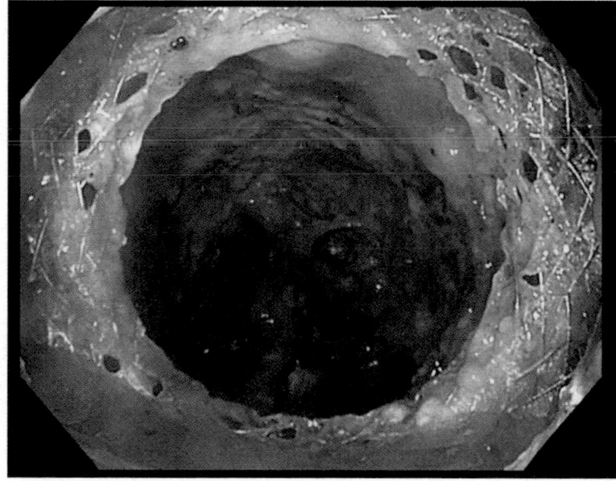

Chapter 31 Lumen-opposing metal stent: gastric port to pancreatic necrosis.

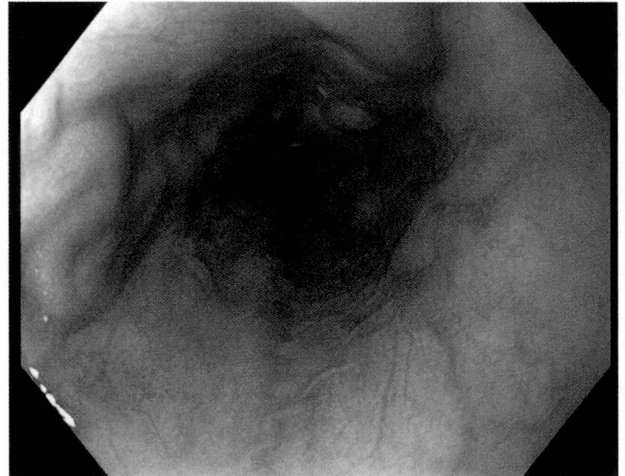

Chapter 39 Esophageal varices: linear vessels in the distal esophagus.

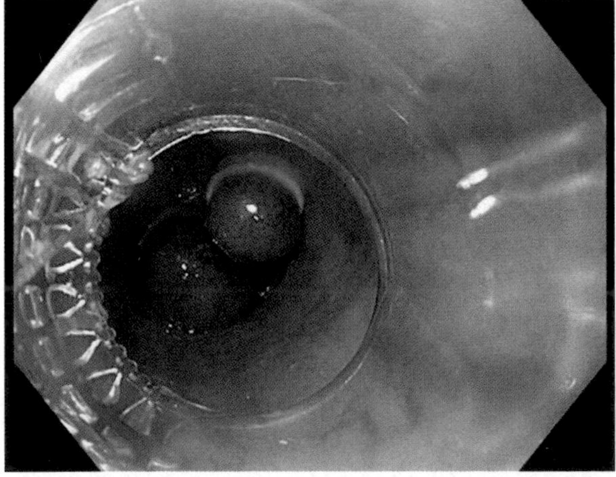

Chapter 39 Esophageal varices after endoscopic band ligation therapy.

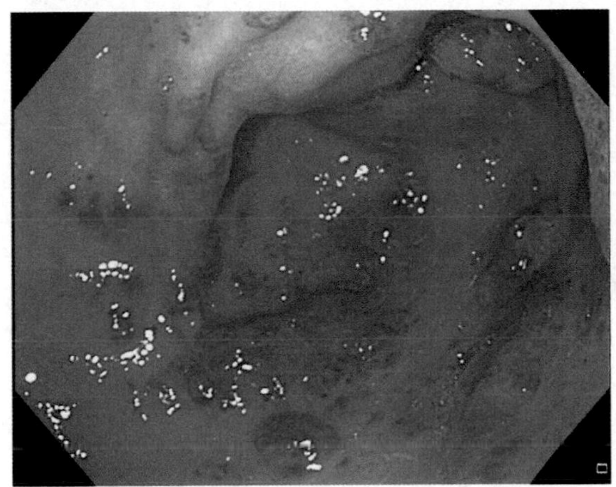

Chapter 42 Gastric antral vascular ectasia (GAVE).

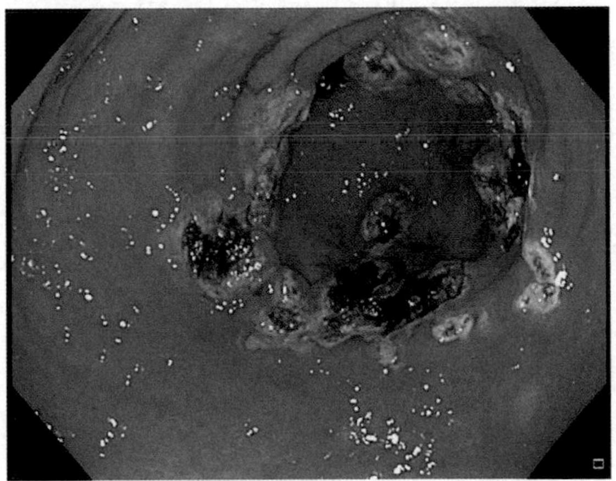

Chapter 42 GAVE: post-treatment with argon plasma coagulation.

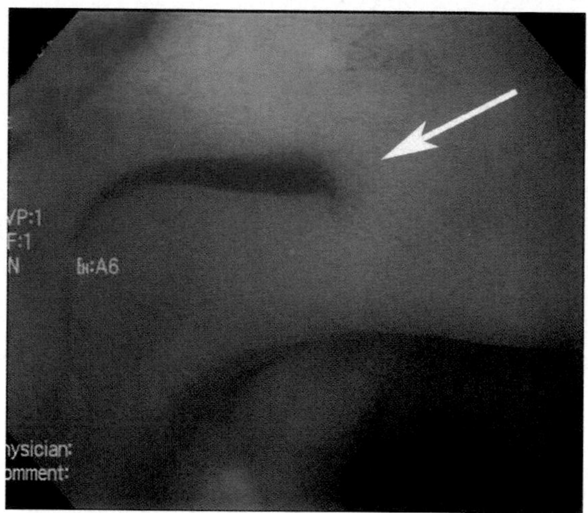

Chapter 42 Vascular ectasia: bleeding vascular ectasia of colon.

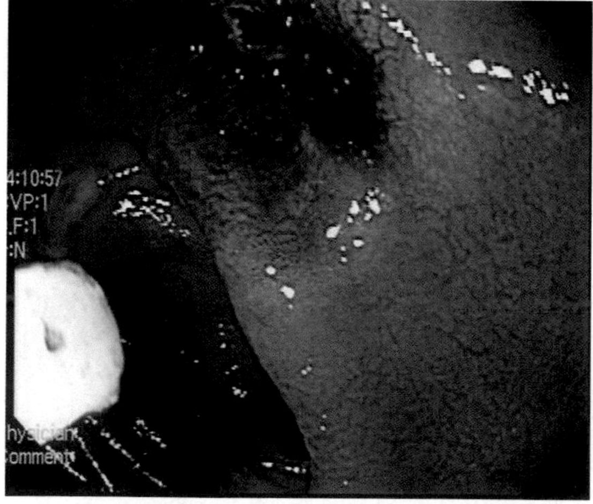

Chapter 42 Vascular ectasia: treatment with argon plasma coagulation.

Table 5.1 Causes of nausea and vomiting

Medications
Nonsteroidal anti-inflammatory drugs (NSAIDs)
Cardiovascular drugs (e.g. digoxin, antiarrhythmics, antihypertensives)
Diuretics
Hormonal agents (e.g. oral antidiabetics, contraceptives)
Antibiotics (e.g. erythromycin)
Gastrointestinal drugs (e.g. sulfasalazine)
Central nervous system disorders
Tumors
Cerebrovascular accident
Intracranial hemorrhage
Infections
Congenital abnormalities
Psychiatric disease (e.g. anxiety, depression, anorexia nervosa, bulimia nervosa, psychogenic vomiting)
Motion sickness
Labyrinthine causes (e.g. tumors, labyrinthitis, Ménière disease)
Miscellaneous causes
Posterior myocardial infarction
Congestive heart failure
Excess ethanol ingestion
Jamaican vomiting sickness
Prolonged starvation
Cyclic vomiting syndrome
Cannabinoid hyperemesis syndrome
Gastrointestinal and peritoneal disorders
Gastric outlet obstruction
Small bowel obstruction
Superior mesenteric artery syndrome
Gastroparesis
Chronic intestinal pseudo-obstruction
Pancreatitis
Appendicitis
Cholecystitis
Acute hepatitis
Endocrine and metabolic conditions
Nausea of pregnancy
Uremia
Diabetic ketoacidosis
Thyroid disease
Adrenal insufficiency
Infectious agents
Viral gastroenteritis (e.g. rotavirus, norovirus)
Bacterial causes (e.g. *Staphylococcus* spp., *Salmonella* spp., *Bacillus cereus, Clostridium perfringens*)
Opportunistic infection (e.g. cytomegalovirus, herpes simplex virus)
Otitis media

syndrome occurs when the duodenum is compressed and obstructed by the superior mesenteric artery as it originates from the aorta and often develops after severe weight loss

Other rare mechanical causes of nausea and vomiting include gastric volvulus and antral webs. Inflammatory conditions (e.g. pancreatitis, appendicitis, and cholecystitis) irritate the peritoneal surface, whereas biliary colic produces nausea by activating the afferent neural pathways. Fulminant hepatitis causes nausea, presumably because of accumulation of emetic toxins and increases in intracranial pressure.

Central nervous system causes

Conditions with increased intracranial pressure, such as tumors, infarction, hemorrhage, infections, or congenital abnormalities, produce emesis with and without nausea. Emotional responses to unpleasant smells or tastes induce vomiting, as can anticipation of cancer chemotherapy. Psychiatric causes of nausea and vomiting include anxiety, depression, anorexia nervosa, and bulimia nervosa. Labyrinthine etiologies of nausea include labyrinthitis, tumors, and Ménière disease. Motion sickness is induced by repetitive movements that result in activating vestibular nuclei.

Endocrinological and metabolic conditions

First-trimester pregnancy is the most common endocrine cause of nausea. This condition, occurring in 50–70% of pregnancies, usually is transitory and is not associated with poor fetal or maternal outcome. However, 1–5% of cases progress to hyperemesis gravidarum, which may produce significant fluid losses and electrolyte disturbances. Other endocrinological and metabolic conditions associated with vomiting include uremia, diabetic ketoacidosis, thyroid disease, hypercalcemia, and adrenal insufficiency.

Infectious causes

Infectious illness produces nausea and vomiting, usually of acute onset. Viral gastroenteritis may be caused by rotaviruses or norovirus. Bacterial infection with *Staphylococcus* or *Salmonella* organisms, *Bacillus cereus*, and *Clostridium perfringens* also produces nausea and vomiting, in many cases via toxins that act on the brainstem. Nausea in immunosuppressed patients may result from gastrointestinal cytomegalovirus or herpes simplex infections. Infections outside the gastrointestinal lumen, such as hepatitis, otitis media, and meningitis, may also elicit nausea.

Miscellaneous causes

Nausea may be a manifestation of posterior wall myocardial infarction or congestive heart failure. Cyclic vomiting syndrome is a condition of unknown etiology characterized by episodes of severe abdominal pain, nausea, and vomiting with intervening asymptomatic periods. Chronic cannabis use may cause cannabinoid hyperemesis syndrome, which is characterized by intermittent nausea, vomiting, and abdominal pain similar in presentation to cyclic vomiting. Acute graft-versus-host disease is the dominant cause of nausea and vomiting in bone marrow transplant recipients.

Management

The first decision in treating the patient with acute or chronic nausea and vomiting is to determine if intravenous fluid resuscitation is needed. Poor skin turgor or orthostatic pulse or blood pressure changes indicate that more than 10% of body fluids have been lost, mandating intravenous fluid resuscitation with careful attention to electrolyte repletion.

If patients can tolerate some oral intake, a liquid diet low in fat and indigestible residue is recommended because such a diet empties from the stomach more readily. Medications that inhibit gastric motor function should be withheld if possible. Patients with diabetes should strive for optimal glycemic control because elevated blood glucose impairs gastric emptying. Nasogastric suction may provide benefit in patients with obstruction or ileus.

When feasible, medical treatment for nausea should be directed at the underlying illness. However, less specific antiemetic therapy is also useful. Antihistamines such as meclizine are useful for labyrinthine disorders, motion sickness, uremia, or postoperative vomiting. Anticholinergic medications such as scopolamine also are effective in motion sickness but produce numerous side effects. Antidopaminergics such as phenothiazines or butyrophenones are commonly prescribed antiemetics that are useful for many causes of nausea and vomiting. This medication class produces many side effects, including sedation, agitation, mood changes, dystonias, parkinsonian symptoms, irreversible tardive dyskinesia, and hyperprolactinemic symptoms (galactorrhea, sexual dysfunction, amenorrhea). Other drug classes that have been suggested as generalized antiemetics include serotonin (5-HT_3) receptor antagonists such ondansetron or granisetron and tricyclic antidepressants.

Gut motility disorders may respond to prokinetic agents. The most widely prescribed prokinetic medication is metoclopramide, which acts via serotonin (5-HT_4) receptor facilitation of gastric cholinergic function as well as by antidopaminergic effects in the stomach and brainstem. This drug enhances gastric emptying and reduces symptoms in gastroparesis but is poorly tolerated by 20% of patients because of significant antidopaminergic side effects. Domperidone is a peripheral dopamine antagonist with prokinetic properties that does not cross the blood–brain barrier and thus is better tolerated. This drug is prescribed throughout much of the world but is not approved for use by the U.S. Food and Drug Administration. The macrolide antibiotic erythromycin stimulates gastric emptying by action on receptors for the hormone motilin, which is the endogenous mediator of fasting gastrointestinal motility. However, erythromycin often is poorly tolerated because it can exacerbate nausea or induce abdominal pain, and its use is hampered by tachyphylaxis. The somatostatin analog octreotide is useful in some cases of intestinal pseudo-obstruction through selective stimulation of contractile activity of the small intestine.

Nondrug therapies can be considered for some conditions of chronic nausea and vomiting. Acupuncture and acupressure have been used to treat nausea of pregnancy, motion sickness, and postoperative nausea. Ginger and pyridoxine have been proposed for nausea of pregnancy. Jejunostomy feedings may improve overall health in patients with advanced gastroparesis, whereas intravenous hyperalimentation may be needed for severe forms of intestinal dysmotility. Surgical resections only rarely benefit patients with nausea and vomiting secondary to dysmotility.

Complications

Chronic nausea and vomiting can produce dehydration, malnutrition, and electrolyte abnormalities. Increased intrathoracic pressure during vomiting produces purpura on the face and neck, whereas retching-induced Mallory–Weiss tears across the esophagogastric junction may present as upper gastrointestinal hemorrhage. The Boerhaave syndrome is a more severe complication that results when vomiting ruptures the esophagus, leading to mediastinitis or peritonitis. In patients with impaired mentation, emesis may cause pulmonary aspiration, producing chemical pneumonitis.

Key practice points

- The differential diagnosis of nausea and vomiting is very broad, including medication side effects, gastrointestinal and intraperitoneal diseases, neurological disorders, metabolic conditions, and infections.
- The timing of vomiting in relation to meals and the character of the vomitus can provide clues to etiology.
- Flat and upright abdominal radiographs provide screening information concerning the presence or absence of intestinal obstruction.
- Contrast radiography of the small intestine can assess for partial intestinal obstruction.
- Upper endoscopy can assess for gastric outlet obstruction and allows diagnostic biopsies of suspicious lesions.
- Medical therapy of nausea and vomiting should be directed at the underlying illness whenever feasible.

Case studies

Case 1

A 55-year-old man presents with a two-month history of persistent nausea and vomiting, abdominal discomfort, and approximately 10-pound weight loss. Symptoms began abruptly with severe nausea and vomiting. These severe symptoms abated after 36 hours, but he has noted persistent mild-to-moderate nausea and vomiting since then. Physical examination is remarkable for dry mucous membranes. Serum laboratories reveal mild hypoalbuminemia, and an abdominal x-ray is normal. Esophagogastroduodenoscopy (EGD) is performed and demonstrates retained food in the gastric fundus and body but is otherwise unremarkable. Gastric emptying study shows delayed gastric emptying.

Discussion

This patient has symptoms of gastroparesis. There is no evidence of gastric outlet obstruction, and evaluation otherwise shows delayed gastric emptying. Although frequently associated with long-standing diabetes, many cases of gastroparesis are idiopathic and/or begin after an episode of infectious gastroenteritis. Patients with gastroparesis should be counseled to adhere to a diet that promotes gastric emptying of foods, including eating foods that are lower in fat or residue and eating smaller, more frequent meals. Some patients will require use of antiemetic or prokinetic agents such as metoclopramide to manage symptoms and improve oral intake.

Case 2

A 30-year-old previously healthy man presents with episodic nausea and vomiting. In between episodes, he is asymptomatic and denies weight loss. Symptoms often abate after taking a hot bath or shower. The history is otherwise notable for frequent cannabis use. Physical examination is unremarkable. Laboratory investigation is normal, and abdominal films taken during an episode do not show any abnormalities. EGD is normal. He is advised to stop cannabis use completely for two to three months.

Discussion and potential pitfalls

This patient presents with symptoms consistent with cannabinoid hyperemesis syndrome. This syndrome is characterized by episodic nausea and vomiting, frequently relieved by hot showers or baths, with few intervening symptoms. Typically, no other etiologies of nausea and vomiting can be identified. It can be difficult to distinguish this syndrome from cyclic vomiting syndrome. Complete cessation of cannabis intake is often needed to manage this condition.

Further reading

Camilleri, M., Parkman, H.P., Shafi, M.A. et al. (2013). Clinical guideline: management of gastroapresis. *Am. J. Gastroenterol.* 108: 18–37.

CHAPTER 6

The Patient with Abdominal Pain

Clinical presentation

History

The location, character, intensity, and timing of pain as well as factors that enhance or minimize the pain are obtained from the history. Symptoms pertinent to past or present illnesses also are evaluated.

Pain localization

Pain from esophagitis, esophageal dysmotility, or esophageal neoplasm usually is substernal and may radiate to the back, jaw, and left shoulder and arm. The usual pain of peptic ulcer disease is epigastric. Radiation of ulcer pain to the back suggests a posterior penetrating duodenal ulcer. Small intestinal disease most commonly produces periumbilical pain, although ileal lesions may elicit hypogastric symptoms. Colonic pain may be perceived in any region of the abdomen or back. Liver capsular distension produces right upper quadrant pain. Gallbladder and bile duct pain is experienced in the epigastrium and right upper quadrant. Pancreatic pain typically is felt in the epigastrium with radiation to the back. Left upper quadrant pain suggests pancreatic disease but may also result from greater curvature gastric ulcers, splenic lesions, perinephric disease, and colonic splenic flexure lesions. Renal pain from acute pyelonephritis or obstruction of the ureteropelvic junction usually is sensed in the costovertebral angle or flank, although upper abdominal pain is not unusual. Ureteral pain may be referred to the testicle or thigh. Uterine lesions produce midline lower abdominal pain, whereas adnexal pain localizes to the ipsilateral lower quadrant. Pelvic pain may radiate to the back.

Migration of pain with disease evolution suggests underlying inflammation. Cholecystitis may begin in the epigastrium and migrate to the right upper quadrant, whereas appendicitis may start in the midline and then move to the McBurney point in the right lower abdomen.

Yamada's Handbook of Gastroenterology, Fourth Edition. John M. Inadomi, Renuka Bhattacharya, Joo Ha Hwang, and Cynthia Ko.

Pain quality

Esophagitis produces burning or warm pain, whereas peptic ulcer pain is dull or gnawing. Pain from small intestinal obstruction or inflammation is colicky or crampy and may be associated with abdominal distension and audible bowel sounds. Pain from appendicitis may be colicky but usually is a constant dull ache. Despite use of the terms *biliary colic* and *renal colic*, obstruction of these organs more often produces a steady rather than colicky pain. Acute cholecystitis leads to squeezing pain, whereas acute pancreatitis results in penetrating or boring pain. Nephrolithiasis evokes a sharp or cutting pain.

Pain intensity

Extremely severe abdominal pain is produced by peptic ulcer perforation, acute pancreatitis, or passage of a renal stone, whereas severe acute pain is evoked by small intestinal obstruction, cholecystitis, and appendicitis. Causes of more moderate acute pain include peptic ulcer disease, gastroenteritis, and esophagitis. Intensity of chronic abdominal pain is more difficult to assess because psychological factors can modify pain perception. Then, indirect questions about interference with sleep or daily function may provide useful information about pain severity.

Pain chronology

Peptic ulcer pain may be intermittent and often occurs in the morning or before meals. Posterior penetration should be considered when peptic ulcer pain becomes constant. Acute cholecystitis commonly develops during sleep and may be preceded by months of intermittent biliary colic. Nocturnal pain rarely occurs in patients with irritable bowel syndrome or functional abdominal pain. Appendicitis typically presents as progressive pain for 10–15 hours without remission. Pain reaching peak intensity within minutes is more characteristic of ulcer perforation, abdominal aortic aneurysm rupture, passage of renal stones, or ruptured ectopic pregnancy. In acute pancreatitis, intestinal obstruction, cholecystitis, or mesenteric arterial occlusion, peak pain intensity is reached in 10–60 minutes. A gradual onset of pain for hours is reported in appendicitis, some cases of cholecystitis, diverticulitis, and mesenteric venous occlusion. The pain of irritable bowel syndrome is chronic and may be most intense after meals. In women, pain at monthly intervals suggests endometriosis or ovulation-related symptoms. Pain after starting medication raises the possibility of acute intermittent porphyria (barbiturates) or pancreatitis (steroids, tetracycline, thiazides).

Alleviating and aggravating factors

Antacids or acid-suppressing medications may relieve the pain of esophagitis or peptic ulcer disease. Ingesting food can relieve discomfort from a duodenal ulcer but may aggravate pain because of gastric body ulcers. The pain of pancreatic disease almost always is intensified by meal ingestion, as is discomfort from intestinal obstruction or mesenteric ischemia. Duodenal obstruction provokes pain within minutes of eating, whereas ileal lesions cause pain one to two hours after a meal. Pain from mesenteric ischemia is intensified after meals due to the inability of the impaired blood supply to satisfy the metabolic demands of the gut. Lactase deficiency may produce discomfort that is specific to consumption of dairy products. Heartburn may be aggravated by reclining or straining. Pancreatic pain is worse in the supine position and is relieved by leaning forward. In contrast, back pain in irritable bowel syndrome may be relieved by hyperextension of the spine. Psoas muscle irritation, as with a psoas abscess in Crohn's disease, often causes the patient to lie supine with the right leg flexed at the hip and knee. The pain of nerve root compressions and other musculoskeletal conditions may worsen with some movements. Abdominal pain in irritable bowel syndrome may be ameliorated by massaging the abdominal wall or by passing feces or flatus. Alternatively, irritable bowel pain is aggravated by eating or stress. Passage of diarrheal stools may reduce cramping in colitis.

Associated symptoms

Abdominal pain usually precedes nausea in conditions that ultimately require surgery, whereas nausea may occur first in disorders not requiring surgery. Diarrhea typically indicates a nonsurgical condition such as gastroenteritis, although appendicitis is an exception to this rule. In elderly patients with acute left-sided pain and bloody stools, ischemic colitis should be considered. Chronic abdominal pain with rectal bleeding suggests colonic neoplasm or inflammatory bowel disease. Abdominal pain with the recent onset of constipation is consistent with colonic obstruction, whereas long-standing constipation is a feature of irritable bowel syndrome. Anorexia and weight loss raise concern for malignancy, whereas high fevers (>39.5 °C) early in the course of a painful condition suggest cholangitis, urinary tract infection, infectious enteritis, or pneumonia.

Late fevers suggest a localized infection such as diverticulitis, appendicitis, or cholecystitis. Jaundice suggests disease of the liver, biliary tree, or pancreas. Many but not all women report abnormal or absent menses with ectopic pregnancy.

Risk factors

Heavy alcohol intake for prolonged periods can lead to acute pancreatitis, whereas analgesic intake predisposes to ulcer disease. Cocaine abuse may cause mesenteric ischemia. A patient with gallstones may present with distal intestinal obstruction secondary to gallstone ileus. Cardiovascular disease predisposes to mesenteric ischemia, whereas prior abdominal surgery increases the likelihood of intestinal obstruction. Patients with cirrhosis and ascites develop spontaneous bacterial peritonitis. During pregnancy, abdominal pain results from appendicitis, pyelonephritis, cholelithiasis, pancreatitis, and adnexal disease. The presence of a gravid uterus may modify the symptom presentation or findings of physical examination. Immunocompromised individuals are susceptible to common causes of abdominal pain as well as neutropenic enterocolitis, opportunistic infections such as cytomegalovirus, and graft-versus-host disease in patients who have undergone bone marrow transplantation. The typical signs of peritonitis may be absent in these patients.

Physical examination

A comprehensive extra-abdominal physical examination is required to provide insight into the cause of abdominal pain. A writhing, diaphoretic, pale patient usually is more ill than one who is resting comfortably, although some individuals with peritonitis may lie motionless to avoid abdominal irritation. Fever or tachycardia may point to an acute infectious or inflammatory process. Hypotension raises concern for an abdominal catastrophe such as a ruptured aneurysm. Scleral icterus or jaundice suggests cholestasis or biliary obstruction. Adenopathy, masses, and hepatomegaly suggest malignancy. A chest examination may reveal pneumonia as the cause of pain, whereas an irregular heart rhythm might suggest new-onset atrial fibrillation as a source of mesenteric arterial embolism. Radiculopathy as a cause of pain is suspected with asymmetrical strength or sensation on neurological examination. Peripheral or autonomic neuropathies are found in some patients with gastrointestinal dysmotility. The presence of occult fecal blood on rectal examination raises the possibility of malignancy, ischemia, ulcer disease, and inflammation. Right-sided tenderness on rectal examination may also be found with appendicitis. Perianal fistulae, fissures, and abscesses suggest Crohn's disease. In women, a pelvic examination is used to evaluate possible adnexal or uterine causes of abdominal pain. Dermatographia is a sign consistent with mast cell activation syndrome.

Abdominal, rectal, genital, and pelvic examinations are mandatory in a patient with acute abdominal pain. Intestinal obstruction is considered if scars are observed on inspection and if auscultation reveals high-pitched bowel sounds. In contrast, a silent distended abdomen suggests ileus secondary to intra-abdominal inflammation or peritonitis. A right upper quadrant friction rub or bruit suggests a possible hepatic tumor, whereas bruits elsewhere may indicate mesenteric insufficiency. Abdominal palpation should begin in an area distant from the reported site of pain to prevent conscious guarding. Involuntary guarding suggests peritonitis. Rebound tenderness suggests peritoneal inflammation but also may be elicited in noninflammatory conditions such as irritable bowel syndrome and thus has been considered an unreliable sign. It is often useful to shake the patient's bed gently from side to side, which may be a more subtle means of detecting peritonitis. Severe pain with little tenderness or guarding is consistent with intestinal infarction or early acute pancreatitis. The Carnett test can distinguish intra-abdominal discomfort from abdominal wall pain. Increased tenderness upon raising the head and tensing the abdomen suggests a superficial abdominal wall source. Discrepancies between tenderness elicited with pressure from the stethoscope and that from the examining hand suggest possible functional abdominal pain.

Fecal occult blood raises concern for malignancy, ischemia, ulcer disease, or inflammatory conditions, whereas perianal fistulae, abscess, or inflammation suggests possible Crohn's disease. Rectal examination also may detect an intra-abdominal inflammatory process such as an appendiceal abscess that is not palpable over the anterior abdominal wall. Inguinal hernias as a cause of intestinal obstruction may be detected on genital examination, whereas pelvic examination of women is essential for diagnosing adnexal masses and pelvic inflammatory disease.

Additional testing

Determining the cause of abdominal pain commonly requires laboratory testing (Figure 6.1). However, diagnostic testing in the patient with chronic functional pain should be directed by alarm findings on exam and screening blood tests to avoid reinforcing the patient's conviction that there is something organically wrong. A complete blood count (CBC) may show leukocytosis, indicating an inflammatory condition, or leukopenia, suggesting a viral syndrome. Microcytic anemia raises the possibility of gut blood loss. The sedimentation rate may be elevated in inflammatory conditions.

Electrolytes, blood urea nitrogen, and creatinine are measured to assess fluid status and renal function. Elevated serum amylase or lipase or both usually are observed early in acute pancreatitis. Perforated ulcers, diabetic ketoacidosis, or mesenteric infarction also may cause hyperamylasemia. Elevated levels of bilirubin or alkaline phosphatase suggest disease of the pancreas or biliary tract, whereas aminotransferase elevations indicate hepatocellular disease. Serum pregnancy testing is performed in women of reproductive potential who present with unexplained abdominal pain. Specific laboratory tests can assist in diagnosing acute porphyria or heavy metal intoxication. Tryptase levels are elevated in mast cell activation syndrome. Urinalysis may show erythrocytes or crystals, suggesting calculi; leukocytes or bacteria, suggesting infection; or bilirubin, suggesting pancreaticobiliary disease. Patients with ascites and abdominal pain should undergo paracentesis to exclude spontaneous bacterial peritonitis. Culdocentesis can aid in assessing intra-abdominal hemorrhage.

Supine and upright (or decubitus) abdominal plain radiography is essential in all patients with acute abdominal pain and can detect pneumoperitoneum from lumenal perforation, calcified gallstones or renal stones, air–fluid levels with intestinal obstruction, generalized or localized distension with ileus, pneumobilia with biliary disease, and a ground-glass appearance with ascites. Barium radiographs may complement the findings of plain films when mechanical obstruction is suspected. Chest radiographs can eliminate pulmonary sources of acute abdominal pain.

Other imaging studies complement findings of the examination, laboratory testing, and plain films. Ultrasound is useful for suspected cholelithiasis, biliary

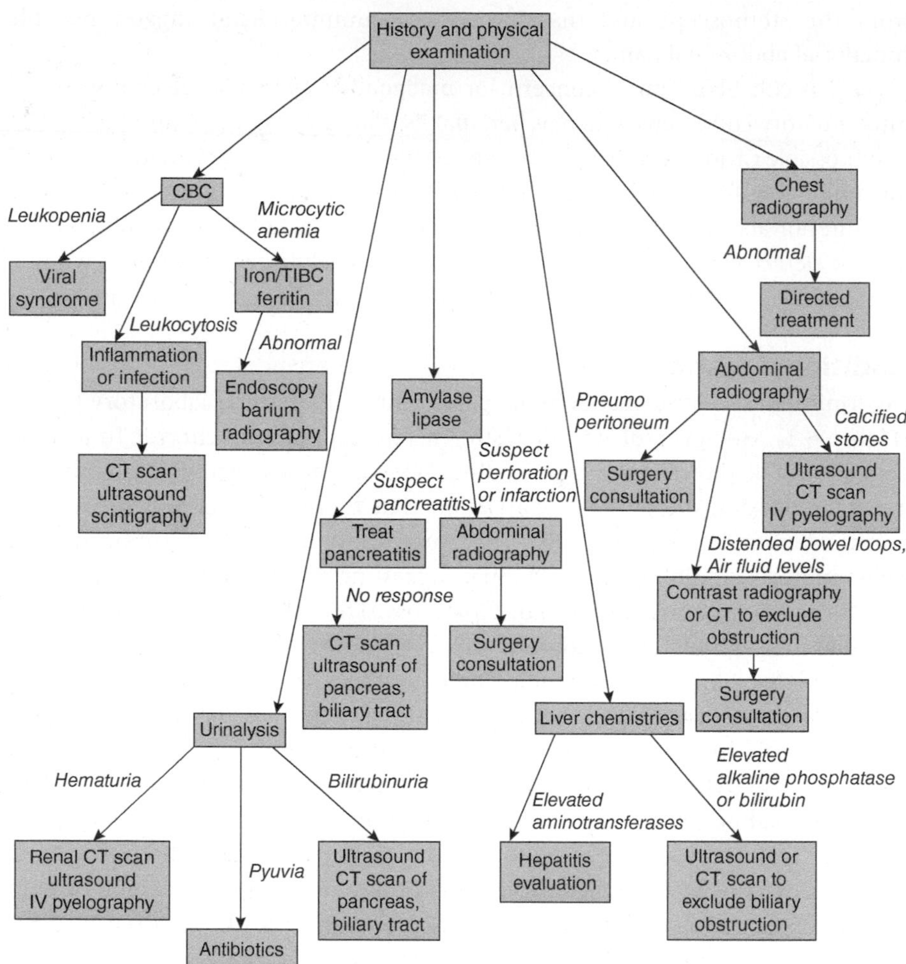

Figure 6.1 Workup of a patient with abdominal pain. CBC, complete blood count; CT, computed tomography; IV, intravenous; TIBC, total iron-binding capacity.

dilation, ovarian cysts, abscess formation, and ectopic pregnancy, whereas computed tomography (CT) is more sensitive for pancreatic disease, retroperitoneal collections, intra-abdominal abscess, some vascular processes, trauma-induced hematomas, and changes in the mesentery or intestinal wall resulting from ischemia or inflammation (as with diverticulitis). Scintigraphy with ^{99m}Tc-iminodiacetic acid derivatives detects cystic duct obstruction from cholecystitis. Angiography or mesenteric resonance angiography may be indicated for suspected vascular occlusion. Ultrasound is sensitive for diagnosing the impending rupture of an abdominal aortic aneurysm, but further study with aortography may delay definitive therapy and should be performed in the operating room, if indicated, because of the risk of exsanguination. Upper endoscopy is performed for chronic epigastric pain that suggests uncomplicated peptic ulcer but is contraindicated with suspected perforation.

Sigmoidoscopy or colonoscopy is helpful with lower abdominal pain secondary to suspected ischemia, infection, volvulus, drug-induced colitis, or inflammatory bowel disease. Magnetic resonance cholangiopancreatography (MRCP) and endoscopic ultrasound (EUS) are sensitive for detecting choledocholithiasis; however, endoscopic retrograde cholangiopancreatography (ERCP) may be required for treatment of cholangitis caused by choledocholithiasis. ERCP, EUS, and MRCP may provide complementary information in diagnosing chronic pancreatitis. Laparoscopy may be performed on an emergency basis in extremely ill patients or electively for chronic abdominal pain where the diagnosis is elusive after extensive diagnostic testing.

Differential diagnosis

The differential diagnosis of abdominal pain includes pathological processes within and outside the abdomen (Table 6.1). Generally, pain from diseases of the hollow organs (e.g. gut, urinary tract, pancreaticobiliary tree) results from obstruction, ulceration, inflammation, perforation, or ischemia. Pain from disorders of solid organs (e.g. liver, kidneys, spleen) is caused by distension from infection, obstruction to drainage, or vascular congestion. In women, the adnexa and uterus are potential sources of pain. Lung or cardiac abnormalities may secondarily cause referred pain in the upper abdomen. Metabolic conditions (e.g. lead poisoning, diabetic ketoacidosis) cause diffuse or localized abdominal pain. Acute intermittent porphyria, a disorder of heme biosynthesis that results in accumulation of toxic intermediates, causes colicky abdominal pain, ileus, and psychiatric disturbances. Familial Mediterranean fever produces painful inflammation of joints, skin, and serosal surfaces in the abdomen and the chest. Mast cell activation syndrome represents an emerging process of immune dysfunction whereby degranulation of mast cells results in inflammation that causes abdominal pain, dermatographia, and other systemic symptoms. Degenerative disk disease, tabes dorsalis, and varicella zoster virus reactivation elicit superficial abdominal wall pain.

The acuity of the clinical presentation restricts the possible differential diagnoses. With acute abdominal pain, the clinician should quickly establish an accurate diagnosis and implement specific measures to reduce pain and treat the underlying cause if possible. Recurrent pain that lasts hours to days with intervening asymptomatic periods represents a diagnostic challenge in some cases. Many such patients are ultimately diagnosed as having a functional abdominal pain syndrome, which is defined as at least six months of nearly continuous pain with poor relationship to physiological events such as eating or defecation, some loss of daily function, no evidence of malingering, and insufficient criteria to satisfy other functional or organic diagnoses. Patients with functional abdominal pain syndrome often exhibit evidence of psychosocial dysfunction, including anxiety, depression, somatization, or hypochondriasis. Functional abdominal

Table 6.1 Causes of abdominal pain

Intra-abdominal
Peritoneal inflammation
Perforated viscus
Spontaneous bacterial peritonitis
Appendicitis
Diverticulitis
Pancreatitis
Cholecystitis/cholangitis
Pelvic inflammatory disease
Familial Mediterranean fever
Visceral mucosal disorders
Peptic ulcer disease
Inflammatory bowel disease
Infectious colitis
Esophagitis
Visceral obstruction
Intestinal obstruction (adhesions, hernia, volvulus, intussusception, malignancy)
Biliary obstruction (stone, tumor, stricture)
Renal colic (stone, tumor)
Capsular distension
Hepatitis
Budd–Chiari syndrome
Pyelonephritis
Tubo-ovarian abscess
Ovarian cyst
Endometritis
Ectopic pregnancy
Vascular disorders
Intestinal ischemia
Abdominal aortic aneurysm
Splenic infarction
Tumor necrosis
Visceral motor and functional disorders
Irritable bowel syndrome
Functional dyspepsia
Esophageal dysmotility
Viral gastroenteritis
Extra-abdominal
Neurological
Radiculopathy
Varicella zoster virus reactivation
Musculoskeletal
Trauma
Fibromyalgia
Cardiothoracic
Pneumonia
Myocardial infarction

Table 6.1 (*cont'd*)

Pneumothorax
Empyema
Pulmonary infarction
Toxic/metabolic
Uremia
Diabetic ketoacidosis
Porphyria
Lead poisoning
Reptile venom, insect bite
Mast cell activation
Addison disease

pain often occurs in individuals with prior childhood abdominal pain or with a history of physical or sexual abuse. Aberrant illness behaviors may be prominent in these patients. Chronic, continuous abdominal pain often has an obvious cause such as disseminated malignancy, chronic pancreatitis, or less serious illnesses with concurrent depression.

Management

Under ideal conditions, therapy is directed at eliminating the cause of abdominal pain. If this is not possible, efforts are aimed at decreasing pain perception and removing factors that exacerbate pain. Patients with pain from fever, vomiting, orthostatic hypotension, tachycardia, rebound, leukocytosis, new hyperbilirubinemia, or impaired mentation may need hospitalization. The threshold for hospital admission is lowered for the very young or old and for immunocompromised individuals.

Specific therapy exists for many conditions such as acid suppressants for gastroesophageal reflux or surgery for appendicitis or cholecystitis, but the diagnosis must be accurate. Some conditions that cause chronic pain may not be curable. Nonsteroidal anti-inflammatory drugs (NSAIDs) are often prescribed for chronic pain. However, because many chronic conditions have little tissue damage or inflammation, it is not surprising that NSAIDs are often ineffective. Opioid agents are useful for managing pain that is secondary to unresectable malignancy, but prescribing them for chronic nonmalignant states is controversial. Regardless of the indication, narcotics are best administered within an integrated treatment program. The use of opioids at regular intervals, rather than on an as-needed basis, is often more effective for treating severe pain. Pain cocktails that incorporate opioids, acetaminophen, and antiemetics allow flexible dosing that prevents mental clouding, respiratory depression, nausea, and constipation. Tricyclic antidepressants have analgesic effects that are independent of their mood-elevating effects. Agents with serotonergic and noradrenergic activity (e.g. amitriptyline, doxepin) exhibit the greatest effects, often at doses lower than required to treat depression. Conversely, although anxiolytics may reduce anxiety, they have little long-term efficacy in managing chronic abdominal pain and may actually worsen symptoms because of depleted brain serotonin levels.

Nonmedical treatments also are useful in treating chronic pain. Patients with pain secondary to unresectable neoplasm may benefit from referral to a multidisciplinary pain clinic. Celiac plexus blockade is effective therapy for selected patients with pancreatic adenocarcinoma but is less likely to control pain from chronic pancreatitis. Local neural blockade of trigger points may provide benefit in some cases of abdominal wall pain. Rhizotomy and cordotomy involve severing the neural pathways that sense pain and are indicated only for conditions in which life expectancy does not exceed six months because of significant complications, including bowel and bladder dysfunction, dysesthesias, and exacerbation of the pain. Transcutaneous electrical nerve stimulation and dorsal column stimulation reduce pain in some chronic conditions, presumably because pain inhibitory nerve fibers are stimulated and endogenous opioid production is activated. Acupuncture may work by similar mechanisms. Unfortunately, these techniques have not shown significant efficacy in treating chronic pain that is secondary to intra-abdominal causes.

Like most chronic illnesses, irritable bowel syndrome and functional abdominal pain have no cure. Thus, efforts should be directed to enhancing the quality of the patient's life. The physician must establish a good working relationship with the patient and acknowledge the reality of the pain and the suffering that it causes. Scheduling of frequent brief visits and directed appropriate diagnostic evaluation are important. The emphasis then shifts from diagnosis to treatment with a realization by the patient that a cure is not possible and an understanding that a major part of the treatment process will be to minimize the impact of the pain on daily life. Psychological or psychiatric consultation is appropriate when the clinician suspects a concurrent, major affective, or personality disorder. Tricyclic agents represent the main form of medication therapy. Meta-analyses of tricyclic agents used to treat functional causes of abdominal pain have shown significant therapeutic benefits compared with a placebo. Most other drug classes provide little or no benefit in this condition. Opioid agents should be avoided in these patients because of drug dependency. Relaxation training, biofeedback, and hypnosis have shown benefit in small trials. Behavioral therapy reduces chronic pain behavior by rewarding the patient's expression of well behavior. Cognitive therapies promote healthy behavior by increasing the patient's awareness of situations that increase pain, with the goal of increasing the patient's control over these situations. Subsets of patients may benefit from formal psychotherapy.

Complications

The potential for complications depends on the cause of the pain. Failure to diagnose peritonitis, a ruptured ectopic pregnancy, or an aortic aneurysm can have fatal consequences. Other inflammatory conditions (e.g. pancreatitis, inflammatory bowel disease, or pelvic inflammatory disease) may require prolonged courses of treatment, producing debilitating symptoms and loss of productivity at home and work. Renal stones may lead to infection and renal insufficiency. The prognosis is excellent for many patients with chronic noninflammatory abdominal pain, including those with irritable bowel syndrome, endometriosis, and nerve root compression syndromes.

Key practice points

- An accurate history needs to be obtained, focusing on details of the abdominal pain, including location, quality, intensity, chronology, alleviating and aggravating factors, and associated symptoms.
- A thorough physical exam should be performed.
- Appropriate laboratory tests should be ordered based on the differential diagnosis.
- Rapid diagnosis of the etiology of the abdominal pain is essential, especially in cases of intestinal perforation, intestinal obstruction, appendicitis, and ruptured aortic aneurysm.

Case studies

Case 1

A 53-year-old man presents to the emergency department with complaints of worsening epigastric pain. The pain initially began four days before and started out as an intermittent dull ache in the epigastric region. The pain would be worse before meals and would improve slightly after a meal. However, over the last five hours the pain has been constant and the patient is very uncomfortable. He denies any nausea or vomiting. He has been taking NSAIDs for the last week because of a knee injury. He has no other medical problems. On physical exam he appears uncomfortable. He has significant tenderness to palpation throughout the entire abdomen and also has rebound and guarding. Labs are significant for a leukocytosis and elevated amylase. An abdominal series radiography with supine and upright views demonstrates evidence of free air within the abdomen. The patient is diagnosed with a perforated viscus and taken to surgery where he is found to have a perforated duodenal ulcer.

Discussion and potential pitfalls

Gastrointestinal perforation requires urgent surgical intervention; therefore, the diagnosis needs to be made rapidly. If a perforation is in the differential an abdominal series radiography with supine and upright or decubitus views should be obtained immediately. However, in gastroduodenal perforations free air may not be appreciated in one-third of cases on abdominal series radiography. If an abdominal series radiography is negative but perforation is still suspected, a CT scan should be performed. Failure to rapidly identify a gastrointestinal perforation leads to increased mortality.

Case 2

A 26-year-old man presents to the emergency department with a three-day history of dull periumbilical pain. Over the past 24 hours, the pain has become progressively worse and has migrated to the right lower quadrant. He also reports nausea, vomiting, and diarrhea over the past 24 hours. On physical exam he has a fever to 38.0 °C, heart rate of 110, and is normotensive. Labs are only notable for a leukocytosis with a left shift. On physical exam the patient has McBurney point tenderness. A CT scan with intravenous (IV) and oral contrast demonstrates appendiceal wall thickening with periappendiceal fat stranding. The patient is diagnosed with acute appendicitis and is managed with surgical intervention with a laparoscopic appendectomy during which an inflamed appendix without evidence of perforation is identified and removed.

Discussion and potential pitfalls

Acute appendicitis is a common cause of acute abdominal pain seen in the emergency department. Classic symptoms include right lower quadrant abdominal pain, anorexia, nausea, and vomiting. However, patients may also present with nonspecific symptoms such as increased flatulence, diarrhea, and indigestion. If the diagnosis is suspected but unclear, a CT scan with IV and oral contrast should be performed. The diagnosis should be made early and managed with surgical intervention.

CHAPTER 7
The Patient with Gas and Bloating

Gas and bloating are common complaints for which patients seek gastroenterology consultation. It is useful to differentiate symptoms of eructation from flatulence, or the symptom of bloating from the physical sign of abdominal distention. Eructation, or belching, is the retrograde expulsion of esophageal and gastric gas from the mouth. Flatulence is the volitional or involuntary release of gas from the anus, particularly gas with an unpleasant odor. Bloating refers to the perception or sensation of fullness in the abdomen, with or without an increase in abdominal girth that defines abdominal distension. Although some conditions lead to increased gas production, many individuals with bloating exhibit normal gut gas volumes. Functional bloating is defined by Rome III criteria as the recurrent sensation of bloating or visible abdominal distension for at least three days/month for three months, without fulfilling criteria for functional dyspepsia, irritable bowel syndrome, or other functional gastrointestinal (GI) disorder. Excessive GI gas has four main sources: swallowed air; carbon dioxide produced through digestion; bacterial fermentation of food residues producing carbon dioxide, hydrogen, and methane; and diffusion of gas from blood in the GI tract.

Clinical presentation

History

Patients with complaints of excess gas should be queried about the timing and duration of symptoms; relationship of symptoms with meals; social habits including smoking, alcohol, ingestion of carbonated drinks, and chewing gum; their medical history including diabetes and hypothyroidism; medications, dietary assessment; family history of celiac disease, inflammatory bowel disease, and food allergies and intolerances; and the presence of associated symptoms including pain, bloating, halitosis, anorexia, early satiety, nausea, belching, loud

---

Yamada's Handbook of Gastroenterology, Fourth Edition. John M. Inadomi, Renuka Bhattacharya, Joo Ha Hwang, and Cynthia Ko.

borborygmi, constipation, and flatulence. Relief of symptoms with defecation or passage of flatus is consistent with a functional disorder, as is the absence of symptoms that awaken the patient from sleep. Conversely, symptoms of fever, weight loss, nocturnal diarrhea, steatorrhea, or rectal bleeding increase the likelihood of organic disease. Medical conditions that predispose to bacterial overgrowth and use of medications that delay gut transit should be elicited. Selected carbohydrate malabsorptive conditions are hereditary, whereas others (e.g. lactase deficiency) are more prevalent in some ethnic groups. Anxiety disorders and other psychiatric conditions predispose to aerophagia and functional bowel disorders.

A detailed dietary history may correlate specific foods with symptoms. Ingestion of fermentable oligo-/di-/mono-saccharides and polyols (FODMAPs), such as legumes, fruits, unrefined starches, dairy, and lactose-containing food should be addressed, as should consumption of diet foods or soft drinks that contain sucrose, sorbitol, or fructose. Gum chewing, smoking, and chewing tobacco predispose to aerophagia.

Physical examination

The physical examination is usually normal in patients with complaints of excess gas; however, patients with functional disease may exhibit anxiety, hyperventilation, and air swallowing. Abdominal distension should be assessed and differentiated from exaggerated lumbar lordosis or ascites. Physical findings suggesting organic disease include sclerodactyly (scleroderma), peripheral or autonomic neuropathy (dysmotility syndromes), or cachexia, jaundice, and palpable masses (malignant intestinal obstruction). Abdominal auscultation can assess for absent bowel sounds with ileus or myopathic dysmotility, high-pitched bowel sounds with intestinal obstruction, or a succussion splash with gastric obstruction or gastroparesis. Abdominal percussion and palpation may reveal tympany and distension in mechanical obstruction or intestinal dysmotility.

Additional testing

Laboratory studies

Normal values for a complete blood count (CBC), electrolytes, glucose, albumin, total protein, and sedimentation rate exclude most inflammatory and neoplastic conditions. In selected patients, calcium and phosphate levels, renal function, liver chemistry values, and thyroid function tests may be indicated. Patients with diarrhea should undergo stool examination for enteric pathogens including bacteria or parasites such as Giardia or *Entamoeba histolytica*. Serum tissue transglutaminase and deaminated gliadin antibodies can screen for celiac disease. Rarely, antinuclear and scleroderma antibodies to screen for collagen vascular disease or antinuclear neuronal antibodies (anti-Hu) for paraneoplastic visceral neuropathy may be indicated.

Structural studies

Supine and upright plain abdominal radiographs may reveal generalized lumenal distension with ileus, diffuse haziness in ascites, and air–fluid levels in mechanical obstruction. Upper endoscopy can be considered to assess for an inflammatory or neoplastic process, and obtain small bowel biopsies to diagnosis celiac disease. Other tests such as ultrasound and computed tomography (CT) can be used to assess for suspected obstruction, pseudo-obstruction, or other intra-abdominal disorders that might predispose the patient to complaints of excess gas.

Functional studies

Gastric emptying scintigraphy or manometry of the esophagus, stomach, and small intestine can be performed when an underlying motility disorder is considered. Radio-opaque markers may be detected using plain abdominal radiographs to document colonic transit. An ingested capsule (SmartPill, Buffalo, NY) that records pressure, temperature, and pH can document gastric and small and large intestinal transit time.

Monosaccharide or disaccharide malabsorption increases hydrogen and methane gas production by intestinal bacteria that can be detected by breath testing. Expired breath samples are obtained before and after ingesting an aqueous solution of the suspected malabsorbed sugar. For example, an increase in breath hydrogen of greater than 20 ppm or methane greater than 10 ppm within 120 minutes of 25 g lactose ingestion distinguishes biopsy-proven, lactase-deficient persons from lactase-sufficient persons with a sensitivity of 90%. Patients can be tested for fructose or sorbitol malabsorption using hydrogen breath testing, but the normal values of these tests are not well established. Glucose (75 mg dose) or lactulose (10–20 mg dose) are the most commonly used sugars for breath hydrogen testing in suspected bacterial overgrowth. Elevated fasting breath hydrogen prior to substrate ingestion and early rises within 30 minutes of sugar ingestion are consistent with small intestinal bacterial overgrowth (SIBO).

Differential diagnosis

Common causes of gas and bloating are listed in Table 7.1.

Carbohydrate maldigestion

Malabsorption of small amounts of carbohydrates, demonstrated by increased breath hydrogen excretion, may produce eructation, bloating, abdominal pain, and flatulence. A diet high in FODMAPS increases maldigestion and provides substrate for intestinal bacteria. Lactase deficiency is the most common form of carbohydrate intolerance, affecting approximately 20% of the population in the United States. Fructose is naturally found in honey and fruits and is used as a sweetener in many commercial soft drinks. Sorbitol is also present in fruits and is used as a sweetener in dietetic candies and chewing gum. Other poorly

Table 7.1 Causes of gas and bloating

Eructation
Involuntary postprandial belching
Magenblase syndrome
Aerophagia (e.g. from gum chewing, smoking, oral irritation)
Gastroesophageal reflux
Biliary colic
Bacterial overgrowth
Intestinal or colonic obstruction
Diverticula of the small intestine
Hypochlorhydria
Chronic intestinal pseudo-obstruction
Cologastric fistula
Coprophagia
Functional bowel disorders
Irritable bowel syndrome
Functional dyspepsia
Idiopathic constipation
Functional diarrhea
Carbohydrate malabsorption
High FODMAP diet (fermentable oligo-, di-, mono-saccharides and polyols) including fructose, lactose, fructans (wheat, onions, garlic), galactans (legumes), polyols (sugar alcohols and fruits with pits/seeds)
Gas-bloat syndrome
Postfundoplication
Miscellaneous causes
Hypothyroidism
Medications (e.g. anticholinergics, opiates, calcium channel antagonists, antidepressants)

absorbed carbohydrates include xylitol and isomalt. The autosomal recessive hereditary syndrome sucrase-isomaltase deficiency typically presents in infancy with malabsorption of sucrose.

Of the complex carbohydrates, only rice and gluten-free wheat are completely absorbed in healthy individuals, whereas up to 20% of the carbohydrates from whole wheat, oat, potato, and cornflour are maldigested and can contribute to gas generation. Nondigestible oligosaccharides (e.g. stachyose, raffinose, and verbascose), abundant in beans and legumes, are avidly fermented by colonic bacteria to produce voluminous quantities of intestinal gas. Fiber intake correlates with flatus production in some individuals, although other studies suggest that fiber only increases the sensation of bloating without increasing gas production.

Small intestinal bacterial overgrowth

SIBO may result from a number of etiologies including mechanical obstruction of the gut from postoperative adhesions, Crohn's disease, radiation enteritis, ulcer disease, malignancy, small intestinal diverticula, and gastric achlorhydria.

Motor disorders of the gut such as diabetic diarrhea are associated with overgrowth because of an impaired ability to clear organisms from the gut. Disorders that increase bacterial delivery to the upper gut (e.g. cologastric fistulae and coprophagia) can overwhelm normal defenses against infection.

Dysmotility syndromes

Conditions that alter gut motor function produce prominent gas and bloating. Bloating is reported by patients with gastroparesis and by those with fat intolerance and rapid gastric emptying. Surgical fundoplication to treat gastroesophageal reflux disease is associated with an inability to belch or vomit secondary to an unyielding wrap of gastric tissue around the distal esophagus. Intestinal pseudo-obstruction leads to gaseous symptoms because of delayed small bowel transit of gas and development of bacterial overgrowth. Bloating also is reported by patients with chronic constipation.

Functional bowel disorders

Irritable bowel syndrome and functional dyspepsia may have symptoms of gas and bloating. The pathogenesis is likely multifactorial, and although some studies illustrate increased gas production and objective abdominal distension in irritable bowel syndrome, others do not. Abnormal gut motor and sensory function contribute to the symptoms of gas and bloating.

Miscellaneous causes

Aerophagia during gum chewing, smoking, or oral irritation produces significant gas symptoms, especially eructation. Patients who have undergone laryngectomy experience eructation from swallowing air for esophageal speech. Patients with intestinal obstructions may infrequently present only with symptoms of gas and bloating. Small bowel malabsorptive conditions including celiac disease may produce gaseous manifestations that may predominate or be part of a larger constellation of symptoms. Individuals with peptic ulcer, gastroesophageal reflux, or biliary colic may belch to relieve their other symptoms. Gaseous complaints may be reported as consequences of endocrinopathies such as hypothyroidism. Many medications (e.g. anticholinergics, opiates, calcium channel antagonists, and antidepressants) produce gas by retarding gut transit.

Management

The evaluation and management of patients presenting with gas and bloating is outlined in Figure 7.1.

Medical

The underlying disorder responsible for symptoms of excess gas should be specifically managed whenever possible. Mechanical obstruction is usually managed surgically. Surgeries to vent the gut may help selected individuals with gas-bloat

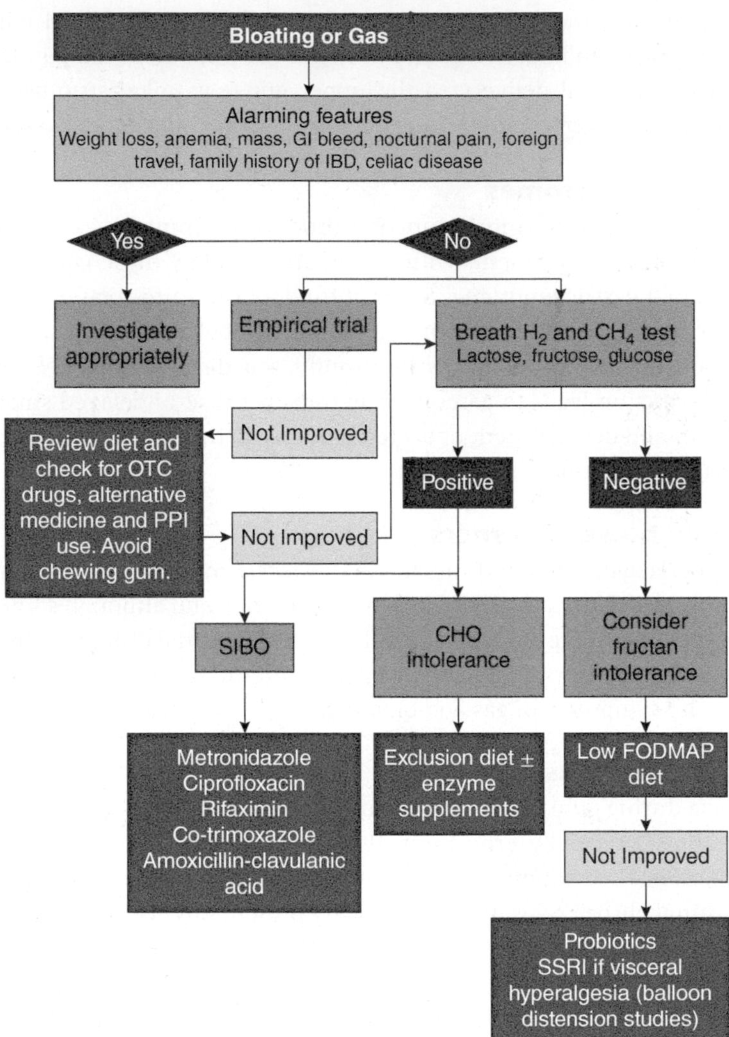

Figure 7.1 Management of the patient with bloating and gas. CHO, carbohydrate; FODMAP, fermentable oligo-/di-/mono-saccharides and polyol; GI, gastrointestinal; IBD, inflammatory bowel disease; OTC, over-the-counter; PPI, proton pump inhibitor; SIBO, small intestinal bacterial overgrowth; SSRI, serotonin selective reuptake inhibitor. (Source: figure 40.5 from Podolsky et al. 2016)

syndrome or intestinal pseudo-obstruction. Lactase deficiency is controlled by excluding lactose from the diet or by supplementing the diet with exogenous lactase. Fructose restriction should be advocated for individuals found to be intolerant. Acid-suppressive medications may reduce eructation associated with gastroesophageal reflux disease. Single or intermittent courses of oral antibiotics such as ciprofloxacin or rifaximin may control SIBO. Probiotics with *Lactobacillus casei* and *L. acidophilus* have been demonstrated to reduce symptoms of SIBO. In addition to SIBO, manipulation of the intestinal microbiome using probiotics containing *Bifidobacterium infantis* can reduce symptoms in patients with irritable bowel syndrome.

For complaints of excess gas for which no organic disorder is defined after appropriate diagnostic testing, attempts are made to decrease intestinal gas and to regulate bowel function. Aerophagia may be controlled by cessation of gum chewing and smoking and improving oral hygiene. The chronic belcher may be aided by self-observation in a mirror to demonstrate aerophagia.

Reducing the amount of fermentable oligosaccharides, disaccharides and monosaccharides, and polyols (FODMAPs) may improve symptoms in appropriate individuals. Common foods high in FODMAPs include wheat, onion, garlic, artichoke, broccoli, dairy, and fruits. In particular, fructans in breakfast cereal, pasta, and bread are implicated in gas and bloating. A low FODMAP diet can reduce symptoms in appropriate patients, and foods to avoid are illustrated in Table 7.2.

Flatulence is best managed by education of the foods that increase gas production such as beans, cabbage, lentils, Brussel sprouts, nuts, and legumes. High-fiber diets can also cause bloating and gas. Bloating associated with bean ingestion can be reduced with alpha-galactosidase (Beano – A.K. Pharma). Bismuth subsalicylate (524 mg four times daily) has been shown to decrease bloating. However, the evidence supporting activated charcoal in reducing symptoms of bloating and gas is variable.

Table 7.2 FODMAP dietary sources

FODMAP	Constituent	Sources
Oligosaccharides	Fructans, galacto-oligosaccharides	Wheat, barley, rye, onion, leek, garlic, shallots, artichokes, beetroot, fennel, peas, chicory, pistachio, cashews, legumes, lentils, chickpeas
Disaccharides	Lactose	Milk, custard, ice cream, yogurt
Monosaccharides	Fructose in excess of glucose	Apples, pears, mangoes, cherries, watermelon, asparagus, snap peas, honey, high-fructose corn syrup
Polyols	Sorbitol, mannitol, maltitol, xylitol	Apples, pears, apricots, cherries, nectarines, peaches, plums, watermelon, mushrooms, cauliflower, artificial sweetener

Source: table 40.5 from Podolsky et al. 2016.

Complications

Few complications occur in patients with gas and bloating caused by functional disease. However, complications from organic disease usually are manifestations of the underlying disease rather than of the gas itself. There have been rare case reports of explosions resulting from ignition by tobacco smoking of feculent gas expelled during eructation in patients with gastrointestinal obstruction and proximal bacterial overgrowth. Similarly, colonic explosions with perforation have been reported in patients undergoing colonoscopy with intracolonic cautery. In general, these vanishingly rare complications result from inadequate bowel cleansing or the use of mannitol or sorbitol purging solutions, both of which generate hydrogen gas.

Case studies

Case 1

A 32-year-old woman complains of excessive belching, in excess of 30 times per day. She denies abdominal pain, nausea, diarrhea, or weight loss. She has no medical problems including diabetes or thyroid disease and denies medication use. Physical examination is normal. CBC, thyroid-stimulating hormone (TSH), and fasting cortisol are normal and antibodies to deaminated gliadin and tissue transglutaminase are negative. The patient is queried further and her symptoms had increased when she tried to stop smoking by using nicotine gum, although she continues to smoke. She is counseled about aerophagia and over time is able to stop smoking and discontinue the gum, which results in substantial reduction in her symptoms.

Discussion

The most common cause of excessive eructation is aerophagia. Aerophagia is commonly exacerbated by smoking or gum chewing but can be primary and is generally a learned behavior. Patients are often unaware of aerophagia, so the use of a mirror to provide objective evidence of episodes of air swallowing can be useful. Self-awareness of this behavior can be therapeutic.

Case 2

A 48-year-old man with a 30-year history of type 1 diabetes complains of excessive gas and flatulence, with cramping abdominal pain and loose stools. He states that there had been a progressive increase in intestinal gas over the past six months despite no change in his diet, good glucose control, and regular exercise. His physical examination confirms reduced proprioception, but the remainder of his examination is normal, including the abdomen. Laboratory tests reveal an elevated blood urea nitrogen and creatinine but a normal HbA1C and thyroid function. Stool is negative for *Giardia* antigen, ova, and parasites examination. Glucose hydrogen breath testing reveals an abnormally elevated baseline level that increases significantly after carbohydrate ingestion. Ciprofloxacin 500 mg orally twice daily for seven days is prescribed, which rapidly improves symptoms.

Discussion

Diabetes is associated with SIBO. Diabetic "enteropathy" is a neuropathy that interferes with normal intestinal motility; it rarely occurs in the absence of peripheral neuropathy so physical findings (reduced proprioception) are key to the diagnosis. The glucose hydrogen breath test is classically used to evaluate for the presence of bacterial overgrowth; however, it is insensitive, and empirical therapy is often employed in lieu of diagnostic testing. Ciprofloxacin has been demonstrated to have greater efficacy in resolving SIBO than trimethoprim, amoxicillin-clavulanic acid and cefoxitin, or norfloxacin. Rifaximin plus neomycin is an alternative, especially for patients with SIBO in the setting of irritable bowel syndrome

Further reading

Podolsky, D.K., Camilleri, M., Fitz, J.G. et al. (eds.) (2016). *Yamada's Textbook of Gastroenterology*, 6e. Oxford: Blackwell.

CHAPTER 8
The Patient with Ileus or Obstruction

Acute ileus is a potentially reversible state of inhibited motor activity in the gastrointestinal tract. Chronic pseudo-obstruction is a functional abnormality of longer duration that simulates mechanical obstruction but has no anatomical cause and may exhibit clinical manifestations similar to ileus. Toxic megacolon is a special form of ileus in which severe transmural inflammation produces colonic atony, systemic toxemia, and a high risk of spontaneous perforation. Obstruction implies complete or partial blockage of the gut at one or more levels.

Clinical presentation

History

Patients with ileus, obstruction, and pseudo-obstruction have symptoms of abdominal pain, nausea, vomiting, abdominal distension, or obstipation. Acute ileus or gastric or duodenal obstruction may be associated with little abdominal pain, whereas distal intestinal or colonic obstructions generally cause greater discomfort. The pain of mechanical obstruction is dull, ill defined, or squeezing. True colic (intermittent waves of pain) may be prominent. Upper and mid-abdominal pain are characteristic of obstruction proximal to the transverse colon, whereas left colonic obstruction is associated with lower abdominal discomfort.

Distension may be pronounced with ileus and with distal obstruction but minimal with gastric obstruction. Copious vomiting of clear liquid characterizes gastric obstruction, whereas marked bilious emesis occurs with duodenal blockage. Distal obstruction and ileus may result in only mild nausea and vomiting. The pain of proximal, not distal, obstruction is often relieved by vomiting. If mechanical obstruction is incomplete or if ileus is mild, pain and distension may be intermittent and aggravated by fiber-rich, poorly digestible foods. Complete obstruction usually produces obstipation and the inability to expel flatus. Conversely, watery diarrhea is noted with partial obstruction and fecal impaction.

Yamada's Handbook of Gastroenterology, Fourth Edition. John M. Inadomi, Renuka Bhattacharya, Joo Ha Hwang, and Cynthia Ko.

A complete family, medication, endocrine, immunological, and metabolic history should be obtained from a patient with ileus, focusing on the potential for thyroid and parathyroid disorders, diabetes, scleroderma, heavy metal intoxication, and porphyria. Prior surgery can cause adhesions, and reports of abdominal wall bulging suggest a hernia. Histories of malignancy, radiation, inflammatory bowel disease, ulcer disease, gallstones, diverticular disease, pancreatitis, motility disorders, and foreign body ingestion suggest specific causes. Exacerbation of pain with menses is consistent with endometriosis.

Physical examination

A patient with obstruction usually appears to be in great distress, whereas a patient with ileus may be more comfortable despite pronounced abdominal distension. Inspection may reveal scars and visible distension. Auscultation usually reveals hypoactive or absent bowel sounds with ileus, whereas obstruction produces louder, high-pitched, hyperactive bowel sounds that may have a musical or tinkling quality. Shaking of the abdomen while listening through a stethoscope may reveal a succussion splash, which is associated with gastric obstruction or gastroparesis. Gentle palpation may detect subtle hernias that are not obvious on inspection. Hepatosplenomegaly, lymphadenopathy, and masses raise concern for malignancy, although tender masses may be present in inflammatory diseases (e.g. Crohn's disease). Tympany accompanies both ileus and obstruction, whereas shifting dullness and a fluid wave characterize ascites.

Rectal examination may detect occult fecal blood with inflammatory, neoplastic, infectious, or ischemic disease. Digital rectal and pelvic examinations may also detect subtle masses not found on abdominal palpation or may reveal obturator or sciatic hernias. Repeated abdominal examinations are essential to assess for development of complications such as perforation. If fever, hypotension, or signs of sepsis or peritonitis develop or if bowel sounds disappear, the viscus may be ischemic and operative intervention may be urgently indicated.

Key practice points

The physical examination can usually differentiate between ileus and obstruction. Ileus will present with absent or rare bowel sounds, whereas the physical examination in obstruction will reveal hyperactive, high-pitched (tinkling) bowel sounds.

Additional testing

Laboratory studies

Blood tests may not identify the cause of mechanical obstruction; in contrast, laboratory studies often indicate the cause of ileus. Abnormal electrolyte (including calcium, phosphate, and magnesium), blood urea nitrogen (BUN), or creatinine values support a clinical impression of dehydration. Leukocytosis may be present with inflammation or infection. Measurement of arterial blood gases may be necessary to evaluate the acid–base balance. With an ischemic or infarcted bowel, elevations in amylase, alkaline phosphatase, creatine phosphokinase, aspartate and alanine aminotransferase, and lactate dehydrogenase may be evident, although these enzymes also increase with hepatic and pancreaticobiliary disease.

Plain radiographic studies

Plain radiographs should be the initial structural studies performed on patients with suspected ileus or obstruction. Chest radiography can detect pneumonia, evaluate cardiorespiratory status, and detect free subdiaphragmatic air, whereas supine and upright abdominal plain films show intra-abdominal gas distribution. With complete occlusion of the small intestine, the lumen is widely distended and the valvulae conniventes are observed to span the lumenal air column; in addition, colonic air is radiographically absent. Upright or decubitus views commonly demonstrate air–fluid levels in a stepladder configuration.

With colonic obstruction, the colon proximal to the blockage dilates and the characteristic incomplete and scalloped indentations of the haustra are visible. With advanced strangulation, the bowel wall becomes edematous, exhibiting a thumbprint pattern on radiographs, and air in the intestinal wall, portal vein, and peritoneal cavity may be observed.

In ileus, lumenal dilation may be generalized, or it may only manifest adjacent to an inflammatory site, producing a sentinel loop, as in appendicitis or pancreatitis. With concurrent peritonitis, the bowel wall may thicken. Colonic gas usually is more prominent in ileus than with small intestinal obstruction. Pure colonic dilation, most pronounced in the cecum, is the defining feature of acute colonic pseudo-obstruction. Stepladder air–fluid levels may be observed with either ileus or obstruction, but they are more well defined and longer with obstruction. A string-of-beads pattern of the air–fluid interfaces is most suggestive of high-grade obstruction of the small intestine. A diffusely hazy pattern with central localization of bowel loops is characteristic of ascites.

Additional structural studies

Computed tomographic scanning is used to define the site of obstruction and to exclude selected underlying disease processes (i.e. inflammation versus neoplasm). Ultrasound is generally not useful because of the obscuring effects of intralumenal gas. Upper endoscopy may identify esophageal, gastric, or duodenal lesions and offers the additional capability of therapeutic dilation of any stricture. Push enteroscopy provides similar diagnostic and therapeutic capabilities to the proximal jejunum. Angiography or magnetic resonance angiography may be useful for patients with suspected mesenteric ischemia and infarction.

Functional studies

Functional testing of gut motility may be considered for patients with prolonged ileus or suspected chronic intestinal pseudo-obstruction. Gastric emptying scintigraphy may document gastroparesis, whereas esophageal or gastroduodenal manometry may show the characteristic hypomotility pattern of visceral myopathy or the random, intense bursts of contractions in visceral neuropathy.

Differential diagnosis

Acute ileus, chronic pseudo-obstruction, and mechanical obstruction have numerous causes (Table 8.1).

Acute ileus

Several conditions have been associated with the development of acute ileus. Ileus is the normal physiological response to laparotomy. Gastric and small intestinal motility recover in the first postoperative day, whereas colonic contractions return in three to five days. Postoperative ileus beyond that time is considered pathological and warrants a search for surgical complications. Other intra-abdominal causes of acute ileus include abdominal trauma and inflammatory gut disorders. Noninflammatory conditions (radiation damage and mesenteric ischemia) and retroperitoneal disorders can also produce acute ileus. Extra-abdominal causes of ileus include reflex inhibition of gut motility by craniotomy, fractures, myocardial infarction, heart surgery, pneumonia, pulmonary embolus, and burns. Medications or metabolic abnormalities may inhibit motor activity.

Chronic intestinal pseudo-obstruction

Chronic intestinal pseudo-obstruction is a consequence of a variety of conditions. Chronic idiopathic pseudo-obstruction often presents after a viral prodrome, suggesting an infectious etiology. Hereditary conditions such as familial visceral myopathies and neuropathies produce pseudo-obstruction at early ages. In addition to gastroparesis, long-standing, poorly controlled diabetes mellitus may disrupt motor function in the small intestine. Rheumatological disorders and some endocrinopathies can lead to chronic pseudo-obstruction. Neuromuscular diseases chronically disrupt motor activity. In selected geographic locations, Chagas disease represents an infectious cause of pseudo-obstruction that occurs after exposure to *Trypanosoma cruzi*. Viral pseudo-obstruction in immunosuppressed patients has been reported as a consequence of infection with cytomegalovirus and other agents. Pheochromocytoma produces chronic intestinal hypomotility, probably because of the motor inhibitory effects of circulating catecholamines. Chronic intestinal pseudo-obstruction can be a paraneoplastic manifestation of small cell lung carcinoma and, less commonly, other malignancies. Paraneoplastic pseudo-obstruction results from malignant invasion of the celiac axis or, alternatively, from plasma cell infiltration of the myenteric plexus, leading to the loss of enteric neural function.

Mechanical obstruction

The causes of mechanical intestinal obstruction may be divided into extrinsic lesions, intrinsic lesions, and intralumenal objects.

Table 8.1 Causes of ileus and obstruction

Acute ileus
Postoperative ileus
Abdominal trauma
Ulcer perforation
Bile or chemical peritonitis
Toxic megacolon
Pancreatitis
Cholecystitis
Appendicitis
Diverticulitis
Inflammatory bowel disease
Radiation therapy
Mesenteric ischemia
Retroperitoneal disorders (e.g. renal calculi, pyelonephritis, renal transplant, hemorrhage)
Extra-abdominal sources (e.g. craniotomy, fractures, myocardial infarction, cardiac surgery, pneumonia, pulmonary embolus, burns)
Metabolic disorders (e.g. electrolyte abnormalities, uremia, sepsis, diabetic ketoacidosis, sickle cell anemia, respiratory insufficiency, porphyria, heavy metal toxicity)
Medications (e.g. anticholinergics, opiates, calcium channel antagonists, chemotherapy, antidepressants)
Chronic intestinal pseudo-obstruction
Hereditary diseases (e.g. familial visceral neuropathy, familial visceral myopathy)
Diabetes mellitus
Rheumatological disorders (e.g. scleroderma, systemic lupus erythematosus, amyloidosis)
Endocrinopathies (e.g. hypothyroidism, hyperparathyroid disease or hypoparathyroid disease, Addison disease)
Neuromuscular diseases (e.g. muscular dystrophy, myotonic dystrophy)
Chagas disease
Infectious pseudo-obstruction
Pheochromocytoma
Paraneoplastic pseudo-obstruction
Mechanical obstruction
Adhesions
Congenital bands (e.g. Ladd bands)
Hernias (e.g. external, internal, diaphragmatic, pelvic)
Volvulus (e.g. colon, small intestine, stomach)
Obstructive lumenal tumors
Inflammatory bowel disease
Diverticulitis
Mesenteric ischemia
Radiation injury
Intussusception
Congenital conditions (e.g. hypertrophic pyloric stenosis, Hirschsprung disease, intestinal atresia/agenesis)
Fecal impaction
Gallstone ileus
Retained barium
Gastric bezoars

Extrinsic lesions

Extrinsic adhesions are the most common cause of small intestinal obstruction in adults, but they rarely occlude the colon. Congenital bands behave similarly and may occur in association with malrotation (Ladd bands). Hernias represent another extrinsic cause of obstruction that may be external (protruding through the abdominal wall), internal, diaphragmatic (usually para-esophageal), or pelvic.

Volvulus is an abnormal torsion of the bowel that produces a closed and obstructed loop of bowel, associated with an impairment of blood flow. Colonic volvulus involves the sigmoid colon in 70–80% and the cecum in 10–20% of cases and manifests as sudden abdominal pain followed by distension. Gastric volvulus occurs with diaphragmatic defects, congenital malformations, and large para-esophageal hernias.

Intrinsic lesions

Intrinsic lesions are less common causes of mechanical obstruction. Benign and malignant tumors can obstruct the lumen or provide a leading point for intussusception. Primary small intestinal malignancies are rare and include lymphoma, adenocarcinoma, and carcinoids, whereas adenocarcinoma represents the most common obstructing colonic neoplasm. Metastatic tumors usually tether and fix the bowel rather than obstruct the lumen. Inflammatory processes and ischemia cause obstructing strictures, whereas blunt trauma may produce an intramural hematoma. In addition to neoplasm, a Meckel diverticulum may initiate intussusception. In children, there usually is no underlying mucosal or submucosal lesion that predisposes to intussusception.

Intralumenal objects

Intralumenal objects represent the least common causes of mechanical obstruction. Fecal impaction may produce colonic obstruction in patients who are dehydrated or immobile, who have underlying constipation, or who take medications that slow colonic transit. Rarely, large gallstones erode through the gallbladder into the gut lumen, where they migrate to obstruct the intestine, usually at the level of the distal ileum. Barium from radiographic procedures may obstruct the colon in patients with underlying colonic motility disorders. Gastric bezoars and ingested foreign bodies may occlude the gut lumen in select cases.

Diagnostic investigation

The diagnostic investigation of a patient with suspected ileus or obstruction is illustrated in Figure 8.1. The history and physical examination may direct the evaluation toward ileus or obstruction. Predisposing historical features modify the risk of either condition, and physical examination can indicate the presence of ileus (absent bowel sounds) or obstruction (hyperactive or high-pitched bowel

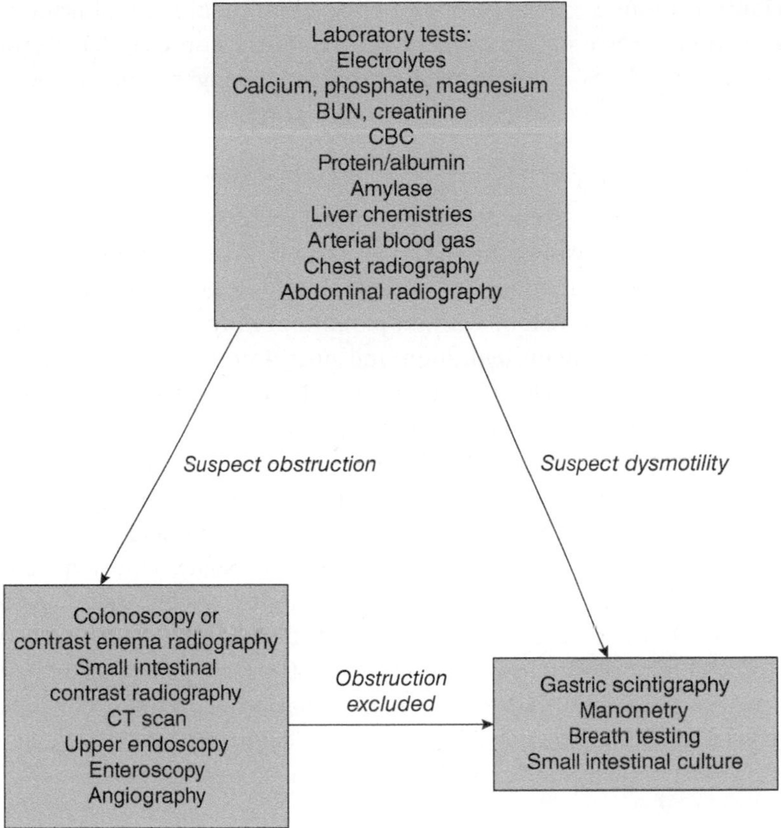

Figure 8.1 Workup of a patient with ileus or obstruction. BUN, blood urea nitrogen; CBC, complete blood count; CT, computed tomography.

sounds). Laboratory abnormalities may reveal the etiology of ileus, and radiographic tests usually differentiate obstruction from ileus.

Obstruction generally requires assessment of the location by computed tomography (CT) scan, and accessible lesions can be identified and possibly sampled for tissue using appropriate endoscopic procedures. Ileus can be treated empirically with medication (see below) or more fully evaluated using gastric scintigraphy (emptying) tests and/or esophageal or gastroduodenal manometry.

Management

Medical

Fluid replacement

Correction of fluid, electrolyte, and acid–base imbalances is guided by the physical findings coupled with laboratory determination of hematocrit, electrolyte, BUN, creatinine, and blood gas levels. With severe hypovolemia, fluid resuscitation should be performed with concurrent monitoring of urine output, central venous pressure, and blood pressure. With gastric outlet obstruction, potassium chloride is often needed after establishing normal urine output because renal potassium losses are high in this condition.

Bowel decompression

Abdominal distension increases gastrointestinal secretion and causes nausea and vomiting, thereby increasing the risk of aspiration. Nasogastric suction is appropriate in ileus and obstruction. The patient should be given nothing by mouth, and intravenous fluids with or without parenteral nutrients should be administered to maintain adequate hydration and nutrition. Drugs that inhibit motor activity should be withheld. Placing a rectal tube or administering tap water enemas may reduce colonic distension in some patients.

In patients with documented ileus who do not have significant cardiovascular disease, the acetylcholinesterase inhibitor neostigmine may promote gas expulsion when administered in a controlled setting with cardiac monitoring. For patients with acute colonic pseudo-obstruction, some clinicians advocate therapeutic colonoscopic decompression, although few objective data support this practice. On the other hand, sigmoid volvulus is effectively treated by gentle endoscopic detorsion with aspiration of retained gas.

For patients with obstruction, endoscopic dilation of adhesions or radiation-induced strictures may be possible. Inoperable colorectal cancer may be endoscopically treated by placing expandable metal intralumenal stents.

Surgical

Complete intestinal obstruction is generally an indication for urgent surgery as soon as resuscitation is completed and nasogastric decompression is achieved because strangulation cannot be excluded using clinical criteria in this setting. If strangulation is discovered, necrotic bowel should be resected. With partial obstruction, immediate surgery and antibiotics are of no proven benefit. However, if fever, peritoneal signs, leukocytosis, or hyperamylasemia develop, laparotomy is indicated. Colonic obstruction nearly always requires surgery; nasogastric suction may have little effect in this setting. If the bowel cannot be cleansed, many surgeons perform a two-stage operation with initial resection of the obstructed segment and placement of a diverting colostomy followed by reanastomosis at a later date to reduce wound infection.

Complications

The most serious complication of obstruction or ileus is bowel infarction, with resulting peritonitis and possible death. Other complications include aspiration pneumonia, electrolyte abnormalities, and malnutrition. All may have serious consequences for unstable patients who have other concurrent disease. Many of the diseases that produce ileus and obstruction have serious sequelae, in addition to those that result from involvement of the bowel.

Case studies

Case 1

A 53-year-old man presents to the emergency department with abdominal pain for six hours. He has no prior history of abdominal pain but awoke from sleep with gradual onset of diffuse upper abdominal pain in a colicky (intermittent) pattern. He mentions associated nausea and emesis of clear fluid. The pain does not radiate, and he has not had a bowel movement or passed gas since its onset. Physical examination reveals an uncomfortable man who is constantly shifting his position on the gurney. The abdomen is distended and high-pitched bowel sounds are present. An appendectomy scar is noted in the right lower quadrant. There is diffuse tenderness to palpation with voluntary guarding but no rebound. His rectal examination is notable for brown, heme-negative stool. His white blood count (WBC) is 16.3 and his Hb is 17.4 g/dl. Plain abdominal radiographs illustrate distended loops of small intestine with air–fluid levels and a transition point in the right lower quadrant. CT scan of the abdomen confirms distended small intestine with abrupt narrowing in the mid-ileum and a paucity of gas in the large intestine.

The surgical service performs a laparoscopic examination, which reveals adhesions in the right lower quadrant and small intestinal obstruction. The adhesions are taken down and the remainder of the bowel appears normal without signs of ischemia. Postoperatively the patient recovers quickly and is discharged in good condition.

Discussion

Obstruction of a hollow viscus such as the small intestine will create colicky pain, which increases and dissipates in a cyclical fashion. The physical examination should be sufficient to diagnose small bowel obstruction. Signs of prior surgery should be sought to determine the likelihood of adhesions causing obstruction. Unlike ileus or chronic pseudo-obstruction, the bowel sounds are hyperactive. Plain abdominal radiographs should be sufficient to illustrate dilated small intestinal loops that are generally fluid-filled with an air interface. CT scans will generally be able to identify the transition point or site of obstruction.

Case 2

A 76-year-old woman recently underwent an open reduction with internal fixation for a hip fracture. A gastroenterologist is consulted to manage increasing abdominal distension with diffuse, continuous, pressure-like abdominal pain that is 3/10 in severity. The patient mentions associated nausea but no emesis. Her past medical history is notable only for diabetes mellitus. Physical examination reveals an obese woman who is in no acute distress. Vital signs are normal and her abdominal examination is notable for a distended abdomen, absence of bowel sounds, and no abdominal tenderness to palpation. WBC is 7.6 and Hb is 7.5 mg/dl. Plain abdominal radiographs reveal gas distension of the entire colon including the rectum, with the cecum 9 cm in diameter.

Discussion

This is a typical presentation of acute colonic pseudo-obstruction in which a patient is admitted to hospital for a nongastrointestinal indication and during the hospital course is noted to have a distended abdomen and dilated large intestine. The abdominal examination differs from acute obstruction in that bowel sounds are absent and tenderness is generally absent to minimal. Significant tenderness is worrisome for perforation, which will usually occur in the cecum due to LaPlace's law, which explains why despite similar colonic wall thickness throughout the colon, the greatest wall tension will occur in the region with the greatest diameter (the cecum).

The patient is managed conservatively, with correction of serum electrolytes, discontinuation of narcotics, and frequent turning. A nasogastric tube is placed and set to intermittent suction, and the patient is not given anything by mouth. The next day her abdomen remains distended and tympanitic, with mild diffuse tenderness but no rebound or guarding. Her plain abdominal radiographs reveal a cecum that is 12 cm in diameter, without thumbprinting or perforation. Based on her increased symptoms and enlarged cecal diameter, intervention is recommended. Intravenous neostigmine is administered under close cardiac monitoring. No bradycardia is noted and the patient responds appropriately with increased flatus and a reduction in abdominal distension. Although slow to recover, she is discharged one week later having had no further episodes of ileus.

Discussion

Neostigmine was shown in a randomized controlled trial to reduce colonic distension, symptoms, and complications of acute colonic pseudo-obstruction. Since this is an acetylcholinesterase inhibitor, contraindications include cardiovascular disease (especially brady-dysrhythmias) and bronchospasm. Infusion of 2 mg neostigmine intravenously should be performed in a telemetry setting and atropine should be available for symptomatic bradycardia.

(Source: Ponec et al. 1999.)

Further reading

Ponec, R.J., Saunders, M.D., and Kimmey, M.B. (1999). Neostigmine for the treatment of acute colonic pseudo-obstruction. *N. Engl. J. Med.* 341 (3): 137–141.

CHAPTER 9

The Patient with Constipation

Constipation is defined as a symptomatic decrease in stool frequency to fewer than three bowel movements per week. Some patients with normal stool frequency report constipation if they pass abnormal stools (Bristol stool form types 1 or 2), experience excessive straining during defecation, have defecatory urgency, or have a sense of incomplete fecal evacuation. Constipation may be primary (due to disordered regulation of colonic and anorectal neuromuscular function or brain-gut neuroenteric function) or secondary as a result of diet, drugs, behavioral, endocrine, metabolic, neurological, or other disorders (Table 9.1). Primary constipation may be further classified as slow-transit (prolonged transit of stool through the colon), evacuation disorders (dyssynergic defecation or Hirschsprung disease), or constipation-predominant irritable bowel syndrome (IBS).

Clinical presentation

History

The evaluation of a patient presenting with constipation is outlined in the American Gastroenterological Association Medical Position Statement on Constipation (Figure 9.1). A thorough history will identify slow-transit constipation from dyssynergic defecation in which incomplete evacuation is the primary symptom; however, dyssynergic defecation can also cause constipation, so these disorders are not mutually exclusive. Lifelong symptoms may suggest a congenital disorder of coloanal motor function or functional disease. Conversely, a recent change in bowel habits or rectal bleeding in adults warrants exclusion of organic obstructive disease including neoplasia. The presence of associated symptoms (e.g. straining, abdominal pain, bloating, or incomplete evacuation) are more common with functional disorders such as IBS. Reports of skin or hair changes, temperature intolerance, or weight gain suggest possible

Yamada's Handbook of Gastroenterology, Fourth Edition. John M. Inadomi, Renuka Bhattacharya, Joo Ha Hwang, and Cynthia Ko.

Table 9.1 Causes of secondary constipation

Anorectal and colonic disorders
Anal fissure
Hemorrhoids
Ulcerative proctitis
Diverticulitis
Colorectal cancer
Strictures
Drugs
Opioids
Anticholinergics
Antidepressants
Antihypertensives (especially calcium channel blockers)
Anti-parkinsonians
Anticonvulsants
Antihistamines
Diuretics
Metal ions (aluminum or calcium antacids; iron or calcium supplements)
Serotonin 5-HT3 antagonists
Endocrine and metabolic disorders
Diabetes mellitus
Hypothyroidism
Hypokalemia
Hypercalcemia
Porphyria
Neuromuscular disorders
Spinal cord lesions
Parkinsonism
Multiple sclerosis
Cerebrovascular disease
Chagas disease
Hirschsprung disease

hypothyroidism, whereas weight loss raises concern for malignancy. Underlying systemic illness (e.g. diabetes or a rheumatological condition) should be identified. A careful history of medication use, including laxative use, is essential. A description of the stool form using a measure such as the Bristol Stool Form Scale provides a common reference from which classification of bowel disorders or comparison of symptoms over time may be described.

Rome IV criteria subdivides functional bowel disorders into IBS (with predominant constipation [IBS-C]; diarrhea [IBS-D]; mixed bowel habits [IBS-M]; unclassified [IBS-U]), functional constipation, functional diarrhea, functional abdominal pain/distention, opioid-induced constipation, and unspecified functional bowel disorder.

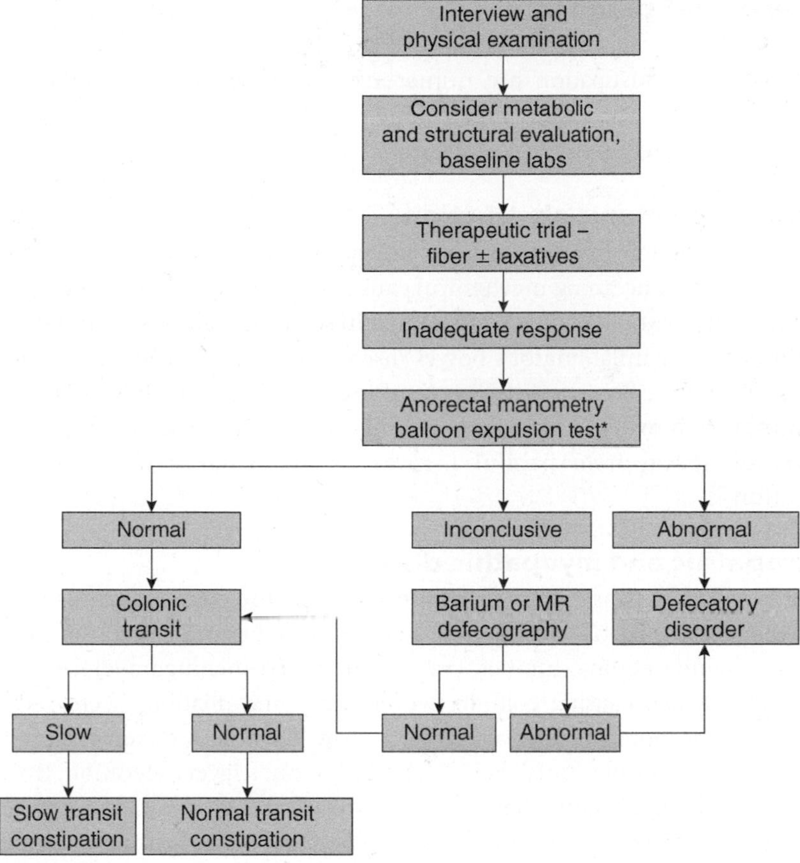

Figure 9.1 Workup of a patient with constipation. MR, magnetic resonance.

Physical examination

A neurological examination can screen for organic conditions that cause secondary constipation. An abdominal examination may reveal abdominal masses, hepatomegaly, or lymphadenopathy that suggest possible obstructing malignancy. Peripheral or autonomic neuropathy may indicate a neuropathic motility disorder. A careful digital rectal examination is critical to detect tumors, strictures, fissures, hemorrhoids, and rectal prolapse. Anorectal neuromuscular function is tested by assessing basal anal tone, adequacy of maximal anal squeeze, and perianal cutaneous sensation, including the anal wink. Long-standing constipation with straining and prolapse may produce anal or perineal nerve damage that leads to reduced anal pressure and fecal incontinence. Examination during attempted defecation maneuvers can suggest rectal prolapse and evidence of rectosphincteric dyssynergia. Pelvic examination in women may demonstrate a rectocele with straining.

Differential diagnosis

The causes of constipation are numerous, including primary and secondary causes, and relate to either impairment of colonic transit or to structural or functional obstruction to fecal evacuation.

Mechanical colonic obstruction

Colonic obstruction may result from mechanical or functional outlet obstruction. The most concerning mechanical cause is colorectal cancer, which typically presents in individuals over age 45 years or in selected high-risk groups including individuals with inflammatory bowel disease or a family history of colorectal cancer. Benign colonic strictures resulting from diverticulitis, ischemia, or inflammatory bowel disease produce similar symptoms. Anal strictures, foreign bodies, or spasm from painful fissures or hemorrhoids may also impede defecation.

Neuropathic and myopathic disorders

Diseases of the extrinsic or enteric innervation of the colon and anus may present with constipation. Constipation may be caused by transection of the sacral nerves or cauda equina, lumbosacral spinal injury, meningomyelocele, or low spinal anesthesia, causing colonic hypomotility and dilation, decreased rectal tone and sensation, and impaired defecation. Colonic reflexes are preserved with high spinal lesions; thus, digital stimulation can trigger defecation. However, patients with spinal injury have reduced meal-induced colonic motor activity and impaired rectal sensation and compliance that can contribute to constipation. Constipation is prevalent with multiple sclerosis, cerebrovascular accidents, Parkinson disease, and dysautonomias, including Shy–Drager syndrome.

Hirschsprung disease is the best characterized enteric nervous system disease that presents with constipation and most commonly presents in infants as obstipation and proximal colonic dilation at birth. The physiological abnormality in Hirschsprung consists of nonrelaxation of the internal anal sphincter with rectal stimulation due to the absence of enteric ganglion cells. Some individuals with very short segment involvement present with constipation in adulthood or, in rare instances, incontinence. Other enteric nervous system diseases include zonal colonic aganglionosis (in which patchy areas of the colon are devoid of neurons either congenitally or secondary to ischemia), chronic intestinal pseudo-obstruction (myopathic and neuropathic), or Chagas disease (resulting from infection with *Trypanosoma cruzi*). Neurofibromatosis, long-standing laxative abuse, and diabetes mellitus may lead to enteric neuronal damage. Idiopathic megacolon is divided into primary and secondary disorders. Primary megacolon is thought to be associated with neuropathic dysfunction. Secondary megacolon and megarectum develop later in life, usually in response to chronic fecal retention.

Rheumatological disorders evoke a generalized slowing of colonic transit. Dermatomyositis and myotonic dystrophy produce myopathic dysfunction. Amyloidosis and scleroderma may produce either myopathic or neuropathic disease. Constipation in systemic lupus erythematosus has multiple mechanisms, including local ischemia secondary to vasculitis.

Metabolic and endocrine disorders

The most common endocrine causes of constipation are diabetes, pregnancy, and hypothyroidism. Although symptoms usually are mild, life-threatening megacolon may develop in myxedema. Other endocrine causes of constipation include hypercalcemia, hypokalemia, porphyria, panhypopituitarism, pheochromocytoma, and glucagonoma.

Medications

Many medications are associated with constipation. Drug classes that directly inhibit colonic transit include antispasmodics, tricyclic antidepressants, antipsychotics, anti-parkinsonian agents, opiates, certain antihypertensives, ganglionic blockers, vinca alkaloids, anticonvulsants, calcium channel antagonists, and cation-containing agents such as iron, aluminum antacids, calcium, barium, and heavy metals (e.g. arsenic, lead, mercury).

Idiopathic and functional causes

No organic abnormality is identified in most patients with constipation. A common cause of constipation in association with abdominal pain is IBS, which is not a diagnosis of exclusion but can be diagnosed by symptom criteria (Rome IV). These patients have normal colonic transit. Those with delayed colonic transit may have a generalized disorder of propulsion in the colon and are given a diagnosis of slow-transit constipation or colonic inertia. Some patients with slow-transit constipation also exhibit dysmotility of the esophagus, small intestine, or bladder that suggests the presence of a systemic disorder of smooth muscle function. Other persons with delayed colonic transit exhibit a functional impediment to defecation at the level of the anorectum. Causes of outlet obstruction include rectal prolapse, rectal intussusception, rectocele, megarectum, and dyssynergic defecation. Dyssynergic defecation is characterized by impaired relaxation or paradoxical contraction of the puborectalis muscle or anal sphincter.

Childhood constipation often manifests as fecal impaction with rectosigmoid dilation. The cause of childhood constipation is uncertain; impaired rectal sensation and altered anal tone are not reliably demonstrable. Many children exhibit evidence of rectosphincteric dyssynergia upon attempted defecation, which may be a learned behavior in response to prior painful defecation problems.

Additional testing

Laboratory studies

If the history or examination suggests systemic or structural anorectal disease, further evaluation may be needed. A microcytic anemia raises concern for colonic neoplasm or inflammatory disease. Other screening tests include measuring serum calcium to exclude hyperparathyroidism and thyroid-stimulating hormone (TSH) levels to exclude hypothyroidism. Specific serological tests can detect rheumatological disease, Chagas disease, or paraneoplastic pseudo-obstruction, whereas other assays are used for catecholamines, urine porphyrins, and glucagon.

Functional studies

Anorectal manometry with balloon expulsion should be performed in patients with chronic constipation who do not respond to empirical medical therapy and should be performed prior to evaluation of colonic transit. Rectosphincteric dyssynergia is suggested by manometric demonstration of increased anal tone with attempted defecation. Rectal sensation is quantified during progressive rectal balloon inflation. Some patients with IBS tolerate balloon distension poorly, whereas individuals with megarectum accommodate large balloon volumes without sensing a need to defecate. Measurement of anal tone during rectal balloon inflation detects a normal volume-dependent relaxation (*rectoanal inhibitory reflex*), the loss of which suggests possible Hirschsprung disease. This diagnosis must be confirmed by deep rectal biopsy because falsely absent rectoanal inhibitory reflexes are present with megarectum if inadequate rectal volumes are delivered. Attempted defecation maneuvers, including expulsion of a rectal balloon, can help to assess for abnormalities of anal relaxation.

If anorectal manometry is normal, the transit of stool through different colonic regions can be quantified by obtaining serial abdominal radiographs after ingesting radio-opaque markers or by newer technology involving a swallowed capsule that measures pH, temperature, and intralumenal pressure to determine intestinal transit time (SmartPill). These studies can distinguish between slow-transit constipation (colonic inertia), in which transit is delayed in all colonic regions, and functional outlet obstruction, where passage is selectively retarded at the level of the anorectum. In some cases, marker elimination is normal, even though the patient denies stool output. Such individuals often exhibit psychological disturbances that contribute to their symptoms.

Defecography involves cinefluoroscopic recording of the attempted defecation of barium paste that is infused into the rectum. Structural abnormalities, including rectoceles and rectal prolapse or intussusception, can be diagnosed by this technique. Defecography also quantifies the anorectal angle at rest and with defecation. Rectosphincteric dyssynergia is characterized by a paradoxical decrease in this angle during defecation, which precludes evacuation of the rectal contrast material.

Structural studies

Endoscopic or radiographic evaluation is performed on any individual with suspected mechanical obstruction as a cause of constipation. In young patients, flexible sigmoidoscopy is sufficient, but if alarm findings such as rectal bleeding, iron deficiency anemia, or weight loss are present, it is important to evaluate the entire colon by colonoscopy because of the increased risk of colorectal neoplasm. Computed tomography (CT) scans or barium enema radiography can show proximal colonic dilation as well as persistent contraction of the denervated segment in Hirschsprung disease. Deep rectal biopsy specimens obtained at least 3 cm above the anal verge are obtained to exclude Hirschsprung disease, when indicated.

Management

Dietary, fiber, and behavioral approaches

After structural and metabolic causes of constipation are excluded and offending medications are withdrawn, dietary and lifestyle changes can be offered. Many persons respond to increasing fluid intake (2 l daily) and increasing dietary or supplemental fiber 20–30 g/day. Bulk-forming agents such as psyllium, methylcellulose, and polycarbophil increase stool volume, improve fecal hydration, and increase colonic bacterial mass, leading to acceleration of colonic transit and reduced straining. In patients with IBS, fiber should be gradually increased to minimize bloating. Establishing routine defecation after meals is recommended to take advantage of the gastrocolonic reflex, the increase in colonic motility that occurs in the initial postprandial hour. Daily exercise, including walking, has been shown to significantly reduce constipation.

Pharmacological therapy

Stool softeners include docusate salts. Docusate salts are anionic surfactants that reduce fecal surface tension, allowing better mixing of aqueous and fatty substances and thereby softening the stool. Mineral oil penetrates and softens the stool but may reduce absorption of vitamins A, D, and K.

Osmotic laxatives are ions or molecules that are not well absorbed, driving retention of water by the intestinal lumen to maintain osmotic balance with plasma, and include hypertonic cationic and anionic (polyethylene glycol [PEG], magnesium hydroxide) or hyperosmotic sugar (sorbitol, lactulose) laxatives. Cationic laxatives increase intralumenal water content by their osmotic effects. The use of magnesium products should be avoided in renal failure. Sorbitol and lactulose are nonabsorbable sugars that are degraded by colonic bacteria to increase stool osmolarity. PEG is a large polymer that is poorly absorbed and is metabolically inert. PEG does not cause electrolyte disturbances and increases stool frequency and improves stool consistency in patients with constipation.

Stimulant laxatives include castor oil, anthraquinones (e.g. cascara, senna, casanthranol, and danthron), ricinoleic acid (castor oil), and phenylmethanes (e.g. sodium picosulfate and bisacodyl). Anthraquinones may produce melanosis coli, whereas danthron has reported hepatotoxic effects.

For patients nonresponsive to lifestyle changes, stool softeners, and laxatives, there are several newer agents approved for patients with either chronic constipation or constipation-predominant IBS. *Chloride channel activators* include lubiprostone that is approved for women with constipation (24 mcg twice daily) and constipation-dominant IBS (8 mcg twice daily). Its main adverse effects include nausea and headache. The *guanylate cyclase agonist* linaclotide activates chloride secretion though the cystic fibrosis transmembrane conductance regulator (CFTR) and is approved for treatment of chronic constipation (145 mcg daily) and IBS-C (290 mcg daily). It has been shown to accelerate colonic transit and reduce bloating and constipation. Plecanatide activates *guanyl cyclase C* (GC-C) receptors, thereby stimulating chloride and bicarbonate secretion and inhibiting sodium absorption. This drug increased stool frequency and reduced straining and bowel discomfort in patients with chronic idiopathic constipation (3 mg daily). The *serotonergic agent* (5-HT4 receptor agonist) prucalopride has demonstrated efficacy for the treatment of chronic constipation at a dose of 2mg daily (1mg daily for renal impairment and creatinine clearance <30mL/min).

Nonpharmacological treatment

Nonmedication treatments are more appropriate for some causes of constipation. Biofeedback techniques using manometry or electromyography are indicated for selected conditions of anorectal dysfunction, including pelvic floor dyssynergia, that do not respond to laxative therapy. With these methods, rectal sensation can be enhanced, and paradoxical anal contractions with defecation can be corrected with learned behaviors.

Surgery is indicated for Hirschsprung disease. Anal myotomy may be beneficial with short segment involvement, whereas resection, bypass, or endorectal pull-through procedures are performed for more typical presentations of the disease. Subtotal colectomy with ileorectal anastomosis may be beneficial in carefully selected patients with severe colonic inertia that is unresponsive to medications. Surgical resection or reduction of large rectoceles is considered in patients when digital pressure on the pelvis or posterior vaginal wall results in improved fecal evacuation. Rectal prolapse may be surgically repaired with suspension or rectopexy, although these operations often have no effect on the underlying defecation problem.

Complications

Chronic constipation may lead to rectal prolapse, hemorrhoidal bleeding, or development of an anal fissure. Fecal impaction may produce colonic obstruction or stercoral ulcers, which can bleed or perforate. Large fecalomas may cause extrinsic ureteral compression, resulting in recurrent urinary infections. Fecal incontinence results from anal sphincter damage or perineal nerve dysfunction from straining or prolapse.

Case studies

Case 1

A 25-year-old woman presents with lifelong constipation described as one bowel movement every week induced by stimulant laxatives, but always with a sensation of incomplete evacuation. Without laxatives she will have a bowel movement perhaps once every other week. She describes abdominal bloating but no associated abdominal pain, and no weight loss or rectal bleeding. Physical examination reveals a well-developed woman with a normal examination of the abdomen and pelvis. Rectal examination has normal squeeze and anal wink is intact. Laboratory values include a normal complete blood count, calcium, and TSH.

Discussion

Chronic constipation in the absence of associated abdominal pain is classified as a separate entity from IBS. In addition to not meeting criteria for IBS, two or more of the following must be present to fulfill the diagnosis of chronic constipation: during at least 25% of defecations, have (i) straining, (ii) lumpy or hard stools, (iii) sensation of incomplete evacuation, (iv) sensation of anorectal obstruction, (v) manual maneuvers to facilitate bowel movement, or (vi) fewer than three defecations per week. In this young woman without alarm features, no structural examination is needed.

While some of the management is similar between IBS and chronic constipation, these are categorized differently due to potential differences in etiology, evaluation, and management. Treatment for this patient starts with dietary and lifestyle changes including adequate hydration, increased fiber consumption, and exercise. Either osmotic or stimulant laxatives may be safely used long term. If these interventions are insufficient to treat her symptoms, the first test to order is an anorectal manometry, preferably with a balloon expulsion test. Inconclusive anorectal manometry may be followed by defecography. Defecatory disorders such as pelvic floor dyssynergia may be treated with biofeedback. Normal manometry may be followed by a colonic transit test. Pharmacological interventions with chloride channel activators or guanylate cyclase agonists may be effective.

Case 2

A 53-year-old woman has a chief complaint of constipation for several years. She has a bowel movement once per week and often requires manual maneuvers to induce a movement. Her physical examination is normal and her laboratory tests including blood counts, albumin, and TSH are normal. She previously consulted another gastroenterologist who performed a colonoscopy, which was normal. You perform anorectal manometry, which is notable for increased anal contraction with attempted defecation. You follow this abnormality with defecography that illustrates paradoxical contraction of the puborectalis muscle and an inability to expel a 50 ml water-filled balloon. You provide her with a diagnosis of dyssynergic defecation, and she is successfully treated with a course of biofeedback therapy.

Discussion

Dyssynergic defecation criteria include: (i) the diagnostic criteria for functional chronic constipation, (ii) dyssynergia during repeated attempts to defecate defined as a paradoxical increase in anal sphincter pressure (anal contraction) or less than 20% relaxation of the resting anal sphincter pressure or inadequate propulsive forces based on manometry, imaging, or electromyography, (iii) one or more of the following: (a) inability to expel an artificial stool (50 ml water-filled balloon) within one minute, (b) prolonged colonic transit time, (b) inability to evacuate or >50% retention of barium during defecography.

Further reading

American Gastroenterological Association (2013). American Gastroenterological Association medical position statement on constipation. *Gastroenterology* 144: 211–217.

CHAPTER 10

The Patient with Diarrhea

The range of normal bowel patterns is broad, but 99% of the population in western societies defecates between three times a week and three times a day. The normal daily stool weight is 100–200 g, although individuals on high-fiber diets may pass 500 g/day. In the United States, a daily stool weight of more than 200 g is considered abnormal.

Clinically, however, a more useful definition of diarrhea is three or more loose or watery bowel movements daily, or an increase in frequency above an individual's baseline.

Patients may describe diarrhea as an increase in frequency or size of bowel movements or stools that are loose or watery in consistency or associated with urgency or incontinence.

Clinical presentation

History

Diarrhea can be acute (≤14 days in duration), persistent (>14 and ≤30 days in duration), or chronic (>30 days in duration). The rationale for this distinction is that most patients presenting with acute diarrhea do not require evaluation or specific treatment other than to ensure adequate hydration; however, severe acute diarrhea (hypovolemia, bloody stool, prolonged fever, >6 stools/24 hours) and persistent diarrhea require more extensive evaluation and management. Acute diarrhea is usually due to infection with bacteria or viruses, although drugs or osmotically active compounds may also be implicated.

Management of acute and persistent diarrhea

To identify the etiology of infection, the patient should be questioned about recent travel, sexual practices, ingestion of well water or poorly cooked food and shellfish, and exposure to high-risk persons in day-care centers, hospitals, mental

Yamada's Handbook of Gastroenterology, Fourth Edition. John M. Inadomi, Renuka Bhattacharya, Joo Ha Hwang, and Cynthia Ko.

institutions, and nursing homes. The characteristics of the diarrhea provide clues to the causative organism. Watery diarrhea with nausea but little pain is most consistent with toxin-producing bacteria, whereas invasive bacteria may produce more pain and bloody diarrhea. Viruses induce watery diarrhea in association with pain, fever, and mild-to-moderate vomiting. Antibiotic-associated colitis must be considered in appropriate circumstances, and new medication or inadvertent use of over-the-counter drugs with laxative effects (e.g. antacids containing magnesium) should be identified.

The differential diagnosis of chronic diarrhea is more extensive and can be categorized into motility, inflammatory, secretory, or osmotic/malabsorption disorders. Frequent passage of voluminous stools that do not abate with food avoidance is consistent with a secretory process, whereas passage of low-volume, loose stools at a normal frequency may be secondary to a motor disturbance. Foul-smelling, bulky, greasy stools suggest fat malabsorption. Soft stools that float or disperse in the toilet water and resolve with fasting are reported by some patients with carbohydrate malabsorption, especially if they occur after ingesting specific foodstuffs such as dairy products or fruits. Fever, bleeding, pain, and weight loss raise concern for a mucosal injury. Severe pain also may be present with pancreatic disease. Fecal incontinence raises the question of a neuropathic disorder.

Identification of risk factors is important in diagnosing the cause of diarrhea (Table 10.1). Diabetes and scleroderma are associated with intestinal dysmotility and bacterial overgrowth. Heat intolerance, palpitations, and weight loss suggest possible hyperthyroidism, whereas flushing and wheezing are reported by some patients with carcinoid syndrome. Chronic diarrhea may be a consequence of selected abdominal surgeries including vagotomy and cholecystectomy. Long-standing ethanol abuse impairs small intestinal function and promotes development of pancreatic exocrine insufficiency. A family history of diarrheal illness warrants evaluation for inflammatory bowel disease, celiac sprue, hereditary pancreatitis, or multiple endocrine neoplasia.

Physical examination

Orthostatic pulse or blood pressure changes, decreased skin turgor, and dry mucous membranes indicate severe diarrhea and the need for intravenous hydration and possible hospital admission. Emaciation, edema, peripheral neuropathy, cheilosis, and glossitis result from malabsorption of essential nutrients. Relevant skin findings include dermatitis herpetiformis associated with celiac disease, pyoderma gangrenosum with inflammatory bowel disease, and sclerodactyly with scleroderma. Arthritis may complicate inflammatory bowel disease or Whipple disease. Resting tachycardia suggests hyperthyroidism, whereas pulmonic stenosis and tricuspid regurgitation are found in carcinoid syndrome. Peripheral or autonomic neuropathy suggests diabetes or intestinal pseudo-obstruction. Neuropsychiatric findings are characteristic of Whipple disease.

Table 10.1 Causes of diarrhea

Osmotic diarrhea	
Nonabsorbed solutes	Magnesium, sulfate, and phosphate laxatives
	Sorbitol, fructose, lactulose
Disaccharidase deficiency	Lactase deficiency
	Isomaltase-sucrase deficiency
	Trehalase deficiency
Small intestinal mucosal disease	Celiac disease
	Tropical sprue
	Viral gastroenteritis
	Whipple disease
	Amyloidosis
	Intestinal ischemia
	Lymphoma
	Giardiasis
	Intestinal radiation
	Mastocytosis
	Eosinophilic gastroenteritis
	Abetalipoproteinemia
	Lymphangiectasia
Pancreatic insufficiency	Chronic pancreatitis
	Pancreatic carcinoma
	Cystic fibrosis
Reduced intestinal surface area	Small intestinal resection
	Enteric fistulae
	Bariatric surgery including jejunoileal bypass
Other medications	Olestra and orlistat
Secretory diarrhea	
Laxatives	Bisacodyl
	Ricinoleic acid
	Dioctyl sodium sulfosuccinate
	Senna and aloe
	Oxyphenisatin
Medications	Diuretics
	Thyroid supplements
	Theophylline
	Colchicine
	Quinidine
	Selective serotonin reuptake inhibitors
Bacterial toxins	*Vibrio cholerae*
	Enterotoxigenic *Escherichia coli*
	Staphylococcus aureus
	Bacillus cereus
	Clostridium perfringens
Hormonally induced	Vasoactive intestinal polypeptide
	Serotonin
	Calcitonin

(continued)

Table 10.1 *(cont'd)*

	Glucagon
	Gastrin
	Substance P
	Prostaglandins
Defective neural control	Diabetic diarrhea
Bile acid diarrhea	Ileal resection
	Crohn's disease
	Bacterial overgrowth
	Post cholecystectomy
Mucosal inflammation	Collagenous colitis
	Lymphocytic colitis
Defective transport	Congenital chloridorrhea
	Villous adenoma
Mucosal injury diarrhea	
Inflammatory bowel disease	Crohn's disease
	Ulcerative colitis
Acute infections	Viruses (rotavirus, Norwalk agent)
	Parasites (*Giardia, Cryptosporidium, Cyclospora*)
	E. coli (enteroinvasive, enterohemorrhagic)
	Shigella
	Salmonella
	Campylobacter
	Yersinia enterocolitica
	Entamoeba histolytica (amebiasis: acute or chronic)
Chronic infections	*Clostridium difficile*
	Nematode infestation
Ischemia	Atherosclerosis
	Vasculitis
Normal-volume diarrhea	
Functional bowel disorders	Irritable bowel syndrome (IBS)
Endocrinopathies	Hyperthyroidism
Proctitis	Ulcerative proctitis
	Infectious proctitis
Fecal incontinence	Surgical and obstetrical trauma
	Hemorrhoids
	Anal fissures
	Perianal fistulae
	Anal neuropathy (diabetes)

An abdominal mass suggests the presence of malignancy, Crohn's disease, or diverticulitis. Localized abdominal tenderness implicates an inflammatory condition. Rectal examination may reveal perianal disease with Crohn's disease, reduced sphincter tone that could lead to incontinence, and occult or gross fecal blood suggestive of mucosal injury.

Additional testing

Stool tests

Evaluation beyond a careful history and physical examination is not necessary in the majority of patients presenting with acute diarrhea. Additional testing should be considered in patients with (i) profuse diarrhea causing hypovolemia, (ii) bloody stool, (iii) fever >38.5 °C that persists >48 hours, (iv) >6 stools/24 hours, (v) elderly patients (>70 years of age), or (vi) immunocompromised patients (DuPont 2009).

Routine stool cultures can detect *Salmonella, Campylobacter,* and *Shigella,* whereas special culture techniques are needed to diagnose Shiga-toxin producing *Escherichia coli, Yersinia,* and *Plesiomonas.* Stool examination for ova and parasites can diagnose *Giardia, Cryptosporidium, Entamoeba histolytica,* or *Strongyloides.* Stool antigen tests also are available for *Giardia.* In individuals with recent antibiotic use or inflammatory bowel disease, stools should be sent for *Clostridium difficile* toxin detection. Newer diagnostic tests use a panel of molecular diagnostics that can identify multiple enteric pathogens including bacteria, viruses, and parasites.

Inflammatory etiologies are characterized by red and white blood cells in the stool. Noninflammatory diarrhea may be further evaluated by stool electrolytes, specifically sodium and potassium. Direct measurement of stool osmolality may be altered by bacterial degradation of carbohydrate so it is not routinely obtained; instead, normal plasma osmolality is assumed (290 mOsm/kg H_2O). A difference of >125 mOsm/kg between stool osmolality and twice the sum of stool sodium plus potassium concentrations suggests an osmotic cause, whereas a gap of <50 mOsm/kg is consistent with secretory diarrhea. Stool Osm gaps between 50 and 125 mOsm/kg are difficult to categorize with certainty. Osmotic diarrhea suggests ingestion of nonabsorbed solutes such as magnesium, phosphate, or sulfate. Stool or urine samples can be analyzed for sulfate, magnesium, phosphate, bisacodyl, castor oil, or anthracene derivatives.

> **Key practice points**
>
> Stool electrolytes are used to differentiate osmotic from secretory diarrheas. Laxative use generally results in an osmotic diarrhea. However, sodium sulfate or sodium phosphate ingestion will not produce an osmotic gap. While direct examination of stool osmolality is difficult, it is helpful in some situations such as factitious diarrhea: stool osmolality >375–400 mOsm/kg H_2O suggests contamination of stool with concentrated urine, while values <200–250 mOsm/kg H_2O are seen when stool is contaminated with dilute urine or water.

Malabsorption is diagnosed by fecal fat detection, generally screened using qualitative tests and verified with quantified fat on a 72-hour collection while the patient is ingesting >100 g fat/day. Fecal fat exceeding 7 g/24 hours is abnormal; however, severe diarrhea (>800 g stool/24 hours) can wash fat from the bowel lumen and result in fat excretion as high as 14 g/24 hours.

Lower endoscopy is indicated if there are signs of mucosal injury or for chronic diarrhea if no other etiology is found with less invasive testing. Random biopsies of the proximal and distal colon should be performed to evaluate for microscopic (collagenous or lymphocytic) colitis even if the endoscopic appearance of the colon is normal. If a small intestinal etiology of malabsorption is suspected, upper endoscopy may be performed to evaluate for inflammation or malabsorption disorders such as celiac disease.

Breath testing also is used to detect bacterial overgrowth as well as lactase deficiency. In selected instances, ^{14}C-triolein breath tests can provide evidence of fat malabsorption, whereas D-xylose testing can screen for small intestinal mucosal disease. Schilling tests help distinguish small bowel disease, bacterial overgrowth, and pancreatic disease as causes of malabsorption. Pancreatic etiologies, including chronic pancreatitis and pancreatic neoplasms, can be evaluated by abdominal cross-sectional radiography, endoscopic retrograde pancreatography, or endoscopic ultrasound. Arteriography or mesenteric resonance imaging may be necessary to confirm the diagnosis of mesenteric ischemia.

Suspected secretory diarrhea should be evaluated by serum gastrin, vasoactive intestinal peptide (VIP), serotonin, calcitonin, histamine, and prostaglandins and urine 5-hydroxyindoleacetic acid to detect endocrine neoplasia. Further evaluation with abdominal computed tomography (CT), endoscopic ultrasound, and somatostatin receptor scintigraphy can localize the tumor(s) and direct therapy. Octapeptide (^{111}In-OTPA) cholecystokinin analog scanning has been used for medullary thyroid carcinoma. Stool α_1-antitrypsin can confirm the presence of protein-losing enteropathy.

Differential diagnosis

High-output diarrhea of more than 200 g daily arises from two pathophysiological mechanisms: increased anion secretion or decreased absorption of water and electrolytes. Increased anion secretion may result from enterotoxins, endogenous hormones or neuropeptides, inflammatory mediators, bile salts, laxatives, and medications. Decreased water and electrolyte absorption develop from enterotoxins, decreased mucosal absorptive surface area, acceleration of transit with inadequate time for absorption, impaired mucosal barrier function, and ingestion of poorly absorbed osmotically active solutes. Conditions that produce high-output diarrhea are divided into osmotic, secretory, and mucosal injury categories, although some diseases produce diarrhea by more than one mechanism. Patients with normal stool output of less than 200 g daily may also complain of diarrhea. Normal-output diarrhea most often results from anorectal disease, hormonally induced hyperdefecation, or functional bowel disorders in which gut sensorimotor defects alter perception and transit of lumenal contents.

Osmotic diarrhea

The majority of ingested food is absorbed before it reaches the colon under normal conditions. In many diarrheal disorders, undigested nutrients act as osmotic agents to draw free water into the intestinal lumen. The most common cause of osmotic diarrhea is lactase deficiency. Other causes of osmotic diarrhea include ingestion of nonabsorbable laxatives, magnesium-containing antacids, medications, and candies or soft drinks that contain fructose and sorbitol. Congenital defects of carbohydrate absorption include sucrase-isomaltase deficiency, trehalase deficiency, and glucose-galactose malabsorption.

Some small intestinal diseases produce osmotic diarrhea from maldigestion or malabsorption. Celiac disease is caused by hypersensitivity to dietary gluten. Patients with this disease may be asymptomatic, exhibit iron deficiency anemia, or develop diarrhea and malabsorptive symptoms. Villous atrophy is the hallmark of celiac disease, but pathology may only reveal increased intraepithelial lymphocytes. Villous atrophy is not specific for celiac disease: tropical sprue is presumed to be an infectious disease that occurs on the Indian subcontinent, Asia, the West Indies, northern South America, central and southern Africa, and Central America. It produces diarrhea and malabsorption due to villous atrophy in persons who have resided in these regions for as little as one to three months. Crohn's disease involving the small intestine may lead to malabsorption and diarrhea. Whipple disease, caused by infection with *Tropheryma whippelii*, is diagnosed by demonstration of characteristic periodic acid–Schiff (PAS)-positive macrophages on examination of small intestinal mucosal biopsies. Congenital or acquired (secondary to trauma, lymphoma, or carcinoma) intestinal lymphangiectasia causes protein-losing enteropathy with steatorrhea as a result of obstructed lymphatic channels. Bacterial overgrowth produces steatorrhea from bile salt deconjugation, brush border injury, and mucosal inflammation. Intestinal infection with *Giardia*, *Cryptosporidium*, *Isospora*, or *Mycobacterium avium* complex produces brush border and intramucosal damage. Systemic mastocytosis and eosinophilic gastroenteritis grossly distort the intestinal mucosa and promote nutrient malabsorption. Short bowel syndrome and fistulae reduce the villous surface area available for nutrient uptake. Other conditions (e.g. postvagotomy diarrhea and thyrotoxicosis) accelerate intestinal transit, leaving inadequate time for nutrient assimilation. Adrenal insufficiency causes generalized disturbances in mucosal absorption.

Pancreaticobiliary disease can also present with osmotic diarrhea due to maldigestion and malabsorption that manifest with steatorrhea. Cirrhosis and bile duct obstruction can produce maldigestion because of the impaired delivery of bile salt to the small intestine, which then leads to poor micelle formation with ingested fats.

Secretory diarrhea

The most common causes of acute secretory diarrhea are enterotoxins released by infectious organisms. Viruses (e.g. rotavirus, Norwalk agent) are also likely to act through toxins. In some acquired immunodeficiency syndrome (AIDS) patients, secretory diarrhea results from defined organisms (*Cryptosporidium, M. avium* complex), but other cases are idiopathic. Laxatives represent the other common cause of secretory diarrhea.

Rare cases of secretory diarrhea result from overproduction of circulating agents that stimulate secretion. Carcinoid syndrome classically presents with watery diarrhea and flushing, which are consequences of secreting serotonin, histamine, catecholamines, kinins, and prostaglandins. Diarrhea is the major symptom in 10% of patients with gastrinoma and exhibits both secretory and osmotic characteristics. Overproduction of VIP by VIPoma tumors produces the syndrome of watery diarrhea, hypokalemia, and achlorhydria (WDHA), in which patients often pass more than 3l of stool daily. Medullary carcinoma of the thyroid, which may be sporadic or part of the multiple endocrine neoplasia (MEN type IIA) syndrome, causes secretory diarrhea because of the release of calcitonin. Glucagonoma causes diarrhea as well as characteristic rashes (migratory necrolytic erythema), glossitis, cheilitis, neuropsychiatric manifestations, and thromboembolism. Systemic mastocytosis produces a mixed secretory and osmotic diarrhea associated with flushing. Villous adenomas larger than 3cm in diameter produce secretory diarrhea, possibly secondary to prostaglandin production.

Other disorders also cause secretory diarrhea. Collagenous and lymphocytic colitis induce active colonic secretion of water and electrolytes. Bile salt diarrhea results from stimulation of colonic secretion. Diabetic diarrhea is multifactorial but has a secretory component. Diabetic diarrhea presents in patients with longstanding diabetes and characteristically is profuse, watery, nocturnal, and associated with severe urgency. Chronic alcoholics may develop severe watery diarrhea, which may be partly secretory. Ten to 25% of long-distance runners develop diarrhea, which is postulated to result from release of gastrin, motilin, VIP, or prostaglandins.

Inflammatory diarrhea

Conditions that injure the small intestinal or colonic mucosa lead to passive secretion of fluids from damaged epithelia and alterations in electrolyte and water absorption. Small intestinal infections that produce mucosal injury diarrhea include yersiniosis, tuberculosis, and histoplasmosis. Chronic mucosal injury diarrhea may result from inflammatory bowel diseases such as Crohn's disease and ulcerative colitis, ischemic colitis, and radiation enterocolitis. Microscopic (lymphocytic and collagenous) colitis is inflammatory but does not present with mucosal ulcerations. Other diseases that manifest as inflammatory diarrhea include eosinophilic gastroenteritis, milk and soy protein allergy,

Behçet syndrome, Cronkhite–Canada syndrome, graft-versus-host disease, and Churg–Strauss syndrome.

Normal-output diarrhea

Patients with stools of normal daily volume may also complain of chronic diarrhea. The most common cause of chronic diarrhea in the United States is diarrhea-predominant irritable bowel syndrome (IBS). Endocrinopathies such as hyperthyroidism alter colonic motor activity, leading to passage of multiple low-volume stools. Proctitis also is a common cause of low-volume, frequent stools. Fecal impaction in institutionalized or hospitalized patients may cause diarrhea from flow of fluid around the obstructing bolus (pseudo-diarrhea).

> **Discussion and potential pitfalls**
>
> IBS is the most common etiology of chronic diarrhea in the United States. In a young person without alarm symptoms or signs such as overt or occult gastrointestinal bleeding, weight loss, or anemia, the presence of diarrhea and abdominal pain relieved with defecation is most likely diarrhea-predominant IBS. Basic laboratory tests to evaluate for anemia and malabsorption and stool examination for chronic infection are generally sufficient to make a positive diagnosis of IBS. Structural examination with colonoscopy is not needed to rule out organic disease. In the correct demographic, serology and/or genetic testing for celiac disease may also be obtained.

Diagnostic investigation

Acute diarrhea

The evaluation of acute diarrhea should focus on infectious etiologies. Stool cultures routinely examine for *Salmonella, Shigella,* and *Campylobacter*. It may be necessary to specify cultures to include enterohemorrhagic *E. coli, Yersinia,* and *Plesiomonas*. Ova and parasites to detect *Giardia, Cryptosporidium, E. histolytica,* or *Strongyloides* may be considered. Stool antigen tests are available for *Giardia*. Newer molecular tests use polymerase chain reaction (PCR) technology to detect multiple pathogens including bacteria, viruses and parasites. In individuals with recent antibiotic use, stools should be sent for *C. difficile* toxin determination. Twenty to 40% of cases of acute infectious diarrheas remain undiagnosed despite laboratory evaluation.

Chronic diarrhea

Most patients with chronic diarrhea require laboratory testing in addition to a thorough history and physical examination. Chronic infections should be excluded by stool examination for ova and parasites, *C. difficile* toxin, and selected bacterial cultures. Newer molecular diagnostic testing with panels of multiple enteric infections may be used if available. If infection is present, directed therapy should be initiated. The next step is to differentiate inflammatory from noninflammatory etiologies of chronic diarrhea. The presence of leukocytes and erythrocytes in the stool confirms inflammatory diarrhea. Flexible sigmoidoscopy or colonoscopy should be performed to evaluate for the presence of mucosal injury, which occurs in inflammatory bowel disease or invasive infections, and biopsies taken even if mucosa is normal to evaluate for microscopic colitis.

In the absence of inflammatory indicators, stool should be examined to rule out the presence of malabsorption. Steatorrhea is a separate entity from diarrhea, but symptoms can overlap; therefore, stool should be examined for fat, initially qualitatively and if positive, verified quantitatively. Serum albumin and globulin may be reduced by malabsorption, malnutrition, or protein-losing enteropathy. Protein and hemoglobin levels tend to be lower with small intestinal versus pancreatic etiologies of malabsorption. Tissue transglutaminase antibodies are positive in many cases of celiac disease, and the diagnosis is excluded by the absence of HLA-DQ2/8 defects.

Discrimination of noninflammatory, nonmalabsorptive diarrhea into osmotic or secretory causes is performed by stool electrolytes. Osm gaps >125 mOsm/kg are consistent with osmotic diarrhea and gaps <50 mOsm/kg are normal, indicating secretory processes; gaps between these values are inconsistently classified and investigation into both categories may be warranted. Secretory diarrhea should be evaluated for evidence of hormone-secreting tumors and other etiologies illustrated in Figure 10.1. Osmotic diarrhea should be evaluated in the manner suggested in Figure 10.2.

Finally, exclusion of structural/organic causes of chronic diarrhea is consistent with motility or functional gastrointestinal disorders including IBS. Note, however, that in the correct setting, an IBS diagnosis can be made positively without the need for invasive testing.

Management

Acute diarrhea

Therapy for diarrhea depends on its severity and its cause. Fluid resuscitation is crucial in cases of severe diarrhea. Oral rehydration solutions maximize intestinal absorption and should be started early in the course of illness. Intravenous crystalloid solutions are indicated for hypotensive patients or those who cannot drink. Serum electrolytes should be closely monitored. Zinc and magnesium losses may be significant with chronic diarrhea, so specific replacement therapy may be needed. Acute infectious diarrhea without bleeding, severe dehydration, or host factors that impair the ability to clear the infection can be treated symptomatically with antidiarrheal agents and rehydration. The antidiarrheal effects of bismuth subsalicylate in traveler's diarrhea may stem from both antimicrobial and antisecretory properties.

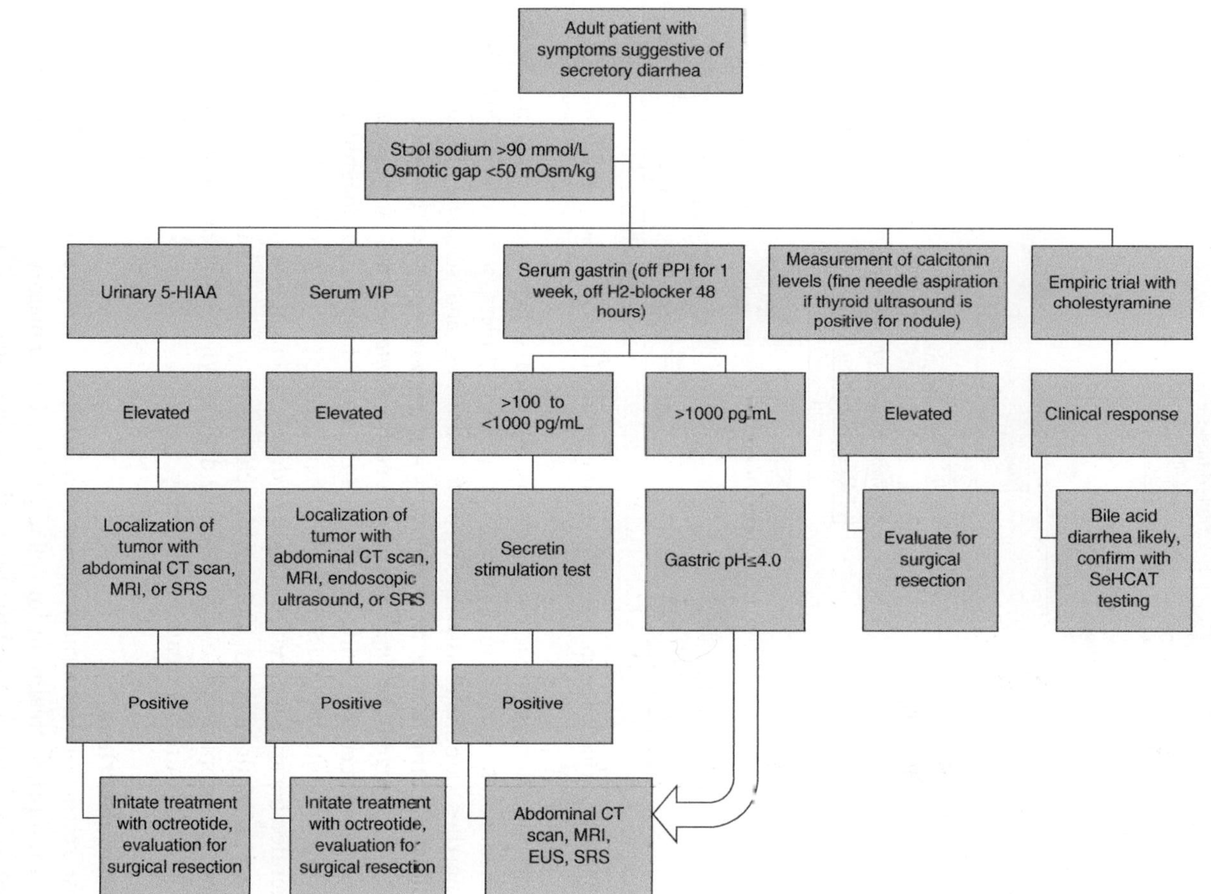

Figure 10.1 Evaluation of secretory diarrhea. 5-HIAA, 5-hydroxyindoleacetic acid; CT, computed tomography; EUS, endoscopic ultrasound; MRI, magnetic resonance imaging; PPI, proton pump inhibitor; SRS, somatostatin-receptor scintigraphy; VIP, vasoactive intestinal peptide. (Source: figure 41.3 from Podolsky et al. 2016.)

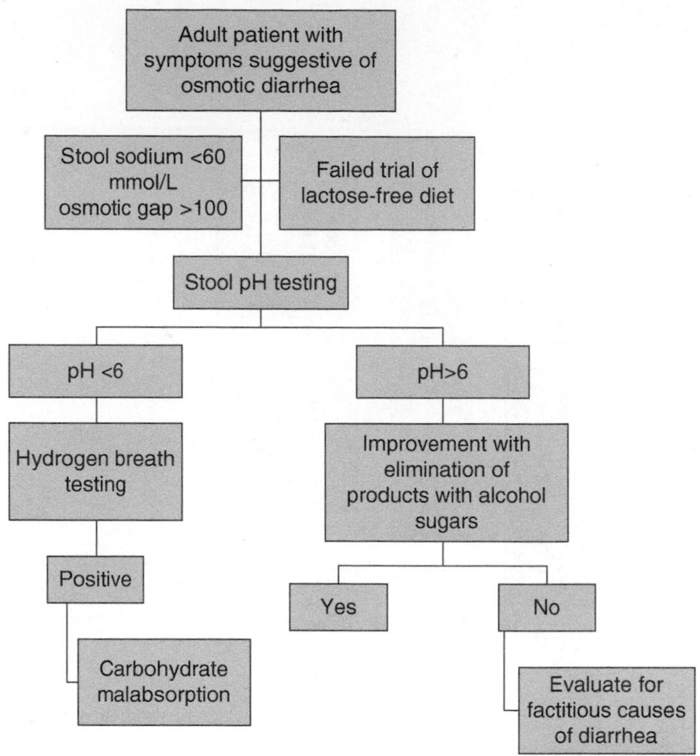

Figure 10.2 Evaluation of osmotic diarrhea. (Source: figure 41.4 from Podolsky et al. 2016.)

Antibiotic therapy of acute infectious diarrhea depends on the causative organism. Antibiotics are indicated for shigellosis, cholera, some cases of traveler's diarrhea, antibiotic-associated colitis, parasites, and sexually transmitted infections. Treatment with an antibiotic is usually recommended for noncholera vibrios, prolonged *Yersinia* infection, early *Campylobacter, Aeromonas,* and *Plesiomonas* infections, and day-care outbreaks of enteropathogenic *E. coli.* Antibiotic treatment of O157:H7 enterohemorrhagic *E. coli* infection is not recommended because it may predispose to development of hemolytic uremic syndrome. Antibiotics also are indicated for chronic diarrhea secondary to bacterial overgrowth, tropical sprue, and Whipple disease. Viral diarrhea and cryptosporidiosis usually are not treated specifically.

Chronic diarrhea

Lactose restriction is indicated for lactase deficiency, whereas a gluten-free diet is the appropriate treatment for celiac disease. Inflammatory bowel diseases are treated with specific anti-inflammatory medications, and pancreatic enzyme replacement is indicated for chronic pancreatitis. For secretory diarrhea secondary to endocrine neoplasia, AIDS, or diabetes, the somatostatin analog octreotide has antisecretory and antimotility effects that reduce diarrhea. Parenteral calcitonin can treat diarrhea from VIPoma and carcinoid tumors.

The α-adrenoceptor agonist clonidine treats diabetic diarrhea and diarrhea associated with opiate withdrawal. Indomethacin is occasionally effective for diarrhea secondary to endocrine tumors and food allergy.

For diseases that do not have a specific treatment, therapy relies on medications that stimulate absorption, inhibit secretion, or retard transit to afford time for improved fluid absorption. The opiate derivatives loperamide, diphenoxylate, codeine, and paregoric are the most common nonspecific treatments for diarrhea and act to retard gut transit by evoking a segmenting motor pattern to promote increased fluid absorption. Cholestyramine binds bile acids and some toxins and may be useful in some cases.

Diarrhea secondary to irritable bowel syndrome (IBS-D) may be controlled with antispasmodic drugs such as hyoscyamine, a tricyclic antidepressant, or a serotonin receptor antagonist in cases refractory to opiate agents. Rifaximin and eluxadoline have US Food and Drug Administration approved indications and have been shown to reduce diarrhea in patients with IBS-D.

Complications

Most cases of diarrhea in the United States result only in loss of productive work and personal time. However, in other regions of the world and in high-risk patients in the United States (e.g. persons with AIDS), diarrhea is a major cause of morbidity and mortality, especially in children. Diarrhea causes up to eight million deaths of children yearly because of severe volume depletion or electrolyte disturbances. This group requires aggressive fluid and electrolyte replacement, intravenously with crystalloid formulations or orally with glucose-electrolyte combinations (e.g. the World Health Organization solution) or commercial formulas (e.g. Pedialyte and Infalyte).

Key practice points

- Diarrhea can be acute (≤14 days in duration), persistent (>14 and ≤30 days in duration), or chronic (>30 days in duration). Most patients with acute diarrhea can be managed with hydration without further investigation. Severe acute diarrhea as well as persistent and chronic diarrhea may require additional evaluation.
- Evaluation of diarrhea begins with stool to evaluate for bacterial or viral infection and for evidence of mucosal injury or inflammation. If inflammatory changes (red or white cells) are present, endoscopic evaluation is indicated to evaluate for inflammatory bowel disease, infections, ischemia, and other ulcerating diseases.
- In the absence of mucosal injury, stool electrolytes are helpful to differentiate between osmotic and secretory causes of diarrhea.
- Fecal fat is used to identify patients with malabsorption.
- Motility and functional disorders such as IBS present without inflammation, malabsorption, or osmotic changes in the stool.

Case studies

Case 1

A 19-year-old man presents with two months of bloody diarrhea. He describes 8–10 watery bowel movements daily that are associated with tenesmus. Associated symptoms include bilateral lower quadrant abdominal pain, fatigue, and low-grade fevers. He has lost 5 kg over the past 10 weeks and has diminished appetite. He has no recent travel and no prior history of prolonged diarrhea. On physical examination, he is pale and appears tired. His blood pressure is 95/60 with a pulse of 96 bpm and a temperature of 38 °C. His examination is notable for dry mucous membranes and bilateral lower quadrant abdominal tenderness, left greater than right, without rebound or guarding. His rectal examination is notable for blood and stool with normal sphincter tone. Laboratory tests include a white blood count of 15.3, Hb 9.1 mg/dl, platelet count 475,000. Liver tests, international normalized ratio, and amylase are normal. Stool tests reveal white and red blood cells, negative *C. difficile* toxin, and negative bacterial cultures and examination for ova and parasites. Abdominal CT scan reveals thickening of the colonic wall from cecum to rectum, with a cecal diameter of 12 cm.

Discussion

This patient has evidence of mucosal injury diarrhea. After elimination of infectious etiologies, the most likely diagnosis is inflammatory bowel disease. The CT findings of pancolonic inflammation favor a diagnosis of ulcerative colitis. The preferred method for evaluating the presence of inflammatory bowel disease is lower endoscopy. With a patient as ill as depicted in this scenario, an unprepped flexible sigmoidoscopy is likely adequate for establishing the diagnosis. Colonoscopy may be hazardous even without evidence of toxic megacolon, and formal assessment of the extent of the patient's disease should be deferred until his condition improves.

Case 2

A 23-year-old woman presents with abdominal pain and diarrhea for more than one year. She complains of multiple episodes of watery to loose bowel movements that occur one to two times per week. There is no blood in her stool, but she describes lower abdominal pain prior to the diarrhea, which is relieved with defecation. She has not lost weight and is eating normally. Between episodes she feels well, and the symptoms never awaken her from sleep. Physical examination reveals a well-developed woman with normal vital signs. Her abdominal examination is notable for minor bilateral lower quadrant tenderness without rebound or guarding and there are no masses or enlarged organs. Laboratory tests include a normal complete blood count, electrolytes, liver tests, and amylase, with an albumin of 4.2 mg/dl. Stool tests are negative for white or red cells, *C. difficile* toxin, and ova and parasites × three evaluations.

Discussion

This patient has no evidence of mucosal injury or inflammation. The most likely diagnoses include IBS, although osmotic diarrhea due to poorly absorbed carbohydrates is possible. An acceptable management strategy would include an elimination diet trial, starting with lactose-containing foods. If this is unsuccessful, symptomatic treatment of diarrhea-predominant IBS with antidiarrheals such as loperamide would be indicated. Persistent symptoms could be evaluated with lower endoscopy with biopsies to evaluate for inflammatory bowel disease and/or serologic tests to identify susceptibility for celiac disease, neither of which is likely based on the normal laboratory tests. If her symptoms persist, a tricyclic antidepressant or a serotonin receptor antagonist can be effective in relieving symptoms. Rifaximin (550 mg orally three times daily for 14 days) has been shown to reduce diarrhea in patients with IBS-D. For refractory symptoms, eluxadoline (100 mg orally twice daily) is indicated for IBS-D.

Further reading

DuPont, H.L. (2009). Bacterial diarrhea. *N. Engl. J. Med.* 361: 1560–1569.

Podolsky, D.K., Camilleri, M., Fitz, J.G. et al. (eds.) (2016). *Yamada's Textbook of Gastroenterology*, 6e. Oxford: Blackwell.

CHAPTER 11
The Patient with an Abdominal Mass

Mass lesions in the abdomen may arise from localized infection or from inflammation, trauma, vascular disease, or neoplasm. These can be difficult to distinguish from the history and physical examination alone, given that the clinical presentation often is nonspecific. Careful radiological or endoscopic characterization of the lesion is important because the etiology determines the clinical management and prognosis.

Clinical presentation

History

The history provides important clues to the etiology of an abdominal mass. Pain related to meals or defecation suggests a lumenal origin, whereas gross or occult fecal bleeding or alterations in bowel function suggest either a primary source within or invasion of a lumenal site. Nausea and vomiting with abdominal distension raise concern for an obstructive process within the proximal gut. Dysuria or hematuria may indicate involvement of the urinary tract either by primary disease or by local irritation, as with Crohn's disease. Jaundice suggests benign or malignant obstruction at the level of the pancreas or bile ducts. Impingement of a large mass on surrounding vasculature may present with lower extremity edema or intestinal ischemia. Ascites may indicate peritoneal metastases from an intra-abdominal malignancy or a worsening of liver function in a cirrhotic patient with hepatocellular carcinoma. High fever points toward an intra-abdominal abscess, whereas unexpected loss of more than 5% of body weight raises suspicion of malignancy. Medications may predispose to selected liver masses (e.g. hepatic adenoma with oral contraceptive use). Paraneoplastic syndromes may suggest specific malignancies: pseudoachalasia may relate to

Yamada's Handbook of Gastroenterology, Fourth Edition. John M. Inadomi, Renuka Bhattacharya, Joo Ha Hwang, and Cynthia Ko.

hepatocellular carcinoma, dermatomyositis may develop with lumenal cancer, seborrheic keratoses (Leser–Trélat sign) or acanthosis nigricans are seen with gastric cancer, and deep venous thromboses (Trousseau syndrome) are found with intra-abdominal adenocarcinoma. A family history of neoplasia or inflammatory bowel disease may suggest these as etiologies.

Physical examination

A general physical examination as well as directed assessment of the mass complements the history. Scleral icterus or jaundice suggests liver infiltration versus biliary obstruction from a bile duct or pancreatic tumor. Temperature higher than 38 °C is consistent with an infectious or inflammatory process such as an intra-abdominal abscess. Lower fevers may accompany some neoplasms. If the mass is tender, as with Crohn's disease, this suggests that the mass is inflammatory. Lymphadenopathy raises concern for metastatic malignancy. Palpable supraclavicular (Virchow) or periumbilical (Sister Mary Joseph) nodes are found with gastric cancer. Rectal examination detects approximately half of all rectal neoplasms. Occult fecal blood is highly predictive of malignancy in a patient with a known abdominal mass.

Additional testing

Laboratory studies

Laboratory tests are important in evaluating selected abdominal masses. A complete blood count can test for anemia due to blood loss or chronic disease or for leukocytosis with inflammation or localized infection such as an abscess. Liver chemistry levels are abnormal with some hepatobiliary neoplasms. Determination of chronic liver chemistry abnormalities with the new onset of a liver mass suggests possible hepatocellular carcinoma arising in pre-existing cirrhosis. Amylase and lipase values may be elevated in some pancreatic cancers. Endocrine neoplasms may secrete hormones that can be detected by specific blood tests or measurement of urinary metabolites. Serum tumor markers may provide adjunctive information in the diagnostic workup. CA-19-9 and CA-242 are reasonably sensitive for detecting pancreatic adenocarcinoma but are not specific. Carcinoembryonic antigen is elevated with colon cancer as well as with benign liver and pancreatic diseases. α-Fetoprotein is secreted by larger hepatocellular carcinomas. Ovarian tumors are suggested by elevations of CA-125.

If ascites is present, cytological examination may reveal malignant cells. Serologies for infections such as echinococcosis may be obtained for suspicious cystic liver masses. A high level of triglycerides in the ascitic fluid indicates chylous ascites possibly due to lymphoma. Hematuria is worrisome for urological malignancy versus bladder or ureteral involvement by intra-abdominal tumors. Aspiration of pus with Gram stain and culture can provide both a diagnosis and treatment of selected intra-abdominal abscesses.

Structural studies

Endoscopy of the gastrointestinal tract is useful in evaluating suspected lumenal masses because of the ability to visualize suspicious lesions directly and to obtain biopsies. Routine upper endoscopy evaluates to the descending duodenum. Enteroscopy can be used to evaluate more distal small intestinal masses. Push enteroscopy can reach lesions in the upper jejunum. When there is no evidence of obstruction, capsule endoscopy may detect unsuspected small bowel tumors in patients with unexplained blood loss. Sigmoidoscopy examines the colon distal to the splenic flexure in optimally prepared patients, whereas colonoscopy visualizes the entire organ as well as the distal ileum. Endoscopic retrograde cholangiopancreatography defines filling defects within the pancreas or biliary tree and can obtain diagnostic brushings in approximately 50% of pancreaticobiliary neoplasms. Endoscopic ultrasound provides additional detail in characterizing tumors of the gut lumen and pancreaticobiliary tree and can determine if local disease extension precludes surgical resection.

Radiological and radionuclide imaging techniques are useful for evaluating suspected masses in the solid organs of the abdomen, pelvis, and retroperitoneum and in regions of the gut lumen that are poorly investigated by endoscopic techniques. Ultrasound is an effective screening examination for imaging the biliary tree and liver. Computed tomography (CT) provides a more detailed and comprehensive evaluation of suspected neoplasia in many organs. Specialized dedicated protocols have been developed to focus on selected regions such as the pancreas. Both techniques are of value in diagnosing intra-abdominal abscess as well. Both modalities can be used to direct needle aspiration or biopsy of suspected lesions. Magnetic resonance imaging (MRI) is especially useful in the study of selected liver masses and can help delineate the presence of hemangiomas, focal nodular hyperplasia, adenomas, and other abnormalities. Magnetic resonance cholangiopancreatography can assess for abnormalities within the bile and pancreatic ducts. Selected nuclear medicine tests are indicated in evaluating certain abdominal masses. Octreoscanning has assumed a crucial role in investigating suspected endocrine neoplasia. ^{111}In-labeled leukocyte scans may define the extent and locations of intra-abdominal abscesses. ^{18}F-fluorodeoxyglucose positron emission tomography is emerging as a promising modality for characterizing selected intra-abdominal malignancies.

Histopathological evaluation

In many instances, tissue must be obtained to distinguish accurately between a malignant and a noncancerous etiology of a radiographically or endoscopically detected mass. For solitary liver lesions, a directed biopsy can be obtained either percutaneously under radiologic guidance or endoscopically by endoscopic ultrasound-guided fine needle aspiration (FNA) or fine needle biopsy (FNB).

If radiographic testing suggests hepatic adenoma, surgical resection is advised rather than biopsy due to the risk of hemorrhage. When multiple liver lesions suggest metastases, CT or ultrasound can be used to direct percutaneous biopsy. For suspected resectable pancreatic cancer, tissue is best obtained using endoscopic ultrasound-guided FNA or FNB. Mucosal masses in the stomach, colon, and rectum often are easily accessible to endoscopy for biopsy. Tissue from submucosal masses may be obtained by FNA/FNB under endoscopic ultrasound guidance or by endoscopic resection.

Differential diagnosis

The differential diagnosis of abdominal masses is broad (Table 11.1). The likelihood of finding unresectable neoplasm also is highly variable, depending on the anatomical site of its origin. Many intra-abdominal masses present with pain, whereas others present with bleeding, systemic symptoms such as weight loss or fever, or obstruction. Others are detected while still asymptomatic as part of a routine healthcare surveillance program.

Liver masses

Both solid and cystic masses may develop in the liver. Causes of single solid hepatic masses include hemangiomas, adenomas, focal nodular hyperplasia, focal fatty infiltration, leiomyomas, teratomas, hepatocellular carcinoma, lymphomas, sarcomas, and solitary metastases from distant cancer. The presence of multiple solid lesions should prompt a search for extrahepatic malignancy, most commonly from the breast, colon, or lung. Cystic masses include benign cysts, bacterial liver abscesses (which may be multiple), amebic abscess, and echinococcal cysts.

Pancreaticobiliary masses

Most solid masses in the pancreas are malignant. Pancreatic adenocarcinoma usually arises from pancreatic ductal epithelium. Other solid pancreatic masses include lymphoma, solid and papillary epithelial neoplasms, and neuroendocrine tumors (insulinomas, gastrinomas, glucagonomas, somatostatinomas, VIPomas). Pancreatic masses with cystic components include pancreatic pseudocysts complicating pancreatitis, mucinous or serous cystadenoma, cystadenocarcinoma, and intraductal papillary mucinous tumors.

Masses of the biliary tree also may be cystic or solid. Cystic lesions include choledochal cysts and Caroli disease, which is characterized by segmental dilation of the intrahepatic bile ducts. Cholangiocarcinoma is the most common malignant tumor of the bile ducts. Other biliary tumors include gallbladder carcinoma, bile duct adenomas, cystadenomas, and granular cell tumors.

Table 11.1 Causes of abdominal masses

Hepatic masses
Hemangioma
Adenoma
Focal nodular hyperplasia
Focal fatty infiltration
Hepatocellular carcinoma
Lymphoma
Sarcoma
Leiomyoma
Teratoma
Metastatic tumor
Abscess
Benign cysts
Echinococcal cyst
Pancreaticobiliary masses
Pancreatic adenocarcinoma
Lymphoma
Neuroendocrine tumors
Pseudocysts
Abscess
Mucinous and serous cystadenoma
Cystadenocarcinoma
Intraductal papillary mucinous tumors
Bile duct adenoma
Choledochocele
Cholangiocarcinoma
Gallbladder carcinoma
Granular cell tumor
Gastrointestinal masses
Adenocarcinoma
Adenoma
Lymphoma
Hyperplastic polyps
Hamartoma
Leiomyoma
Leiomyosarcoma
Leioblastoma
Kaposi sarcoma
Carcinoid
Colitis cystica profunda
Lipoma
Liposarcoma
Angioma
Neuroma
Schwannoma
Inflammatory mass (Crohn's disease, appendicitis)
Abscess

(continued)

Table 11.1 (*cont'd*)

Miscellaneous masses
Renal cell carcinoma
Renal cyst
Transitional cell carcinoma of the renal pelvis
Renal lymphoma
Mesenteric cyst
Cystic teratoma
Mesothelioma
Hematoma
Abdominal aortic aneurysm
Ovarian carcinoma
Ovarian cyst
Uterine fibroma
Uterine carcinoma
Tubo-ovarian abscess
Ectopic pregnancy

Gastrointestinal masses

Masses involving the lumenal gastrointestinal tract are prevalent. Adenocarcinoma accounts for 95% of gastric cancers. Lymphoma is the second most common cell type. Small intestinal masses more commonly are benign and include adenomas, hamartoma, fibromas, and angiomas. Adenocarcinoma, leiomyosarcoma, and lymphoma are malignancies that arise from the small intestine. The most common colorectal masses are benign polyps, including nonadenomatous (hyperplastic, hamartoma) and adenomatous growths. Polyps may be sporadic, occur in those with risk factors such as a positive family history or long-standing colitis, or arise as part of a hereditary polyposis syndrome.

Adenocarcinomas constitute the majority of colorectal cancers, although lymphoma and Kaposi sarcoma also occur. Benign colonic masses may be due to perforation of an inflamed appendix, selected infections (e.g. amebiasis), or inflammation from Crohn's disease. The appearance of colorectal cancer can be mimicked by colitis cystica profunda, a benign disease characterized by submucosal mucus-filled cysts. Carcinoids arise most commonly in the appendix, followed by the ileum, rectum, and stomach. Gastrinomas may originate in the pancreas or in the proximal bowel wall. Tumors originating from smooth muscle (leiomyoma, leiomyosarcoma) or fat (lipoma, liposarcoma) may be seen throughout the digestive tract. Less common cell types include neurofibromas, schwannomas, and leioblastomas.

Miscellaneous masses

Miscellaneous lesions may present as abdominal masses. Renal masses may be infectious, neoplastic, or congenital. The most common malignancy is renal cell carcinoma. Other neoplasms include transitional cell carcinoma of the renal pelvis with parenchymal invasion, lymphoma, and renal oncocytoma. Renal cysts most commonly are benign but may harbor carcinoma, especially in patients with von Hippel–Lindau or tuberous sclerosis. Cystic masses in the mesentery include mesenteric cysts, cystic teratomas, and cystic mesotheliomas. A hematoma is considered in any patient with a history of blunt abdominal trauma. Abdominal aortic aneurysms may be detected as pulsatile abdominal masses. Gynecological masses involving the ovaries or uterus may be palpable on abdominal examination.

Management

Management of an intra-abdominal mass depends on the nature of the mass and whether it is malignant, has disseminated, and is no longer surgically resectable. In general, solitary neoplasms are best cured by surgical removal. Additional benefit may be obtained with adjuvant chemotherapy with or without concomitant radiotherapy in some settings, as with certain colorectal carcinomas. Intra-abdominal carcinomas with local or distant spread that preclude resection may be subjected to systemic chemotherapy with variable, often disappointing results. Other multifocal neoplasms such as lymphomas may be more responsive to cytotoxic chemotherapy. Some endocrine tumors may respond to hormonal suppression using chronic therapy with the somatostatin analog octreotide. Abdominal abscesses should be drained percutaneously or surgically, and therapy should be directed at the underlying cause (e.g. active Crohn's disease). Pancreatic pseudocysts can be drained percutaneously, endoscopically, or surgically. Finally, endoscopy can be used to remove large polyps (including some with superficial carcinoma) using a snare and retrieval technique.

Complications

The complications associated with an abdominal mass depend on its location and histological characteristics. Lumenal obstruction results from gut mucosal tumors, whereas biliary obstruction is a consequence of bile duct or pancreatic masses. Certain masses such as hepatic adenomas may rupture and produce life-threatening hemorrhage. Abscesses may not respond to antibiotic therapy and may have lethal outcomes if not appropriately drained. Similarly, many malignant tumors are fatal, especially if dissemination has already occurred when diagnosed.

Key practice points

- Mass lesions in the abdomen may arise from localized infection or from inflammation, trauma, vascular disease, or neoplasm.
- Cross-sectional imaging is essential in localizing the mass and can provide additional information regarding the etiology of the mass.
- Mass lesions in the pancreas are often malignant.
- A biopsy may be indicated if it will change management of the lesion.

Case studies

Case 1

A 58-year-old woman presents to her physician with complaints of a new fullness in her mid-abdomen and progressive fatigue. She denies any symptoms of abdominal pain, nausea, vomiting, or altered bowel movements. She has not seen any blood in her stool. On physical exam, she has a nontender abdomen but there is a firm mobile mass palpable just to the left of the umbilicus. Labs are notable for a hematocrit of 30, mean corpuscular volume (MCV) of 70, low serum iron, elevated total iron-binding capacity (TIBC), and low ferritin. CT scan demonstrated a 5 cm mass adjacent to the small bowel. Surgery is performed to remove the mass. Histology demonstrates a tumor with spindle cell morphology that stains positively for CD117 (C-KIT). In addition, there are >5 mitoses per high-power field. The tumor is diagnosed as a gastrointestinal stromal tumor (GIST) with features that are high risk for malignancy due to the size, location (small bowel), and mitotic rate. The patient is referred to an oncologist for consideration of adjuvant therapy with imatinib.

Discussion and potential pitfalls

GISTs are mesenchymal neoplasms that can occur anywhere along the GI tract. A majority of GISTs occur in the stomach, with the next most common location being the small bowel. GISTs are often asymptomatic but can also present with vague abdominal pain, obstructive symptoms (nausea and vomiting), GI bleeding due to ulceration, and fatigue due to iron deficiency anemia from chronic blood loss. The risk of malignant potential depends on the tumor size, mitotic rate, and location. GISTs and leiomyomas can be difficult to differentiate based on histology alone so immunohistochemistry (IHC) for CD117 (C-KIT) is recommended. However, in ~5% of cases IHC for CD117 can be negative due to a platelet-derived growth factor receptor-α (PDGFR-α) mutation.

Case 2

A 45-year-old man is referred to a gastroenterologist for evaluation of abdominal pain and symptoms of chronic flushing and diarrhea. The patient states that the flushing episodes typically last for one to five minutes and involve the face, neck, and upper chest. He cannot identify any particular triggers to the flushing episodes. In addition, he experiences watery diarrhea three to four times daily. On physical exam, he appears healthy with normal vital signs. His abdomen is nontender and no masses are palpable. Laboratory studies demonstrate an elevated urinary 5-hydroxyindoleacetic acid (HIAA) 250 mg in a 24-hour urine collection and an elevated serum chromogranin A. In addition, a 24-hour stool collection is consistent with a secretory diarrhea. A CT scan is performed that demonstrates a 3 cm vascular mass in the terminal ileum and multiple metastatic lesions in the liver. The patient is diagnosed with metastatic carcinoid. He is treated with depot octreotide with monthly intramuscular injections and loperamide for management of his symptoms. The patient is also referred to oncology for consideration of chemotherapy.

Discussion and potential pitfalls

Carcinoid tumors are neuroendocrine tumors. Patients who present with carcinoid syndrome (chronic flushing and/or diarrhea) usually have metastatic disease to the liver. Carcinoid tumors may occur anywhere in the GI tract and can also originate from the lungs and rarely the kidneys or ovaries. Occasionally localization of the tumor can be challenging using conventional imaging methods such as CT or MRI. In cases where localization of the tumor is difficult, somatostatin receptor scintigraphy can be performed because more than 90% of carcinoids have somatostatin receptors, which can be imaged using radiolabeled octreotide.

CHAPTER 12

The Patient with Jaundice or Abnormal Liver Biochemical Tests

Evaluating suspected liver disease requires understanding the diverse tests of liver function and serum markers of hepatobiliary disease. Measurements of hepatic function evaluate the liver's ability to excrete substances and assess its synthetic and metabolic capacity.

Serum markers of hepatic function

Bilirubin

Serum bilirubin determination measures capabilities for hepatic conjugation and organic anion excretion. Hyperbilirubinemia can occur from increases in the unconjugated or conjugated bilirubin fractions. Increased production of bilirubin because of hemolysis and defective conjugation produces unconjugated hyperbilirubinemia, whereas hepatocellular disorders and extrahepatic obstruction cause conjugated hyperbilirubinemia. A third form of bilirubin, seen with prolonged cholestasis, is covalently bound to albumin. The presence of this albumin-bound bilirubin explains the slow resolution of jaundice in convalescing patients with resolving liver disease. The urine bilirubin level is elevated in conjugated, not unconjugated, hyperbilirubinemia.

Albumin

Total serum albumin is a useful measure of hepatic synthetic function. With a half-life of 20 days, albumin is a better index of disease severity in chronic rather than acute liver injury. Hypoalbuminemia may result from increased catabolism of albumin, decreased synthesis, dilution with plasma volume expansion, and increased protein loss from the gut or urinary tract. Prealbumin has a shorter half-life (1.9 days) than albumin and therefore has been proposed as a useful measure of hepatic synthetic capacity after acute injury (e.g. acetaminophen overdose).

Yamada's Handbook of Gastroenterology, Fourth Edition. John M. Inadomi, Renuka Bhattacharya, Joo Ha Hwang, and Cynthia Ko.

Clotting factors

Prothrombin time detects the activity of vitamin K-dependent coagulation factors (II, VII, IX, and X). Synthesis of these factors requires adequate intestinal vitamin K absorption and intact hepatic synthesis. Therefore, prolonged prothrombin times result from hepatocellular disorders that impair synthetic functions and from cholestatic syndromes that interfere with lipid absorption. Parenteral vitamin K administration distinguishes these possibilities. Improvement in prothrombin time by 30% within 24 hours of vitamin K administration indicates that the synthetic function is intact and suggests vitamin K deficiency. Prolonged prothrombin time is a poor prognostic finding that signifies severe hepatocellular necrosis in acute hepatitis and the loss of functional hepatocytes in chronic liver disease. Individual clotting proteins have been proposed as useful clinical guides in severe acute hepatitis. Factor VII is the best indicator of liver disease severity and prognosis.

Miscellaneous tests of hepatic function

Serum bile acid determination has been proposed for assessing suspected liver disease, although poor diagnostic sensitivity in mild disease has prevented widespread application. However, the finding of normal levels of fasting serum bile acids in a patient with unconjugated hyperbilirubinemia supports a diagnosis of Gilbert syndrome in questionable cases. Plasma clearance of sulfobromophthalein, an organic anion, may help distinguish between Dubin–Johnson syndrome and Rotor syndrome. Serum globulin determinations can also give useful diagnostic information. Levels in excess of 3 g/dl are observed primarily in autoimmune liver disease, whereas selective increases in levels of immunoglobulin A (IgA) and IgM are noted in alcoholic cirrhosis and primary biliary cirrhosis (PBC), respectively. Elevated serum ammonia levels may be noted with severe acute or chronic liver disease and can correlate roughly with hepatic encephalopathy. Breath tests of antipyrine clearance and aminopyrine demethylation measure impaired hepatic drug metabolism.

Serum markers of hepatobiliary dysfunction or necrosis

Aminotransferases

Aspartate aminotransferase (AST; serum glutamic oxaloacetic transaminase, [SGOT]) and alanine aminotransferase (ALT; serum glutamic pyruvic transaminase, [SGPT]) are markers of hepatocellular injury. Because AST is also found in muscle, kidney, heart, and brain, ALT elevations are more specific for liver processes. The highest elevations occur in viral, toxin-induced, and ischemic hepatitis, whereas smaller (<300 IU/ml) elevations are observed in alcoholic hepatitis and other hepatocellular disorders. An AST/ALT ratio greater than two suggests alcoholic liver disease and/or the presence of cirrhosis, whereas a ratio less than one characterizes viral infection and biliary obstruction. When evaluating a patient with liver disease, decreases in AST and ALT levels usually suggest resolving injury, although decreasing aminotransferase levels may also be an ominous indicator of overwhelming hepatocyte death in fulminant liver failure, especially when associated with progressive increases in prothrombin time.

Alkaline phosphatase

Alkaline phosphatase originates in the bile canalicular membranes. Elevations of this enzyme are prominent in cholestasis and infiltrative liver disease; smaller increases are observed in other liver diseases. Alkaline phosphatase activity also occurs in bone, placenta, intestine, kidney, and some malignancies. Low levels of alkaline phosphatase may be observed in acute hemolysis complicating Wilson disease as well as in hypothyroidism, pernicious anemia, and zinc deficiency. Evaluation of alkaline phosphatase elevation is outlined in Figure 12.1.

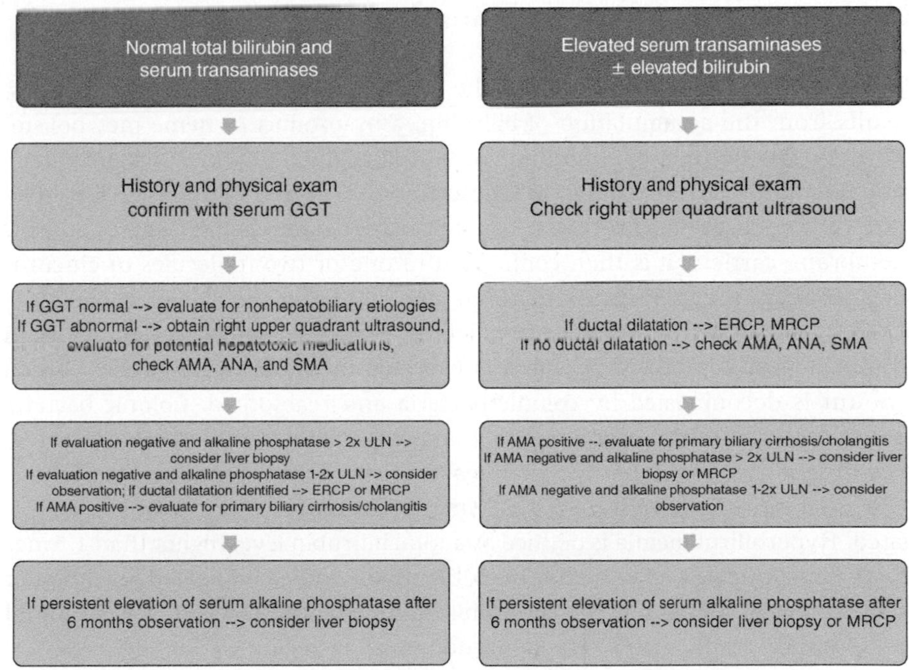

Figure 12.1 Evaluation of elevated serum alkaline phosphatase. ACG clinical guideline: evaluation of abnormal liver chemistries. AMA, antimicrobial antibody; ANA, antinuclear antibody; ERCP, endoscopic retrograde cholangiopancreatography; GGT, γ glutamyltransferase; MRCP, magnetic resonance cholangiopancreatography; SMA, smooth muscle antibody; ULN, upper limit of normal. (Source: Kwo et al. 2017.)

Miscellaneous markers of hepatobiliary dysfunction

Serum levels of γ glutamyl-transferase (GGT), 5′-nucleotidase, and leucine aminopeptidase (LAP) are elevated in cholestatic syndromes and may help distinguish hepatobiliary from bony sources of alkaline phosphatase elevations. Levels of GGT are also elevated with pancreatic disease, myocardial infarction, uremia, lung disease, rheumatoid arthritis, nonalcoholic fatty liver disease, and diabetes. Alcohol, anticonvulsants, and warfarin induce hepatic microsomal enzymes, producing striking increases in GGT level. Levels of LAP may be elevated in normal pregnancy. The hepatic mitochondrial enzyme glutamate dehydrogenase is elevated in alcoholic patients and in patients with liver disease secondary to congestive heart failure. The lactate dehydrogenase concentration is frequently obtained as a "liver function test," but it has limited specificity for liver processes.

Consideration must always be given to potential nonhepatic causes of abnormal liver chemistries, as outlined in Table 12.1. Abnormalities in liver chemistry levels may result from cholestasis, hepatocellular injury, and infiltrative diseases of the liver.

Cholestatic disorders and jaundice

Jaundice, a yellow discoloration of the sclera, skin, and mucous membranes, results from the accumulation of bilirubin, a by-product of heme metabolism. Of the 250–300 mg of bilirubin produced daily, 70% results from the reticuloendothelial breakdown of senescent erythrocytes. Bilirubin is cleared by the liver in a three-step process. It is first transported into hepatocytes by specific membrane carriers. It is then conjugated to one or two molecules of glucuronide. Finally, the conjugated bilirubin moves to the canalicular membrane, where it is excreted into the bile canaliculus by another carrier protein. Once in the bile, most conjugated bilirubin is excreted in the feces, although a small amount is deconjugated by colonic bacteria and reabsorbed. Colonic bacteria also reduce bilirubin to urobilinogens that are reabsorbed and excreted in urine. Any disturbance of this pathway can lead to hyperbilirubinemia and jaundice.

Normal bilirubin levels are 0.4 ± 0.2 mg/dl, and more than 95% is unconjugated. Hyperbilirubinemia is defined as a total bilirubin level higher than 1.5 mg/dl, an unconjugated level higher than 1.0 mg/dl, and a conjugated level higher than 0.3 mg/dl. Generally, the serum bilirubin level must exceed 2.5–3.0 mg/dl for jaundice to be visible. Hyperbilirubinemia is separated into two classes: unconjugated (>80% of total bilirubin) and conjugated (>30% of total bilirubin). With prolonged jaundice, circulating bilirubin may bind covalently to albumin, which prevents its elimination until the albumin is degraded. Therefore, with certain cholestatic disorders, measurable hyperbilirubinemia persists after the disease is resolved. Conjugated bilirubin is cleared by renal glomeruli; in renal failure, bilirubin levels may increase.

Table 12.1 Nonhepatic causes of abnormal liver chemistries

Test	Nonhepatic causes	Discriminating tests
Albumin	Protein-losing enteropathy	Serum globulins, a_1-antitrypsin clearance
	Nephrotic syndrome	Urinalysis, 24-hour urinary protein
	Malnutrition	Clinical setting
	Congestive heart failure	Clinical setting
Alkaline phosphatase	Bone disease	GGT, SLAP, 5′-NT
	Pregnancy	GGT, 5′-NT
	Malignant disease	Alkaline phosphatase electrophoresis
Serum aspartate aminotransferase	Myocardial infarction	MB-CPK
	Muscle disorders	Creatine kinase, aldolase
Bilirubin	Hemolysis	Reticulocyte count, peripheral smear, urine bilirubin
	Sepsis	Clinical setting, cultures
	Ineffective erythropoiesis	Peripheral smear, urine bilirubin, hemoglobin electrophoresis, bone marrow examination
	"Shunt" hyperbilirubinemia	Clinical setting
GGT	Alcohol, drugs	History
Ferritin	Systemic disease, chronic inflammation	Clinical setting
Prothrombin time	Antibiotic and anticoagulant use, steatorrhea, dietary deficiency of vitamin K (rare)	Response to vitamin K, clinical setting

GGT, γ-glutamyltransferase; MB-CPK, MB isoenzyme of creatine phosphokinase; 5′-NT, 5′-nucleotidase; SLAP, serum leucine aminopeptidase (LAP).

Conjugated hyperbilirubinemia

Causes of conjugated hyperbilirubinemia are listed in Table 12.2.

Congenital forms

Rotor syndrome is a rare, asymptomatic, autosomal recessive disorder that manifests as mild conjugated hyperbilirubinemia (2–5 mg/dl) in childhood. It is unclear whether the primary defect involves impaired hepatocyte secretion or impaired storage of bilirubin; although oral cholecystograms appear normal, biliary scintigraphy shows absent or delayed secretion. Dubin–Johnson syndrome is an asymptomatic autosomal recessive disorder from the impaired secretion of bilirubin, which produces serum bilirubin levels of 2–5 mg/dl. The results of scintigraphy and oral cholecystography are abnormal, whereas histological examination of the liver reveals darkly pigmented tissue. Patients with progressive familial intrahepatic cholestasis (PFIC) present with watery diarrhea, cholestasis, fat-soluble vitamin deficiency, jaundice, and occasionally pancreatitis caused by defective hepatic secretion of bile acids at the canalicular membrane.

Table 12.2 Causes of conjugated hyperbilirubinemia

Congenital conjugated hyperbilirubinemias
Rotor syndrome
Dubin-Johnson syndrome
Intrahepatic cholestasis
Familial and congenital
Progressive familial intrahepatic cholestasis types 1–3
Benign recurrent intrahepatic cholestasis
Cholestasis of pregnancy
Choledochal cysts, Caroli disease
Congenital biliary atresia
Hepatocellular conditions
Alcohol-related disorders
Viral hepatitis
Autoimmune hepatitis
Cirrhosis
Drug-related hepatitis
Wilson disease
Hereditary hemochromatosis
Infiltrative conditions
Granulomatous
Carcinoma
Hematological malignant disease
Amyloidosis
Cholangiopathies
Primary biliary cirrhosis
Idiopathic adult ductopenia
Autoimmune (overlap) cholangiopathies
Infections
Bacterial
Fungal
Parasitic
HIV related
Miscellaneous causes
Postoperative sepsis
Pregnancy
Total parenteral nutrition
Cholestasis after liver transplantation
Drug hepatotoxicity
Extrahepatic cholestasis
Inside bile ducts
Calculi
Parasites
Stricture
Cholangiocarcinoma
Sclerosing cholangitis
Choledochal cysts
Outside duct wall
Tumor in porta hepatis
Tumor in pancreas
Pancreatitis, acute or chronic

PFIC exists in different forms; all are autosomal recessive disorders, which have been mapped to several cloned transporters (FIC1, BSEP, MDR3). Choledochal cysts and Caroli disease are congenital malformations of the bile ducts and can manifest as jaundice or cholangitis and, eventually, cholangiocarcinoma. Choledochal cysts often are resectable, whereas Caroli disease (type IV choledochal cyst) usually requires liver transplantation for cure because of its diffuse intrahepatic nature.

Familial forms

Benign recurrent intrahepatic cholestasis (BRIC) presents with intense pruritus and elevated alkaline phosphatase levels, with mild increases in levels of aminotransferases and serum bilirubin (<10 mg/dl). Attacks, which begin from age 8 to 30, can last weeks to months, only to recur every several months to years. Liver biopsies reveal centrilobular cholestasis, which appears to be related to altered bile acid transport and enterohepatic circulation. BRIC is a milder form of PFIC-1 and, similarly, is caused by mutations in the FIC1 gene. Cholestasis of pregnancy is an autosomal dominant trait that manifests in the third trimester as pruritus. This benign condition must be distinguished from acute fatty liver of pregnancy, toxemia, acute cholecystitis, and acute or chronic hepatitis.

Acquired forms

Acquired disorders constitute the largest group of diseases that manifest conjugated hyperbilirubinemia. Many of these conditions are associated with cholestasis and can exhibit symptoms of pruritus, hypercholesterolemia, and steatorrhea. Intrahepatic cholestasis may result from liver disease (e.g. fulminant hepatitis, chronic hepatitis with significant hepatocellular dysfunction, and the recovery phase of acute hepatitis), infections, and medications. Hyperbilirubinemia occurs in alcoholic patients with acute fatty liver, alcoholic hepatitis, and cirrhosis. Of patients with alcoholic hepatitis, 10–20% present with a predominantly cholestatic condition, which may have a poor prognosis if bilirubin levels exceed 10 mg/dl or if encephalopathy, renal failure, or coagulopathy develop. Primary hepatic malignancy, lymphoma, and metastatic carcinoma cause hyperbilirubinemia late in their courses, whereas cholangiocarcinoma and other biliary obstructing lesions produce early jaundice. Bone marrow transplant patients may develop jaundice because of chemotherapy-induced veno-oclusive disease and acute or chronic graft-versus-host disease. Postoperative jaundice may result from anesthesia, intrahepatic cholestasis, transfusions, hypotension, hypoxia, and hemolysis.

Rheumatological disorders (e.g. rheumatoid arthritis, systemic lupus erythematosus, and scleroderma) elevate alkaline phosphatase levels but rarely produce jaundice. Sjögren syndrome has an increased occurrence of antimitochondrial antibodies (AMAs) and is associated with PBC, which produces jaundice late in its course. Congestive heart failure, shock, and trauma may produce hyperbilirubinemia, whereas renal failure can exacerbate hyperbilirubinemia from any cause. Furthermore, obstructive jaundice increases the risk of renal insufficiency, especially in the postoperative period. Infections can cause jaundice by bile duct obstruction (e.g. ascariasis), cholestasis (e.g. tuberculosis), or by sepsis and endotoxemia. Infections with Legionella, *Escherichia coli*, Klebsiella, Pseudomonas, Proteus, Bacteroides, and Streptococcus produce conjugated hyperbilirubinemia. Two-thirds of patients with acquired immunodeficiency syndrome have elevated levels of aminotransferases or alkaline phosphatase because of hepatitis, infectious sclerosing cholangitis, papillary stenosis, acalculous cholecystitis, malignancy, or medication effects, and all of these disorders may elevate bilirubin levels.

Hepatotoxicity accounts for 3.5% of adverse drug effects. Oral contraceptives induce intrahepatic cholestasis that leads to jaundice in up to four of 10,000 patients. Nonsteroidal anti-inflammatory drugs can cause hepatitis, cholestasis, granulomatous liver disease, and hypersensitivity reactions. Acetaminophen can produce dose-dependent hepatotoxicity, a condition that occurs at lower doses in individuals who consume significant quantities of alcohol. Alcohol induces expression of cytochrome P450 and leads to increased metabolism of acetaminophen to its hepatotoxic metabolite. Alcoholic patients also may have reduced glutathione stores secondary to chronic malnutrition. Isoniazid produces jaundice in 1% of patients. Chemotherapeutic agents delivered into the hepatic arterial circulation may cause a syndrome similar to sclerosing cholangitis. Numerous other medications affect the liver; when identified, the offending medication should be discontinued. Total parenteral nutrition causes hyperbilirubinemia because of intrahepatic cholestasis, infection, and the development of gallstones.

The common extrahepatic obstructive causes of jaundice include stones, blood, and malignant and benign strictures. Gallstone disease represents the most common cause of obstructive jaundice in the United States, although biliary parasitic infection is a common problem in certain areas of the world. The most common malignant causes include pancreatic carcinoma, cholangiocarcinoma, and lymphoma. Pancreatitis may produce swelling of the pancreatic head, leading to common bile duct obstruction. Primary sclerosing cholangitis (PSC) is most commonly associated with inflammatory bowel disease. With obstructive jaundice, alkaline phosphatase levels are elevated concurrently. For hyperbilirubinemia to develop, the bile ducts must be largely obstructed. Ductal dilation may not be detectable on radiographs for 72 hours or in chronic liver disease, such as PSC.

Unconjugated hyperbilirubinemia

Hemolysis and ineffective erythropoiesis

Hemolysis and ineffective erythropoiesis lead to overproduction of bilirubin that exceeds the conjugative capability of the liver. Hemolysis may result from sickle cell anemia, thalassemia, glucose-6-phosphate dehydrogenase deficiency, paroxysmal nocturnal hemoglobinuria, ABO blood group incompatibility, or medications. Severe hemolysis rarely elevates serum bilirubin levels above 5 mg/dl, although hepatocyte dysfunction or Gilbert syndrome can magnify the hyperbilirubinemia. Iron deficiency, vitamin B12 deficiency, lead toxicity, sideroblastic anemia, and dyserythropoietic porphyria produce unconjugated hyperbilirubinemia due to ineffective erythropoiesis. Resorption of large hematomas may also increase production of unconjugated bilirubin.

Neonatal jaundice

Physiological neonatal jaundice is noticed in the first five days of life in term infants; unconjugated bilirubin levels peak near 6 mg/dl by day 3 and then decrease to normal within 14 days because of the increased activity of uridine diphosphate glucuronosyltransferase (UGT), the hepatic enzyme responsible for bilirubin conjugation. Higher levels of unconjugated bilirubin may persist up to one month in preterm infants. Nonphysiological causes in neonates include ABO blood group incompatibility between mother and infant, glucose-6-phosphate dehydrogenase deficiency, pyruvate kinase deficiency, and hypothyroidism. Lucey–Driscoll syndrome is transient unconjugated hyperbilirubinemia resulting from a UGT inhibitor in the mother's blood. Breast milk jaundice, which may produce bilirubin levels up to 20 mg/dl, results from an inhibitor of UGT activity in breast milk. Severe unconjugated hyperbilirubinemia produces kernicterus in infants, which manifests as lethargy, hypotonia, and seizures.

Uridine diphosphate glucuronosyltransferase deficiencies

Gilbert syndrome, which is inherited in an autosomal dominant manner, is the most common cause of unconjugated hyperbilirubinemia; it affects 3–8% of the population. One-half of the patients have mild associated hemolysis, and some have splenomegaly. Gilbert syndrome results from a partial defect of bilirubin conjugation (50% of normal). However, affected patients are asymptomatic and occasionally exhibit jaundice (bilirubin levels up to 6 mg/dl) with intercurrent illness, fasting, stress, fatigue, and ethanol use, or during the premenstrual period. Type I Crigler–Najjar syndrome is an autosomal recessive disorder characterized by the absence of UGT activity. Untreated patients develop profound unconjugated hyperbilirubinemia and die by 18 months. Treatment consists of phototherapy, plasmapheresis, or liver transplantation, which is curative. Type II Crigler–Najjar syndrome (Arias disease) is an autosomal dominant condition characterized by 10% of normal UGT activity, which often leads to jaundice by age one year. Treatment of type II Crigler–Najjar usually is unnecessary unless it affects the very young who are at risk for developing kernicterus.

Other causes of unconjugated hyperbilirubinemia

Probenecid and rifampin decrease hepatic bilirubin uptake. Sulfonamides, aspirin, contrast dye, and some parenteral nutritional formulations displace bilirubin from albumin and thereby reduce its transport into the hepatocyte. Penicillin, quinine, and methyldopa induce hemolysis.

Disorders with hepatocellular injury

Hepatocellular injury may result from a diverse group of diseases. Acute viral hepatitis in the United States most commonly results from infection with hepatitis A, B, or C viruses. Hepatitis D complicates the course of infection in chronic hepatitis B carriers. Hepatitis E occurs primarily in developing countries, where it is well recognized as a cause of fulminant hepatic failure, particularly in pregnant women. Other viral causes of hepatitis include cytomegalovirus, herpes simplex virus, Epstein–Barr virus, and varicella zoster virus. Chronic infection with either hepatitis B or C viruses may also produce chronic hepatitis or cirrhosis. Chronic ethanol consumption produces a broad range of liver diseases, including fatty liver, alcoholic hepatitis, and cirrhosis. Hereditary liver diseases that produce hepatocellular injury are Wilson disease, hemochromatosis, and α1-antitrypsin deficiency. Congestive and ischemic disease in the liver is caused by congestive heart failure, constrictive pericarditis, hypotension, portal vein thrombosis or hepatic vein outflow obstruction from Budd–Chiari syndrome, inferior vena cava occlusion, or veno-occlusive disease. Significant liver disease during pregnancy, such as acute fatty liver of pregnancy and hepatocellular damage secondary to toxemia, usually occurs in the third trimester. Medication-induced and toxin-induced causes of injury are very common and require a high index of suspicion and careful questioning.

Infiltrative diseases

Malignant diseases, including primary tumors (e.g. hepatocellular carcinoma, cholangiocarcinoma), metastases, lymphoma, and leukemia, may produce infiltrative liver disease.

Clinical presentation

History

An accurate history is critical for a patient whose laboratory studies provide evidence of liver disease. The presenting symptoms provide important diagnostic clues. Pruritus is a common and early symptom in patients with cholestasis. Although classically associated with PBC and PSC, pruritus also is reported in extrahepatic biliary obstruction and hepatocellular disease. Many conditions that produce abnormal liver chemistry levels are painless, but acute biliary obstruction from stones can produce intense right upper quadrant pain. Concurrent high fever raises concern for cholangitis. Acute hepatitis produces less well-defined right upper quadrant discomfort with profound fatigue, whereas hepatic tumors may cause subcostal aching.

A family history is useful in diagnosing and evaluating hereditary hemolytic states, BRIC, hemochromatosis, Wilson disease, and α1-antitrypsin deficiency.

Exposure to ethanol and industrial and environmental toxins should be identified. A detailed medication history, including over-the-counter and herbal remedies, is critical. In particular, the use of episodic or intermittent medications, such as steroid tapers for asthma or antibiotics, may require specific questioning. Alcoholic patients should be questioned about acetaminophen use because hepatotoxicity can occur in these persons with therapeutic dosing as a result of cytochrome P450 induction. Intravenous drug abuse, sexual contact, and blood transfusions are associated with a risk for viral hepatitis B or C, whereas sudden worsening of liver chemistry levels in a chronic hepatitis B carrier suggests possible hepatitis D superinfection. Waterborne outbreaks of viral hepatitis have been reported in South East Asia and India, underscoring the importance of obtaining a travel history. Risk factors for hepatitis A include recent ingestion of raw or undercooked oysters or clams, male homosexuality, or exposure through day care.

Other diseases associated with liver disorders should be ascertained. Right-sided congestive heart failure, hypotension, and shock are recognized causes of abnormal liver chemistry findings. Chronic pancreatitis may produce abnormal liver tests as a result of stenosis of the common bile duct. PSC affects 10% of patients with inflammatory bowel disease, in particular those with ulcerative colitis. Obesity, hyperlipidemia, diabetes, and corticosteroid use are risk factors for nonalcoholic fatty liver disease. Hematological disorders (e.g. polycythemia rubra vera, myeloproliferative disorders, and paroxysmal nocturnal hemoglobinuria) associated with hypercoagulable states predispose to hepatic vein thrombosis. Hemoglobinopathies (e.g. sickle cell anemia, thalassemia) lead to pigment stone formation. Rashes, arthritis, renal disease, and vasculitis may develop with viral hepatitis. The presence of hypogonadism, heart disease, and diabetes suggests possible hemochromatosis. Concurrent lung disease may occur with α 1-antitrypsin deficiency, and central nervous system findings are associated with Wilson disease. Patients with leptospirosis will present with hepatic and renal abnormalities. Renal cell carcinoma manifests as abnormal liver chemistry levels in the absence of metastases. Recent surgery should be noted because anesthetic exposure, perioperative hypotension, and blood transfusions all may affect the liver. Recent biliary tract surgery raises concern for bile duct stricture. Cirrhosis is a late complication of jejunoileal, but not gastric, bypass surgery for morbid obesity.

Physical examination

Physical findings are of discriminative value for a patient with abnormal liver chemistry findings. Fever suggests an infectious cause or hepatitis. Jaundice is visible when the serum bilirubin concentration exceeds 2.5–3.0 mg/dl. Spider angiomas, palmar erythema, parotid enlargement, gynecomastia, a Dupuytren contracture, and testicular atrophy are stigmata of chronic liver disease, usually cirrhosis, though many of these signs have low specificity. Hyperpigmentation is seen with hemochromatosis and PBC. Ichthyosis and koilonychia are manifestations of hemochromatosis. Xanthomas and xanthelasma appear in chronic cholestasis. Kayser–Fleischer rings and sunflower cataracts suggest Wilson disease. Conjunctival suffusion raises the possibility of leptospirosis. A liver span greater than 15 cm suggests passive congestion or liver infiltration. Splenomegaly is found with portal hypertension or infiltrative processes. Abdominal tenderness suggests an inflammatory process (e.g. cholecystitis, cholangitis, pancreatitis, hepatitis), whereas a palpable, nontender gallbladder (i.e. the Courvoisier sign) raises the possibility of an obstructive malignancy. A Murphy sign (i.e. inspiratory arrest during deep, right upper quadrant palpation) is highly suggestive of acute cholecystitis. A pulsatile liver suggests tricuspid insufficiency, and hepatic bruits or rubs raise the possibility of hepatocellular carcinoma. Occult or gross fecal blood on rectal examination suggests possible inflammatory bowel disease or neoplasm.

Additional testing and diagnostic investigations

Disease-specific markers

Viral serology

The hepatitis A IgM antibody (anti-HAV IgM) is initially detectable at the onset of clinical illness and persists for 120 days. Anti-HAV IgG is a convalescent marker that may persist for life. Hepatitis B surface antigen (HBsAg) precedes aminotransferase elevations and symptom development and persists for one to two months in self-limited infections. The antibody to core antigen (anti-HBc) is detected two weeks after the appearance of HBsAg and initially is of the IgM class. The antibody to HBsAg (anti-HBs) appears sometime after the disappearance of HBsAg and may persist for life. During the period between the disappearance of HBsAg and the appearance of anti-HBs, anti-HBc IgM may be the only marker of recent hepatitis B infection. Measurement of hepatitis B e antigen and antibody, as well as a polymerase chain reaction (PCR) assay for serum hepatitis B DNA levels, can be used to quantify the degree of active viral replication in some patients with chronic hepatitis B infection. Enzyme-linked immunosorbent assays (ELISAs) are screening tests for detecting exposure to hepatitis C. Recombinant immunoblot assays can be used as supplements to ELISAs if a false-positive result with the ELISA is suspected. Both tests may produce negative findings for up to six months after acute infection; therefore, if hepatitis C is a diagnostic possibility, hepatitis C viremia should be determined by a PCR assay of hepatitis C RNA. Hepatitis D infection occurs only in patients with HBsAg positivity and can be measured by hepatitis D viral RNA and antihepatitis D antibodies. Persistence of anti-HDV IgM predicts progression to chronic hepatitis D infection. Acute hepatitis E can be detected by ELISA for antihepatitis E. A subset of patients in whom the tests for the above viral markers have negative results will exhibit positive serological findings for cytomegalovirus, herpes simplex, coxsackievirus, or Epstein–Barr virus.

Immunological tests

Markers that may be detected in autoimmune liver disease include antinuclear antibody (ANA, homogeneous pattern) and the anti-smooth muscle antibodies (ASMAs). ASMAs are detected in 70% of patients with autoimmune chronic active hepatitis but may also be present in 50% of patients with PBC. The presence of anti-liver/kidney microsomal antibodies (anti-LKM1) with reduced titers of antiactin antibodies or ANAs identifies a subset of patients with autoimmune chronic active hepatitis, a disease that follows an aggressive course in young women. AMAs are present in 90% of patients with PBC. Antibodies to the Ro antigen and to anticentromeric antibodies are observed with PBC, especially in patients with sicca syndrome or scleroderma.

Copper storage variables

Ceruloplasmin is a copper transport protein in the plasma that circulates in low concentrations in Wilson disease; low levels (<20 mg/dl) are measured in 90% of homozygotes and 10% of heterozygotes. Reduced levels may also occur with severely depressed synthetic function caused by other end-stage liver diseases. Alternative diagnostic tests for Wilson disease include urinary copper, which exceeds 100 mg per 24 hours in nearly all patients, and free serum copper, which is markedly elevated. Urinary copper also is elevated in patients with cholestasis or cirrhosis. Although the gene for Wilson disease has been identified (ATP7B), the lack of a dominant mutation has limited the role of genetic tests for the disease.

Iron storage variables

Serum iron level and total iron-binding capacity (transferrin) are useful measures in diagnosing hemochromatosis. Transferrin is normally 20–45% saturated. A transferrin saturation higher than 45% will identify more than 98% of patients with hemochromatosis. Elevations in serum iron with normal transferrin saturation occur in alcoholic liver disease. Serum ferritin more closely correlates with hepatic and total body iron stores, although ferritin may be elevated in inflammatory disease because it is an acute-phase reactant. The identification of a single recessive mutation in the HFE gene (C282Y), which is responsible for the majority of hemochromatosis, has eliminated the need for a liver biopsy in diagnosing many cases. A liver biopsy may be required for older patients with high ferritin levels to quantify tissue iron and to determine the extent of fibrosis, which will guide the need for screening for hepatocellular carcinoma.

α1-Antitrypsin

α1-Antitrypsin is a hepatic glycoprotein that migrates in the α1-globulin fraction in serum protein electrophoresis. Homozygotes for the Pi ZZ variant of this protein (normal is Pi MM) exhibit decreased serum α1-antitrypsin activity, which predisposes to development of chronic liver and pulmonary disease. Hepatocytes that cannot excrete the Z protein accumulate periodic acid–Schiff (PAS)-positive, diastase-resistant globules, as seen in liver biopsy specimens. Phenotyping is more accurate for diagnosis than determination of serum levels of the protein. Whether heterozygotes (Pi MZ) can develop liver disease in the absence of other hepatic insults remains controversial.

Percutaneous liver biopsy

As a general rule, direct forms of liver injury tend to cause predominant centrizonal necrosis; immunologically mediated forms of hepatocyte injury are localized to the periportal region; and cholestatic injury is recognized by the accumulation of canalicular bile and feathery degeneration of hepatocytes in the absence of a significant inflammatory infiltrate. Clinical applications of liver biopsy include evaluating persistently abnormal liver chemistry levels, establishing the diagnosis in unexplained hepatomegaly, and evaluating suspected systemic disease or carcinoma involving the liver. Contraindications to liver biopsy are an uncooperative or unstable patient, ascites, right-sided empyema, and suspected hemangioma. Impaired coagulation function is a relative contraindication. For patients with ascites or an increased risk of bleeding, a transjugular approach is an alternative to the percutaneous approach.

Management

Liver disease is classified into three groups: cholestatic, hepatocellular, and infiltrative. Screening the patient by determining levels of AST and ALT activity, serum alkaline phosphatase, serum total and direct bilirubin, serum protein and albumin, and prothrombin time can direct the subsequent evaluation into one of these groups.

Cholestatic liver disease usually results in increased serum bilirubin and alkaline phosphatase levels with normal to mildly elevated aminotransferase levels, although transient profound aminotransferase elevations may occur in early biliary obstruction. Figure 12.2 illustrates the suggested evaluation of patients presenting with jaundice or suspected cholestatic liver disease. In extrahepatic cholestasis, the serum bilirubin level increases by 1.5 mg/dl per day and reaches a maximum of 35 mg/dl in the absence of renal dysfunction or hemolysis. In partial biliary obstruction, the bilirubin level may remain normal in the face of an elevated alkaline phosphatase concentration. The most direct approach to evaluating suspected cholestasis is performing ultrasound to assess bile duct size. If malignancy or pancreatic disease is suspected, a computed tomography (CT) scan may provide better anatomical definition of the desired structures. If biliary dilation is detected, endoscopic retrograde cholangiopancreatography (ERCP) or percutaneous transhepatic cholangiography (PTC) can further define

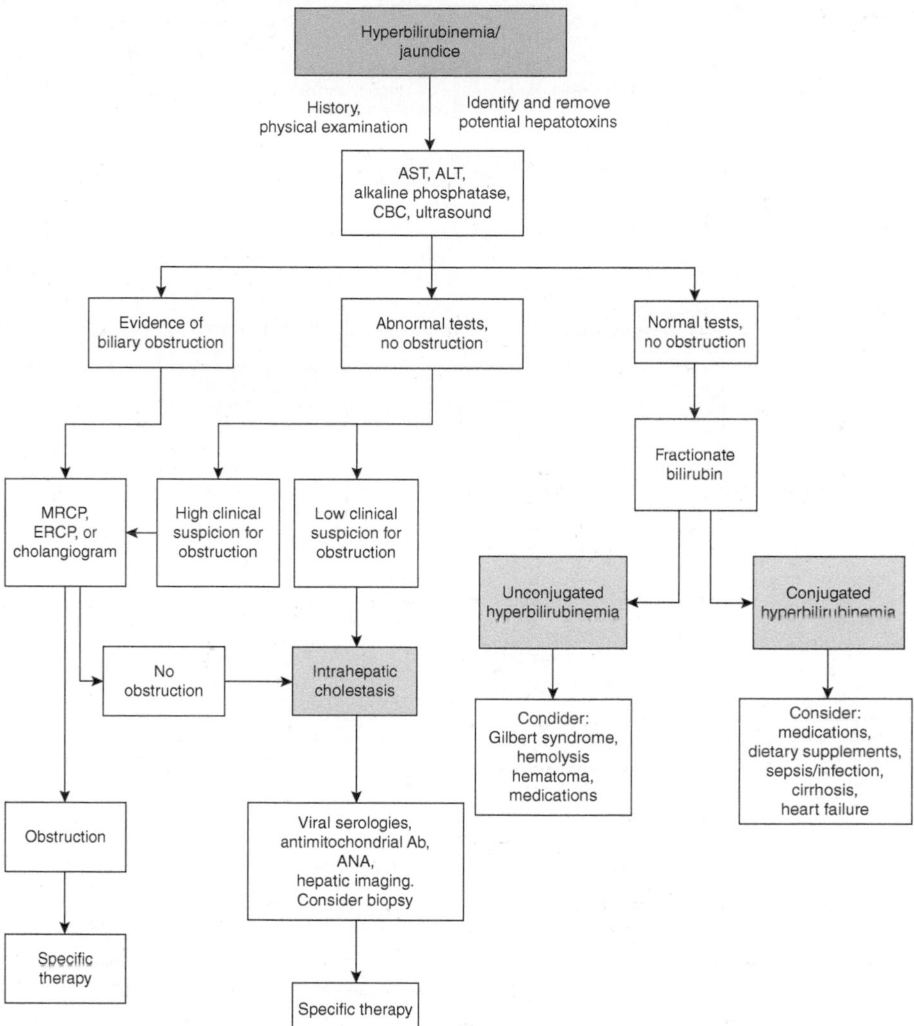

Figure 12.2 Diagnostic approach to the patient with cholestatic liver tests. ALT, alanine aminotransferase; ANA, antinuclear antibody; AST, aspartate aminotransferase; CBC, complete blood count; ERCP, endoscopic retrograde cholangiopancreatography; MRCP, magnetic resonance cholangiopancreatography.

and potentially be used to treat the abnormality. In some cases of extrahepatic obstruction, bile duct size will be normal; in these cases, ERCP or PTC may still be indicated because of a high clinical suspicion. In questionable cases, percutaneous liver biopsy may provide a definitive diagnosis. However, intrahepatic cholestasis cannot always be distinguished from extrahepatic cholestasis on liver biopsy specimens.

Hepatocellular injury is suggested by elevations in aminotransferase levels, and suggested management is outlined in Figure 12.3. Alkaline phosphatase and

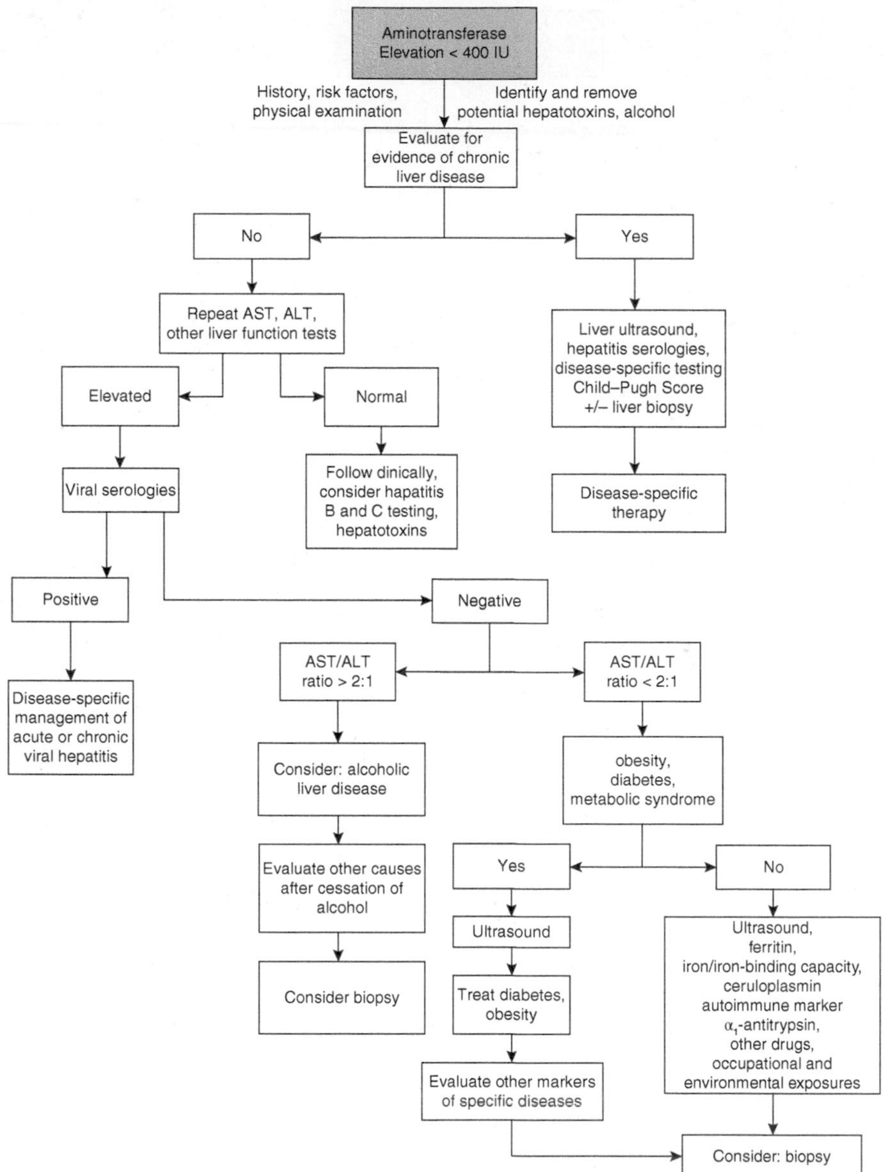

Figure 12.3 Diagnostic approach to the patient with elevated aminotransferases. ALT, alanine aminotransferase; AST, aspartate aminotransferase.

bilirubin elevations may also be elevated in hepatocellular disease, depending on the cause and severity of the clinical condition. Prolongation of prothrombin time and decreases in serum albumin levels indicate significant hepatic synthetic dysfunction. In patients with acute malaise, anorexia, nausea, jaundice, tender hepatomegaly, and elevated levels of aminotransferases, serum should be screened for viral markers to exclude hepatitis A, B, or C infection, depending on the patient risk factors. With disease duration of more than six months, additional studies (e.g. serum protein electrophoresis, ferritin or iron studies, and measurement of serum ceruloplasmin) should be added to the viral serological studies to exclude hereditary liver disease. Eosinophilia suggests possible drug hypersensitivity. For a patient with prominent systemic symptoms that suggest autoimmune disease, the clinician should perform serum protein electrophoresis; measure quantitative immunoglobulins in the blood; and measure the presence of ANA, AMA, and ASMA. A hepatocellular pattern is observed with ischemic and congestive liver disease, but measures to improve hepatic blood flow in these conditions can produce brisk reductions in aminotransferases to near normal levels within 48–72 hours. With congestive liver disease, the prothrombin time may be prolonged out of proportion to other signs of liver disease. Hepatic vein thrombosis (Budd–Chiari syndrome) may be suggested by increased caudate lobe size on CT scanning and usually is confirmed by Doppler ultrasound, CT, or magnetic resonance imaging that shows hepatic vein outflow obstruction and narrowing of the inferior vena cava.

Most acute elevations in aminotransferase levels do not require further evaluation unless they are severe or progressive. If aminotransferase levels remain high for longer than six months without an identifiable cause, a liver biopsy is indicated for diagnosis and to offer prognostic information about possible progression to cirrhosis. Many persons with persistently high aminotransferase levels are obese or use ethanol, and the usual finding on liver biopsy is fatty liver disease in the absence of serological diagnosis. However, the unexpected finding of chronic active hepatitis in a subset of these patients provides support for biopsy even in asymptomatic individuals.

Key practice points

- Liver chemistries provide information regarding liver function and serve as markers of hepatobiliary disease.
- The pattern of liver test abnormalities can direct the diagnosis toward a cholestatic, hepatocellular, or infiltrative process.
- Based on the pattern of laboratory test abnormality, additional serological, imaging, and biopsy studies can be obtained to clarify the diagnosis.

Case studies

Case 1

A 67-year-old woman is referred to the hepatology clinic with concerns for possible cirrhosis. Her physical examination notes the absence of hepatosplenomegaly, but she has pitting edema of her lower extremities. Her laboratory tests are notable for normal AST and ALT at 30 and 28, alkaline phosphatase 110, and bilirubin 1.1 mg/dl; however, her serum albumin is low at 2.8 g/dl with an elevated international normalized ratio (INR) of 1.8. Her complete blood count is unremarkable, with platelets of 250,000/μl. On review of her medical history, you note she has long-standing diabetes complicated by severe gastroparesis. You suspect she may have protein in her urine, and urine tests confirm nephrotic range proteinuria for which she is started on an angiotensin-converting enzyme (ACE) inhibitor. You further suspect that she is malnourished as a result of her gastroparesis, and you provide her with vitamin K supplementation. Follow-up laboratory values after several months reveal improved serum albumin to 3.6 and INR of 1.1.

Discussion and potential pitfalls

While albumin and INR are the two most important measures of liver function, it is important to recognize that there are many alternative etiologies for abnormalities in these values. Protein losses due to proteinuria, protein-losing enteropathy, and malnutrition can result in marked hypoalbuminemia. The use of antibiotics and anticoagulants can prolong the prothrombin time, as can persistent cholestasis, steatorrhea, and malnutrition.

Case 2

You are asked to see a 21-year-old man who has been diagnosed with Wilson disease and would like to transfer care to your medical center. He is being maintained on trientene. His diagnosis of Wilson disease was made in the setting of abnormal liver tests. Liver biopsy was nonspecific but showed advanced fibrosis. The patient's ceruloplasmin was borderline low, and a subsequent 24-hour urine showed a markedly elevated copper quantitation. Upon review of his labs, you note his alkaline phosphatase is elevated at 490 U/l. This raises your suspicion that the diagnosis of Wilson disease is incorrect. You obtain a magnetic resonance cholangiopancreatography scan, which shows classic changes of PSC.

Discussion and potential pitfalls

The diagnosis of Wilson disease is challenging, and it is typically a combination of tests and a high level of suspicion that results in the diagnosis. Classic diagnostic features include low serum ceruloplasmin, high urinary copper, and elevated quantitative tissue copper. Kayser–Fleischer rings may be noted on ophthalmological exam. Less specific but more readily available diagnostic clues include elevated serum bilirubin, hemolytic anemia, and low serum alkaline phosphatase. It is important to note that prolonged cholestasis, which often accompanies PBC and PSC, can result in significant elevations of urinary copper and hepatic copper quantitation.

Further reading

Kwo, P.Y., Cohen, S.M., and Lim, J.K. (2017). ACG clinical guideline: Evaluation of abnormal liver chemistries. *Am. J. Gastroenterol.* 112: 18–35.

CHAPTER 13

The Patient with Ascites

Ascites is the pathological accumulation of fluid within the peritoneal cavity. It is important to establish a cause for its development and to initiate a rational treatment regimen to minimize the complications of ascites. Most cases of ascites in the United States result from liver disease, although disorders involving other organ systems may produce abdominal fluid accumulation in certain situations (Table 13.1).

Pathogenesis

Chronic parenchymal liver disease

Portal hypertension is a prerequisite for ascites formation in patients with liver disease. In general, ascites is a complication of chronic liver diseases (e.g. cirrhosis), but some acute diseases such as acute alcoholic hepatitis or fulminant hepatic failure may result in ascites. In this setting, a high (>1.1 g/dl) serum-ascites albumin gradient (SAAG) indicates acute portal hypertension and a mechanism of fluid formation similar to that in chronic liver disease.

Three theories have been proposed to explain fluid accumulation. The underfill theory postulates that an imbalance of Starling forces produces intravascular fluid loss into the peritoneum, with resultant hormonally mediated renal sodium retention. The overfill theory proposes that primary renal sodium retention produces intravascular hypervolemia that overflows into the peritoneum. The more recent peripheral arterial vasodilation theory proposes that portal hypertension leads to vasodilation and reduced effective arterial blood volume, which increases renal sodium retention and promotes fluid accumulation. In the vasodilation theory, the underfill mechanism is operative in early, compensated cirrhosis, whereas the overflow mechanism operates in advanced disease (Figure 13.1).

Yamada's Handbook of Gastroenterology, Fourth Edition. John M. Inadomi, Renuka Bhattacharya, Joo Ha Hwang, and Cynthia Ko.

Table 13.1 Causes of ascites

Causes of ascites
Chronic parenchymal liver disease (cirrhosis and alcoholic hepatitis)
"Mixed" (portal hypertension plus another cause, e.g. cirrhosis and peritoneal carcinomatosis)
Heart failure
Malignancy
Tuberculosis
Fulminant hepatic failure
Pancreatic
Nephrogenous ("dialysis ascites")
Miscellaneous[a]

[a] Includes biliary ascites and chylous ascites resulting from lymphatic tears, lymphoma, and cirrhosis.

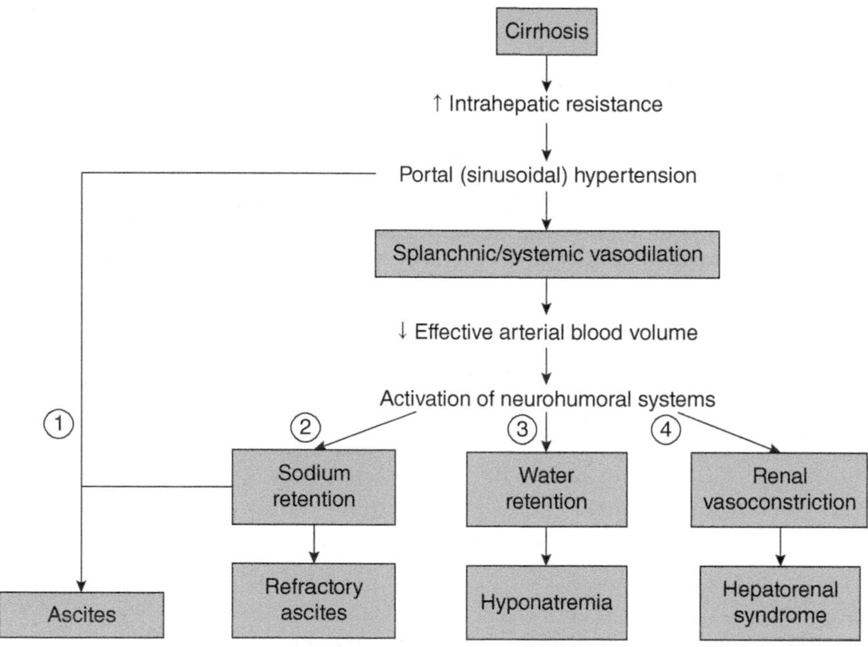

Figure 13.1 Common pathogenesis of ascites, hyponatremia, and hepatorenal syndrome. Ascites (1) results from increased sinusoidal pressure and sodium retention. Sinusoidal pressure increases because of increased intrahepatic resistance. Sodium retention results from splanchnic and systemic vasodilation that leads to decreased effective arterial blood volume and subsequent upregulation of sodium-retaining hormones. With progression of cirrhosis and portal hypertension, vasodilation is more pronounced, leading to further activation of the renin-angiotensin-aldosterone and sympathetic nervous systems. The resulting increase in sodium and water retention can lead to refractory ascites (2) and hyponatremia (3), respectively, while the resulting increase in vasoconstrictors can lead to renal vasoconstriction and hepatorenal syndrome (4). (Source: Yamada et al. 2008.)

Cardiac disease

Ascites is an uncommon complication of both high-output and low-output heart failure. High-output failure is associated with decreased peripheral resistance; low-output disease is defined by reduced cardiac output. Both lead to decreased effective arterial blood volume and, subsequently, to renal sodium retention. Pericardial disease is a potential cardiac cause of ascites.

Renal disease

Nephrotic syndrome is a rare cause of ascites in adults. It results from protein loss in the urine, leading to decreased intravascular volume and increased renal sodium retention. Nephrogenous ascites is a poorly understood condition that develops with hemodialysis; its optimal treatment is undefined and its prognosis is poor. Continuous ambulatory peritoneal dialysis is an iatrogenic form of ascites that takes advantage of the rich vascularity of the parietal peritoneum to eliminate endogenous toxins and control fluid balance. Urine may accumulate in the peritoneum in newborns or as a result of trauma or renal transplantation in adults.

Pancreatic disease

Pancreatic ascites develops as a complication of severe acute pancreatitis, pancreatic duct rupture in acute or chronic pancreatitis, or leakage from a pancreatic pseudo-cyst. Many patients with pancreatic ascites have underlying cirrhosis. Pancreatic ascites may be complicated by infection or left-sided pleural effusion.

Biliary disease

Most cases of biliary ascites result from gallbladder rupture, which usually is a complication of gangrene of the gallbladder in elderly men. Bile also can accumulate in the peritoneal cavity after biliary surgery or biliary or intestinal perforation.

Malignancy

Malignancy-related ascites signifies advanced disease in most cases and has a dismal prognosis. Exceptions are ovarian carcinoma and lymphoma, which may respond to debulking surgery and chemotherapy, respectively. The mechanism of ascites formation depends on the location of the tumor. Peritoneal carcinomatosis produces exudation of proteinaceous fluid into the peritoneal cavity, whereas primary hepatic malignancy or liver metastases are likely to induce ascites by producing portal hypertension, either from vascular occlusion by the tumor or arteriovenous fistulae within the tumor. Chylous ascites can result from lymph node involvement with a tumor.

Infectious disease

In the United States, tuberculous peritonitis is a disease typically seen in Asian, Mexican, and Central American immigrants, and as a complication of acquired immunodeficiency syndrome (AIDS). One-half of patients with tuberculous peritonitis have underlying cirrhosis, usually secondary to ethanol abuse. Exudation of proteinaceous fluid from the tubercles lining the peritoneum induces ascites formation. Coccidioides organisms cause infectious ascites formation by a similar mechanism. For sexually active women who have a fever and inflammatory ascites, chlamydia-induced, and the less common gonococcus-induced, Fitz-Hugh–Curtis syndrome should be considered.

Chylous ascites

Chylous ascites is a result of the obstruction of or damage to chyle-containing lymphatic channels. The most common causes are lymphatic malignancies (e.g. lymphomas, other malignancies), surgical tears, and infectious causes, but it can occur in patients with cirrhosis alone.

Other causes of ascites formation

Serositis with ascites formation may complicate systemic lupus erythematosus. Meigs syndrome (ascites and pleural effusion due to benign ovarian neoplasms) is a rare cause of ascites formation. Most cases of ascites caused by ovarian disease are from peritoneal carcinomatosis. Ascites with myxedema is secondary to hypothyroidism-related cardiac failure. Mixed ascites occurs in about 5% of cases when the patient has two or more separate causes of ascites formation, such as cirrhosis and infection or malignancy. A clue to the presence of a second cause is an inappropriately high white cell count in the ascitic fluid.

Clinical presentation

History

The history can help to elucidate the cause of ascites formation. Increasing abdominal girth from ascites may be part of the initial presentation of patients with alcoholic liver disease; however, the laxity of the abdominal wall and the severity of underlying liver disease suggest that the condition can be present for some time before it is recognized. Patients who consume ethanol only intermittently may report cyclic ascites, whereas patients with nonalcoholic disease usually have persistent ascites. Other risk factors for viral liver disease should be ascertained (i.e. drug abuse, sexual exposure, blood transfusions, and tattoos). A positive family history of liver disease raises the possibility of a heritable condition (e.g. Wilson disease, hemochromatosis, or α1-antitrypsin deficiency) that might also present with symptoms referable to other organ systems (diabetes, cardiac disease, joint problems, and hyperpigmentation with hemochromatosis; neurological disease with Wilson disease; pulmonary complaints with α1-antitrypsin deficiency). Patients with cirrhotic ascites may report other complications of liver disease, including jaundice, pedal edema, gastrointestinal hemorrhage, or encephalopathy. The patient with long-standing, stable cirrhosis who abruptly develops ascites should be evaluated for possible hepatocellular carcinoma.

Information concerning possible nonhepatic disease should be obtained. Weight loss or a prior history of cancer suggests possible malignant ascites, which may be painful and produce rapid increases in abdominal girth. A history of heart disease raises the possibility of cardiac causes of ascites. Some alcoholics with ascites have alcoholic cardiomyopathy rather than liver dysfunction. Obesity, diabetes, and hyperlipidemia are risk factors for nonalcoholic fatty liver disease, which can cause cirrhosis on its own or can act synergistically with other insults (e.g. alcohol, hepatitis C). Tuberculous peritonitis usually presents with fever and abdominal discomfort. Patients with nephrotic syndrome usually have anasarca. Patients with rheumatological disease may have serositis. Patients with ascites associated with lethargy, cold intolerance, and voice and skin changes should be evaluated for hypothyroidism.

Physical examination

Ascites should be distinguished from panniculus, massive hepatomegaly, gaseous overdistension, intra-abdominal masses, and pregnancy. Percussion of the flanks can be used to help determine if a patient has ascites. The absence of flank dullness excludes ascites with 90% accuracy. If dullness is found, the patient should be rolled into a partial decubitus position to test whether there is a shift in the air–fluid interface determined by percussion (shifting dullness). The fluid wave has less value in detecting ascites. The puddle sign detects as little as 120 ml of ascitic fluid, but it requires the patient to assume a hands-and-knees position for several minutes and is a less useful test than flank dullness.

The physical examination can help to determine the cause of ascites. Palmar erythema, abdominal wall collateral veins, spider angiomas, splenomegaly, and jaundice are consistent with liver disease. Large veins on the flanks and back indicate blockage of the inferior vena cava that is caused by webs or malignancy. Masses or lymphadenopathy (e.g. Sister Mary Joseph nodule, Virchow node) suggest underlying malignancy. Distended neck veins, cardiomegaly, and auscultation of an S3 or pericardial rub suggest cardiac causes of ascites, whereas anasarca may be observed with nephrotic syndrome.

Additional testing and diagnostic investigations

Blood and urine studies

Laboratory blood studies can provide clues to the cause of ascites. Abnormal levels of aminotransferases, alkaline phosphatase, and bilirubin are seen with liver disease. Prolonged prothrombin time and hypoalbuminemia are also observed with hepatic synthetic dysfunction, although low albumin levels are noted with renal disease, protein-losing enteropathy, and malnutrition. Hematological abnormalities, especially thrombocytopenia, suggest liver disease. Renal disease may be suggested by electrolyte abnormalities or elevations in blood urea nitrogen and creatinine. Urinalysis may reveal protein loss with nephrotic syndrome or bilirubinuria with jaundice. Specific tests (e.g. α-fetoprotein) or serological tests (e.g. antinuclear antibody) may be ordered for suspected hepatocellular carcinoma or immune-mediated disease, respectively.

Ascitic fluid analysis

Abdominal paracentesis is the most important means of diagnosing the cause of ascites formation. It is appropriate to sample ascitic fluid in all patients with new-onset ascites, as well as in all those admitted to hospital with ascites, because there is a 10–27% prevalence of ascitic fluid infection in the latter group. Paracentesis is performed in an area of dullness either in the midline between the umbilicus and symphysis pubis, because this area is avascular, or in one of the lower quadrants. Needles should not be inserted close to abdominal wall scars with either approach because of the risk for bowel perforation; puncture sites too near the liver or spleen should be avoided as well. In 3% of cases, ultrasound guidance may be needed. The needle is inserted using a Z-track insertion technique to minimize postprocedure leakage, and 25 ml or more of ascitic fluid is removed for analysis.

Analysis of ascitic fluid should begin with gross inspection. Most ascitic fluid from portal hypertension is yellow and clear. Cloudiness raises the possibility of infectious processes, whereas a milky appearance is seen with chylous ascites. A minimum density of 10,000 erythrocytes per μl is required to provide a red tint to the fluid, which raises the possibility of malignancy if the paracentesis is atraumatic. Pancreatic ascitic fluid is tea colored or black. The ascitic fluid cell count is the most useful test. The upper limit of the neutrophil cell count is 250 cells/μl, even in patients who have undergone diuresis. If paracentesis is traumatic, only one neutrophil per 250 erythrocytes and one lymphocyte per 750 erythrocytes can be attributed to blood contamination. With spontaneous bacterial peritonitis (SBP), the neutrophil count exceeds 250 cells/μl and represents more than 50% of the total white cell count in the ascitic fluid. Chylous ascites may produce increases in ascitic lymphocyte counts. If infection is suspected, ascitic fluid should be inoculated into blood culture bottles at the bedside and sent for bacterial culture. Gram stain is insensitive for detecting bacterial infection, and results should not be considered reliable if negative because 10,000 organisms per milliliter are needed for a positive Gram stain, whereas spontaneous peritonitis may occur with only one organism per milliliter. Similarly, the direct smear has only 0–2% sensitivity for detecting tuberculosis. Ascites fluid culture for tuberculosis is only 40% sensitive, and the sensitivity of peritoneal biopsy is

64–83%. If tuberculosis is strongly suspected, laparoscopic rather than blind biopsy of the peritoneum is indicated, because it requires direct visualization of the peritoneal surface with a laparoscope and is almost 100% sensitive. Certain infections can reduce ascitic fluid glucose levels (usually related to perforation of the gastrointestinal tract), but because glucose concentrations usually are normal with SBP, this measure has limited utility. Similarly, the yield of testing of ascitic fluid pH and lactate levels is low.

The SAAG provides important information about the cause of ascites (Table 13.2). Calculating the gradient involves subtracting the albumin concentration in the ascitic fluid from the serum value. A patient can be diagnosed with portal hypertension with 97% accuracy if the serum albumin minus ascitic albumin concentration is 1.1 g/dl or higher. Causes of high-gradient ascites include cirrhosis, alcoholic hepatitis, cardiac ascites, massive liver metastases, Budd–Chiari syndrome, portal vein thrombosis, veno-occlusive disease, acute

Table 13.2 Etiology of ascites and classification by SAAG and ascites protein level

	SAAG	Ascites protein
Main etiological factors of ascites		
Cirrhosis or alcoholic hepatitis	High	Low
Congestive heart failure	High	High
Peritoneal malignancy	Low	High
Peritoneal tuberculosis	Low	High
Other etiologies of cirrhosis (account for <2% of all cases)		
Massive hepatic metastases	High	Low
Nodular regenerative hyperplasia	High	Low
Fulminant liver failure	High	Low?
Budd–Chiari syndrome (late)	High	Low
Budd–Chiari syndrome (early)	High	Low
Constrictive pericarditis	High	High
Veno-occlusive disease	High	High
Myxedema	High	High
Nephrogenous (dialysis) ascites	High	High
Mixed ascites (cirrhosis + peritoneal malignancy)	High	Variable
Pancreatic ascites	Low	High
Serositis (connective tissue disease)	Low	High
Chlamydial/gonococcal	Low	High
Biliary	Low	High?
Ovarian hyperstimulation syndrome	Low?	High
Nephrotic syndrome	Low	Low

Those assessments followed by a question mark are theoretical and have not been confirmed by data in the literature.

Source: Yamada et al. 2008.

fatty liver of pregnancy, myxedema, and some mixed ascites. Conversely, a gradient less than 1.1 g/dl signifies ascites that is not caused by portal hypertension. Low-albumin gradient ascites may result from peritoneal carcinomatosis, tuberculosis, pancreatic or biliary disease, nephrotic syndrome, or connective tissue disease. Previous means of assessing the cause included measuring total ascitic fluid protein and ascitic fluid-to-serum lactate dehydrogenase ratios. Although sometimes still used to distinguish "exudative" from "transudative," the accuracy of these measures is only 55–60%.

Detecting malignancy in ascitic fluid can be a diagnostic challenge. Although nearly 100% of patients with peritoneal carcinomatosis have positive results on cytological analysis of the peritoneal fluid, patients with liver metastases, lymphoma, and hepatocellular carcinoma usually have negative cytological results. Peritoneal biopsy is rarely needed for peritoneal carcinomatosis. The value of ascitic fluid levels of carcinoembryonic antigen and humoral tests of malignancy in detecting malignant ascites is undefined. Other ascitic fluid tests may be ordered, depending on the clinical scenario. In uncomplicated cirrhotic ascites, the ascitic fluid amylase level is low, with an ascitic fluid-to-serum ratio of 0.4. With pancreatic ascites, the levels may exceed 2000 IU/l and amylase ratios may increase to six. With milky ascitic fluid, a triglyceride level is obtained. Chylous ascites triglyceride levels exceed 200 mg/dl versus 20 mg/dl in cirrhotic ascites. Brown ascitic fluid and a bilirubin level higher in the ascitic fluid than in the serum suggest a biliary or bowel perforation.

Management

Initial management of ascites involves diagnostic evaluation to confirm the etiology. Sampling and analysis of the ascitic fluid for cell count, total protein, albumin, and cytology can lead to the appropriate diagnosis (Table 13.3). Subsequent testing and management hinges on initial fluid results (Figure 13.2).

Ascites unrelated to portal hypertension

In patients with peritoneal carcinomatosis, peripheral edema responds to diuretic administration, but the ascites does not. The mainstay for treating these patients is periodic therapeutic paracentesis. Peritoneovenous shunts may be used in selected cases, but in most instances, the short life expectancy does not warrant this aggressive intervention. Nephrotic ascites will respond to sodium restriction and diuretics. Tuberculous peritonitis requires specific antituberculosis agents. Pancreatic ascites may resolve spontaneously, respond to octreotide therapy, or require endoscopic stenting or surgery if a ductal leak is present. Postoperative lymphatic leaks may require surgical intervention or peritoneovenous shunting. Nephrogenous ascites may respond to vigorous dialysis.

Table 13.3 Tests performed in diagnostic paracentesis

Routine analysis of ascitic fluid
Gross appearance
Total protein
Albumin (with simultaneous estimation of serum albumin) so that the ascites–serum albumin gradient can be calculated by subtracting the ascetic fluid value from the serum value
White blood cell count and differential
Bacteriological cultures
Focused analysis of ascetic fluid
Cytology (to exclude malignant ascites)
Amylase (if pancreatic ascites is suspected)
Acid-fast bacilli smear, culture, and adenosine deaminase determination (if peritoneal tuberculosis is suspected)
Glucose and lactic dehydrogenase (if secondary peritonitis is suspected in a patient with ascites PMN >250/mm^3)
Triglycerides (if the fluid has a milky appearance, i.e. chylous ascites)
Red blood cell count (if the fluid is bloody)

PMN, polymorphonuclear leukocytes.
Source: Yamada et al. 2009

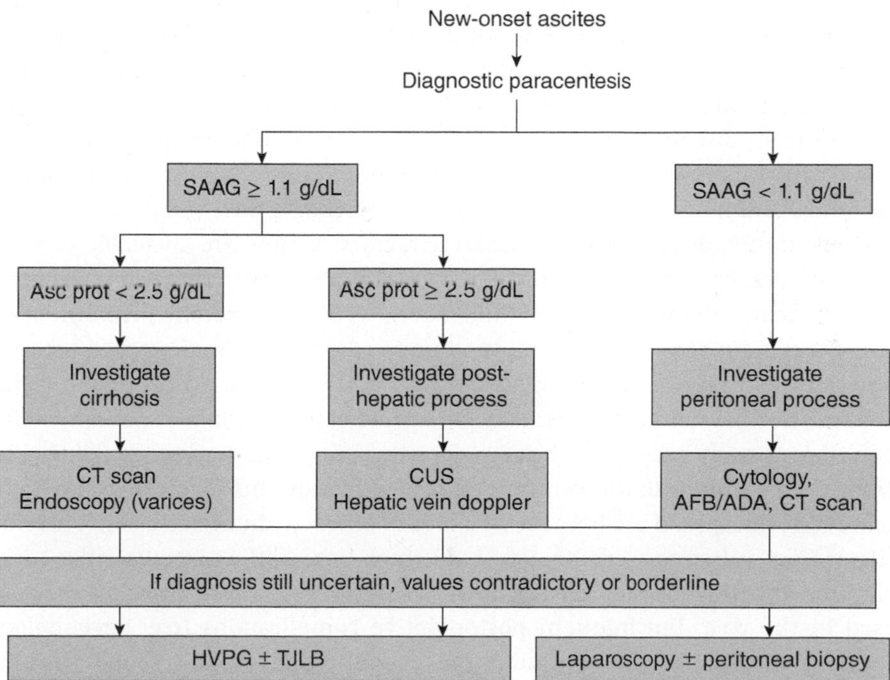

Figure 13.2 Approach to the patient with new-onset ascites. ADA, adenosine deaminase; AFB, acid-fast bacilli; Asc prot, ascites total protein levels; CT, computed tomography; CUS, cardiac echosonography; HVPG, hepatic venous pressure gradient; SAAG, serum-ascites albumin gradient; TJLB, transjugular liver biopsy.

Ascites related to portal hypertension

For patients with ascites secondary to portal hypertension, restricting dietary sodium to a daily intake of 2 g is essential. Fluids do not need to be restricted unless the serum sodium is less than 120 mEq/l. If single-agent diuretic therapy is planned, a daily dose of 100 mg spironolactone is the best choice. For patients who experience spironolactone side effects (e.g. painful gynecomastia), 10 mg/d of amiloride may be given. The physician should expect a slow response to spironolactone because of its long half-life; weight loss may not be evident for two weeks. It is often reasonable to add a loop diuretic (e.g. furosemide) at 40 mg/d to maximize natriuresis. Doses may be increased slowly to maxima of 400 mg/d of spironolactone and 160 mg/d of furosemide. If diuresis is still suboptimal, metolazone or hydrochlorothiazide may be added, although the hyponatremic and hypovolemic effects of such triple-drug regimens mandate close physician follow-up, often on an inpatient basis.

There should be no limit to the amount of weight that can be diuresed daily if pedal edema is present. Once the dependent edema has resolved, diuretics should be adjusted to achieve a daily weight loss of 0.5 kg. Urine sodium levels may be used to direct diuretic therapy. Patients with urine sodium excretion less than potassium excretion are likely to require higher diuretic doses. If urine sodium excretion exceeds potassium excretion, the total daily sodium excretion is likely to be adequate (i.e. >78 mmol/d) in 95% of circumstances. Development of encephalopathy, a serum sodium level less than 120 mEq/l that does not respond to fluid restriction, or serum creatinine higher than 2 mg/dl are relative indicators for discontinuing diuretic therapy. Because concurrent use of nonsteroidal anti-inflammatory drugs promotes renal failure, inhibits the efficacy of diuretics, and may cause gastrointestinal hemorrhage, their use is discouraged. Various nonmedical means to treat refractory ascites are available. Large-volume paracentesis, with removal of 5 l of fluid, can be performed in 20 minutes. If greater than 5 l of ascites fluid is removed, it is generally recommended that the patient receive intravenous albumin (8 g/l ascites removed) to prevent paracentesis-induced changes in electrolytes and creatinine. Transjugular intrahepatic portosystemic shunts (TIPSs) are effective in many patients with diuretic-resistant ascites. Peritoneovenous shunts (e.g. Denver and LeVeen) drain ascitic fluid into the central venous circulation; however, they have not achieved widespread use because of a lack of efficacy, shunt occlusion, and side effects (e.g. pulmonary edema, variceal hemorrhage, diffuse intravascular coagulation, and thromboembolism). Surgical portocaval shunt procedures were used in the past, but frequent postoperative complications (e.g. encephalopathy) have tempered enthusiasm for the techniques. Liver transplantation cures both refractory ascites and underlying cirrhosis and should be considered for patients without contraindications. The management of ascites in cirrhosis is outlined in Figure 13.3.

First-Line
- Cessation of alcohol use, when present
- Sodium-restricted diet and diet education
- Dual diuretics, usually spironolactone and furosemide, orally with single daily dosing
- Discontinue nonsteroidal anti-inflammatory drugs
- Evaluation for liver transplantation

Second-Line
- Discontinue beta blockers, angiotensin-converting enzyme inhibitors, and angiotensin receptor blockers
- Consider adding midodrine especially in the profoundly hypotensive patient
- Serial therapeutic paracenteses
- Evaluation for liver transplantation
- TIPS

Third-Line
- Peritoneovenous shunt

Figure 13.3 Treatment options for patients with cirrhosis and ascites. TIPS, transjugular intrahepatic portosystemic shunt. (Source: Runyon 2013.)

Complications

Infection

SBP is defined as ascitic fluid infection with pure growth of a single organism and an ascitic fluid neutrophil count higher than 250 cells/μl without evidence of a surgically remediable intra-abdominal cause. SBP occurs only in the setting of liver disease, for all practical purposes, although it has been reported with nephrotic syndrome. Ascites is a prerequisite for SBP, but it may not be detectable on physical examination. Infection usually occurs with maximal fluid accumulation. *Escherichia coli, Klebsiella pneumoniae,* and Pneumococcus organisms are the most common isolates in SBP; anaerobes are the causative organism in 1% of cases. Approximately 85% percent of patients with SBP present with symptoms, most commonly fever, abdominal pain, and changes in mental status, although the clinical manifestations may be subtle.

Antibiotics should be initiated when an ascitic fluid neutrophil count higher than 250 cells/μl is documented before obtaining formal culture results. The most accepted antibiotic for SBP is cefotaxime, the third-generation cephalosporin to which 98% of offending bacteria are sensitive, though ceftriaxone, amoxicillin-clavulanic acid, and fluoroquinolones have been used in trials with seemingly equivalent results. When susceptibility testing is available, a drug with a narrower spectrum may be substituted. A randomized trial comparing 5–10 days of therapy showed no difference, supporting a shorter antibiotic course. The treatment course generally is five to seven days. A repeat paracentesis that demonstrates a reduction in neutrophil counts 48 hours after initiating antibiotic treatment indicates that the antibiotic choice was appropriate. If the correct antibiotics are given in a timely manner, the mortality rate of SBP should not exceed 5%; however, many patients succumb to other complications of the underlying liver disease. Renal function is a major cause of death in patients with SBP. It is therefore recommended to give intravenous albumin (1.5 g/kg on day 1, 1 g/kg on day 3), which is of greatest benefit in patients with a bilirubin >4 and creatinine >1. Oral quinolones and trimethoprim-sulfamethoxazole are given as prophylactic agents after an initial episode of SBP because of a reported one-year recurrence rate of 69% in the absence of prophylaxis.

SBP is not the only infectious complication of ascites. Monomicrobial bacter-ascites is defined as the presence of a positive result from ascitic fluid culture of a single organism with a concurrent fluid neutrophil count lower than 250 cells/μl. One series of patients with bacterascites demonstrated a predominance of Gram-positive organisms, whereas another showed flora similar to SBP. Because of the high mortality rate of untreated bacterascites (22–43%), antibiotic treatment is warranted for many patients. Alternatively, paracentesis may be repeated for cell count and culture. Culture-negative neutrocytic ascites is defined as ascitic fluid with a neutrophil count higher than or equal to 250 cells/μl with negative fluid culture results in patients who have received no prior antibiotics. Spontaneously resolving SBP is the likely explanation of culture-negative neutrocytic ascites; however, empirical antibiotics generally are given. A decline in ascitic neutrophil counts on repeat paracentesis indicates an appropriate response to therapy.

If there is no response to antibiotics, cytological analysis and culture of the ascitic fluid for tuberculosis may be indicated. Secondary bacterial peritonitis manifests as a polymicrobial infection with a very high ascitic fluid neutrophil count from an identified intra-abdominal source such as appendicitis, diverticulitis, or intra-abdominal abscess. In contrast to SBP, secondary peritonitis usually requires surgical intervention. Gut perforation is suspected with two of the following three criteria: ascitic protein concentration higher than 1 g/dl, glucose level lower than 50 mg/dl, and lactate dehydrogenase level higher than 225 mU/ml. In patients with secondary peritonitis but no perforation, repeat paracentesis 48 hours after initiating antibiotic treatment will usually demonstrate increasing neutrophil counts. Polymicrobial bacterascites with an ascitic neutrophil count less than or equal to 250 cells/μl is suggestive of inadvertent gut perforation by the paracentesis needle. It is usually treated with broad-spectrum antibiotics that include coverage for anaerobes. Alternatively, the decision to treat may be deferred until the results of a repeat paracentesis are obtained.

Abdominal wall hernias

Umbilical and inguinal hernias are common in patients with ascites. These hernias may produce skin ulceration or rupture (flood syndrome), or they may become incarcerated. More than half of these patients will need surgery. If the patient is a candidate for liver transplantation, hernia repair should be delayed until the time of transplant. A more aggressive surgical approach is needed for ulceration, rupture, or incarceration because of the risk for systemic infection, but surgery should be performed after preoperative paracentesis or TIPS to control the ascites. The mortality of rupture is significant (11–43%), and it increases in patients with jaundice or coagulopathy.

Hepatic hydrothorax

Pleural effusions (usually right-sided) are prevalent in patients with cirrhotic ascites. Left-sided effusions are more common with tuberculosis or pancreatic disease. Hepatic hydrothorax is postulated to result from a defect in the diaphragm, which preferentially permits fluid passage into the thorax when negative pressure is generated by normal inspiration. Infection of this fluid is unusual, except in a patient with concurrent SBP. Treatment of hepatic hydrothorax is often challenging because it often does not respond to diuretics. TIPS placement is often successful, whereas pleurodesis and peritoneovenous shunts often lead to complications.

Hepatorenal syndrome

Hepatorenal syndrome is the final stage of functional renal impairment in patients with cirrhosis and portal hypertension; it occurs almost exclusively in patients with refractory ascites. It is characterized by peripheral vasodilation and a creatinine clearance less than 40 ml/min (or serum creatinine level higher than 1.5 mg/dl) with normal intravascular volume and the absence of intrinsic renal disease or other renal insults. Urine sodium content is typically less than 10 mmol/l. Treatment initially involves withdrawing diuretics and nephrotoxins, followed by infusing saline and/or albumin. Vasoactive agents, octreotide, midodrine, and vasopressin, as well as TIPS, have been used with encouraging results in largely uncontrolled studies. Liver transplantation is the only definitive cure and should be undertaken for all appropriate candidates.

Further reading

Runyon, B.A. (2013). Introduction to the revised American Association for the Study of Liver Diseases practice guideline management of adult patients with ascites due to cirrhosis 2012. *Hepatology* 57: 1651–1653.

Yamada, T., Alpers, D.H., Kalloo, A.N. et al. (eds.) (2008). *Principles of Clinical Gastroenterology*, 443 and 445. Oxford: Wiley.

Yamada, T., Alpers, D.H., Kalloo, A.N. et al. (eds.) (2009). *Textbook of Gastroenterology*, 5e, 2305. Oxford: Blackwell.

CHAPTER 14
The Patient Requiring Nutritional Support

Most people can ingest the necessary fluids, nutrients, vitamins, and minerals to maintain health. However, certain patients cannot satisfy their nutritional requirements with oral intake alone because of disease or surgical procedures. It is possible to supplement or provide the complete fluid and nutrition needs of these patients with enteral or intravenous solutions. In healthy adults, 30–35 ml of fluid is required for each kilogram of body weight. An additional 360 ml/day is required for each degree centigrade of fever. In anabolic conditions, 300–400 ml more water is needed. Fluids may need to be restricted with volume overload or hyponatremia. Electrolyte requirements are affected by renal and gastrointestinal disease. Potassium and phosphate supplementation is required for diarrhea or vomiting and to compensate for intracellular shifts during intravenous nutrition. Sodium is restricted for heart failure, renal disease, and portal hypertension, whereas potassium, phosphate, and magnesium are reduced with renal failure. Levels of magnesium, iron, copper, selenium, and zinc should be monitored and supplemented as indicated.

Healthy adults require 20–25 kcal/kg of body weight to satisfy daily caloric requirements. With the stress of disease or surgery, this need increases to 30–40 kcal/kg/day. For nonstressed patients, the recommended dietary protein allowance is 0.8 g/kg daily. This increases to 1.5–2.0 g/kg daily for catabolic patients. There are nine amino acids that cannot be synthesized by human tissues and must be part of any protein-calorie supplement. Sufficient carbohydrates and fats must be provided to ensure that oral or intravenous proteins or amino acids are used for protein synthesis and not for energy from gluconeogenesis. For patients requiring long-term nutritional support, multivitamin supplementation may be necessary to prevent deficiency syndromes.

Yamada's Handbook of Gastroenterology, Fourth Edition. John M. Inadomi, Renuka Bhattacharya, Joo Ha Hwang, and Cynthia Ko.

Clinical presentation

History and physical examination

Patients with conditions such as Crohn's disease or pancreatitis exhibit historical features and physical findings characteristic of the illnesses. Persons with protein-calorie malnutrition have weight loss and clinical evidence of deficiencies of essential nutrients, vitamins, and minerals. Loss of greater than 15% of body weight usually indicates significant malnutrition. Development of dependent edema may cause the clinician to underestimate the amount of muscle mass lost. Affected patients may report fatigue resulting from anemia, neuropathy secondary to vitamin B_{12} deficiency, impaired night vision with vitamin A deficiency, or easy bruising resulting from decreased vitamin K levels. The physical examination may detect muscle wasting and edema as well as signs specific for nutritional deficiencies. Pallor indicates anemia, whereas cheilosis and stomatitis are observed with B vitamin deficiencies.

Additional testing

Laboratory tests are important in assessing nutritional status and also are used during nutritional replenishment to test for the adequacy of supplementation and for complications of nutritional support. Low albumin, prealbumin, and transferrin levels are observed with malnutrition. Electrolyte abnormalities such as hypokalemia and alkalosis are consequences of chronic vomiting or diarrhea, whereas prerenal azotemia or renal failure may result from chronic fluid loss. Electrolytes (including magnesium, calcium, and phosphate), renal function, and albumin are monitored during enteral or parenteral supplementation. Because many regimens produce hyperglycemia or liver injury, serum glucose levels and liver chemistries are monitored during nutritional support.

Management

Implementation of nutritional support

The goal of nutritional support is to decrease morbidity and mortality by providing nutrients or modifying nutrient metabolism. A calorie count by the dietary staff may provide an assessment of nutrient intake. Allowance must be made for fecal losses in patients with malabsorption. Next, nutrient expenditure must be determined. The resting energy expenditure may double in highly catabolic conditions (e.g. burns). Finally, the degree of protein and calorie malnutrition is estimated using objective variables, including serum albumin, creatinine height index, serum transferrin, total circulating lymphocyte counts, delayed cutaneous hypersensitivity skin testing, serum transthyretin, body mass index, and skinfold thickness. However, none of these measures is reliable by itself, and there is no gold standard for determining nutritional status. Scales based on weight, dietary intake, symptoms, and functional capacity have been devised to correlate nutritional status with clinical outcome after surgery.

General rules of nutritional supplementation have been proposed. For patients who are not eating, enteral feeding is provided within 7–10 days for well-nourished, noncatabolic patients; in 1–5 days for catabolic or malnourished patients; and in 1–2 days for catabolic and malnourished patients. If parenteral nutrition is required, this should be initiated in 14–21 days, 1–10 days, and 1–7 days for each category of patients, respectively.

When initiating a nutritional program, energy and protein goals must be set. For patients who are not critically ill, optimal calorie support is obtained if energy equal to 100–120% of the total daily energy expenditure is received. A crude calculation of the energy goal for a given patient is to estimate the basal energy expenditure (20 kcal/kg/day) and multiply by a stress factor for the severity of illness, which ranges from 1.0 for mild disease to 2.0 for severe burns. An additional 0–20% of the basal energy expenditure is added for activity level, and if weight gain is desired, an additional 500–1000 kcal/day is included. A positive nitrogen balance is desired to incorporate amino acids into new protein. To achieve this goal, ingesting 25–35 kcal/g of protein is required. Individuals with renal or liver failure may require less protein, whereas highly catabolic patients, such as those with burns, may require more.

Oral rehydration therapy

Prolonged vomiting or diarrhea can result in loss of excessive amounts of fluid and electrolytes. Oral rehydration therapy enhances sodium and water absorption by stimulating intestinal sodium/glucose cotransport. Various solutions are currently available and include a glucose component (70–150 mmol/l) with variable concentrations of sodium and other electrolytes. In some severe diarrheal conditions, making the solution hypotonic by replacing the glucose with rice solids or other polymeric forms can decrease stool output. In a patient with short bowel syndrome, sodium concentrations greater than 90 mEq/l produce a net sodium and fluid balance.

Enteral nutrition

Enteral nutrition may be administered by several routes. Oral supplementation can be provided by increasing meal portions, adding high-calorie foods, or giving commercial nutritional supplements. Whole foods may include a standard diet or diets modified in consistency (liquid, pureed, or soft) or content (low residue, low fat, low sodium, low protein, high fiber). Nasogastric or nasoenteric formulas may be provided for patients who require short-term nutritional support (<6 weeks) and who cannot eat.

If nutritional support is required for more than four weeks, a gastrostomy or jejunostomy is indicated and may be placed endoscopically, radiographically, or surgically. Gastrostomy feedings generally are delivered in bolus fashion four to six times daily, although they may be given continuously if there is esophageal reflux of feedings or if gastric emptying is delayed. Jejunostomy feedings are indicated for patients undergoing gastric surgery, who have duodenal obstruction, or in whom pulmonary aspiration is a significant risk. Jejunostomy feedings require continuous infusion to prevent diarrhea and abdominal pain and to ensure adequate nutrient absorption.

Standard formulas are appropriate for most patients, although high-protein formulas may be needed for those with extensive trauma or healing wounds. Formulas containing fiber can be given if diarrhea is a problem. Disease-specific preparations are available for patients with renal, hepatic, or pulmonary disease. Renal formulas are low in protein, high in essential amino acids, and low in electrolytes, whereas hepatic formulas are low in sodium, low in aromatic amino acids, and high in branched-chain amino acids. Pulmonary preparations are high in fat and low in carbohydrates because metabolism of carbohydrate generates carbon dioxide. Elemental formulas contain nitrogen as free amino acids and have very little fat. Such preparations are best for those with pancreatic insufficiency or for individuals who require an extremely low-fat diet.

Parenteral nutrition

Intravenous nutritional supplementation is provided by a peripheral (peripheral parenteral nutrition [PPN]) or central (total parenteral nutrition [TPN]) vein. PPN is reserved for patients whose nutritional status is nearly normal and in whom the goal of nutritional supplementation is to maintain lean body mass for a relatively short period of time. Such patients include those undergoing elective surgery who will not be given oral nutrition for three to seven days. PPN also benefits inpatients who ingest inadequate nutrients or calories, by preventing a negative nitrogen balance during their hospitalization. The limiting factor for PPN is phlebitis induced by hypertonic solutions. Successful PPN mandates solutions with osmolarity less than 900 mOsm and glucose concentrations less than 10%. To meet the nutritional needs of most patients, combinations of hypertonic glucose, amino acids, and lipid emulsions are given with vitamins, minerals, and trace elements. These solutions provide the best nutritional support, if half of the caloric needs are met by the lipid infusion.

For patients who require long-term intravenous nutritional support (>10 days), TPN is preferred. TPN requires the central venous placement of a large-bore catheter, which permits rapid dilution of the hypertonic TPN formulation to prevent phlebitis or hemolysis. Temporary central venous access may be provided by peripherally inserted central catheter (PICC) lines or catheters aseptically placed into the subclavian or internal jugular veins. In patients who need TPN beyond their inpatient stay, permanent catheters (e.g. Hickman, Broviac) are surgically or radiographically placed for home TPN administration. TPN solutions are tailored to the specific needs of the patient. Standard TPN formulations provide 510–1020 kcal/l depending on the glucose concentration. Emulsified lipids are given two to three times weekly to prevent essential fatty acid deficiency in patients requiring TPN for more than one week. Commercially available multiple vitamin supplements are included that contain all the water-soluble and fat-soluble vitamins except vitamin K, which must be given separately.

Mineral and trace elements usually are included in standard TPN solutions but also may be given as additives. Iodine may be included if TPN is to be given long term. Iron is not routinely included because it is incompatible with the lipid emulsion. Medications including acid-suppressive agents can be included in TPN formulations, as clinically indicated. Patients with renal disease can receive TPN formulations rich in essential amino acids and with few or no nonessential amino acids to minimize the nitrogen load. Formulas for hepatic encephalopathy are high in branched-chain amino acids (leucine, isovaline, valine), which are oxidized outside the liver and block hepatic and muscle protein breakdown.

TPN has been beneficial in several clinical settings. The most unequivocal indication for home TPN is intestinal failure from any cause. TPN is also the primary therapeutic modality that leads to closure of enterocutaneous fistulae in 30–50% of patients. If spontaneous closure does not occur after 30–60 days, continuation of TPN is unlikely to be successful. TPN is commonly used in managing inflammatory bowel disease, although bowel rest with TPN does not represent primary therapy, nor does it decrease the need for surgery in patients with colitis. TPN corrects disease-associated vitamin, mineral, and nutrient deficiencies in severe Crohn's ileitis. It is indicated for patients with complicated acute pancreatitis, if enteral feeding exacerbates abdominal pain or if ascites, fistulae, or pseudocysts are present. Lipid emulsions are given cautiously and should be reduced if serum triglyceride levels exceed 400 mg/dl.

Differential diagnosis

Causes of nutrient deficiency

A variety of clinical conditions mandate nutritional support (Table 14.1). Many patients have diminished nutritional intake as a consequence of oral and upper gastrointestinal problems such as poorly fitting dentures, esophagitis, ulcer disease, or neoplasm of the head and neck. Medications can induce dyspepsia or suppress appetite. Similarly, anorexia is common in depression. Neurological disease, as with a stroke, can produce dysphagia or aspiration that prevents adequate oral intake. Volitional food consumption is impossible with obtundation from any cause. Decreased intake is most likely to affect nutrients that have small body stores, such as folate, water-soluble vitamins, and protein. All of these patient subsets exhibit normal gut absorptive function and can be supplemented with oral or enteral formulas.

Other clinical conditions without impairment of food intake are associated with nutrient deficiencies. Malabsorptive conditions may produce profound

Table 14.1 Physical signs of deficiencies of specific nutrients

Hair
Thin, sparse (protein, zinc, biotin)
Flag sign (transverse pigmentation) (protein, copper)
Easy pluckability (protein)

Nails
Spoon-shaped (i.e. koilonychia) (iron)
No luster, transverse ridging (protein, energy)

Skin
Dry, scaling (i.e. xerosis) (vitamin A, zinc)
Seborrheic dermatitis (essential fatty acids, zinc, pyridoxine, biotin)
Flaky paint dermatosis (protein)
Follicular hyperkeratosis (vitamin A, vitamin C, essential fatty acids)
Nasolabial seborrhea (niacin, pyridoxine, riboflavin)
Petechiae, purpura (vitamins C, K, A)
Pigmentation, desquamation (niacin)
Pallor (folate, iron, cobalamin, copper, biotin)

Eyes
Angular palpebritis (riboflavin)
Blepharitis (B vitamins)
Corneal vascularization (riboflavin)
Dull, dry conjunctiva (vitamin A)
Bitot spot (vitamin A)
Keratomalacia (vitamin A)
Fundal capillary microaneurysms (vitamin C)
Ophthalmoplegia (Wernicke encephalopathy) (thiamine)

Mouth
Angular stomatitis (B vitamins, iron, protein)
Cheilosis (riboflavin, niacin, pyridoxine, protein)
Atrophic lingual papillae (niacin, iron, riboflavin, folate, cobalamin)
Glossitis (niacin, pyridoxine, riboflavin, folate, cobalamin)
Decreased taste and smell (vitamin A, zinc)
Swollen, bleeding gums (vitamin C)

Glands
Parotid enlargement (protein)
Sicca syndrome (vitamin C)
Thyroid enlargement (iodine)

Heart
Enlargement, tachycardia, high-output failure (i.e. beriberi) (thiamine)
Small heart, decreased output (protein, energy)
Cardiomyopathy (selenium)
Cardiac arrhythmias (magnesium, potassium)

Extremities
Edema (protein, thiamine)
Muscle weakness (protein, energy, selenium)
Bone and joint tenderness (vitamins C, A)
Osteopenia, bone pain (vitamin D, calcium, phosphorus, vitamin C)

(*continued*)

Table 14.1 *(cont'd)*

Neurological
Confabulation, disorientation (i.e. Korsakoff psychosis) (thiamine)
Decreased position and vibration sense, ataxia (cobalamin, thiamine)
Decreased tendon reflexes (thiamine)
Weakness, paresthesias (cobalamin, pyridoxine, thiamine)
Mental disorders (cobalamin, niacin, thiamine, magnesium)
Other
Delayed wound healing (vitamin C, protein, zinc, essential fatty acids)
Hypogonadism, delayed puberty (zinc)
Glucose intolerance (chromium)

nutrient deficiency, especially those that impair the effective small intestinal mucosal absorptive surface area (e.g. celiac disease, short bowel syndrome, Whipple disease). Affected patients also lose endogenous stores of minerals, vitamins, and proteins that are not reabsorbed from gastric, pancreaticobiliary, and small intestinal secretions. When steatorrhea is present, divalent cations (calcium, magnesium, zinc) are lost because they combine with unabsorbed fatty acids to form nonabsorbable soaps.

Drugs may induce malabsorption by several mechanisms. Cholestyramine binds fats and fat-soluble vitamins, whereas neomycin precipitates bile salts. Sulfasalazine inhibits folate absorption and colchicine inhibits enterocyte release of fat-soluble vitamins. In addition to suppressing appetite, chronic ingestion of large amounts of ethanol is toxic to intestinal enterocytes, causing decreased transport of glucose, amino acids, folate, and thiamine.

Protein-calorie malnutrition occurs in conditions with increased catabolism, such as Crohn's disease or high-dose corticosteroid use. Likewise, increased caloric and fluid needs are observed with pregnancy, lactation, sepsis, trauma, and burns. Additional deficiencies in Crohn's disease include those of calcium, vitamin D, iron, vitamin B_{12}, zinc, and potassium. Other causes of intestinal failure that result in malabsorption include radiation enteritis, intestinal pseudo-obstruction with bacterial overgrowth, chronic adhesive peritonitis, and mucosal diseases without effective treatment (collagenous sprue). Advanced liver disease may alter the plasma amino acid profile. Increased fluid and electrolyte losses occur in the absence of malabsorption in patients with diarrhea, vomiting, enterocutaneous fistulae, gastric suctioning, and renal wasting.

Mineral deficiency states

Major mineral deficiencies elicit a range of clinical manifestations. Sodium deficiency results from increased losses caused by vomiting, diarrhea, diuresis, salt-wasting renal disease, fistulae, or adrenal insufficiency. Among hospitalized patients, hyponatremia commonly results from excess free water caused by cardiac, renal, or hepatic insufficiency. Severe sodium depletion with dehydration produces nausea and vomiting, exhaustion, cramps, seizures, and cardiorespiratory collapse.

Pseudohyponatremia results from excess lipid, glucose, blood urea nitrogen, mannitol, or glycerin in the serum. Potassium depletion results from gastrointestinal or urinary losses (diuretics, alkalosis, mineralocorticoid excess, renal tubular acidosis). Hypokalemia also results from potassium shifts from the extracellular to the intracellular compartment during alkalosis or after insulin or glucose administration or periodic paralysis. Symptoms of potassium depletion include confusion, lethargy, weakness, cramps, myalgias, cardiac arrhythmias, glucose intolerance, nausea, vomiting, diarrhea, ileus, and gastroparesis. Hypocalcemia is caused by vitamin D deficiency, failed vitamin D synthesis or action, hypoparathyroidism, hypomagnesemia, acute pancreatitis, osteoblastic malignancies, malabsorption, and medications (e.g. aminoglycosides, cisplatin, calcitonin, furosemide, phosphates, and anticonvulsants). Manifestations of hypocalcemia include a positive Chvostek or Trousseau sign, tetany, hyperreflexia, paresthesias, seizures, mental status changes, increased intracranial pressure, bradycardia, heart block, and choreoathetotic movements. Chronic calcium deficiency causes rickets in children and osteomalacia in adults. Eighty to 85% of phosphorus stores are in bone.

Hypophosphatemia occurs in 2–3% of hospitalized patients because of decreased intestinal absorption (antacids, malabsorption, vitamin D deficiency, hypoparathyroidism), increased renal excretion (proximal tubule disease, alkalosis, diuretics, hyperparathyroidism, burns, corticosteroids), and intracellular shifts (respiratory alkalosis, carbohydrate administration). Severe hypophosphatemia produces hemolysis, encephalopathy, seizures, paresthesias, muscle weakness, rhabdomyolysis, decreased glucose utilization, and reduced oxygen delivery. Similarly, 70% of magnesium stores are in bone. Magnesium absorption decreases in malabsorption syndromes. Excessive urinary loss results from hypercalcemia, volume expansion, tubular dysfunction, alcoholism, diabetes, hyperparathyroidism, hypophosphatemia, and medications (e.g. diuretics, aminoglycosides, cyclosporine, amphotericin, cisplatin, digoxin). Shifts into the intracellular space result from refeeding, treating diabetic ketoacidosis, pancreatitis, and correcting acidosis in renal failure. Patients with hypomagnesemia present with tremors, myoclonic jerks, ataxia, tetany, psychiatric disturbances, coma, ventricular arrhythmias, hypotension, or cardiac arrest.

Trace mineral deficiencies also are prevalent. Iron deficiency results from gastrointestinal bleeding, excessive menstrual loss, and malabsorption (e.g. celiac sprue, achlorhydria). Clinical manifestations of iron deficiency stem from anemia and include weakness, light-headedness, decreased exercise tolerance, and tachycardia. Zinc deficiency results from malabsorption, cirrhosis, alcoholism, nephrotic syndrome, sickle cell anemia, pregnancy, pica, pancreatic insufficiency, use of penicillamine, and chronic diarrhea of any cause. Clinical manifestations of zinc deficiency include growth retardation, scaling skin, alopecia, diarrhea, apathy, night blindness, poor wound healing, and dysgeusia. Copper deficiency in adults is rare and occurs with parenteral nutrition without copper supplements and during penicillamine therapy. Clinical manifestations of copper deficiency include microcytic anemia, leukopenia, neutropenia, and skeletal abnormalities. Selenium deficiency occurs with small bowel causes of malabsorption, fistulae, alcoholism, cirrhosis, acquired immunodeficiency syndrome, and cancer, and with parenteral nutritional formulas without supplemental selenium. Symptoms of selenium deficiency include myositis, weakness, and cardiomyopathy.

Only 2% of dietary chromium is absorbed. Chromium deficiency occurs with short bowel syndrome and in patients who receive poorly supplemented parenteral nutritional formulas. Clinical manifestations include hyperglycemia, insulin insensitivity, encephalopathy, peripheral neuropathy, and weight loss. Iodine deficiency usually is caused by inadequate intake and results in hypothyroidism, thyroid hyperplasia, and hypertrophy. Iodine supplements are rarely needed in parenteral nutritional solutions, presumably because sufficient iodine is present as a contaminant or is absorbed from the skin.

Vitamin deficiency states

In general, deficiencies of fat-soluble vitamins (A, D, E, and K) take years to develop because large stores are present in adipose tissue. Vitamin D is made endogenously in sun-exposed skin. Vitamins that undergo enterohepatic circulation (e.g. A and D) may be lost in malabsorptive conditions. Blood values for fat-soluble vitamins are difficult to interpret because of adipose stores and plasma-binding proteins. Vitamin A or its carotenoid precursors are present in animal products (e.g. liver, kidney, dairy products, eggs) and in green and yellow vegetables. Vitamin A deficiency results from decreased intake and fat malabsorption, although impaired carotenoid conversion in mucosal disease, inability to store the vitamin in liver disease, and increased urinary losses (e.g. as from tuberculosis, cancer, pneumonia, urinary tract infection) may contribute. Vitamin A deficiency produces night blindness, xerophthalmia, follicular hyperkeratosis, altered taste and smell, increased cerebrospinal fluid pressure, and increased infections.

Vitamin D from fish liver oils, eggs, liver, and dairy products is absorbed by the small intestine. Cholecalciferol (vitamin D_3) is synthesized on ultraviolet exposure of the skin. Vitamin D deficiency results from inadequate exposure to the sun, steatorrhea, severe liver or kidney disease, Crohn's disease, or small bowel resection. Manifestations of deficiency include hypocalcemia, hypophosphatemia, bone demineralization, osteomalacia in adults, rickets in children, and bony fractures. Vitamin E is a fat-soluble antioxidant and a free radical scavenger found in plants and vegetable oils. Deficiency is rare in humans but may occur with malabsorption in aβ-lipoproteinemia, cystic fibrosis, cirrhosis, and malabsorption, and from ingesting excess mineral oil. Vitamin E deficiency elicits hemolysis and a progressive neurological syndrome (areflexia, gait disturbance, decreased vibratory and proprioceptive sensation, and gaze paresis). Vitamin K is abundant in the diet and is synthesized by intestinal bacteria. Deficiency results from malabsorption of fat, diminished liver function or bile secretion, or antibiotic inhibition of bacterial production. Vitamin K deficiency prolongs prothrombin time and increases the risk of hemorrhage.

In contrast to fat-soluble vitamins, water-soluble vitamins are not stored in large quantities in the body. Blood levels of water-soluble vitamins reflect body stores and fall before clinical manifestations of vitamin deficiency develop. Thiamine (vitamin B_1) is readily available in the diet, and deficiency presents in alcoholics or in patients with malabsorption, severe malnutrition, or prolonged fever, or on chronic hemodialysis. Thiamine deficiency causes beriberi, which is characterized by easy fatigability, weakness, paresthesias, and high-output congestive heart failure. Other manifestations include peripheral neuropathy, cerebellar dysfunction, subacute necrotizing encephalomyelopathy, and Wernicke encephalopathy (with mental changes, ataxia, nystagmus, paresis of upward gaze). Thiamine deficiency may also play a role in Korsakoff syndrome. Riboflavin (vitamin B_2) is present in milk, eggs, and leafy green vegetables. Deficiency occurs in conjunction with other B vitamin deficiencies in alcoholism and malabsorption. Riboflavin deficiency produces angular stomatitis, cheilosis, glossitis, seborrhea-like dermatitis, pruritus, photophobia, and visual impairment.

Niacin (vitamin B_3) and its precursor, tryptophan, are found in animal proteins, beans, nuts, whole grains, and enriched breads and cereals. Niacin deficiency occurs rarely as a complication of alcoholism, malabsorption, carcinoid syndrome, or Hartnup disease. Niacin deficiency causes pellagra, which presents with a scaly, hyperpigmented dermatitis localized to sun-exposed surfaces, diarrhea, and central nervous system dysfunction (irritability and headache progressing to psychosis, hallucinations, and seizures). Pyridoxine (vitamin B_6) is present in animal protein and whole-grain cereals. Pyridoxine deficiency most commonly occurs during treatment with pyridoxine antagonists (isoniazid, hydralazine, and penicillamine) but also occurs in alcoholics and malabsorption. Pyridoxine deficiency produces peripheral neuropathy, seborrheic dermatitis, glossitis, angular stomatitis, cheilosis, seizures, and sideroblastic anemia. Folate is abundant in vegetables, legumes, kidney, liver, and nuts. Folate deficiency is caused by poor intake or altered small bowel mucosal function in alcoholics, by malabsorption, and during use of sulfasalazine or anticonvulsants. Folate deficiency elicits macrocytic anemia, thrombocytopenia, leukopenia, glossitis, diarrhea, fatigue, and possibly neurological findings. Cobalamin (vitamin B_{12}) is found in animal tissues. Cobalamin deficiency occurs in some vegetarians and also is caused by pernicious anemia, gastrectomy, ileal disease or resection, or bacterial overgrowth, in which bacteria bind dietary cobalamin so that it cannot be absorbed. Clinical findings of deficiency include macrocytic anemia, anorexia, loss of taste, glossitis, diarrhea, dyspepsia, hair loss, impotence, and neurological disease (i.e. peripheral neuropathy, loss of vibratory sensation, incoordination, muscle weakness and atrophy, irritability, and memory loss).

Ascorbic acid (vitamin C) is present in fruits (especially citrus) and vegetables. Scurvy develops after two to three months of a diet deficient in ascorbic acid. Other causes of deficiency include alcoholism, malabsorption, and Crohn's disease. Vitamin C deficiency produces weakness, irritability, aching joints and muscles, and weight loss, which progress to perifollicular hyperkeratotic papules, petechiae, and swollen, hemorrhagic gums. Biotin deficiency occurs in persons whose diet is high in egg whites, which contain a biotin-binding glycoprotein, and in patients who take hyperalimentation solutions without biotin supplements. Biotin deficiency produces anorexia, nausea, dermatitis, alopecia, mental depression, and organic aciduria.

Essential fatty acid deficiency

Essential fatty acids are long-chain compounds that cannot be synthesized by mammals (i.e. linoleic, linolenic, and arachidonic acids). Because humans synthesize arachidonic acid from exogenous linoleic acid, only linoleic acid (and, to a lesser degree, linolenic) is required in the diet. Vegetable oils are rich dietary sources. Parenteral nutritional lipid emulsions consist of soybean or safflower oil, which are predominantly linoleic acid. Essential fatty acid deficiency, caused by fat-free hyperalimentation, appears within three to six weeks as scaly dermatitis, alopecia, coarse hair, hepatomegaly, thrombocytopenia, diarrhea, and growth retardation.

Protein-calorie malnutrition

From 20 to 60% of inpatients may have protein-calorie malnutrition. Healthy adults die of starvation after 60–90 days if no proteins or calories are provided, which may decrease to 14 days in hypermetabolic conditions. Protein-calorie malnutrition produces weakness, impaired immune responses, skin breakdown, infection, apathy, and irritability. If malnutrition is severe, full recovery of cardiac and skeletal muscle function may not occur.

Complications

Enteral nutrition

The major complications of enteral feedings are pulmonary aspiration, nausea and vomiting, abdominal pain, diarrhea, metabolic abnormalities, and infection (pneumonia, gut infections). Aspiration is rare if feedings are delivered distal to the ligament of Treitz. During gastric feedings, the upper body should be elevated at least 30° above the horizontal. Diarrhea results from excessive infusion rates, concurrent use of antibiotics and antacids, sorbitol-containing elixir, inadequate fiber supplementation, too much lipid with fat malabsorption, hypertonic formulations, vitamin or mineral deficiency, or hypoalbuminemia. If no remediable cause of diarrhea is found, loperamide elixir, diphenoxylate with atropine, or tincture of opium may be given. Complications of gastrostomies and jejunostomies include wound infections, leakage, tube migration, ileus, fever, peritonitis, and necrotizing fasciitis.

Parenteral nutrition

Potential complications of intravenous nutrition include mechanical, infectious, and metabolic problems. Pneumothorax, hemorrhage, brachial plexus injury, air or guidewire embolism, cardiac tamponade, and death may result from inserting a central venous catheter. Catheters can become occluded by blood, fibrin, intravenous lipid, or precipitated drugs. Vascular catheters are responsible for one-third of nosocomial bacteremias and half of candidemias. Skin flora are the most common pathogens and include *Staphylococcus aureus*, *Staphylococcus epidermidis*, *Klebsiella pneumoniae*, *Pseudomonas aeruginosa*, *Enterobacter* species, and *Candida albicans*. Early metabolic complications of TPN include electrolyte abnormalities, hyperglycemia or hypoglycemia, hyperlipidemia, acid–base disturbances, hypercapnia, and fluid overload (Table 14.2). Lipid emulsions can cause pulmonary dysfunction, impaired function of the

Table 14.2 Metabolic complications associated with TPN

Early
Electrolyte abnormalities
Sodium
Potassium
Calcium
Magnesium
Phosphate
Refeeding syndrome
Hyperglycemia
Hypoglycemia
Elevated urea nitrogen
Adverse reactions to lipid emulsions
Hyperlipidemia
Poor lipid clearance
Thrombocytopenia
Hypercapnia
Hyperammonemia
Fluid overload
Hyperosmolar nonketotic hyperglycemic coma
Acidosis
Alkalosis
Delayed
Lipid overload syndrome
Essential fatty acid deficiency
Metabolic bone disease
Liver dysfunction
Gallbladder disease
Mineral deficiency or excess
Zinc
Copper
Chromium
Selenium
Molybdenum
Iron
Manganese

immune system, pancreatitis, delayed platelet aggregation, and hypersensitivity reactions. Delayed metabolic consequences include liver dysfunction, bone demineralization, essential fatty acid deficiency, and mineral deficiency or excess. Liver abnormalities occur frequently with long-term TPN, including calculous and acalculous cholecystitis, hepatic steatosis, steatohepatitis, fibrosis, and cirrhosis. TPN-induced liver abnormalities may be minimized by not exceeding the caloric needs of the patient, especially the glucose component.

Key practice points

- Healthy adults require 20–25 k/kg of body weight to satisfy daily caloric requirements.
- Loss of greater than 15% of body weight usually indicates significant malnutrition.
- Laboratory tests are important in assessing nutritional status and also are used during nutritional replenishment to test for the adequacy of supplementation and for complications of nutritional support.
- When initiating a nutritional program, energy and protein goals must be set.
- Jejunostomy feedings require continuous infusion to prevent diarrhea and abdominal pain and to ensure adequate nutrient absorption.
- Blood values for fat-soluble vitamins are difficult to interpret because of adipose stores and plasma-binding proteins.

Case studies

Case 1

A 27-year-old man with refractory Crohn's disease is admitted to the hospital due to a partial small bowel obstruction. The patient has been experiencing severe diffuse abdominal pain, nausea, and vomiting for the past 48 hours. He vomits immediately after any attempt at oral intake. The patient has a history of a stricture involving the terminal ileum that required resection two years before. He has had multiple small bowel strictures requiring surgical intervention. The patient is currently being treated with adalimumab and azathioprine for his Crohn's disease. He is noted to have an albumin of 2.4 g/dl and a sedimentation rate of 94 mm/h. Physical exam demonstrates a diffusely tender abdomen and multiple surgical scars across the abdomen. Computed tomography (CT) scan demonstrates a small bowel obstruction with dilated loops of small bowel. Surgery has evaluated the patient and is recommending conservative management with placement of a nasogastric tube for decompression, intravenous hydration, and TPN given the low albumin, active inflammation, and likelihood that the patient will not receive any enteral nutrition while the small bowel obstruction is being monitored.

Discussion and potential pitfalls

TPN in Crohn's disease patients admitted to hospital who either require bowel rest or are unable to tolerate oral intake should be considered early. Due to the catabolic state of inflammation in Crohn's disease and the fact that many Crohn's patients have nutritional deficiencies, TPN should be initiated within one to five days. Furthermore, TPN can also be used to correct nutritional deficiencies prior to surgery. Once TPN is initiated, routine monitoring should include fluid intake and output measurements, serum electrolytes, aminotransferases, bilirubin, and triglycerides. Patients receiving TPN are at increased risk of bloodstream infection, and patients with Crohn's disease on immunosuppressive therapies are at even greater risk and should be monitored carefully for signs of infection.

Case 2

A 50-year-old man presents to the emergency department with a one-day history of sudden-onset severe periumbilical pain, nausea, and vomiting. He admits to heavy alcohol consumption prior to the onset of abdominal pain. On physical examination, he is afebrile, pulse is 120 bpm, respiratory rate is 22. He is tachypneic and anxious. His abdomen is tender to palpation with no bowel sounds appreciated. His labs are notable for a white blood count of 22 K cells/ml, hematocrit of 56%, blood urea nitrogen of 26 mg/dl, amylase 2000 U/l, and lipase of 1947 U/l. The patient is diagnosed with acute pancreatitis. He is aggressively hydrated with normal saline. A CT scan performed 48 hours after admission demonstrates significant necrosis of the pancreatic gland with absence of perfusion in 70% of the gland. He is determined to have severe acute pancreatitis, and early enteral nutrition is initiated through a nasojejunal feeding tube.

Discussion and potential pitfalls

Enteral feeding should be initiated as soon as severe acute pancreatitis has been diagnosed because this has demonstrated reduced infectious complications, decreased hospital days, and a trend toward improving mortality. Benefit has been demonstrated when enteral nutrition is initiated within 36–48 hours of presentation. Enteral nutrition should be performed through a nasojejunal feeding tube.

Further reading

McClave, S.A., DiBaise, J.K., Mullin, G.E., and Martindale, R.G. (2016). Nutrition therapy in the adult hospitalized patient. *Am. J. Gastroenterol.* 111: 315–334. https://doi.org/10.1038/ajg.2016.28.

CHAPTER 15
The Patient Requiring Endoscopic Procedures

Introduction and background

Utility of endoscopy

Gastrointestinal endoscopy has transformed all aspects of diagnosing and treating patients with diseases of the gastrointestinal tract. Each endoscopic procedure has a specific set of indications and contraindications. In general, an endoscopic procedure is indicated only when the results are expected to influence the course of patient management. In some cases, however, the attendant risks of endoscopy may outweigh the benefits. Before proceeding with endoscopic intervention, a patient should give a complete history and have a complete physical examination to establish the indication for the study and exclude the presence of any contraindications. Many procedures require bowel cleansing or prolonged fasting; therefore, the clinician must be aware of comorbid conditions, such as diabetes, heart failure, or renal dysfunction, which may require adjusting the instructions for patient preparation. All patients should be counseled on the risks and benefits of endoscopy; written and verbal informed consent are mandatory.

Principles of moderate sedation

Most endoscopic procedures require moderate (conscious) sedation to permit a safe and complete examination. The optimal agents and dosages vary, but all carry the risk of cardiopulmonary complications. All patients should be monitored for changes in blood pressure, heart rate, and respiratory rate throughout the course of sedation. Many centers use pulse oximetry and electrocardiographic monitoring, but it is uncertain if routine use of these more expensive monitoring procedures improves treatment outcomes. No electronic monitoring can replace clinical judgment; therefore, if significant cardiopulmonary signs or symptoms arise, the procedure should be aborted. The benzodiazepine antagonist flumazenil and the opiate antagonist naloxone can be used to reverse the effects of benzodiazepines and narcotics, respectively, in patients with

Yamada's Handbook of Gastroenterology, Fourth Edition. John M. Inadomi, Renuka Bhattacharya, Joo Ha Hwang, and Cynthia Ko.

complications of oversedation, but they should not be used routinely to reverse sedation. Slow titration of the initial dose of the sedative agent is the best way to avoid oversedation.

Antibiotic prophylaxis

The role of preprocedure antibiotics to prevent endocarditis or bacteremia in patients with vascular or other prostheses is undefined. Based on the documented risks of bacteremia with given procedures and the risks of establishing an infection in certain pre-existing conditions, the American Society of Gastrointestinal Endoscopy provides guidelines for antibiotic prophylaxis before endoscopic procedures (Table 15.1). In many circumstances, no definitive

Table 15.1 Recommendations for antibiotic prophylaxis

Risk group	Procedure	Antibiotic prophylaxis
High risk of endocarditis (prosthetic valve, prior endocarditis, systemic pulmonary shunt, or synthetic vascular graft <1 year old)	Stricture dilation, sclerotherapy Esophagogastroduodenoscopy (EGD) or colonoscopy	Recommended with an antibiotic regimen that is active against enterococci, such as penicillin, ampicillin, piperacillin, or vancomycin (low quality of evidence)
Moderate risk of endocarditis (rheumatic valvular disease, mitral valve prolapse with insufficiency, hypertrophic cardiomyopathy, and most congenital malformations)	Stricture dilation, sclerotherapy EGD or colonoscopy	Not recommended (low quality of evidence)
Low risk of endocarditis (coronary bypass surgery, pacemakers, and implantable defibrillators)	All endoscopic procedures	Not recommended
Prosthetic joints	All endoscopic procedures	Not recommended
Obstructed biliary system or pancreatic pseudo-cyst	Endoscopic retrograde cholangiopancreatography (ERCP)	Recommended to prevent cholangitis
Cirrhosis and ascites	Stricture dilation, sclerotherapy	Insufficient data (endoscopist's discretion)
	EGD or colonoscopy	Not recommended
Peritoneal dialysis	Lower GI endoscopy	Suggested to prevent peritonitis (low quality of evidence)
All patients	Percutaneous gastrostomy	Recommended

recommendations can be made, and the decision is made at the clinician's discretion. Antibiotics can be costly, and many have a substantial risk of allergic reactions. These issues must be considered when contemplating the use of prophylactic antibiotics.

Coagulation disorders

Although coagulation abnormalities are not absolute contraindications to endoscopy, the use of endoscopic biopsy can be associated with an increased risk of bleeding. Before any therapeutic intervention, including percutaneous gastrostomy tube placement and electrocoagulation for polypectomy or hemostasis, attempts should be made to correct coagulation disorders. Prolongation of prothrombin time unrelated to the administration of warfarin may require parenteral vitamin K therapy. If there is no response to vitamin K or if emergency therapy is necessary, coagulation factors should be supplemented with fresh-frozen plasma. Antiplatelet agents (e.g. aspirin) should ideally be withheld for 7–10 days before and after these therapeutic measures, although there is no evidence that routine endoscopy including polypectomy is associated with an increased risk of bleeding complications in patients using daily aspirin. Depending on the underlying medical condition, warfarin can often be withheld for five to seven days before the procedure and reinstituted one to two days after therapy.

If medical conditions prohibit discontinuation, one of two potential management pathways can be used. In the first, the patient is hospitalized, warfarin is discontinued, and heparin is initiated. When the prothrombin time normalizes, the patient is prepared for the procedure, and heparin is discontinued four hours before the intervention. Heparin can be restarted four hours after the procedure, and warfarin can be reinstituted 12–24 hours after heparin if no procedure-related hemorrhage occurs. Alternatively, warfarin may be stopped five days prior to the procedure and subcutaneous low molecular weight heparin (e.g. dalteparin) initiated, once or twice daily, according to the patient's weight. The last low molecular weight heparin dose is given the night before the procedure and then restarted the evening of the procedure and continued for five days, whereas warfarin is restarted the evening of the procedure and continued as previously taken. This second approach avoids hospitalization because the subcutaneous low molecular weight heparin is self-administered in an outpatient setting.

Upper gastrointestinal endoscopy

Indications and contraindications

Many symptoms attributable to diseases of the esophagus, stomach, and duodenum are best assessed by esophagogastroduodenoscopy (EGD) or upper gastrointestinal endoscopy. The American Society of Gastrointestinal Endoscopy has established consensus guidelines for the appropriate use of EGD (Table 15.2). Therapeutic endoscopy is often indicated for control of variceal and nonvariceal bleeding, dilation of strictures, removal of some foreign bodies, palliation of advanced malignancies with stents or tumor ablation, and placement of a percutaneous gastrostomy tube. The advent of longer endoscopes has expanded the capability of upper gastrointestinal endoscopy in diagnosing and potentially treating diseases of the small intestine. Enteroscopy is indicated when investigating chronic bleeding presumed secondary to a source in the small intestine or if visualization or sampling the small intestine is warranted by radiological abnormalities.

The major contraindications to upper gastrointestinal endoscopy include perforation, hemodynamic instability, cardiopulmonary distress, and inadequate patient cooperation. Coagulation disorders are relative contraindications to therapeutic intervention. Percutaneous gastrostomy tube placement is contraindicated if the stomach is inaccessible because of a prior gastrectomy or interposed bowel, liver, or spleen.

Table 15.2 Indications for upper gastrointestinal endoscopy

Diagnostic
Upper abdominal distress despite an appropriate trial of therapy
Upper abdominal distress associated with signs or symptoms of organic disease (weight loss, anorexia)
Refractory vomiting of unknown cause
Dysphagia or odynophagia
Esophageal reflux symptoms unresponsive to therapy
Upper gastrointestinal bleeding
When sampling of duodenal or jejunal tissue or fluid is indicated
To obtain a histological diagnosis for radiographically demonstrated gastric or esophageal ulcers, upper intestinal tract strictures, or suspected neoplasms
To screen for varices so that patients with cirrhosis can be identified as possible candidates for prophylactic medical or endoscopic therapy
To assess acute injury after caustic ingestion
When management of other disease processes is affected by the presence of upper gastrointestinal pathological conditions (e.g. use of anticoagulants)
Therapeutic
Treatment of variceal and nonvariceal upper gastrointestinal bleeding
Removal of foreign bodies
Removal of selected polypoid lesions
Dilation of symptomatic strictures
Palliative treatment of stenosing neoplasms
Placement of percutaneous feeding gastrostomy tube
Surveillance
Follow-up of selected gastric, esophageal, or stomal ulcers to document healing
Barrett esophagus
Familial adenomatous polyposis
Adenomatous gastric polyps
Follow-up of varices eradicated by endoscopic therapy

Patient preparation and monitoring

Patients should not ingest solid food for six to eight hours or liquids for four hours before elective upper gastrointestinal endoscopy. If delayed gastric emptying is suspected, a liquid diet can be instituted 24 hours before the procedure and the fasting interval increased to 8–12 hours. For complete gastric outlet obstruction, evacuation of the stomach with a nasogastric tube may be necessary. If an emergency endoscopic procedure is required for gastrointestinal bleeding, measures should be taken to avoid aspiration. Evacuation of the stomach with an orogastric tube before the procedure, attentiveness to oral suction during the procedure, and prophylactic endotracheal intubation in an obtunded patient protect the patient's airway.

Moderate (conscious) sedation is typically performed using a combination of a short-acting benzodiazepine (e.g. midazolam) along with a short-acting opiate (e.g. fentanyl), although the synergistic cardiopulmonary depressant effects of this combination may increase the rate of cardiopulmonary complications. Throughout the procedure, a trained assistant should work together with the endoscopist to monitor the oral secretions as well as the overall clinical condition of the patient.

Performance of the procedure

The endoscope is introduced under direct visualization by passing the instrument into the posterior pharynx and instructing the patient to swallow. Direct visualization is preferred because it is less traumatic and provides a view of the larynx. A standard EGD involves a complete inspection of the esophagus, the stomach, and the first two portions of the duodenum. A pediatric colonoscope or push enteroscope can be advanced into the proximal jejunum. Enteroscopy can also be performed with overtubes with inflatable balloons on the tip of the overtube and the tip of the enteroscope to aid advancement of the endoscope into the small bowel.

Endoscopic biopsy or brush cytology studies may provide a pathological diagnosis. For some disease processes (e.g. infections caused by *Helicobacter pylori* and causes of malabsorption in the small intestine), random biopsies of normal-appearing mucosa may be indicated. Upper gastrointestinal endoscopy also provides the capability of therapeutic intervention. Dysphagia from esophageal strictures or achalasia can be relieved with endoscopic dilation using pneumatic balloon or sequential bougienage techniques. The safest means of bougienage dilation involves passage of the dilator over a guidewire placed endoscopically into the distal stomach. Although fluoroscopy reduces the complication rate of dilation, radiation exposure and resource limitations have precluded its routine use in many centers. Acute or chronic nonvariceal hemorrhage can be controlled with electrocoagulation, heater probe application, injection therapy, or laser photocoagulation. Large or bleeding esophageal varices may be treated with injection sclerotherapy or band ligation. Mucosal polyps can be excised with electrocoagulation using hot biopsy forceps or with snare polypectomy. Deep tissue sampling and excision of mucosal lesions may be accomplished with submucosal injection and endoscopic mucosal resection (EMR). Large stenosing esophageal or gastric malignancies can be ablated with laser photocoagulation or electrocoagulation. Esophageal malignancies can also be palliated by deploying metallic expandable stents.

Complications

Diagnostic upper gastrointestinal endoscopy is usually very safe, and rates of serious complications are low. Most complications are related to oversedation, emphasizing the need for preprocedural patient assessment and vigilant patient monitoring throughout the period of sedation. The high rate of wound infections associated with gastrostomy tube placement can be substantially reduced by prophylactic antibiotics. The benefit of prophylactic antibiotics for other indications remains unproven.

Video capsule endoscopy

Indications and contraindications

Wireless capsule endoscopy or video capsule endoscopy (VCE) uses a wireless, short focal length lens to capture two images per second as the capsule traverses the gastrointestinal tract. The video images are transmitted by radiotelemetry to an array of aerials attached to the body via a recording belt. The primary indication for VCE is for evaluating obscure gastrointestinal bleeding. However, indications continue to evolve, and it has been used for evaluating small bowel tumors and small intestinal Crohn's disease. Contraindications to VCE include esophageal stricture and intermittent or partial small bowel obstruction. Relative contraindications include dementia, gastroparesis, and the presence of a pacemaker because of potential interference as the capsule traverses the chest. No cases of complications in patients with pacemakers who have undergone VCE have been reported.

Performance of the procedure

The procedure is generally performed in ambulatory patients after an overnight fast with or without a polyethylene glycol preparation. An eight-lead sensor array is fastened to the abdomen in a designated pattern that allows image capture and continuous triangulation of the capsule location in the abdomen. The images are stored on a small portable recorder carried on the belt and are subsequently downloaded for interpretation. Patients may proceed with normal activities and can consume clear liquids two hours after capsule ingestion and food four hours after capsule ingestion. The capsule itself is disposable and is passed by normal excretion.

Complications

The primary risk of VCE is capsule retention, which occurs in up to 25% of patients but requires surgical intervention in less than 1%. Retained capsules rarely cause obstructive symptoms, and most cases can be observed for extended periods during which most capsules will pass spontaneously, thereby avoiding surgery.

Lower gastrointestinal endoscopy

Indications and contraindications

Diseases or symptoms referable to the colon and rectum are best evaluated by colonoscopy or flexible sigmoidoscopy. All patients older than 40 years with symptoms referable to any portion of the colon are best evaluated by total colonoscopy. The American Society of Gastrointestinal Endoscopy has established recommendations for using colonoscopy (Table 15.3) that are intended as guidelines. They should not replace the clinical judgment of the clinician.

As with any endoscopic procedure, colonoscopy is contraindicated if a perforation is suspected. Lower gastrointestinal endoscopy is specifically contraindicated

Table 15.3 Indications for colonoscopy

Diagnostic
Fecal occult blood
Hematochezia in the absence of a convincing anorectal source
Melena, if an upper intestinal source is excluded
Unexplained iron deficiency
Abnormality on barium enema that is probably significant (filling defect, stricture)
To exclude the presence of synchronous cancer or polyps in a patient with confirmed colorectal neoplasia
Chronic, unexplained diarrhea
Selected patients with altered bowel habits at risk of colonic neoplasia
Inflammatory bowel disease, if establishing a diagnosis or determining the extent of disease will alter management decisions
Therapeutic
Excision of polyps
Bleeding from vascular ectasias, neoplasia, polypectomy site, or ulceration
Foreign body removal
Decompression of acute colonic pseudo-obstruction or volvulus
Balloon dilation of stenotic lesions
Palliative treatment of inoperable stenosing or bleeding neoplasms
Surveillance
Prior history of colorectal cancer or adenomatous polyps
Family history of hereditary nonpolyposis colon cancer
Family history of colorectal cancer in a first-degree relative (<age 55) or in several family members
Long-standing (>7–10 years) chronic ulcerative pan-colitis with biopsies to detect dysplasia; colitis limited to the left side may require less intensive surveillance

in fulminant colitis and the suppurative phase of acute diverticulitis. Recent myocardial infarction is a relative contraindication to colonoscopy and should delay elective procedures for several weeks.

Performance of the procedure

Flexible sigmoidoscopy involves introducing the instrument to the descending colon or splenic flexure, whereas total colonoscopy involves passing the instrument to the cecum. Although experienced endoscopists may reach the cecum in 90–98% of examinations, a significant number of patients have colonic anatomies that preclude safe completion of the procedure. Therefore, the well-trained endoscopist should be willing to abandon a colonoscopic study that appears unreasonably traumatic.

As with upper gastrointestinal endoscopy, colonoscopy provides the capability of obtaining biopsy specimens to establish the diagnosis of endoscopic abnormalities and to sample normal-appearing mucosa if occult conditions (e.g. microscopic colitis) are suspected. Therapeutic colonoscopic techniques include polypectomy with hot biopsy forceps or with snare polypectomy using electrocoagulation to promote hemostasis. Acute and chronic bleeding from angiodysplasias can be treated with electrocoagulation, heater probe application, and laser photocoagulation. Less common procedures include through-the-scope pneumatic balloon dilation of discrete benign strictures, decompressive colonoscopy with tube placement for acute pseudo-obstruction, and palliative laser ablation of inoperable neoplasms.

Complications

The overall risk of serious complications, including perforation and uncontrolled hemorrhage, is approximately 1 in 500 for diagnostic colonoscopy. Therapeutic maneuvers increase the risk of complications, although there are wide variations in reported rates. Hemorrhage after polypectomy is common. It may occur in up to 1–2% of patients and often occurs up to 7–10 days after the procedure when residual necrotic tissue and scar tissue are sloughed. The risk of perforation is also increased in therapeutic maneuvers. The transmural burn syndrome represents a localized, contained perforation that may be associated with localized pain, fever, and leukocytosis 6–24 hours after polypectomy or after any therapy that uses electrocoagulation. Many patients can be treated conservatively with parenteral broad-spectrum antibiotics, but any patient with signs of frank perforation should undergo surgical exploration.

Endoscopic retrograde cholangiopancreatography

Indications and contraindications

Endoscopic retrograde cholangiopancreatography (ERCP) is indicated for evaluating patients with suspected biliary or pancreatic disorders when noninvasive imaging with ultrasonography or computed tomographic (CT) scanning is equivocal and when therapeutic intervention is necessary (Table 15.4). Various

Table 15.4 Indications for endoscopic retrograde cholangiopancreatography (ERCP)

Suspected biliary disorders
Unexplained jaundice or cholestasis
Postcholecystectomy complaints
Postbiliary surgery complaints
Acute cholangitis
Acute gallstone pancreatitis
Evaluation of bile duct abnormalities in other imaging studies
Sphincter of Oddi manometry
Suspected pancreatic disorders
Chronic upper abdominal pain consistent with pancreatic origin
Unexplained weight loss
Steatorrhea
Unexplained recurrent pancreatitis
Evaluation of pancreatic abnormalities in other imaging studies
To obtain pancreatic duct brushings or pure pancreatic juice
Before therapeutic intervention
Endoscopic sphincterotomy
Endoscopic biliary drainage
Endoscopic pancreatic drainage
Endoscopic cystgastrostomy
Balloon dilation of pancreaticobiliary strictures
Preoperative mapping for pancreatic or biliary resections

abdominal symptoms can be attributed to the pancreaticobiliary system, and the decision to proceed with ERCP should be made by a clinician experienced in caring for patients with these disorders. ERCP has a role in the preoperative evaluation of selected patients undergoing laparoscopic cholecystectomy, pancreatic resection, or surgical pseudo-cyst drainage. Many of the available therapeutic options, including endoscopic sphincterotomy, stone extraction, endoscopic cystgastrostomy, and biliary or pancreatic stent placement, also require the availability of surgical support. Thus, the treatment of patients undergoing ERCP often requires the combined expertise of the endoscopist and a surgeon.

In addition to the standard contraindications for all endoscopic procedures, ERCP is relatively contraindicated in the presence of an obstructed biliary system or a documented pancreatic pseudo-cyst, unless immediate endoscopic or surgical drainage is planned. Any procedure performed under these conditions should be accompanied by administration of prophylactic antibiotics (see Table 15.1). Therapeutic interventions, particularly endoscopic sphincterotomy, are contraindicated in patients with severe coagulopathy.

Patient preparation and monitoring

All patients undergoing ERCP should be prepared in the same manner as patients undergoing EGD. Attention should be given to several factors specific to ERCP. First, because the endoscope used for ERCP is equipped with side-viewing rather than with forward-viewing optics, special attention should be given to patients with dysphagia. Passing the instrument through the esophagus is done blindly, increasing the risk of perforation if there is a Zenker diverticulum or esophageal stricture. The ductal injection of contrast material can result in significant systemic absorption, as demonstrated occasionally by the appearance of a postinjection nephrogram. Although anaphylactic reactions have not been reported, erythema and rash can occur, and some clinicians choose to pretreat patients who have histories of reactions to contrast agents with antihistamines and corticosteroids 12 and 2 hours before the procedure. Because ERCP involves radiographic imaging of the upper abdomen, any residual gastrointestinal contrast agent should be evacuated with purgatives. Immediately before sedating the patient, abdominal radiographs should be obtained to ensure that all contrast material is gone and to establish the location of soft tissue shadows and calcifications.

The sedation of patients undergoing ERCP is similar to the procedure for patients undergoing upper gastrointestinal endoscopy. Patient movement should be minimized to obtain optimal imaging. Because the patient is in the prone position on the fluoroscopic table rather than in the left decubitus position used for upper gastrointestinal endoscopy, special attention should be given to removing oral secretions.

Performance of the procedure

ERCP involves passing a side-viewing endoscope into the second portion of the duodenum and visualizing the major papilla. Both the pancreatic and biliary system can be cannulated with specialized catheters that are advanced through the duodenoscope. After selective cannulation of the pancreatic or biliary system, radiological contrast dye is injected under fluoroscopic guidance until the entire ductal system is visualized. Care should be taken to avoid injecting air because bubbles may be mistaken for biliary or pancreatic stones. Overinjection of dye into the pancreas leads to staining of the parenchyma, a pattern termed *acinarization*, which is associated with an increased risk of ERCP-induced pancreatitis. Abdominal radiographs are obtained during the injection and periodically as the contrast dye drains from the duct. After one ductal system is examined, the alternate system is cannulated and injected. For some disorders, only cholangiography or pancreatography is necessary. Biliary manometry can be performed in specialized centers as part of the ERCP examination with a specialized water-perfused manometry catheter positioned across the sphincter of Oddi. The ampulla of Vater may not be easily accessible in patients whose anatomy has been altered by a Billroth II or Roux-en-Y gastrojejunostomy.

ERCP is a nonoperative method of treating many pancreaticobiliary disorders. Endoscopic sphincterotomy is often performed to facilitate biliary stone extraction. The procedure involves cannulation of the common bile duct with a papillotome, a specialized catheter with an exposed wire that extends across the most distal portion of the catheter. Positioning the wire across the papilla and applying electrical current produces a cut through the papilla. After sphincterotomy, stones may pass spontaneously but extraction with balloon catheters or baskets placed through the endoscope and into the bile duct is often necessary. If endoscopic stone extraction fails, a nasobiliary tube or endoscopic stent can be placed while the patient awaits definitive surgical therapy. Sphincterotomy also relieves obstruction caused by sphincter of Oddi dyskinesia or papillary stenosis. Specialized centers may perform sphincterotomy of the minor papilla to treat pancreas divisum.

Biliary or pancreatic strictures can also be treated with ERCP. Inoperable, malignant obstruction of the extrahepatic bile ducts is best relieved by endoscopic placement of a plastic or metallic stent, in many cases after sphincterotomy. Occasionally, patients with primary sclerosing cholangitis will have dominant strictures of the extrahepatic bile ducts, which are amenable to pneumatic balloon dilation followed by stent placement. For most benign biliary strictures, however, surgical therapy is preferred because of superior long-term patency. Transpapillary placement of a pancreatic stent has been used to treat symptomatic pancreatic ductal strictures and pseudo-cysts in patients with chronic pancreatitis.

Complications

Acute pancreatitis is the most common complication of ERCP. Sixty to 80% of patients undergoing ERCP develop asymptomatic elevations in serum amylase and lipase levels, but clinically overt pancreatitis is much less common. Retrospective series report an incidence of 1–2%, but prospective series suggest that symptomatic acute pancreatitis occurs in 4–7% of patients undergoing ERCP. The risk is increased by acinarization of the pancreas, repeated attempts at cannulation, and sphincter of Oddi manometry. Conservative management leads to resolution for most patients, but severe necrotizing pancreatitis occurs in a small subset of patients. Placement of a temporary pancreatic duct stent following free-cut sphincterotomy or sphincterotomy for sphincter of Oddi dysfunction reduces the risk of ERCP-induced pancreatitis.

Endoscopic sphincterotomy has an overall complication rate of 5–8%, equally divided among bleeding, perforation, cholangitis, and pancreatitis. One to 2% of patients undergoing sphincterotomy require surgical intervention for related complications; the mortality rate for sphincterotomy is 0.5–1%. Attempted biliary drainage with endoprosthesis placement has an 8% risk of cholangitis, but most of these episodes occur when drainage is unsuccessful or incomplete. Stent occlusion and cholangitis are delayed complications that occur in 40% of patients in a mean of five to six months after endoprosthetic insertion.

Endoscopic ultrasound

Indications and contraindications

Endoscopic ultrasound (EUS) provides the capability of obtaining high-resolution ultrasound images within the upper and lower gastrointestinal tracts. Specialized endoscopes with ultrasound probes at the tips and oblique-viewing optics can generate acoustic images of gastrointestinal wall layers and surrounding

Table 15.5 Indications for endoscopic ultrasound (EUS)

Tumor staging (esophageal, gastric, pancreatic, ampullary, distal bile duct, rectal, non-small cell lung)
Neuroendocrine tumor localization
Evaluation of submucosal mass lesions
Suspected chronic pancreatitis
Detection of distal bile duct stones
Fine needle aspiration of adjacent lymph nodes or mass lesions
Evaluation of anal sphincters
Suspected enterocutaneous fistula
Direct endoscopic cystgastrostomy for pancreatic pseudo-cysts

strictures. The increased availability of the instruments and clinical experience with the technique have expanded the list of clinical indications for EUS (Table 15.5). Focal intramural and extramural mass lesions and wall thickening are easily identified by EUS. Localization to a specific wall layer (i.e. mucosa, submucosa, muscularis, serosa, extralumenal) often helps to identify the histological origin of the lesion. EUS is useful in detecting anal sphincter defects in patients with incontinence and has been used to localize enterocutaneous fistulae in Crohn's disease. EUS is also of value in identifying and staging several tumors, including esophageal carcinoma, gastric carcinoma, gastric lymphoma, ampullary carcinoma, distal bile duct carcinoma, pancreatic carcinoma, and rectal carcinoma. It is both sensitive and specific in determining the local extent of the tumor (T stage) and the presence of regional lymph nodes (N stage), but it is not a reliable means of establishing distant metastatic disease (M stage). EUS is superior to CT and magnetic resonance imaging studies and to transabdominal ultrasound for pancreatic imaging, and it is the most accurate means for defining vascular invasion by tumors in the peripancreatic bed. Similarly, EUS can localize pancreatic islet cell tumors not detected by conventional imaging studies. Evidence suggests that the sensitivity of EUS is equivalent to that of ERCP for detecting common bile duct stones and chronic pancreatitis.

The introduction of instruments to obtain ultrasound-directed fine needle aspiration has further expanded the role of EUS. Sampling of pancreatic mass lesions has proved useful, particularly in patients with unresectable disease who are candidates for palliative radiation therapy or chemotherapy. EUS-directed transesophageal aspiration of mediastinal lymph nodes has proved superior to other nonsurgical methods of staging non-small cell lung cancer and often provides information critical to the decision to pursue surgical or nonsurgical therapy in these patients. The same instrumentation used in tissue sampling has launched EUS into therapeutics. EUS-guided needle injection of the celiac ganglia has been used to control chronic pain caused by chronic pancreatitis or pancreatic cancer. EUS can direct needle placement and detect pericystic blood vessels in patients undergoing endoscopic cystgastrostomy, thereby improving the safety profile of the procedure. Future refinements in endosonographic image quality and performance will probably expand the diagnostic and therapeutic capabilities of EUS.

Because EUS is a specialized form of upper and lower gastrointestinal endoscopy, contraindications are identical to those for diagnostic endoscopy in their respective locations in the gastrointestinal tract.

Patient preparation and monitoring

Preparation of the patient for EUS of the upper gastrointestinal tract is identical to that for EGD. Similarly, EUS of the rectum or colon requires bowel cleansing in accordance with the techniques used for flexible sigmoidoscopy or colonoscopy, respectively. The principles of sedation and monitoring are also based on the standard practices for upper and lower gastrointestinal endoscopy.

Performance of the procedure

There are two principal types of echoendoscopes. The linear or curved array instruments provide 100° sector images parallel to the longitudinal axis of the endoscope, whereas radial scanning instruments provide 360° images perpendicular to the longitudinal axis of the endoscope. Although upper echoendoscopes usually have oblique-viewing optics, echocolonoscopes are also available with forward-viewing optics. The ultrasound frequency can be altered on most of the available instruments. Higher frequency imaging (12–20 MHz) provides increased resolution, and lower frequency imaging (5.0–7.5 MHz) provides increased depth of penetration. Because images from linear or curved array instruments are oriented along the axis of the endoscope, specialized needles can be advanced through the working channel and directed under real-time ultrasound guidance into a lesion for tissue aspiration.

EUS provides high-resolution images of the bowel wall and, in most structures, identifies five echolayers that correlate with the mucosa, muscularis mucosae, submucosa, muscularis propria, and serosa or adventitia. Directing the instrument to a focal submucosal mass or to an area of wall thickening can identify the layer from which the abnormality originates. The pancreas can be visualized from the duodenum or posterior wall of the stomach, whereas the bile duct and gallbladder can be identified from the duodenum. The major vascular structures of the splanchnic circulation can also be identified from the duodenum or stomach. Flow within these structures can be assessed by the color flow and pulse Doppler modes available on curved array instruments.

Complications

EUS has a safety profile similar to that of diagnostic upper and lower gastrointestinal endoscopy. The larger diameter of the echoendoscope makes traversing lumenal strictures more hazardous, which is problematic for esophageal tumors. Patients with significant dysphagia should undergo preliminary forward-viewing endoscopy or barium swallow radiography, so that the severity of lumenal narrowing can be assessed. Although pancreatitis following EUS fine needle aspiration has been reported, EUS-directed biopsy is relatively safe, with a complication rate of 1–2%.

Key practice points

- Moderate (conscious) sedation requires careful monitoring by an assistant to assess for any cardiopulmonary complications.
- Antibiotic prophylaxis for endoscopic procedures should be based on the documented risks of bacteremia with given procedures and the risks of establishing an infection in certain pre-existing conditions.
- Management of periprocedural anticoagulation should be based on the risk of bleeding with the planned procedure and risk of thromboembolic events if anticoagulation is held.

Further reading

ASGE Standards of Practice Committee (2018 Feb). Guidelines for sedation and anesthesia in GI endoscopy. *Gastrointest. Endosc.* 87 (2): 327–337. https://doi.org/10.1016/j.gie.2008.09.029.

ASGE Standards of Practice Committee (2016). Management of antithrombotic agents for patients undergoing GI endoscopy. *Gastrointest. Endosc.* 83: 3–16. https://doi.org/10.1016/j.gie.2015.09.035.

ASGE Standards of Practice Committee (2015). Antibiotic prophylaxis for GI endoscopy. *Gastrointest. Endosc.* 81: 81–89. https://doi.org/10.1016/j.gie.2014.08.008.

ASGE Standards of Practice Committee (2014). Routine laboratory testing before endoscopic procedures. *Gastrointest. Endosc.* 80: 28–33. https://doi.org/10.1016/j.gie.2014.01.019.

ASGE Standards of Practice Committee (2015). Bowel preparation before colonoscopy. *Gastrointest. Endosc.* 81: 781–794. https://doi.org/10.1016/j.gie.2014.09.048.

PART 2
Specific Gastrointestinal Diseases

CHAPTER 16
Motor Disorders of the Esophagus

Introduction

Dysphagia can be classified as oropharyngeal dysphagia, which includes disorders of the oral and pharyngeal phases of swallowing, and esophageal dysphagia, which results from achalasia and other distal esophageal disorders.

Oropharyngeal dysphagia

Clinical presentation

Neuromuscular diseases of the hypopharynx and upper esophagus cause oropharyngeal dysphagia, in which the patient cannot initiate swallowing or propel the food bolus from the hypopharynx into the esophageal body. A careful history can distinguish oropharyngeal dysphagia from esophageal dysphagia, which is characterized by the sensation of food blockage after successful initiation of swallowing. Patients with oropharyngeal dysphagia usually localize symptoms to the cervical region. Patients may describe nasal regurgitation, tracheal aspiration, drooling, or the need to dislodge impacted food manually. Gurgling, halitosis, and a neck mass suggest a Zenker diverticulum, whereas hoarseness may reflect nerve dysfunction or intrinsic vocal cord muscular disease. Dysarthria and nasal speech suggest muscle weakness of the soft palate and pharyngeal constrictors. Physical examination may demonstrate focal neurological deficits with cerebrovascular accidents, a palpable neck mass with a hypopharyngeal diverticulum, ptosis, end-of-day weakness with myasthenia gravis, and paucity of movement with Parkinson disease.

Yamada's Handbook of Gastroenterology, Fourth Edition. John M. Inadomi, Renuka Bhattacharya, Joo Ha Hwang, and Cynthia Ko.

Diagnostic investigation

Video-esophagography

Videofluoroscopy records the complex and rapid sequence of events in the mouth, pharynx, and upper esophagus during a swallow. Motility disturbances manifest as delayed initiation and prolonged duration of swallowing or a disturbance in the sequence of muscle movements. Contrast retention in the pharyngeal recesses is caused by altered mucosal sensitivity, decreased muscle tone, or alterations in recess shape or size. Misdirected swallows with laryngeal penetration or aspiration can be seen with neurological or muscular disorders. Delayed upper esophageal sphincter (UES) opening and cricopharyngeal bars also may be noted.

Manometry

Intralumenal esophageal manometry obtains measurements from the oropharynx and proximal esophagus, including the strength of pharyngeal contraction, the completeness of UES relaxation, and the timing of these events.

Endoscopy

Endoscopy can be performed transorally or transnasally to identify tumors, webs, or hypopharyngeal diverticula.

Differential diagnosis

Hypopharyngeal diverticula

Acquired hypopharyngeal (Zenker) diverticula occur between the oblique fibers of the inferior pharyngeal constrictor and the transverse cricopharyngeus muscle and result from delayed or failed cricopharyngeus relaxation, premature cricopharyngeus contraction, or restrictive cricopharyngeus myopathy with poor compliance.

Neurological disorders

The most common cause of acute oropharyngeal dysphagia is a cerebrovascular accident. Symptoms usually appear abruptly and are associated with other neurological deficits. Degenerative neuronal changes with progressive bulbar palsy and pseudo-bulbar palsy produce tongue and pharyngeal paralysis. Polio and the postpolio syndrome alter pharyngeal clearance. Patients with amyotrophic lateral sclerosis present with choking attacks and aspiration pneumonias secondary to dysfunction of the tongue as well as the pharyngeal and laryngeal musculature. Hypopharyngeal stasis, aspiration, and UES dysfunction are prevalent in Parkinson disease. Swallowing abnormalities, including difficult initiation and UES abnormalities, occur in patients with multiple sclerosis. Rare neurological causes of oropharyngeal dysphagia include brainstem tumors, syringobulbia, tetanus, botulism, lead poisoning, alcoholic neuropathy, carcinoma, chemotherapy, and radiation therapy.

Primary muscle disorders

Polymyositis and dermatomyositis produce poor pharyngeal and proximal esophageal contraction, pooling in the valleculae, and decreased UES tone. Myotonic and oculopharyngeal dystrophy are the two forms of muscular dystrophy that affect the swallowing mechanism. Myotonic dystrophy presents with myopathic facies, swan neck, myotonia, muscle wasting, frontal baldness, testicular atrophy, and cataracts. Oculopharyngeal dystrophy presents with ptosis and dysphagia but does not have other gastrointestinal manifestations. Myasthenia gravis affects striated esophageal musculature, producing dysphagia in two-thirds of patients that worsens with the duration of a meal. Hyperthyroidism and hypothyroidism affect swallowing, as do sarcoidosis, systemic lupus erythematosus, and the stiff man syndrome.

Treatment and prevention

The first step in managing a patient with oropharyngeal dysphagia is to recognize and correct reversible causes of symptoms, including Parkinson disease, myasthenia gravis, hyperthyroidism or hypothyroidism, and polymyositis. The treatment for hypopharyngeal diverticula is endoscopic or surgical cricopharyngeal myotomy, which reduces resting UES tone and resistance to UES flow. Endoscopic dilation with a large caliber bougie may be effective for a cricopharyngeal bar, but the role of myotomy in this condition is less clear. The results of videofluoroscopy can be used to modify the properties of meals and the mechanics of food ingestion in some patients with neuromuscular etiologies of oropharyngeal dysphagia. In patients who cannot safely obtain adequate nutrition, enteral feedings through a nasoenteric tube or gastrostomy may be necessary.

Esophageal dysphagia: Achalasia

Introduction

Achalasia is characterized by aperistalsis of the smooth muscle esophagus and failure of the lower esophageal sphincter (LES) to relax completely with swallowing. Achalasia may be primary or secondary due to neoplastic infiltration of the LES or para-neoplastic syndromes.

Clinical presentation

Patients with achalasia report solid-food dysphagia, and most also have liquid dysphagia. Many complain of regurgitation of undigested food eaten hours or days previously. Symptoms may be intermittent and insidious in onset, and the duration of symptoms prior to diagnosis averages two years. The patient may have learned special maneuvers such as throwing the shoulders back, lifting the neck, performing a Valsalva maneuver, and drinking carbonated beverages to promote swallowing. Chest pain is reported by two-thirds of patients and may be so severe as to cause decreased food intake and weight loss, but it tends to improve as the disease progresses.

Diagnostic investigation

Radiographic studies

Barium swallow radiography is the initial screening test for achalasia and may show a dilated intrathoracic esophagus with impaired contrast transit, a loss of peristalsis, impaired LES relaxation, and a characteristic tapering of the distal esophagus ("bird's beak").

Esophageal manometry

High-resolution manometry coupled with esophageal pressure topography (HREPT) has greatly improved our understanding of esophageal motility disorders and increased the accuracy of diagnosis of achalasia in addition to other esophageal outflow obstructive disorders. HREPT allows calculation of the integrated relaxation pressure (IRP) that is a function of LES pressure as the esophagus shortens with swallows due to longitudinal muscle contraction. It includes the dimension of time between initiation of the swallow until the arrival of the peristaltic contraction (or 10 seconds in the absence of peristalsis). According to the Chicago Classification of HREPT, the criteria for classic achalasia are an IRP ≥ 15 mmHg and absent peristalsis; achalasia with esophageal compression has an IRP ≥ 15 mmHg and at least 20% of swallows associated with pan-esophageal pressurization to >30 mmHg; and spastic achalasia has an IRP ≥ 15 mmHg and a nonperistaltic esophageal contractions with ≥20% of swallows, and the latency between upper esophageal sphincter relaxation and distal esophageal contraction is <4.5 seconds (Table 16.1).

Key practice points

The advent of high-resolution manometry with esophageal pressure topography has revolutionized the categorization of achalasia by differentiating the contractile function of the esophageal body. All forms have an IRP (mean esophagogastric junction [EGJ] pressure persisting for four seconds after a swallow) that is greater than 15 mmHg; in addition:

Type I: Classic achalasia requires absent peristalsis

Type II: Achalasia with esophageal compression includes at least 20% of swallows associated with pan-esophageal pressurization to >30 mmHg

Type III: Spastic achalasia has spastic contractions with >20% of swallows and the latency (lag) between UES relaxation and distal esophageal contraction is <4.5 seconds.

Upper gastrointestinal endoscopy

Upper gastrointestinal endoscopy is insensitive for the diagnosis of achalasia but is necessary to exclude malignancy that could cause pseudo-achalasia. Typically, endoscopy reveals esophageal dilation, atony, and erythema, friability, and

Table 16.1 Clinical achalasia syndromes within and beyond Chicago Classification, version 3.0[a]

Syndrome	Median integrated relaxation pressure (IRP)	Esophageal contractility	Qualifications/notes
Chicago Classification (CC): type I achalasia	Greater than upper limit of normal (ULN)	Absent contractility	Most published treatment trials excluded end-stage cases
CC: type II achalasia	Greater than ULN	Absent peristalsis	Most common presenting achalasia sub-type
		Pan-esophageal pressurization with ≥20% of swallows	Often misdiagnosed before high-resolution manometry (HRM) because of esophageal shortening and pseudo-relaxation
CC: type III achalasia	Greater than ULN	Absent peristalsis	Often mistaken for spasm before HRM
		Premature contractions with ≥20% of swallows	Obstructive physiology includes the distal esophagus
CC: esophagogastric junction (EGJ) outflow obstruction	Greater than ULN	Sufficient peristalsis to exclude type I, II, or III achalasia	Can be early or incomplete achalasia (12–40%)
			Can resolve spontaneously
			Can be artifact; further imaging of EGJ may clarify diagnosis
CC: absent contractility	Less than ULN	Absent contractility	Abnormal functional luminal imaging probe (FLIP) distensibility index or esophageal pressurization with swallows or multiple repetitive swallows (MRS) supports an achalasia diagnosis
CC: distal esophageal spasm	Normal or increased	≥20% premature contractions (distal latency [DL] <4.5 seconds)	May be evolving type III achalasia
CC: jackhammer	Normal or increased	≥20% of swallows with distal contractile integral (DCI) >8000 mmHg/s/cm	May be evolving type III achalasia if DL <4.5 seconds with ≥20% swallows
Opioid effect:	Greater then ULN	Normal, hypercontractile, or premature	Can mimic EGJ outflow obstruction, type III achalasia, distal esophageal spasm (DES), or jackhammer
mechanical obstruction:	Normal or increased	Absent, normal, or hypercontractile	Endoscopic ultrasound (EUS) or computed tomography (CT) imaging of the EGJ may clarify the etiology

[a] Apart from the achalasia sub-types, these syndromes are not specific for achalasia and may have distinct pathophysiology, but instances occur in which they are optimally managed as if they were achalasia.
Source: Kahrilas et al. (2017).

ulcerations from chronic stasis. The LES may be puckered, but passage of the endoscope into the stomach should not be difficult in the absence of malignancy. Careful examination of the gastric cardia is mandatory to rule out secondary causes of achalasia.

Differential diagnosis

Pseudo-achalasia, caused by neoplasia, presents with identical manometric findings as primary achalasia. The most common is adenocarcinoma of the EGJ; however, pancreatic carcinoma, small cell and squamous cell lung carcinoma, prostate carcinoma, and lymphoma may also cause secondary achalasia either by direct compression of the distal esophagus or by malignant cell infiltration of the esophageal myenteric plexus. Other tumors (e.g. Hodgkin disease, lung carcinoma, and hepatocellular carcinoma) produce achalasia by a paraneoplastic mechanism.

Infectious causes of secondary achalasia include Chagas disease, which is caused by the protozoan *Trypanosoma cruzi* that is endemic in South America. After an acute septic phase, chronic destruction of ganglion cells in the gut, urinary tract, heart, and respiratory tract develops over years. The presence of megaureter, megaduodenum, megacolon, or megarectum is helpful in distinguishing Chagas disease from primary achalasia. Complement fixation and polymerase chain reaction tests are available to confirm the diagnosis. Other causes of secondary achalasia include infiltrative diseases (with amyloid, sphingolipids, eosinophils, or sarcoid), diabetes, intestinal pseudo-obstruction, pancreatic pseudo-cysts, von Recklinghausen disease, multiple endocrine neoplasia type IIB, juvenile Sjögren syndrome, postfundoplication dysphagia, and familial adrenal insufficiency with alacrima.

Treatment and prevention

Achalasia is not curable, and no treatment can restore normal esophageal body peristalsis or complete LES relaxation. Treatment therefore rests with measures to reduce LES pressure sufficiently to enhance gravity-assisted esophageal emptying.

Medication therapy

Endoscopic therapy has largely eclipsed the use of medications to treat achalasia. If patients refuse endoscopic or surgical interventions, there are medications with limited effectiveness to reduce dysphagia caused by achalasia. Sublingual isosorbide dinitrate reduces LES pressures by 66% for 90 minutes. Sublingual nifedipine 30–40 mg/day is significantly better than placebo in symptom relief and lowers LES pressure by 30–40% for an hour or more. Sildenafil transiently decreases LES pressure in achalasia. Medication therapy has significant limitations, including a short duration of action and tachyphylaxis.

Pneumatic dilation

Pneumatic dilation using balloons >30 mm diameter can disrupt the LES circular muscle and produce symptom relief in 32–98% of cases. A postdilation LES pressure of less than 10 mmHg is associated with remission up to two years; however, 20–40% of patients will have symptom recurrence. The most common complication of pneumatic dilation is esophageal perforation that occurs in 1–5% of cases.

Endoscopic therapy: Injection

Botulinum toxin, a potent inhibitor of neural acetylcholine release, reduces LES pressure and relieves symptoms for up to six months in patients with achalasia when directly injected into the LES during endoscopy (80 units total divided into four quadrant injections). Because of incomplete symptom control and the requirements for costly repeat injections, botulinum toxin is best reserved for elderly or frail patients who are poor risk for more definitive therapy.

Surgery

Surgical therapy of achalasia usually involves a longitudinal incision of the muscle layers of the LES (i.e. Heller myotomy). Good to excellent responses to myotomy occur in 62–100% of patients. Thoracoscopic and laparoscopic procedures are associated with similar benefits and less morbidity than open approaches. Comparisons between surgical and endoscopic myotomy are limited: current data indicate similar relief of dysphagia but a higher incidence of gastroesophageal reflux symptoms after per-oral endoscopic myotomy (POEM).

Complications and their management

Achalasia is associated with squamous cell carcinoma, which results from chronic stasis and occurs in 2–7% of patients, usually those who have had unsatisfactory treatment or no treatment. Surgery may be associated with symptomatic gastroesophageal reflux that occurs in 10% of cases, which may be further complicated by strictures. Rarely, refractory cases mandate more aggressive operations, including esophageal resection with gastric pull-up or colonic interposition.

Key practice points: Achalasia treatment

1. Type II achalasia with esophageal pressurization has the highest rate of response to any therapy; Type III spastic achalasia has the lowest response rate.
2. Surgical myotomy provides long-standing relief from dysphagia; per-oral endoscopic myotomy is an emerging therapy that may also provide long-term remission.
3. Pneumatic dilatation has proven efficacy but has substantial risk of perforation.
4. Patients in whom surgery or dilation is not performed can be treated using endoscopic injection of botulin toxin, but the effect is transient.

Other motor disorders of the esophagus

In addition to the three achalasia sub-types, the Chicago Classification recognizes EGJ outflow obstruction as another syndrome in which LES dysfunction can cause dysphagia. With EGJ outflow obstruction, the IRP is greater than normal, but the "absent peristalsis" criterion for achalasia is not met. Peristalsis may be fragmented or even normal. EGJ outflow obstruction is a heterogeneous group with a spectrum of potential etiologies, including incompletely expressed or early achalasia or an isolated disorder of impaired LES relaxation. Alternatively, EGJ outflow obstruction may also be secondary to esophageal wall stiffness from an infiltrative disease or cancer, eosinophilic esophagitis, vascular obstruction, sliding, or para-esophageal hiatal hernia, abdominal obesity, or the effects of opiates.

Jackhammer esophagus is characterized by high-amplitude contractions (distal contractile integral >8000 mmHg/s/cm in ≥20% of swallows) with normal or increased IRP. Diffuse esophageal spasm (DES) is diagnosed by a distal latency time <4.5 seconds in ≥20% of swallows; however, many patients progress to achalasia, suggesting that these disorders represent a spectrum of disease.

Scleroderma is a disease that results in smooth muscle atrophy with fibrosis involving the esophagus, intestine, heart, kidneys, skin, and synovium. Two forms of scleroderma are possible: progressive systemic sclerosis with diffuse scleroderma, and the CREST syndrome (calcinosis, Raynaud phenomenon, esophageal dysfunction, sclerodactyly, and telangiectasia). Scleroderma causes hypotensive LES pressures with low amplitude esophageal contractility with low to absent peristaltic activity of the distal esophageal body. The proximal esophageal motor function is generally spared.

Clinical presentation

The major symptoms of spastic disorders are dysphagia and chest pain. Intermittent dysphagia for solids and liquids is present in 30–60% of patients with spastic disorders and may be exacerbated by large boluses of food, medications, or foods of extreme temperatures. Dysphagia is usually not severe enough to produce weight loss. Features that suggest an esophageal rather than a cardiac cause include pain that is nonexertional, continues for hours, interrupts sleep, is meal related, and is relieved by antacids. Associated heartburn, dysphagia, or regurgitation may favor an esophageal cause. Heartburn may not reflect excessive acid reflux into the esophagus but rather may result from hypersensitivity to normal amounts of esophageal acid.

Scleroderma presents primarily with heartburn and dysphagia.

Diagnostic investigation

Endoscopic and radiographic studies

Upper endoscopy is useful in evaluating patients with dysphagia to exclude structural lesions or esophagitis. Barium swallow radiography may define corkscrew esophagus, rosary bead esophagus, pseudo-diverticula, or curling in some patients with DES. Unlike achalasia, "bird's beak" deformities are not observed.

Manometry and ambulatory pH monitoring

Ambulatory pH testing is probably the most useful functional test in patients with unexplained chest pain of presumed esophageal origin to evaluate for symptomatic gastroesophageal reflux. High-resolution esophageal pressure topography is sometimes helpful in the evaluation of chest pain. EGJ outflow obstruction can be diagnosed, in addition to DES that may result from a myenteric neuronal defect that places the affected individuals along the continuum of achalasia.

Scleroderma is diagnosed by hypotensive or absent LES pressure, hypotensive to absent distal esophageal peristalsis, with normal proximal esophageal peristalsis.

Treatment and prevention

Spastic motor disorders of the esophagus are not life-threatening or progressive in most cases. Treatment should attempt to reduce symptoms without exposing the patient to potential therapeutic complications. Gastroesophageal acid reflux disease can be diagnosed by ambulatory pH monitoring or an empiric trial of acid suppression treatment with proton pump inhibitors that can be continued if symptoms resolve. If reflux is not present, the most important step is to reassure the patient that there is no serious heart condition or other disease. When reassurance fails, medical, mechanical, and surgical treatment options are available. Behavioral modification and biofeedback have shown some efficacy in selected refractory cases.

There is no specific treatment for scleroderma involvement of the esophagus; however, gastroesophageal reflux disease is universal and should be treated appropriately based on symptoms and presence of complications.

Medications

Small trials suggest that some patients with outflow obstruction, DES, or jackhammer esophagus experience relief with smooth muscle relaxants such as nitrates, calcium channel blockers, and hydralazine. The antidepressant trazodone has been illustrated in clinical trials to improve global well-being as well as esophageal symptoms, possibly secondary to effects on visceral pain perception. Botulinum toxin injected at the gastroesophageal junction reduced symptoms in one investigation of patients with nonachalasic esophageal spasm.

Mechanical dilation

Therapeutic bougienage probably does not produce symptomatic benefits greater than sham dilation. However, pneumatic dilation has reduced symptoms in some patients with DES and hypertensive LES, especially if dysphagia is prominent.

Surgery

For patients with dysphagia or intractable pain caused by spastic motor esophageal dysfunction, a Heller myotomy to include the LES and the spastic portions of the esophageal body may reduce symptoms in more than 50% of cases. However, the risk of the procedure coupled with the uncertain therapeutic response mandates a cautious approach to surgery.

Essentials of diagnosis

1. Videofluoroscopy and manometry with high-resolution esophageal pressure topography are key tests for evaluating motor disorders of the esophagus.
2. Upper endoscopy is indicated to exclude secondary causes of achalasia.
3. Ambulatory pH testing is most helpful in patients with noncardiac chest pain syndrome.

Further reading

Kahrilas, P.J. (2010). Esophageal motor disorders in terms of high-resolution esophageal pressure topography: What has changed? *Am. J. Gastroenterol* 105: 981–987. PMID 20179690.

Kahrilas, P.J., Katzka, D., and Richter, J.E. (2017). AGA clinical practice update: expert review use of per-oral endoscopic myotomy in achalasia. *Gastroenterology* 153: 1205–1211.

CHAPTER 17
Gastroesophageal Reflux Disease and Eosinophilic Esophagitis

The passage of gastric contents retrograde into the esophagus is a normal physiological event. The development of symptoms, signs, or complications of this process is termed *gastroesophageal reflux disease* (*GERD*). In addition to the esophagus, other structures affected by GERD include the pharynx, larynx, and respiratory tract. A minority of patients with GERD have reflux esophagitis, a term used to describe mucosal damage and inflammation.

Clinical presentation

The most common symptom of GERD is heartburn, which is described as substernal burning that moves orad from the xiphoid. Heartburn generally occurs after meals and may be relieved by acid-neutralizing agents. The frequency and severity of heartburn correlate poorly with endoscopically defined esophagitis. Patients with GERD may also present with substernal chest discomfort that mimics cardiac-related angina pectoris. Regurgitation of bitter or acid-tasting liquid is common. Water brash is the spontaneous appearance of salty fluid in the mouth from reflex salivary secretion in response to esophageal acid. Solid food dysphagia in a patient with GERD may be caused by either peptic strictures or adenocarcinoma from Barrett metaplasia. Note that odynophagia is not a common symptom associated with erosive esophagitis.

Extraesophageal manifestations of GERD include otolaryngological and pulmonary complications. Acid damage to the oropharynx may produce sore throat, earache, gingivitis, poor dentition, and globus, whereas reflux damage to the larynx and respiratory tract causes hoarseness, wheezing, bronchitis, asthma, and pneumonia. Vagally mediated bronchospasm may be initiated by acidification of the esophagus alone; thus, tracheal penetration by the refluxate is not required for the development of asthma with GERD.

Yamada's Handbook of Gastroenterology, Fourth Edition. John M. Inadomi, Renuka Bhattacharya, Joo Ha Hwang, and Cynthia Ko.

Diagnostic investigation

A history of classic heartburn is sufficient for diagnosing GERD and provides an adequate rationale for initiating therapy. The proton pump inhibitor (PPI) test, which evaluates symptom response to proton pump inhibition, is likewise as sensitive and specific as more invasive tests for diagnosing GERD. Diagnostic studies should be considered for patients with atypical symptoms, symptoms unresponsive to therapy, or warning signs of GERD complications or malignancy (e.g. dysphagia, gastrointestinal hemorrhage, weight loss, and anemia).

Upper gastrointestinal endoscopy

Upper gastrointestinal endoscopy is used to document reflux-induced mucosal injury and complications of GERD. Endoscopic findings in patients with GERD include normal mucosa, erythema, edema, friability, exudate, erosions, ulcers, strictures, and Barrett metaplasia. Histological hallmarks of esophagitis are increased height of the esophageal papillae and basal cell hyperplasia. Acute injury to the vascular bed, edema, and neutrophilic (and sometimes eosinophilic) infiltration indicate esophageal damage. Chronic inflammation is characterized by the presence of macrophages and granulation tissue. With severe injury, fibroblasts may deposit enough collagen to form a stricture. Long-standing acid damage also promotes aberrant repair of the mucosa by specialized columnar epithelium that contains goblet cells (i.e. Barrett metaplasia).

Ambulatory esophageal pH monitoring

Traditionally, ambulatory 24-hour pH monitoring is performed with a nasally inserted pH probe positioned 5 cm above the lower esophageal sphincter (LES). The patient is given an event marker to use with a recording device that is triggered to correlate symptoms with changes in esophageal pH. Maximal sensitivity (93%) and specificity (93%) are obtained by quantitating the percentage of time during which the pH is less than 4, using threshold values of 10.5% in the upright position and 6% in the supine position. Patients who exihibit esophageal acid exposure within physiological limits but have heartburn that correlates with acid reflux events may have a hypersensitive esophagus. Esophageal pH monitoring also can be used to correlate atypical symptoms, such as chest pain with acid reflux.

Wireless pH monitoring can also be used to obtain prolonged measurements of esophageal acid exposure. A miniature probe that is attached to the esophageal mucosa transmits data to a receiver worn by the patient. This system affords the ability to study the patient under conditions of more normal eating and physical activity, and to record esophageal pH over several days.

Impedance

Intralumenal electrical impedance is a technique that measures the conductance of the esophageal contents. This test relies on the electrical properties of liquids (low impedance and high conductance) and gases (high impedance and low conductance) to differentiate between liquid and gas reflux (belching). More importantly, impedance allows detection of nonacidic reflux that would otherwise not be detectable by esophageal pH monitoring, thereby allowing characterization of esophageal reflux as either acid or nonacid in content.

Esophageal manometry

Esophageal manometry generally is reserved for patients being considered for surgical antireflux procedures. Although GERD is a condition of disordered motility, the major finding is increased transient LES relaxation (TLESR). Manometric assessment of esophageal body peristalsis also is important preoperatively because documentation of abnormal peristalsis may influence the type of antireflux surgery chosen.

Key practice point

Tests that quantify the amount of acid refluxing into the esophagus are often inaccurate in classifying abnormal from normal (physiological) reflux. For this reason, a classic symptom of heartburn, especially with response to acid suppression with a PPI, is as reliable a test as pH monitoring. Esophageal manometry does not improve the accuracy because substantial variation in the frequency of TLESRs occurs between asymptomatic individuals, and 30–50% of patients with documented GERD have normal LES pressures.

Management of GERD

The course of GERD is highly variable; most patients require continuous medical therapy with acid suppression; however, some patients respond to intermittent (medication used daily for a predetermined duration) or on-demand (medication taken only when symptoms occur) strategies of medication, while others can discontinue medical therapy altogether after resolution of heartburn and acid regurgitation.

Lifestyle modification

The modification of lifestyle is an integral part of the initial management of GERD. The head of the bed should be elevated to enhance nocturnal esophageal acid clearance. Smoking and alcohol, which have deleterious effects on LES pressure, acid clearance, and epithelial function, should be avoided. Reducing meal size and limiting the intake of fat, carminatives, and chocolate limit gastric distension, lower TLESR incidence, and prevent LES pressure reductions. Caffeinated and decaffeinated coffee, tea, and carbonated beverages should be avoided because they stimulate acid production. Tomato juice and citrus products may exacerbate symptoms because of osmotic effects. Medications that reduce LES pressure should be limited whenever possible.

Key practice points: Lifestyle modifications for patients with gastroesophageal reflux

- Elevate the head of the bed 6 in.
- Stop smoking
- Stop excessive ethanol consumption
- Reduce dietary fat
- Reduce meal size
- Avoid bedtime snacks
- Reduce weight (if overweight)
- Avoid specific foods
  - Chocolate
  - Carminatives (e.g. spearmint, peppermint)
  - Coffee (caffeinated, decaffeinated)
  - Tea
  - Cola beverages
  - Tomato juice
  - Citrus fruit juices
- Avoid specific medications (if possible)
  - Anticholinergics
  - Theophylline
  - Benzodiazepines
  - Opiates
  - Calcium channel antagonists
  - β-Adrenergic agonists
  - Progesterone (some contraceptives)
  - α-Adrenergic antagonists

Medication therapy for GERD

PPIs are the most effective drugs to treat erosive esophagitis or symptomatic GERD. These H^+, K^+-adenosine triphosphatase antagonists produce superior acid suppression compared with H_2 receptor antagonists. While many retrospective studies raise concerns about adverse events associated with PPIs such as bone fracture, drug interaction, magnesium deficiency, *Clostridioides difficile* infection, or pneumonia, the absolute incidence of these events is exceedingly low and these associations have not been proven causal. In fact, the only adverse association with an annual incidence >1% is spontaneous bacterial peritonitis in cirrhotics. However, these concerns highlight the need to use the lowest dose of acid suppression necessary to achieve therapeutic goals.

For patients with intermittent or mild symptoms, antacids, and H_2 receptor antagonists provide rapid, safe, and effective relief from GERD symptoms. High-dose regimens may heal erosive disease; however, the required doses often induce significant side-effects (e.g. diarrhea with magnesium antacids and constipation with aluminum antacids) that make compliance difficult. Gaviscon (aluminum hydroxide and magnesium carbonate), an antacid-alginate combination, decreases reflux by producing a viscous mechanical barrier but it may also adversely affect bowel function. Sucralfate, the basic salt of aluminum hydroxide and sucrose octasulfate, acts topically to increase tissue resistance, buffer acid, and bind pepsin and bile salts, but its efficacy in treating patients with GERD is limited. H_2 receptor antagonists (e.g. cimetidine, ranitidine, famotidine, and nizatidine) are safe and effective for treating mild disease.

Prokinetic agents have been used as primary or adjunctive therapy for GERD. Cisapride, an agent that acts on serotonin 5-HT_4 receptors to facilitate myenteric acetylcholine release, promotes gastric emptying and increases LES pressure and was approved for treating GERD. However, it has been withdrawn from the market because of increased risk of cardiac arrhythmias. Emerging motility therapies include γ-aminobutyric acid (GABA) B agonists and mGluR5-negative allosteric modulators (inhibitors). These drugs have been shown in clinical trials to reduce TLESRs and reduce GERD symptoms; however, none is available at the time of this printing.

Treatment strategy for GERD

Most patients with heartburn self-medicate with over-the-counter antacids, H_2 receptor antagonists, or PPIs. Those who do not respond to therapy or those who initially respond but relapse may seek medical attention. In such individuals, the clinician should consider alternative causes of heartburn, including nonacid reflux, functional heartburn, and malignancy (Figure 17.1). The first step is to determine the presence of "alarm" symptoms or signs such as bleeding, anemia, dysphagia, or weight loss that may suggest the presence of upper gastrointestinal malignancy. Upper endoscopy is indicated if any of these factors is present. In the absence of alarm features, it is reasonable to assess whether an adequate trial of acid suppression has been attempted because most other disorders respond variably to acid suppression. PPIs are the most potent class of medications used to treat GERD; therefore, the use of these drugs is advocated. Note that most PPIs reduce symptoms of GERD most effectively if taken 30–60 minutes before ingesting a meal.

If symptoms are not relieved, ambulatory esophageal pH monitoring may differentiate individuals with persistent acid reflux who may require higher doses of acid suppression from individuals without abnormal esophageal acid exposure (Figure 17.2). The latter group comprises patients with nonacid reflux, which can be diagnosed by esophageal impedance testing, patients with esophageal acid hypersensitivity (pH within physiological limits but positive symptom

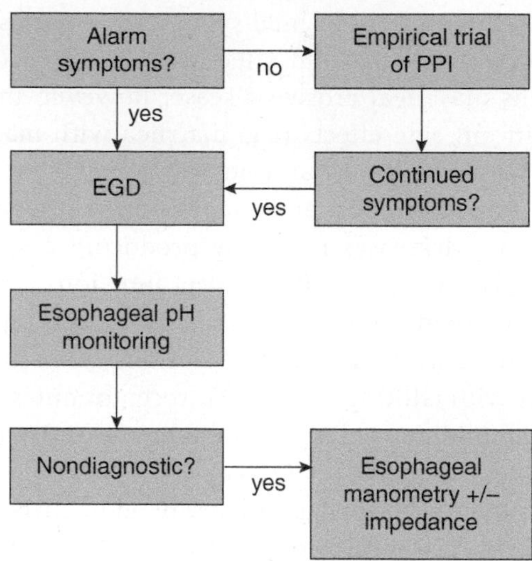

Figure 17.1 Evaluation of heartburn. EGD, esophagogastroduodenoscopy; PPI, proton pump inhibitor.

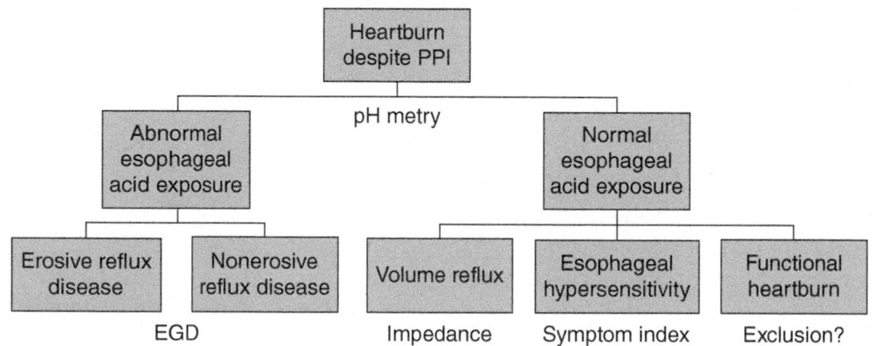

Figure 17.2 Evaluation of heartburn refractory to acid suppression. EGD, esophagogastroduodenoscopy; PPI, proton pump inhibitor.

index) and patients who have functional heartburn (normal acid exposure, absence of nonacid reflux, and poor correlation between symptoms and reflux [symptom index]).

Potential pitfalls

Dyspepsia (discomfort in the upper abdomen) without heartburn or acid regurgitation should be managed differently from GERD and generally requires upper gastrointestinal endoscopy to examine the disorders under this differential diagnosis.

Evaluation for the presence of *Helicobacter pylori* is reasonable for patients presenting with dyspepsia; however, *H. pylori* is not a cause of GERD and eradication will not alleviate heartburn.

Baclofen and other agents that reduce TLESRs may be a reasonable therapy for nonacid reflux. Hypersensitivity may respond to greater acid suppression. Functional heartburn management remains problematic but therapy aimed at decreasing esophageal sensation may be useful (e.g. trazodone, tricyclics).

Surgical treatment of GERD

Antireflux surgery has been demonstrated to be an effective and safe treatment of GERD. A five-year randomized clinical trial comparing laparoscopic antireflux surgery versus esomeprazole in patients with chronic GERD reported no difference in rates of long-term remission from symptoms (Long-Term Usage of Esomeprazole vs Surgery for Treatment of Chronic GERD, or LOTUS). Mortality during the study was low (four deaths in the esomeprazole group and one death in the surgical group) and not attributed to treatment, and the percentages of patients reporting serious adverse events were similar in the esomeprazole group (24.1%) and in the surgical group (28.6%).

Complications and their management

Strictures caused by gastroesophageal reflux are characterized by progressive dysphagia over months to years. Although strictures may be defined radiographically, endoscopy is required in all cases to exclude malignancy. Esophageal bougienage dilation may be performed without (Maloney, Hurst) or with (Savary) endoscopic guidance, or may be accomplished using through-the-scope balloon dilation. Hemorrhage may occasionally develop from esophageal erosions and ulcers. Perforation of an esophageal ulcer is a serious complication that may cause life-threatening mediastinitis.

Barrett esophagus is an acquired condition in which squamous epithelium is replaced by specialized columnar epithelium in response to chronic acid exposure. The clinical consequence of intestinal metaplasia is the development of esophageal adenocarcinoma. Barrett metaplasia is present in 5–15% of patients with GERD who undergo endoscopy. The management of patients with Barrett esophagus is described in detail in Chapter 18. Hemorrhage may occasionally develop from esophageal erosions and ulcers. It may be chronic, with production of iron deficiency anemia, or acute. Perforation of an esophageal ulcer is a serious complication that may cause life-threatening mediastinitis.

Alkaline reflux esophagitis

Alkaline reflux esophagitis develops from prolonged contact of esophageal epithelium with nonacidic gastric or intestinal contents, usually in patients who have undergone ulcer surgery with vagotomy or, less commonly, in patients with achlorhydria who have not undergone surgery. Factors responsible for mucosal damage include deconjugated bile salts and pancreatic enzymes. Medications that may be effective include bile salt-binding agents (e.g. cholestyramine, colestipol, sucralfate) and mucosal coating agents (e.g. antacids). When medications fail, a Roux-en-Y gastrojejunostomy may divert intestinal contents away from the esophagus. Alternatively, fundoplication may be performed in patients with intact stomachs or adequate gastric remnants.

Eosinophilic Esophagitis

Eosinophilic esophagitis is a chronic, immune-mediated motility disturbance characterized by eosinophil-predominant inflammation. The pathogenesis is believed to be an interaction between genetic, environmental, and host-immune response factors, and is more prevalent in males. Prior definitions separated EoE from "proton pump inhibitor responsive esophageal eosinophilia"; however, newer guidelines have reclassified both as forms of eosinophilic esophagitis.

Clinical Presentation

Eosinophilic esophagitis presents with solid food dysphagia, chest and/or abdominal pain and food impaction. Males are more commonly affected and many have evidence of atopy.

Diagnostic Investigation

Eosinophilic esophagitis usually presents with solid food dysphagia, the differential diagnosis for which is broad and includes peptic strictures, Schatzki rings, motility disorders and neoplasia in addition to eosinophilic esophagitis. Individuals suspected to have eosinophilic esophagitis should undergo upper gastrointestinal endoscopy and assessment for food allergen using delayed skin patch testing.

Upper endoscopy is the primary tool for diagnosing eosinophilic esophagitis. There is a validated endoscopic scoring system to assess the presence of edema, rings, exudates, furrows, and strictures that are characteristic of eosinophilic esophagitis. Histopathological criteria for eosinophilic esophagitis include >15 eosinophils per high power field in both proximal and distal esophageal biopsies (compared with up to seven eosinophils per high power field in distal esophageal biopsies found in GERD). Eosinophilic micro-abscesses, dilated intercellular space, increased mast cells and IgE-bearing cells are also found in eosinophilic esophagitis.

Treatment

Dietary management of eosinophilic esophagitis

Some patients with eosinophilic esophagitis respond to avoidance of a specific food allergen. The six-food elimination diet requires avoidance of the most common triggers including cow milk, soy, wheat, egg, peanut/tree nuts and seafood/shellfish, and provides a similar response rate as skin test-directed diet (74–81%); however, adherence to this diet is difficult.

Medication to treat eosinophilic esophagitis

There is a defined subgroup of patients in whom the esophageal eosinophilia responds to PPIs, termed *PPI-responsive esophageal eosinophilia*. In addition, GERD is common among patients with eosinophilic esophagitis and can contribute to the inflammation causing symptoms. For these reasons, PPI therapy is the first-line treatment of eosinophilic esophagitis.

Systemic and topical glucocorticoids have been demonstrated to successfully alleviate symptoms. Fluticasone administered by swallowing drug from a metered-dose inhaler (440–880 mcg twice daily) or budesonide 1 mg mixed with sucralose (Splenda) to create a slurry swallowed twice daily have been shown in clinical trials to induce remission.

Drugs targeted to the eosinophilic inflammation have been tested; however, symptom response has been variable despite achieving reductions in eosinophilic tissue inflammation using IL-5 specific antibodies (mepolizumab, reslizumab). Trials of antibodies directed toward other cytokines, adhesion molecules, or eosinophil-active chemokines are ongoing.

Complications and their management

Strictures caused by eosinophilic esophagitis can also be safely treated by endoscopic dilation using through-the-scope balloons or wire-guided bougie. Gradual dilation is recommended with a target diameter of 15–18 mm with each session increasing by no more than 3 mm after resistance is encountered.

Case Studies

Case 1

A 34 year-old man presents with chronic heartburn described as a burning sensation behind his sternum rising to his throat associated with regurgitation of acidic contents. He was prescribed PPIs that only partially relieve his heartburn and regurgitation; however, he discontinued this drug due to fear about infections. Upper endoscopy reveals a 2 cm hiatal hernia, but is otherwise normal without esophagitis. Ambulatory esophageal pH is notable for 8.7% of total time pH <4 and impedance reveals multiple non-acid reflux events that correlate with symptoms of regurgitation.

You discuss the low absolute risk of PPIs and reinitiate omeprazole 40 mg daily plus baclofen 20 mg orally three times daily and his symptoms greatly improve.

Discussion

The risks of long-term PPI use are greatly exaggerated. The absolute risk of bone fracture, magnesium deficiency, *C. difficile* infection, renal disease, dementia, or pneumonia is <1% annually, with the exception of spontaneous bacterial peritonitis among patients with cirrhosis, which is estimated to be 3–16% excess risk per year. This patient displays non-acidic in addition to acid reflux disease. Baclofen (10–20 mg three times daily) is an effective drug to reduce TLESRs that lead to reflux episodes. Non-acid reflux may also be effectively treated using surgical antireflux procedures.

Case 2

A 19 year-old man presents to the emergency department with symptoms of food impaction. He describes similar symptoms in the past, but this is the first time he has not been able to regurgitate the food bolus. He has no heartburn and between these episodes of dysphagia feels completely well. Endoscopy reveals a 1 cm × 2 cm piece of chicken that is removed with a snare from the lower esophagus (using an esophageal overtube to protect the airway). No stricture is noted, but the proximal and mid-esophagus is notable for linear furrows and multiple concentric rings. Biopsies from both regions of the esophagus reveal 30 eosinophils per high power field. You prescribe omeprazole 40 mg twice daily and repeat the endoscopy in eight weeks, but the eosinophil count does not improve. You change therapy to budesonide slurry (4 × 0.5 mg/2 ml pulmonary respules mixed with sucralose to a volume of 8 ml) twice daily and repeated endoscopy confirms <5 eosinophils per high power field.

Discussion

Eosinophilic esophagitis affects young men more frequently than other groups. The endoscopic appearance of linear furrows, concentric rings and narrowed lumen are suggestive of the diagnosis. Greater than 15 eosinophils per high power field in the correct clinical context is diagnostic of this disorder. The initial therapy should consist of acid suppression with PPIs because some patients respond to this intervention. Non-response to acid suppression can be managed by either topical steroids (budesonide or swallowed fluticasone 880 mcg–1.5 mg twice daily) or elimination diet in which the most common food triggers are avoided (dairy, soy, wheat, eggs, nuts, seafood) and endoscopy is repeated to evaluate histologic response.

Further reading

Furuta, G.T. and Katzka, D.A. (2015). Eosinophilic esophagitis. *N. Engl. J. Med.* 373 (17): 1640–1648.

Galmiche, J.P., Hatlebakk, J., Attwood, S. et al. (2011). Laparoscopic antireflux surgery vs esomeprazole treatment for chronic GERD: The LOTUS randomized clinical trial. *JAMA* 305 (19): 1969–1977.

CHAPTER 18
Esophageal Neoplasia

Adenocarcinoma

Barrett esophagus, which is replacement of esophageal squamous mucosa with specialized columnar epithelium, is the only known risk factor for esophageal adenocarcinoma (EAC). The mechanism by which reflux of gastric contents into the esophagus induces the metaplastic response is unknown. The annual rate of cancer development among patients with Barrett esophagus is about 0.12–0.33%.

Genomic instability is common in dysplastic Barrett mucosa. Aneuploid cell populations and deletions or alterations of tumor suppressor genes, particularly chromosomal regions 17p (*p53*), 5q (*APC,MCC*), 18q (*DCC*), and 13q (*RB1*), are often observed in the mucosa of patients who develop carcinoma. Abnormalities of cell proliferation, as evidenced by the expression of proliferating cell nuclear antigen (PCNA) and Ki-67, are noted in Barrett tissue and EAC. Microsatellite instability, a marker of defective mismatch repair, has also been detected in patients with Barrett esophagus and EAC.

Clinical presentation

Barrett esophagus does not produce symptoms and the endoscopic appearance of Barrett mucosa correlates poorly with the severity of reflux symptoms, which is why screening to detect Barrett esophagus is difficult. The clinical manifestations of EAC include progressive dysphagia, nausea, vomiting, weight loss, and anemia. Symptoms attributable to adenocarcinoma occur in advanced stages when the tumor is large enough to interfere with swallowing. Based on the pathogenesis of EAC and Barrett esophagus, chronic heartburn, acid regurgitation, and chest pain due to gastroesophageal reflux are common.

Yamada's Handbook of Gastroenterology, Fourth Edition. John M. Inadomi, Renuka Bhattacharya, Joo Ha Hwang, and Cynthia Ko.

Diagnostic investigation

Endoscopic studies

Barrett esophagus is diagnosed using upper gastrointestinal endoscopy with biopsy, and requires the presence of circumferential or islands (tongues) of salmon-colored mucosa proximal to the esophagogastric junction in which there is histological confirmation of intestinal metaplasia. The Prague C and M criteria describe the circumferential ("C") and maximum ("M") length of columnar-appearing mucosa. Biopsy specimens should be targeted to all erosions, nodules, and strictures that may indicate the presence of dysplasia, as well as randomly obtained from flat-appearing columnar mucosa.

Histological evaluation

The interpretation of biopsy samples from patients with Barrett esophagus requires the expertise of an experienced gastrointestinal pathologist. There is a high degree of inter-observer variation in distinguishing low-grade dysplasia (LGD) from no dysplasia due to misinterpretation of regenerative changes from reflux-induced inflammation. It may be difficult or impossible to distinguish high-grade dysplasia (HGD) from invasive carcinoma if biopsy samples fail to include the lamina propria; therefore, large-capacity or jumbo forceps should be used when sampling areas of Barrett esophagus. Flow cytometry has been used to identify aneuploid or tetraploid cell populations and shows considerable promise in predicting the development of EAC. Other markers of cell proliferation such as PCNA, Ki-67, tritiated thymidine uptake, and ornithine decarboxylase may be predictive; however, the ability of these tests to affect clinical practice positively has not been established.

> **Diagnostic pitfalls**
>
> Currently the US definition of Barrett esophagus requires endoscopically abnormal (columnar) mucosa in conjunction with histological confirmation of specialized intestinal metaplasia (presence of goblet cells). The British Society of Gastroenterology criteria allow the definition of Barrett esophagus to include other types of metaplastic epithelium, including gastric and junctional (cardiac) epithelium. Because the natural history of Barrett esophagus with regard to cancer risk is still poorly defined, limiting the definition of Barrett esophagus to the entity for which most data are available (intestinal metaplasia) has been accepted by US national society guidelines.

Management

Screening and surveillance

Identification of the link between Barrett esophagus and EAC has led to the implementation of endoscopic screening and surveillance programs (Table 18.1). The strategy proposed by several national societies includes screening patients with multiple risk factors for EAC (age 50 years or older, male sex, white race,

Table 18.1 Management of Barrett esophagus

Barrett esophagus with:	Recommendation
No dysplasia	Endoscopic surveillance with biopsies every three to five years
Low-grade dysplasia (LGD)	Endoscopic surveillance with biopsies every six months × 2, every 12 months thereafter; or endoscopic eradication therapy if LGD is confirmed after 8–12 weeks of high-dose proton pump inhibitor
High-grade dysplasia (HGD)	Endoscopic eradication therapy (endoscopic mucosal resection, radiofrequency ablation, photodynamic therapy)
Esophageal adenocarcinoma (EAC)	Endoscopic excision (T1a) or surgical esophagectomy

chronic symptoms of gastroesophageal reflux disease, hiatal hernia, elevated body mass index, intra-abdominal distribution of body fat, family history of Barrett esophagus or EAC) to detect Barrett esophagus using upper gastrointestinal endoscopy. If intestinal metaplasia is histologically confirmed in a region of the esophagus that has columnar-appearing mucosa, surveillance with high-resolution white-light endoscopy should be performed at intervals dependent on the presence and degree of dysplasia. Current guidelines suggest taking systematic four-quadrant biopsy specimens every 2 cm along the length of Barrett metaplasia. In addition, any endoscopic abnormalities such as erosions, nodules, or strictures should be biopsied because these may harbor dysplasia or cancer.

Patients with no dysplasia are recommended to undergo surveillance at an interval between three and five years. Patients in whom LGD is diagnosed should have surveillance with four-quadrant biopsies every 1 cm performed every six months ×2, and every 12 months thereafter, or be considered for endoscopic eradication therapy if LGD is confirmed by repeated endoscopy with biopsies after eight weeks treatment with high-dose proton pump inhibitor therapy. HGD must be confirmed on review by an experienced pathologist. Confirmation of HGD prompts a recommendation for endoscopic eradication therapy, which should be initiated with removal of all visible lesions (ulcers, nodules, masses) associated with dysplasia by endoscopic mucosal resection or endoscopic submucosal dissection, which are both therapeutic and diagnostic by confirming the absence of invasive cancer. Radiofrequency ablation or cryotherapy can be applied to the remaining flat Barrett segment. Invasive cancer should be staged using endoscopic ultrasound. T1a lesions are amenable to endoscopic excision; more advanced cancers should be treated by surgical resection.

Case–control studies illustrate a potential survival benefit from endoscopic surveillance of patients with Barrett esophagus; however, prospective studies to confirm the efficacy of surveillance are lacking.

Molecular markers for the presence of Barrett esophagus, dysplasia, and cancer are under development; however, markers have not been validated to predict which patients with Barrett esophagus are at risk for progression. Furthermore, advanced imaging techniques such as chromoendoscopy have not been shown to improve the clinical outcomes of patients with Barrett esophagus and are not recommended for routine use at this time.

Diagnostic pitfalls

LGD has been a source of controversy regarding the risk of cancer. While some studies report increased incidence of adenocarcinoma, other studies illustrate cancer risk to be low and similar to the risk among patients with no dysplasia. One of the reasons for the difference may be the poor inter- and intra-observer correlation in the diagnosis of LGD. Inflammation, which is a necessary component of gastroesophageal reflux disease, can cause morphologically similar changes to dysplasia. For this reason, patients diagnosed with LGD should be treated with a high-dose proton pump inhibitor therapy for 8–12 weeks and undergo repeated endoscopy with biopsies. If LGD is confirmed, endoscopic eradication therapy can be considered.

Squamous Cell Carcinoma

Squamous cell carcinoma (SCC) is the most common malignant tumor of the esophagus worldwide. Men have a threefold higher risk than women and in the United States, African-Americans have a fivefold increased risk for SCC relative to whites. The geographic variation in the prevalence of SCC shows the importance of environmental factors in its pathogenesis. Alcohol and tobacco consumption increase the risk for SCC in a dose-dependent manner. This effect appears to be synergistic because the risk for patients who smoke and drink excessively is much higher than the risk for patients who use either substance alone. Deficiencies of vitamins A, C, E, and B_{12}, folic acid, and riboflavin are risk factors for cancer.

Achalasia is associated with a 30-fold increase in the rate of SCC (absolute risk 3.4 per 1000 patient-years). Synchronous or metachronous esophageal SCC develops at an annual rate of 3–7% in patients with SCC of the head and neck. Tylosis, a rare autosomal dominant condition characterized by hyperkeratosis of the palms and soles, is highly linked with esophageal SCC. Lye ingestion that causes an esophageal stricture has been associated with development of squamous cell tumors. Other factors associated with esophageal SCC include ionizing radiation, celiac disease, human papillomavirus, Plummer–Vinson syndrome, and esophageal diverticula.

Clinical presentation

Patients with esophageal SCC present with progressive dysphagia. Odynophagia and weight loss may occur as well as nausea, vomiting, hematemesis, and back pain. Involvement of adjacent mediastinal strictures may result in chronic cough caused by a tracheo-esophageal fistula, hoarseness caused by recurrent laryngeal nerve involvement, and, rarely, massive gastrointestinal hemorrhage due to invasion into the aorta.

A generalized loss of muscle mass and subcutaneous fat is often evident. In patients with early disease, the physical examination findings may be normal but patients with metastatic disease may exhibit hepatomegaly, bony pain, and supraclavicular adenopathy.

Diagnostic investigation

Endoscopic studies

Solid food dysphagia should be evaluated with upper endoscopy. Early cancers can be detected as elevated plaques or small erythematous erosions. All mucosal abnormalities should undergo biopsy for histological examination. Because a sampling error occasionally leads to false-negative results, any lesion that highly suggests malignancy should be rebiopsied.

Radiographic studies

The diagnostic evaluation of patients with dysphagia traditionally began with esophageal radiological imaging. The sensitivity of barium swallow radiography for detecting early lesions is only 75%, which limits its usefulness as a screening test. Fluoroscopic examination can often detect motility abnormalities or proximal diverticula that may not be appreciated in endoscopic studies. However, some malignancies produce a smooth symmetrical stricture, which precludes barium radiographs from reliably distinguishing tumors from benign peptic strictures. For these reasons, endoscopy has become the first-line evaluation for patients presenting with dysphagia.

Staging of EAC and SCC

Esophageal cancer should be staged on the basis of the depth of invasion (T stage), the nodal status (N stage), and the presence of distant metastatic disease (M stage). Staging helps determine the therapeutic approach and assess the prognosis (Table 18.2). The tools for staging include computed tomography (CT) combined with positron emission tomography (PET) scan, and endoscopic ultrasound. Although a sensitive means of documenting aortic invasion or pulmonary and hepatic metastases, CT has low accuracy in determining nodal involvement and magnetic resonance imaging does not provide an advantage over CT. Endoscopic ultrasound is superior to CT for determining the T and N stages in all types of esophageal tumors, and is therefore an important tool for predicting resectability. Endoscopic ultrasound has accuracy rates of about 90 and 85% for establishing the T and N stages of a tumor, respectively.

Table 18.2 TNM staging system for cancer of the esophagus (American Joint Committee on Cancer criteria)

Primary tumor (T)			
TX	Primary tumor cannot be assessed		
T0	No evidence of primary tumor		
Tis	Carcinoma in situ		
T1	Tumor invades lamina propria (T1a) or submucosa (T1b)		
T2	Tumor invades muscularis propria		
T3	Tumor invades adventitia		
T4	Tumor invades adjacent structures		
Lymph node (N)			
NX	Regional lymph nodes cannot be assessed		
N0	No regional lymph node metastasis		
N1	Regional lymph node metastasis		
Distant metastasis (M)			
MX	Presence of distant metastasis cannot be assessed		
M0	No distant metastasis		
M1	Distant metastasis		
M1a	Metastasis in celiac (lower esophagus) or cervical lymph nodes (upper esophagus)		
M1b	Other distant metastasis (lower or upper esophagus) or nonregional lymph nodes (mid-esophagus)		
Stage grouping			
0	Tis		
I	T1	N0	M0
IIA	T2	N0	M0
	T3	N0	M0
IIB	T1	N0	M0
	T2	N1	M0
III	T3	N1	M0
	T4	N1	M0
IV	Any T	Any N	M0
IVA	Any T	Any N	M1
IVB	Any T	Any N	M1a

Source: reproduced with permission from Edge et al. (2010).

Treatment of EAC and SCC

Therapeutic approaches for esophageal SCC and EAC are similar. Endoscopic excision may be performed for cancer confined to the mucosa (T1a). Surgical resection is the primary therapy for patients with tumors that extend beyond the mucosa, but are confined to the esophagus. However, because of the advanced stage at which most esophageal cancers are diagnosed, surgical exploration is indicated in only 60% of patients, of whom only two-thirds are able to undergo resection. Overall, the one- and five-year survival rates are 18 and 5%, respectively. Although curative resection is unlikely for T3 or N1 lesions, palliative resection can provide one to two years of symptom-free survival. Locally advanced (T4) or metastatic (M1) disease is not amenable to curative resection, and the poor long-term survival of these patients makes surgical palliation an unfavorable option.

High rates of recurrence have prompted trials of perioperative chemotherapy and radiation therapy to improve systemic and regional control of the tumor. Combination chemoradiotherapy, either neoadjuvant or peri-operative, is superior to radiotherapy alone. Definitive chemoradiotherapy has been shown to be equivalent to surgical therapy in patients with SCC; however, surgery with chemoradiotherapy is still favored for patients with EAC.

There are several accepted surgical approaches to treating esophageal cancer including transhiatal esophagectomy and transthoracic esophagectomy. The choice of procedure depends on tumor location, lymph node status, the patient's body habitus and performance status, and the preference of the surgeon and institution. With the increase in incidence of EAC in the distal esophagus, transhiatal resection and primary anastomosis has become the most common mode of therapy. Complications include anastomotic leak or stricture, pulmonary disease (e.g. pneumonia, pulmonary emboli), recurrent laryngeal nerve injury, and cardiac disease (e.g. myocardial infarction, arrhythmia, and congestive heart failure).

Palliative therapy for esophageal cancer is primarily achieved with endoscopic placement of self-expanding metal stents to treat esophageal obstruction. In addition, coated stents may be placed across tracheo-esophageal fistulae to allow patients to swallow saliva and food without aspirating. Complications associated with stents include stent migration, chest pain, perforation, and bleeding. Endoscopic therapy using laser, argon plasma coagulation, or bipolar electrocautery may also help to relieve obstruction. Photodynamic therapy consists of administering a photosensitizer, followed by local exposure of the tumor to light of a specific wavelength (630 nm). Tumor destruction occurs as a result of singlet oxygen production that leads to ischemia and necrosis. Systemic chemotherapy with paclitaxel, docetaxel, gemcitabine, irinotecan, and oxaliplatin has shown response rates up to 60%, including increased survival and quality of life.

Essentials of treatment

- Stage T1a: endoscopic resection
- Stage T1b – III: neoadjuvant chemoradioation followed by esophagectomy. Alternatives include perioperative chemotherapy and esophagectomy, or definitive chemoradiation for patients who are not candidates for surgery
- Metastatic disease: test tumor for HER2/Neu amplification: if positive treat with Trastuzumab-based regimen; if negative treat with multi-agent chemotherapy based on patient's performance status (5-FU and cisplatin, or paclitaxel, docetaxel, gemcitabine, irinotecan, oxaliplatin)
- Palliative: radiation therapy, endoscopic stent

Other Malignant Neoplasms

Epithelial tumors

A variant of SCC characterized by a prominent spindle cell component has been variably termed *carcinosarcoma, pseudo-sarcoma, spindle cell carcinoma*, or *polypoid carcinoma*. These lesions are large and polypoid and may be solitary or multiple. Men are affected more often than women, and most are middle-aged or elderly at the time of presentation. Another variant of SCC is termed *verrucous carcinoma* because the primary lesion grows slowly and invades local tissues with only rare metastases. Adenoid cystic carcinomas are rare tumors resemble salivary adenoid cystic carcinoma and develop in elderly males. Adenosquamous carcinomas or adenoacanthomas combine features of the two common forms of esophageal cancer. Mucoepidermoid carcinoma, also composed of glandular and squamous elements, develops in the middle-to-distal esophagus and has a poor prognosis. Melanoma of the esophagus may be primary or metastatic, although the esophagus is a less common site of metastatic gastrointestinal disease than the stomach, small intestine, or colon.

Neuroendocrine tumors of the esophagus include small cell carcinomas, carcinoids, and choriocarcinomas. Small cell carcinoma of the esophagus may be a primary esophageal tumor or it may represent a metastatic lesion from the lung. Neoplasia may be associated with a paraneoplastic phenomenon, including inappropriate antidiuretic hormone secretion and hypercalcemia.

Nonepithelial tumors

Malignant nonepithelial tumors of the esophagus include leiomyosarcomas, metastatic cancers, and lymphomas. Metastatic lesions are most commonly due to melanoma, followed by breast cancer; less common etiologies include gastric, renal, liver, prostate, testicular, bone, skin, lung, and head and neck cancer. Primary esophageal lymphoma may be of the Hodgkin or non-Hodgkin type and is more common among immunocompromised patients.

Benign Esophageal Tumors

Leiomyomas are the most common benign esophageal tumor. Most are asymptomatic but large tumors may cause dysphagia or chest pain. They occur most commonly in the distal esophagus and occur twice as frequently in men as women. Large benign leiomyomas may be difficult to distinguish from rare malignant leiomyosarcomas.

Granular cell tumors are smooth, sessile, small polypoid lesions that generally occur in the distal esophagus. They are derived from neural or Schwann cells, and malignant transformation is rare. Fibrovascular polyps are rare and may prolapse into the larynx causing dysphagia, nausea, vomiting, or bleeding from ulceration. Lymphangiomas are easily compressed during endoscopy and translucent, differentiating them from leiomyomas that are opaque and firm. Lipomas and fibromas can also form in the esophagus and have no malignant potential. Squamous cell papillomas are small, sessile, polypoid lesions discovered incidentally during endoscopic examination for unrelated symptoms. Papillomas usually are solitary and are located in the distal third of the esophagus. They may be associated with chronic irritation from gastroesophageal reflux disease or may result from infection with human papillomavirus. Cancer development has not been documented in these neoplasms.

Further reading

Edge, S.B., Byrd, D.R., Compton, C.C. et al. (2010). *AJCC Cancer Staging Manual*, 7e. New York: Springer.

Shaheen, N.J., Falk, G., Iyer, P.G., and Gerson, L.B. (2016). ACG clinical guideline: diagnosis and management of Barrett's esophagus. *Am. J. Gastroenterol.* 111: 30–50.

Wani, S., Rubenstein, J.H., Vieth, M., and Bergman, J. (2016). American Gastroenterological Association clinical practice update: diagnosis and management of low-grade dysplasia in Barrett's esophagus. *Gastroenterology* 151: 822–835.

CHAPTER 19
Disorders of Gastric Emptying

Disorders of gastric motility can be classified as those with delayed or accelerated emptying, and disorders with motor and sensory abnormalities. While there are variety of disorders that are associated with gastroparesis (delayed gastric emptying), accelerated emptying is clinically relevant only among patients who have undergone surgical intervention that includes vagotomy and gastric drainage. This chapter focuses on the disorders of delayed or accelerated gastric emptying and a separate chapter (Chapter 21) focuses on disorders with motor and sensory abnormalities including functional dyspepsia.

Disorders with Delayed Gastric Emptying (Gastroparesis)

Clinical presentation

Symptoms of gastroparesis include nausea, vomiting, early satiety, postprandial fullness and in some patients, upper abdominal pain. Late postprandial vomiting of undigested food (>one hour after meals) is typical of gastroparesis, in contrast to rumination syndrome in which regurgitation occurs during or within one hour of a meal. The character of abdominal pain in gastroparesis is usually burning, vague, or cramping.

Diagnostic investigation

Laboratory studies

Laboratory studies may assist in determining the severity and chronicity of the patient's disorder. Hypokalemia and contraction alkalosis result from severe vomiting, whereas anemia and hypoproteinemia are consistent with long-standing malnutrition. Specific serological tests may suggest rheumatological diseases such as systemic lupus erythematosus or scleroderma, whereas antineuronal antibody tests can screen for paraneoplastic dysmotility syndromes. Blood tests also can detect diabetes, uremia, or thyroid and parathyroid disease.

Yamada's Handbook of Gastroenterology, Fourth Edition. John M. Inadomi, Renuka Bhattacharya, Joo Ha Hwang, and Cynthia Ko.

Radiographic and endoscopic studies

Patients should undergo structural evaluation to exclude mechanical obstruction. Abdominal radiography screen for obstruction of the small intestine. Ultrasound can detect biliary disease. Upper gastrointestinal endoscopy is appropriate if gastric outlet obstruction secondary to peptic ulcer disease or malignancy is suspected.

Functional testing

Gastric scintigraphic quantitation of gastric emptying is the standard for diagnosing gastroparesis. Solid-phase gastric-emptying scintigraphic images using ^{99m}Tc-sulfur colloid mixed with a solid food such as scrambled eggs exhibit a biphasic emptying profile: an initial lag phase followed by a linear emptying phase, which persists until all digestible residues have been expelled by the stomach. In normal controls, 95% of a solid meal is emptied within four hours of ingestion. The result of a gastric emptying scan should be used in patient management in conjunction with the clinical presentation because some profoundly symptomatic patients will exhibit normal emptying, whereas other asymptomatic individuals may show pronounced gastric retention.

The SmartPill is an ingestible capsule that simultaneously measures pressure, temperature and pH, and transmits this information to a portable recording device wirelessly. With regard to gastric emptying, this technology can measure gastric emptying (and total gastrointestinal transit time) as well as pressure patterns and motility indices for the stomach (and small and large intestine). The "gastric residence time" of the SmartPill can differentiate normal from delayed gastric emptying and has a correlation with scintigraphy of approximately 85%.

Other tests of upper gut function are performed in selected cases in referral centers. Electrogastrography (EGG) noninvasively measures gastric electrical activity. EGG detects disruptions in slow-wave rhythm that are too rapid (tachygastria) or too slow (bradygastria) as well as abnormal electrical responses to meal ingestion in some patients with nausea and vomiting. Abnormal EGGs are demonstrated in approximately 70% of patients with delayed gastric emptying; thus the technique has been proposed as another means of testing gastric emptying.

Antroduodenal manometry involves the peroral or transnasal placement of a catheter that monitors pressure changes during a six to eight-hour period. Specifically, fasting motility should illustrate the migrating motor complex, while the characteristic fed motor pattern should be seen one to two hours after a meal.

Essentials of diagnosis and potential pitfalls

While gastric emptying studies are the standard for the diagnosis of gastroparesis, the accuracy of these tests is suboptimal. Even a four-hour solid-phase test can be normal in patients who are known to have emptying delays; conversely, the test can be abnormal in normal controls. While more accurate, gastroduodenal manometry and EGG have limited clinical utility and should be considered research tools at this time.

Differential Diagnosis

Diabetic gastroparesis

Patients with long-standing insulin-dependent diabetes may develop gastroparesis. Motor abnormalities that contribute to delays in gastric emptying include impaired fundic relaxation, loss of antral contractions, gastric dysrhythmias, antroduodenal dyscoordination, and visceral hypersensitivity. The degree of hyperglycemia can exacerbate delays in gastric emptying in diabetics.

> **Essentials of diagnosis and potential pitfalls**
>
> Diabetic gastroparesis is due to a neuropathy and generally coincides with other complications of diabetes mellitus including retinopathy, nephropathy, and peripheral neuropathy. Orthostatic hypotension may be present as a manifestation of autonomic neuropathy. While generally a complication of type 1 diabetes, gastroparesis can also occur in patients with type 2 diabetes. Note that hyperglycemia itself (blood glucose >230 mg/dl) decreases antral contractility, induces gastric dysrhythmias and delays gastric emptying; however, this is a reversible phenomenon and not necessarily indicative of neuropathy.

Postsurgical gastroparesis

A minority of patients who have undergone gastric surgery for peptic ulcer disease or malignancy experience nausea, vomiting, and early satiety secondary to postoperative stasis. Abnormalities in antral peristalsis and fundus tone have been demonstrated in this condition. This condition is most common following vagotomy to treat peptic ulcer disease, but may also occur after other surgeries including Roux-en-Y operations, and gastroplasty or gastric bypass operations for morbid obesity.

Post-Nissen fundoplication gastric motor dysfunction may result in either rapid or delayed gastric emptying. Rapid emptying occurs if there is acceleration of gastric emptying due to the fundic wrap preventing receptive relaxation, leading to increased intragastric pressure; the most common symptom is early satiety. Conversely, some patients experience similar symptoms of nausea, vomiting, and postprandial fullness due to postprandial antral hypomotility or a delay in gastric emptying, possibly due to inadvertent vagal nerve injury. A separate but equally prevalent complication of fundoplication is gas bloat syndrome, which refers to postoperative symptoms of pain, bloating, and an inability to belch that is a function of the wrap itself.

Medication-induced delays in gastric emptying

Many prescription and over-the-counter medications delay gastric emptying (Table 19.1). Nonmedicinal compounds, including tobacco, marijuana, and intoxicating quantities of ethanol, also inhibit gastric motor function. Total

Table 19.1 Effects of medications on gastric emptying

Delay gastric emptying
Ethanol (high concentration)
Aluminum hydroxide antacids
Anticholinergics
β-Adrenergic receptor agonists
Calcitonin
Calcium channel antagonists
Dexfenfluramine
Diphenhydramine
Glucagon
Interferon-α
L-Dopa
Octreotide
Opiates
Progesterone
Proton pump inhibitors
Sucralfate
Tetrahydrocannabinol
Tobacco/nicotine
Tricyclic antidepressant
Accelerate gastric emptying
β-Adrenergic receptor antagonists
Clonidine
Domperidone
Erythromycin/other macrolides
Nizatidine
Metoclopramide
Naloxone
Tegaserod

parenteral nutrition has been associated with delayed gastric emptying, which may relate in part to the induction of hyperglycemia.

Idiopathic gastroparesis

Many patients with gastroparesis have no identifiable etiology for their disease and are referred to as idiopathic gastroparesis. This disorder is more common among young women. A potential cause is viral injury to the gastric nerves or muscles, based on the observation that this commonly occurs in previously healthy individuals who display delays in gastric emptying following an acute episode of nausea, vomiting, and diarrhea. The prognosis tends to be favorable in this disorder, with slow resolution of symptoms.

Rheumatological disorders

Scleroderma produces dysphagia, heartburn, nausea, vomiting, bloating, abdominal pain, and bowel disturbances as a result of diffuse dysmotility that involves the esophagus, stomach, small intestine, and colon. In most patients, gastroduodenal manometry demonstrates diffuse low-amplitude contractions that are consistent with myopathic involvement. However, a subset of patients with early disease exhibits high-amplitude, uncoordinated contractile activity, which indicates neuropathic disease.

Chronic idiopathic intestinal pseudo-obstruction

This refers to a condition in which recurrent symptoms suggestive of intestinal obstruction are present in the absence of mechanical obstruction. Patients with this disorder may have associated gastric dysmotility and ineffective peristalsis with prominent nausea, vomiting, abdominal pain and distension. The presence of bladder dysfunction or orthostatic hypotension suggests diffuse neuromuscular disease. Pseudo-obstruction may be familial, it may occur after a viral prodrome, or it may be a paraneoplastic consequence of certain malignancies such as small cell lung carcinoma.

Eating disorders

Anorexia nervosa is characterized by distorted body image and fear of obesity with compulsive dieting and self-imposed starvation. Gastrointestinal (GI) symptoms include early satiety, epigastric fullness, abdominal bloating, nausea, and vomiting. Motility studies often reveal reduced gastric emptying, primarily for solids. Causes of gastroparesis with anorexia nervosa include central nervous system inhibition and malnutrition, but no specific gastric pathology has been demonstrated.

Bulimia nervosa is not characterized by altered body image, but rather recurrent episodes of binge eating followed by self-induced vomiting, use of laxatives or diuretics, dieting or fasting, or vigorous exercise to prevent weight gain. Studies are not consistent, but the majority exhibit delayed solid emptying. Rumination syndrome is the effortless regurgitation of recently ingested food into the mouth with subsequent mastication and re-ingestion. This is usually is not associated with delayed emptying, although small reductions in postprandial antral motor activity have been documented.

Cyclic vomiting syndrome

Cyclic vomiting syndrome is a disorder of unknown etiology that is characterized by intermittent symptomatic periods that begin abruptly and last for three to four days followed by prolonged asymptomatic intervals of variable duration. Some patients with cyclic vomiting syndrome exhibit delayed gastric emptying, which suggests underlying gastric motor dysfunction although motility may also be normal. Metabolic derangements, mitochondrial disorders, atopy, and migraine headaches are associated with distinct subsets, suggesting a heterogeneous pathogenesis. Chronic marijuana use may cause similar symptoms (cannabinoid hyperemesis) and the typical relief of nausea with hot showers or bathing may also be experienced with cyclic vomiting.

Neurological disorders

Altered gastric motility or emptying has been demonstrated after cerebrovascular accidents, with migraines, and after high cervical spinal injury. Gastric stasis may occur with disorders of autonomic function (e.g. Shy–Drager syndrome, Parkinson disease, Guillain–Barré syndrome, and multiple sclerosis). Gastroparesis is common in Parkinson disease.

Endocrinological and metabolic disorders

Hypothyroidism causes gastroparesis and, because it is easily treated (with thyroxine supplementation), should be ruled out in patients with gastroparesis unless another etiology is known. Hyperthyroidism can cause rapid gastric emptying, but normal or even delayed emptying may be found. Hypothyroidism, hyperthyroidism, and hypoparathyroidism are associated with intestinal pseudo-obstruction. Nausea, vomiting, and anorexia are frequently reported by patients with end-stage renal disease, even after adequate dialysis, but only a minority of these patients exhibit abnormal gastric emptying.

Table 19.2 summarizes the diagnostic investigation of suspected gastroparesis.

Treatment and prevention

Dietary and nonmedicinal therapies

Nonmedicinal therapies are included in the initial recommendations for the treatment of gastroparesis. Medications that inhibit gastrointestinal motility should be discontinued if possible. Ingesting several small meals four to five times per day may produce fewer symptoms than two to three large meals. Solid foods

Table 19.2 Diagnostic investigation of suspected gastroparesis

1. **Initial investigation**
   History and physical examination
   Blood tests: complete blood count (CBC), glucose, potassium, creatinine, total protein, albumin, calcium, amylase, lipase, pregnancy test
   Radiological tests: plain abdominal series to evaluate for bowel obstruction
2. **Evaluate for organic disorders**
   Upper endoscopy: to evaluate for mucosal lesions or gastric outlet obstruction
   Biliary ultrasound: if abdominal pain is a significant symptom
3. **Evaluate for delayed gastric emptying**
   Solid-phase gastric emptying scintigraphic test (four-hour test) or pH/pressure capsule (SmartPill)
   If gastroparesis is present, screen for secondary causes: thyroid function tests, antinuclear antibody, glycosylated hemoglobin (HbA1C)
4. **Treatment**
   Prokinetic and/or antiemetic agent
5. **Refractory symptoms**
   Electrogastrography (EGG)
   Wireless motility capsule
   Antroduodenal manometry
   Computed tomography (CT) enterography

with large amounts of indigestible residue should be avoided. Hyperglycemia should be treated because it delays gastric emptying of solid foods. Because lipids induce cholecystokinin (CCK) release and delay gastric emptying, a low-fat diet may also reduce symptoms. Alcohol, which reduces antral contractility, and carbonated beverages, which release carbon dioxide gas that increases distension should be avoided. While cannabis may reduce acute nausea, chronic use may lead to cannabinoid hyperemesis that requires abstention to alleviate symptoms.

Prokinetic medication therapy

Medication therapy for gastroparesis focuses on agents that promote gastric emptying (Table 19.3). Metoclopramide (10–20 mg 30 minutes prior to meals and at bedtime) is an antiemetic that enhances gastric emptying by increasing acetylcholine and blocking dopamine receptors, but a sustained prokinetic effect is not always attained and side-effects including fatigue, drowsiness, and acute dystonic reactions (facial spasm, oculogyric crisis, trismus, torticollis) are common. Some cases of irreversible tardive dyskinesia also have been observed after long-term use (>three months).

Erythromycin (100–125 mg orally three times daily) is a potent stimulant of gastric emptying through its action on gastroduodenal receptors for motilin. Tachyphylaxis limits the beneficial effects of erythromycin with long-term use. Clonidine (α2-adrenergic agonist) can reduce symptoms and accelerate gastric emptying in diabetic gastroparesis.

Domperidone is a benzimidazole that functions as a peripheral dopamine receptor antagonist that stimulates upper GI motility by increasing gastroduodenal contractions and coordination. It does not cross the blood–brain barrier, reducing the central nervous system side-effects seen with metoclopramide. The drug is not marketed in the United States but is available in most other countries. Bethanechol is a cholinergic muscarinic receptor agonist and enhances amplitude of contractions throughout the GI tract. The 5-HT_4 receptor agonists cisapride and tegaserod accelerate gastric emptying. Substantial concerns of adverse events led to withdrawal of both from the US market; however, they may be used through limited-access

Table 19.3 Drugs with prokinetic effects on the stomach

Medication	Mechanisms of action	Dosage
Metoclopramide	Dopamine receptor antagonist	5–20 mg four times daily
Erythromycin	Motilin receptor agonist	100–250 mg four times daily
Clonidine	α2-adrenergic agonist	0.1 mg twice daily
Domperidone	Peripheral dopamine receptor antagonist	10–30 mg four times daily
Bethanechol	Muscarinic receptor agonist	25 mg four times daily
Cisapride	5-HT_4 receptor agonist	10–20 mg four times daily

protocols from industry. Prucalopride (1–2 mg daily) is a 5-HT4 receptor agonist recently approved for chronic idiopathic constipation that accelerates gastric emptying and can reduce symptoms in patients with idiopathic gastroparesis.

Antiemetic medication therapy

Antiemetic drugs without prokinetic properties may serve useful adjunctive roles in managing gastroparesis. Antidopaminergic agents such as prochlorperazine, trimethobenzamide, and promethazine may provide symptom control. 5-HT_3 receptor antagonists such as ondansetron and granisetron, and the neurokinin-3 receptor antagonist aprepitnat do not affect gastric emptying but are commonly used for symptom control despite lack of long-term effectiveness data. Antihistamines including diphenhydramine, dimenhydranate, or meclizine reduce tachygastria and reduce symptoms in motion sickness, which has been extrapolated for use in other gastric emptying disorders. Anticholinergics such as scopolamine are advocated by some clinicians, although there have been no studies proving their efficacy.

Other effective medication therapy

Drugs that do not impact gastric emptying may provide symptom relief due to overlap with related syndromes and mechanisms. Tricyclic antidepressants reduce nausea in many patients with diabetic gastropathy and have also been used in some diabetics with delayed gastric emptying. Mirtazapine (15 mg/daily) through central adrenergic and serotonergic activity provides symptom relief in patients with functional dyspepsia that may overlap with gastroparesis. Buspirone (7.5–15 mg twice daily) enhances gastric accommodation and reduces postprandial symptoms in patients with functional dyspepsia.

Endoscopic, radiographic, and surgical therapies

For patients resistant to diet and drug therapy, endoscopic and surgical treatments may be offered. Endoscopic injection of botulinum toxin into the pylorus reportedly improves gastric emptying and symptoms of gastroparesis, presumably by reducing resistance to outflow into the duodenum. Gastric peroral endoscopic myotomy (G-POEM) is an experimental endoscopic therapy to treat functional pyloric obstruction through pyloromyotomy. Case reports are promising, but large, longer-term studies need to confirm effectiveness. Endoscopic, radiographic, or surgical placement of a gastrostomy tube can provide intermittent decompression if the stomach becomes filled with gas or fluid. Placement of a feeding jejunostomy allows the patient to continue receiving enteral nutrition when food ingestion is precluded by severe nausea and vomiting. In rare cases, home total parenteral nutrition can be given to maintain caloric and fluid sustenance.

Surgical implantation of a gastric electrical neurostimulator using high-frequency (12 cycles/minute), low-energy pulses (not to be confused with "gastric pacing" that employs low-frequency, high-energy pulses) may reduce nausea and vomiting in selected patients with diabetic or idiopathic gastroparesis. Pancreatic transplantation can stabilize the loss of neuronal function in a patient with severe diabetic complications; moreover, symptoms are improved with transplantation. Gastric resection is usually of limited benefit, although total gastrectomy reportedly reduces symptoms specifically in patients with severe gastroparesis caused by prior vagotomy.

Complications and their management

Complications of gastroparesis include heartburn from delayed gastric acid clearance, hemorrhage secondary to Mallory–Weiss tears or stasis-induced mucosal irritation, and weight loss. Bezoar development may supervene and exacerbate symptoms of fullness and early satiety. In patients with gastroparesis, endoscopy may detect a bezoar. Endoscopic disruption of organized bezoars improves symptoms in some individuals.

Disorders with Rapid Gastric Emptying

Clinical presentation

The clinical entity characterized by rapid gastric emptying is dumping syndrome, which is largely a complication of gastric surgery. Early dumping syndrome that occurs within 30 minutes after ingesting a meal is characterized by bloating, crampy abdominal pain and diarrhea as well as vasomotor symptoms such as flushing, palpitations, diaphoresis, light-headedness, and tachycardia. Late dumping syndrome occurs two to three hours after eating and presents with weakness, palpitations, diaphoresis, tremulousness, confusion, and syncope.

Diagnostic investigation

The diagnosis of dumping syndrome is based on eliciting a characteristic constellation of symptoms in a patient who has undergone gastric surgery. Diagnostic testing usually is not necessary, but postprandial hypoglycemia and accelerated gastric emptying of both liquids and solids may be found.

Differential diagnosis

Postsurgical dumping syndrome

Any surgical procedure involving gastrectomy or vagotomy may produce the dumping syndrome. The physiology is complex and variable between patients, but can be ascribed to loss of gastric receptive relaxation, decreased gastric capacity, absence of controlled emptying due to bypass or ablation of the pyloric sphincter, or loss of duodenal feedback inhibition (in the case of bypassed duodenum in gastrojejunostomy). Early dumping is believed to result from accelerated gastric emptying of liquids and rapid intestinal filling with hypertonic fluid leading to fluid shifts and reduction in plasma volume. Late dumping may be caused by hyperinsulinemic response to the acute carbohydrate load.

Other causes of rapid emptying

Gastric emptying of fatty liquid meals is accelerated in patients with pancreatic insufficiency and marked steatorrhea. Liquid emptying may be accelerated in some individuals with duodenal ulcer disease. Patients with Zollinger–Ellison syndrome exhibit rapid liquid and solid emptying. Many newly diagnosed diabetics have accelerated rather than delayed gastric emptying. Patients with hyperthyroidism may have accelerated emptying, as do some morbidly obese individuals. In most instances, these findings of accelerated emptying probably do not cause symptoms and are not clinically important.

Management and prevention

Dietary management

Dietary recommendations for patients with dumping syndrome include ingesting small, frequent meals of foods high in proteins and fats and low in carbohydrates with minimal fluid intake during the meal. Because liquid emptying is more rapid while sitting after vagotomy some patients may benefit from lying down (supine) immediately after eating. Viscous guar and pectin have been recommended to thicken ingested liquids.

Medication therapy

Octreotide (50–100 mcg subcutaneously 30 minutes before meals) reduces symptoms of early and late dumping syndrome. Octreotide delays gastric emptying and inhibits the release of enteric hormones and insulin secretion that may cause the symptoms of dumping syndrome. Side effects include iatrogenic diabetes, malabsorption with worsening of diarrhea and cholelithiasis. Oleic acid may activate the "jejunal brake" and slow intestinal transit and decrease diarrhea in patients with dumping syndrome.

Surgical therapy

Revisional surgery for the dumping syndrome include Roux-en-Y gastrojejunostomy, constructing an antiperistaltic jejunal loop between the stomach and intestine, and retrograde electrical pacing of the small intestine. Efficacy of these procedures is not ensured.

> **Key practice points**
>
> The symptoms of accelerated gastric emptying are generally described as "dumping" syndrome, which has been traditionally categorized by whether symptoms occur within 30 minutes (early) or several hours (late) after meals. Treatment is limited but consists of dietary changes to smaller, more frequent meals, lying down after meals, and octreotide to delay gastric emptying.

Case studies

Case 1

A 47-year-old woman presents to your office with nausea and vomiting after most meals. Her medical history is significant for type 1 diabetes mellitus that is poorly controlled. A combination of ondansetron and metoclopramide improved her symptoms; however, their effects seem to be waning despite increasing doses of both medication. On physical examination, she has normal bowel sounds and no abdominal tenderness. Her neurological examination is notable for absent proprioception. Laboratory tests reveal a fasting glucose of 278 and a HbA1C of 12.3. A four-hour solid-phase gastric emptying test is markedly prolonged.

You prescribe erythromycin 125 mg three times daily, 30 minutes before meals and stress to her the importance of improving her glucose control. Her symptoms improve for several months, but she has recurrent postprandial nausea and vomiting. Her HbA1C is now normal. You discontinue the erythromycin and write a prescription for domperidone 20 mg three times daily to be filled by a compounding agency.

Discussion

Diabetic gastroparesis is a form of neuropathy; thus, it occurs when other evidence of neuropathy is present, and in this woman's case identified by the loss of proprioception. Erythromycin in low (125–250 mg) doses has been illustrated to improve emptying and reduce symptoms from diabetic gastroparesis. However, tachyphylaxis is common and adjunctive medical therapy is commonly necessary. If this patient were to return with more symptoms, antiemetic therapy would be reasonable for symptom relief. Difficult cases may require placement of a venting gastrostomy and feeding jejunostomy.

Case 2

A 58 year-old man who recently underwent a subtotal gastrectomy with Bilroth II anastomosis for gastric adenocarcinoma complains of light-headedness, weakness, and diarrhea shortly after meals. He says that these symptoms do not occur in between meals and he did not have them prior to his surgery. With the exception of a well-healed abdominal incision, his examination is normal. His laboratory tests are notable for a potassium of 3.1 and a blood urea nitrogen (BUN) and creatinine of 19 and 1.6 mg/dl, respectively.

You council him to eat smaller but more frequent meals and lie down after eating. His symptoms do not improve and he loses 10 pounds over the next four weeks. You prescribe octreotide 50–100 mcg subcutaneously 30 minutes before meals, which reduce his nausea and vomiting and he regains weight to his baseline.

Discussion

The most likely diagnosis in this patient with this constellation of symptoms shortly after gastric surgery is dumping syndrome. The "early dumping" syndrome is believed to be due to loss of gastric receptive relaxation (due to vagotomy), reduced gastric capacity, loss of controlled emptying due to loss of pyloric sphincter, and loss of duodenal feedback inhibition of gastric emptying. No specific diagnostic tests are reliable; therefore clinical recognition is necessary to pursue empirical therapy.

Case 3

An 18 year-old man comes to your office with symptoms of nausea and vomiting for four months. He has upper abdominal discomfort but no change in bowel movements and is eating normally without a change in his weight. He states that hot showers improve his symptoms and he frequently takes five or more daily. His physical examination is normal as are his laboratory tests including a complete blood count and comprehensive metabolic profile.

Discussion

You should inquire about marijuana use in this patient, who has the typical presentation of cannabinoid hyperemesis syndrome. While cannabinoids in marijuana have an antiemetic effect acutely, their long-term use contributes to recurrent vomiting. The treatment consists of education to discontinue marijuana.

CHAPTER 20
Acid Peptic Disorders

Acid peptic disorders include ulcer disease and gastroesophageal reflux disease, which is discussed in Chapter 17. The majority of ulcers are caused by nonsteroidal anti-inflammatory drugs (NSAIDs) or infection with *Helicobacter pylori*; however, cigarette use and stress are also established causes of ulcers.

Causes of acid peptic disease

Helicobacter pylori

H. pylori is a curved, Gram-negative rod that produces urease. Chronic *H. pylori* infection causes most cases of histological gastritis and peptic ulcer disease and predisposes to development of gastric carcinoma. Evidence suggests that *H. pylori* is transmitted by fecal–oral routes. In the United States, the age-adjusted prevalence rates are higher among African-Americans and immigrants from Latin-American and Asia.

H. pylori colonizes the antrum, body, and fundus of the stomach and causes active chronic gastritis, which is characterized by histological increases in mucosal neutrophils and round cells. *H. pylori* infection affects 90% of patients with duodenal ulcers and 70–90% of those with gastric ulcers. The etiological role of this organism is supported by numerous studies showing that *H. pylori* eradication prevents ulcer recurrences.

H. pylori is a predisposing factor for developing gastric adenocarcinoma and gastric lymphoma of mucosa-associated lymphoid tissue (MALT) and is a WHO recognized carcinogen; regression of this low-grade lymphoma may occur after *H. pylori* is eradicated.

Nonsteroidal anti-inflammatory drugs

Symptomatic ulcers occur in 5% of NSAID users and the annual incidence of serious complications of NSAIDs is 2–4% annually. Risk factors for complications of NSAID associated ulcers include age greater than 60 years, multiple NSAID

Yamada's Handbook of Gastroenterology, Fourth Edition. John M. Inadomi, Renuka Bhattacharya, Joo Ha Hwang, and Cynthia Ko.

use, other comorbidities, and a prior history of peptic ulcer with or without complications. Gastric erosions are diagnosed by endoscopy in 30–50% of patients on chronic NSAID therapy, although these lesions are usually superficial and are not associated with subsequent ulcer development or symptoms. Dyspepsia in patients who take NSAIDs is more common in the first few weeks of therapy and declines with time. A minority (26%) of patients with dyspepsia have ulcers; conversely, 40% of patients with NSAID-induced ulcers are asymptomatic.

In addition to gastric and duodenal ulcers, complications of NSAID include ulceration and strictures of the small intestine; acute colitis; exacerbations of inflammatory bowel disease; and colonic ulcers, strictures, or perforation.

Additional factors associated with ulcer disease

Tobacco smokers are twice as likely as nonsmokers to develop ulcers. Epidemiological studies in areas affected by natural disaster, such as the 1995 Hanshin-Awaji earthquake in Japan, report a significant rise in the diagnosis of peptic ulcer disease, supporting stress as a factor contributing to ulcer development. In a US study, emotional stress was associated with a relative risk of 1.4–2.9 for developing ulcers. Note that alcohol, diet (including spicy foods), and caffeine have not been demonstrated to cause a higher ulcer risk.

Diseases associated with duodenal ulcers

Specific diseases are associated with increases in peptic ulcer disease. Stress ulcers and mucosal erosions occur in patients with acute multisystem failure in the intensive care unit, especially those who are on mechanical ventilation or have a coagulopathy. Cirrhosis and renal failure predispose to development of peptic ulcer disease by unknown mechanisms. The prevalence of peptic ulcer disease is increased threefold with chronic pulmonary disease, although the role of tobacco smoking in this association is uncertain. Peptic ulcer is more common among transplant recipients and in patients suffering from head injury or severe burns. Patients with cystic fibrosis have an increased risk of peptic ulcer disease because of reduced bicarbonate secretion. α_1-Antitrypsin deficiency may lead to peptic ulcer disease because of a lack of protease inhibitors. Seasonal variations have been reported for peptic ulcer disease development, as have regional and geographic differences.

Clinical presentation

Dyspepsia, defined as a symptom or set of symptoms that most physicians consider to originate from the gastroduodenal area is the most common presenting symptom of peptic ulcer disease. This symptom complex includes postprandial heaviness, early satiety, and epigastric pain or burning. About 10% of patients with peptic ulcer disease, especially those with NSAID-related disease, present with complicated ulcers (hemorrhage, perforation, or obstruction) in the absence of a history of abdominal pain. Nausea, vomiting, and weight loss are also common symptoms of peptic ulcer disease.

> **Essentials of diagnosis and potential pitfalls**
>
> **NSAID ulcers:** Patients who develop NSAID-associated ulcer hemorrhage may have no prior symptoms. Thus, the absence of dyspepsia in NSAID users does not eliminate the possibility of ulcer complications and prophylaxis should be considered in high-risk individuals. The risk of NSAID-associated hemorrhage or perforation is increased among patients with a previous history of complicated or uncomplicated peptic ulcer disease, use of multiple or high-dose NSAIDs, advanced age, and concurrent anticoagulant or steroid use.
>
> ***H. pylori* ulcers:** the presence of ***H. pylori*** should be assessed using a test that detects active infection, such as a urea breath test, stool antigen test or endoscopic biopsy. Serological testing is not advised, especially to document eradication after therapy.

Diagnostic investigation

Endoscopy

Esophagogastroduodenoscopy (EGD) has emerged as the preferred test because biopsy specimens can be obtained to document the presence of *H. pylori* infection and to exclude malignancy in gastric ulcers. Gastric ulcers should be examined by repeat upper gastrointestinal endoscopy 8–12 weeks after initiating appropriate therapy to ensure they completely heal and are not malignant in etiology. However, gastric ulcers that clearly develop in association with NSAID use do not always need to be biopsied.

H. pylori testing

A variety of methods may be used to document *H. pylori* infection. Endoscopic biopsies, stool antigen and hydrogen breath tests can document active infection whereas serology cannot distinguish current from prior infection.

Invasive tests

Biopsy specimens obtained by endoscopy are examined using traditional stains such as Giemsa, Warthin–Starry silver, or hematoxylin–eosin stains. Newer molecular tests are available to diagnose *H. pylori*. Biopsy tests may give false-negative results in patients who are bleeding acutely, on proton pump inhibitors (PPIs), or who have recently taken antibiotics.

Noninvasive tests

Enzyme-linked immunosorbent assays are available for detecting serum immunoglobulin G (IgG) antibodies to *H. pylori*, with sensitivities of 80–95% and specificities of 75–95%. Titers frequently remain elevated after successful eradication;

therefore, serological testing is a poor means of assessing active *H. pylori* infection and is not recommended for documenting eradication after therapy. Breath tests may be performed using either ^{13}C-urea (nonradioactive isotope) or ^{14}C-urea (radioactive isotope) labels, which are orally administered. Breath tests have 90–100% sensitivities and specificities for active *H. pylori* infection; however, false-negative results can be produced by intake of PPIs, bismuth compounds, histamine receptor antagonists, and antibiotics. It is recommended that these drugs be held for two to fourweeks prior to examination by breath tests. Fecal antigen tests use an enzymatic immunoassay (HpSA) to detect active infection of *H. pylori* through antigen identification in stool specimens with high levels of sensitivity and specificity.

Differential diagnosis

The differential diagnosis of uninvestigated dyspepsia is discussed in Chapter 6. The most common diagnosis among patients presenting with chronic epigastric pain is functional dyspepsia (60–75% prevalence), which is discussed in Chapter 21. Duodenal ulcers are generally associated with epigastric pain that occurs while fasting and is relieved by eating that may induce weight gain. Gastric ulcers classically cause epigastric pain provoked by eating and are associated with anorexia, early satiety and weight loss. However, sufficient variation in presentation make these characterizations nonspecific for the ulcer location.

Esophageal diseases such as esophagitis or esophageal dysmotility present with epigastric pain that radiates substernally and to the back, jaw, left shoulder, and arm. Small intestinal disease including inflammatory bowel disease can cause epigastric but more commonly para-umbilical pain. Liver capsular distension produces right upper quadrant pain. Gallbladder and bile duct pain is experienced in the epigastrium and right upper quadrant. Pancreatic pain typically is felt in the epigastrium with radiation to the back. Left upper quadrant pain suggests pancreatic disease but may also result from splenic lesions, perinephric disease, and colonic splenic flexure lesions. Cholecystitis may begin in the epigastrium and migrate to the right upper quadrant. Mesenteric ischemia can present with epigastric pain, as can malignancy of the stomach or small intestine. Appendicitis generally causes right lower quadrant abdominal pain but should be considered in any differential diagnosis of abdominal pain.

Nongastrointestinal disease can present with upper abdominal pain. Renal pain from acute pyelonephritis or obstruction of the ureteropelvic junction is usually described as flank pain, but upper abdominal pain is not unusual. Pneumonia, especially basilar in location, can present with abdominal pain that is sufficiently severe to prompt exploratory laparotomy.

Management and prevention

Most gastric and duodenal ulcers are treated medically with drugs that suppress acid secretion, neutralize gastric acid, have cytoprotective effects, and eradicate *H. pylori*. Endoscopy is indicated for control of hemorrhage and possibly gastric outlet obstruction. Interventional radiology can treat ulcer bleeding refractory to endoscopic therapy. Surgery is required for hemorrhage not controlled by endoscopic or radiological methods and for other complications such as perforation and obstruction.

Medical therapy for ulcers

Histamine$_2$ receptor antagonists

Histamine$_2$ receptor antagonists inhibit basal, histamine-stimulated, pentagastrin-stimulated, and meal-stimulated acid secretion in a linear, dose-dependent manner with a maximal 90% inhibition of vagal-stimulated and gastrin-stimulated acid production and near-total inhibition of nocturnal and basal secretion. Side-effects from these agents are rare but include cardiac rhythm disturbances with intravenous therapy, antiandrogenic effects resulting in gynecomastia and impotence (caused by cimetidine), hyperprolactinemia with galactorrhea, central neural effects (e.g. headache, lethargy, depression, memory loss), and hematological effects (e.g. leukopenia, anemia, thrombocytopenia, and elevations in hepatic aminotransferases). Cimetidine (and less commonly ranitidine) binds to hepatic cytochrome P450 enzymes and strongly inhibits the metabolism of theophylline, phenytoin, lidocaine, quinidine, and warfarin.

Proton pump inhibitors

PPIs include omeprazole, esomeprazole, lansoprazole, dexlansoprazole, rabeprazole, and pantoprazole. These substituted benzimidazoles inhibit H^+, K^+-adenosine triphosphatase activity in the gastric parietal cell canalicular membrane, leading to nearly complete inhibition of basal and stimulated acid secretion. PPIs have far greater effects on daytime (meal-stimulated) acid secretion than H_2 receptor antagonists. The optimal time for drug ingestion for most is 30 minutes to 1 hour before meals because PPIs bind only to activated proton pumps, which are maximally stimulated by food. The exception is dexlansoprazole, which is approved for use without regard to timing of dose. PPIs are well tolerated but have been associated with side effects, including headache, constipation, nausea, abdominal pain, and diarrhea. Adverse events have been associated with PPI use, including *Clostridium difficile* infection, pneumonia, bone fracture, renal impairment, and hypomagnesemia; however, the absolute risks of these complications are very low and should not prevent PPI use in appropriate patients. Finally, symptomatic (heartburn) rebound acid hypersecretion has been observed with discontinuation of PPI.

Cytoprotective agents

Sucralfate is a sucrose salt that binds to tissue proteins and forms a protective barrier that decreases exposure of the epithelium to acid, bile salts, and pepsin. Sucralfate may also stabilize gastric mucus and have trophic effects on the mucosa. Adverse effects of sucralfate include constipation and, in renal failure, the possibility of aluminum toxicity. The drug also binds several drugs, limiting their absorption.

Misoprostol is a prostaglandin E_1 analog that inhibits gastric acid secretion, stimulates bicarbonate and mucus secretion, enhances mucosal blood flow, and inhibits cell turnover. The major limitation on its use relates to dose-related diarrhea that occurs in 10–30% of patients. The use of misoprostol is contraindicated in women who may be pregnant.

Treatment of peptic ulcer disease induced by *H. pylori*

Patients diagnosed with peptic ulcers should be tested for *H. pylori* infection and if present, the organism should be eradicated. Numerous regimens have documented efficacy: among the most common are triple therapy with a twice-daily dose PPI with clarithromycin (500 mg twice daily) and a second antibiotic (e.g. amoxicillin 1 g twice daily or metronidazole 500 mg twice daily) for two weeks. Levofloxacin 500 mg twice daily may be substituted for clarithromycin in the face of clarithromycin resistance. Persistent infection can usually be eradicated with quadruple therapy consisting of a 14-day course of bismuth subsalicylate (two tablets, four times daily), metronidazole (250–375 mg four times daily), and tetracycline (500 mg four times daily), plus a PPI twice daily. An alternative quadruple therapy is amoxicillin (1 g twice daily), clarithromycin (500 mg twice daily), metronidazole (500 g twice daily) with twice daily PPI for 14 days. Shorter courses have been proposed to enhance compliance but the eradication rates decrease significantly if treatment is less than 10 days.

Essentials of treatment

Urea breath or stool antigen testing should be performed one month after completing therapy to document *H. pylori* eradication in patients with complicated ulcer disease, or who had gastric MALT lymphoma or early gastric cancer, or persistent or recurrent symptoms. Testing should be conducted with the patient off acid suppression therapy for at least one week. After successful eradication of *H. pylori*, the recurrence rate of gastric and duodenal ulcers is less than 10%. In contrast, peptic ulcer disease recurs within two years in 50–100% of patients who remain infected with *H. pylori* in the absence of acid suppression.

Treating and preventing peptic ulcer disease related to NSAIDs

Whenever possible, a patient with an NSAID-induced ulcer should discontinue NSAIDs, in which case antisecretory therapy with H_2 receptor antagonists, PPIs, or cytoprotective agents will generally induce ulcer healing within eight weeks.

If NSAIDs must be continued for their analgesic or anti-inflammatory effects, a number of regimens have demonstrated efficacy. H_2 receptor antagonists in conventional doses may heal duodenal ulcers but gastric ulcers generally are resistant to healing if NSAIDs are continued. In randomized clinical trials, PPIs have effectively healed both duodenal and gastric ulcers in the presence of continued NSAID use (95% rate of healing within eight weeks). Misoprostol has efficacy equal to PPIs in healing ulcers associated with NSAID use.

Management of refractory ulcers

Duodenal ulcers are considered refractory if eight weeks of therapy fail to heal the ulcer, while refractory gastric ulcers are defined by lack of response to 12 weeks of treatment. Causes of refractory ulcers include nonadherence to medication, surreptitious NSAID use, tobacco use, untreated *H. pylori* infection, gastric acid hypersecretion (gastrinoma), and malignancy. Rare causes of chronic ulceration are Crohn's disease, amyloidosis, sarcoidosis, eosinophilic gastroenteritis, and infections (e.g. tuberculosis, syphilis, and cytomegalovirus). Adherence with prescribed therapy should be evaluated, and any NSAID consumption should be examined. Endoscopic follow-up is indicated with performance of multiple biopsies to exclude malignancy and nonpeptic causes of ulcer. High doses of PPIs can heal 90% of refractory ulcers after eight weeks, reducing the need for surgical intervention. However, surgery should be considered for diagnosing and treating patients who do not respond to this aggressive regimen.

Serum gastrin should be measured to exclude Zollinger–Ellison syndrome (ZES), a disorder of acid hypersecretion caused by gastrin release from a neuroendocrine tumor (gastrinoma, islet cell tumor, non-β islet cell tumor); however, hypergastrinemia has many causes (Table 20.1). ZES may be sporadic or part of a multiple endocrine neoplasia type I (MEN1) that is associated with parathyroid and pituitary neoplasia in addition to pancreatic tumors. A fasting serum gastrin level >10 times the upper limit of normal in the presence of a gastric pH ≤2 is virtually diagnostic of ZES. If the fasting serum gastrin is <10 times the upper limit of normal and the gastric pH is ≤2, additional testing is necessary to establish the diagnosis of ZES: secretin test positive (≥120 pg/ml increase) or elevated basal acid output (>15 mEq/h). Rarely, pernicious anemia, in the setting of achlorhydria, may produce gastrin levels that exceed 1000 pg/ml.

Complications and their management

Complications of peptic ulcer disease include hemorrhage, perforation, penetration, and stricture with obstruction. Acute hemorrhage is best treated initially with endoscopic hemostasis (hemoclips, thermocoagulation) after adequate resuscitation. Massive hemorrhage not responsive to endoscopic therapy should be referred for interventional radiological therapy (embolization) or surgical

Table 20.1 Differential diagnosis of hypergastrinemia

Associated with gastric acid hyposecretion/achlorhydria
Chronic atrophic gastritis/pernicious anemia
Acid-reducing medication (proton pump inhibitor [PPI])
Chronic renal failure
Helicobacter pylori infection
Peptic ulcer surgery (acid reducing)
Associated with gastric acid hypersecretion
H. pylori infection
Gastric outlet obstruction
Antral G-cell hyperfunction/hyperplasia
Chronic renal failure
Short bowel syndrome
Retained gastric antrum
Zollinger–Ellison syndrome

therapy. Strictures have traditionally been treated surgically, but endoscopically deployed self-expanding metal stents may be useful in some cases.

Perforation or penetration occurs in 7% of patients and is increasing in incidence secondary to increased NSAID use. Penetration differs from perforation in that the ulcer erodes into an adjacent organ instead of the peritoneal cavity. Duodenal ulcers usually perforate anteriorly and gastric ulcers perforate along the anterior wall of the lesser curvature. Radiation of ulcer pain to the back suggests a posterior penetrating duodenal ulcer. Gastric ulcers penetrate into the left lobe of the liver or the colon, causing a gastrocolic fistula, whereas duodenal ulcers penetrate into the pancreas, producing pancreatitis. Inflammation, edema, and scarring near the gastroduodenal junction can cause outlet obstruction, which occurs in 2% of patients with peptic ulcer disease, producing symptoms of heartburn, early satiety, weight loss, abdominal pain, and vomiting. Surgery is generally indicated to treat ulcer perforation, although over-the-scope clipping devices have now allowed many ulcers to be successfully treated endoscopically. If *H. pylori* is the etiology of the ulcer, eradication of *H. pylori* prevents recurrent ulcers and ulcer complications.

Key practice points

- NSAIDs and *H. pylori* infection cause the majority of gastrointestinal ulcers.
- Upper endoscopy is the preferred method for diagnosing ulcers and their etiology.
- Treatment depends on whether *H. pylori* is detected: *H. pylori*-positive patients should receive triple or quadruple eradication therapy, while patients testing negative should receive acid suppression, usually in the form of PPIs.
- *H. pylori* detection using a test that detects active infection is recommended (stool antigen test or urea breath or tissue-based test).

- Complications of peptic ulcers include hemorrhage, perforation, and obstruction. Endoscopy is the first-line therapy for hemorrhage, with interventional radiology and surgery for refractory bleeding. Perforating ulcers are generally treated surgically; however, endoscopic devices are emerging to treat these complications. Strictures and obstructions may be treated by endoscopic stents or surgery.

Case Studies

Case 1

A 56 year-old man is admitted with hematemesis and melena. He has a medical history significant for osteoarthritis and coronary artery disease for which he is taking ibuprofen 800 mg three times daily and aspirin 81 mg daily. He describes the onset of epigastric pain three days prior to admission but no antecedent symptoms of dyspepsia. His physical examination is notable for hypotension, tachycardia, and epigastric tenderness without rebound or guarding. Rectal exam confirms melena. Laboratory tests reveal a hemoglobin of 7.8, a hematocrit of 23.5 and a platelet count of 173,000.

He is admitted to the intensive care unit where resuscitation is initiated with 3 l of normal saline. Intravenous PPI is administered. His hemoglobin drops to 7.0 despite transfusion with two units of packed red blood cells. A nasogastric tube is placed with aspiration of 500 cc of bright red blood. He is intubated for airway protection and during the induction he becomes hypotensive, but responds to dopamine and norepineprhine infusion. Resuscitation with colloid and crystalloid continue and you perform an upper endoscopy that reveals a 1 cm ulcer in the antrum with a nonbleeding visible vessel. You place a hemoclip across the visible vessel, which prompts active bleeding. Injection of epinephrine around the bleeding site slows the hemorrhage and placement of two additional hemoclips results in cessation of bleeding.

Discussion

Hemorrhage is a complication of peptic ulcer disease that should be initially assessed and treated endoscopically. Patients with complications of peptic ulcer may not have antecedent symptoms of dyspepsia. NSAIDs are the likely etiology of ulcer in this patient: risk factors for NSAID-associated hemorrhage or perforation include a previous history of peptic ulcer disease, use of multiple or high-dose NSAIDs, advanced age, and concurrent anticoagulant or steroid use. *H. pylori* should still be evaluated and treated if present: serology is sufficient in this case, but documentation of eradication must be performed using tests that detect active infection such as stool antigen or urea breath tests.

Endoscopic therapy for bleeding peptic ulcer consists of mechanical (hemoclips) or thermal (bipolar cautery, heater probe) therapy. Injection therapy is inferior to mechanical or thermal therapy but may be used as adjunctive therapy to gain initial control of bleeding.

Case 2

A 64 year-old woman comes to your office with symptom of epigastric pain associated with nausea and intermittent vomiting. Her pain is reduced after meals and she has not lost weight. She states she has had similar symptoms intermittently most of her adult life, which are temporarily alleviated with a combination of antacids and H2 receptor antagonists. Her primary care provider obtained an *H. pylori* serology, which was positive. She was prescribed clarithromycin, amoxicillin, and omeprazole eradication therapy, but only took the antibiotics because she is fearful of the side effects of PPIs. Her physical examination is normal without abdominal tenderness, and her laboratory tests are unrevealing.

You perform an upper endoscopy that reveals a 1 cm clean-based duodenal ulcer. Biopsies of the gastric antrum and body are notable for chronic active gastritis and special stains reveal *H. pylori* organisms. You prescribe quadruple therapy with bismuth, metronidazole, tetracycline, and a PPI based on her previous course of antibiotics. You also take the time to educate her about the very low risk of bone adverse events with PPIs in contrast to the high benefit she will achieve by treating peptic ulcer, preventing recurrence and reducing the risk of gastric cancer.

Discussion

Chronic *H. pylori* infection is one of the most common causes of peptic ulcer disease. The frequent recurrence after discontinuation of acid suppression is typical, and the histopathological findings are classic for the inflammation caused by this bacteria. The heightened concern about the adverse events associated with PPIs has not only reduced unnecessary use, but also reduced their use for diseases where their efficacy has been has been established. It should be noted that the absolute risk of any of these proposed adverse effects (*C. difficile* infection, pneumonia, bone fracture, renal impairment, and hypomagnesemia) is far less than 1%, with the exception of the risk of spontaneous bacterial peritonitis among cirrhotics taking PPIs compared with non-PPI users.

CHAPTER 21
Functional Dyspepsia

Dyspepsia is a syndrome characterized by persistent or recurrent upper abdominal pain or discomfort. This discomfort can be accompanied by postprandial fullness, early satiety, nausea, and bloating. Patients with dyspepsia who are evaluated and have no definable structural or biochemical abnormality are classified as having a diagnosis of functional dyspepsia. Functional dyspepsia can be diagnosed using the Rome IV criteria and can be further sub-classified as postprandial distress syndrome or epigastric pain syndrome (Table 21.1). Many patients have an overlap syndrome with characteristics of both postprandial distress and epigastric pain.

Although only a minority of individuals with dyspepsia seek medical care, it is estimated that functional dyspepsia and related functional gastrointestinal disorders account for a substantial proportion of visits to primary care providers and referrals for gastroenterology consultation. Patients may seek medical attention because of symptom severity, fear of serious underlying disease, and/or underlying depression, anxiety, or other psychosocial factors.

Aspirin and nonsteroidal anti-inflammatory drugs cause acute dyspepsia but their roles in chronic dyspepsia are less well established. There is no evidence that tobacco or ethanol use are causes of functional dyspepsia. Similarly, it is unlikely that food intolerance is a major contributor to the pathogenesis of functional dyspepsia. Coffee stimulates gastric acid production and may elicit dyspeptic symptoms, but it is unknown if it acts via gastric irritation or induction of gastroesophageal reflux.

Patients with functional dyspepsia have a higher prevalence of anxiety, depression, neuroticism, and somatization than nondyspeptic patients. However, it is unclear whether these disorders represent a cause or a consequence of dyspeptic symptoms. Acute stress elicits gastric motor responses similar to those observed with functional dyspepsia. As in studies of irritable bowel syndrome, the prevalence of prior physical or sexual abuse is higher in patients with functional dyspepsia. Symptoms may also begin after an episode of infectious gastroenteritis.

Yamada's Handbook of Gastroenterology, Fourth Edition. John M. Inadomi, Renuka Bhattacharya, Joo Ha Hwang, and Cynthia Ko.

Table 21.1 Rome IV criteria for functional dyspepsia

Functional dyspepsia
One or more of the following: bothersome postprandial fullness, bothersome early satiation, bothersome epigastric pain, or bothersome epigastric burning
AND
No evidence of structural disease that is likely to explain symptoms
Criteria fulfilled for the last three months with symptom onset at least six months before diagnosis
Postprandial distress syndrome
One or both of the following at least three days per week: bothersome postprandial fullness or bothersome early satiation
No evidence of organic, systemic, or metabolic disease that is likely to explain symptoms
Criteria fulfilled for the last three months with symptom onset at least six months before diagnosis
Epigastric pain syndrome
At least one of the following symptoms at least one day per week: bothersome epigastric pain and/or bothersome epigastric burning
No evidence of organic, systemic, or metabolic disease that is likely to explain symptoms
Criteria fulfilled for the last three months with symptom onset at least six months before diagnosis

Clinical presentation

Dyspepsia can present with symptoms of epigastric pain or burning, early satiety, or postprandial fullness. It is often aggravated by food or associated with nausea, vomiting, or bloating. Symptoms of early satiety and postprandial fullness are more prominent in patients with postprandial distress syndrome, while epigastric discomfort or burning is more prominent with epigastric pain syndrome. Patients with overlap syndrome may have features of both epigastric pain and postprandial distress.

Symptoms suggestive of organic causes of dyspepsia should be sought. For example, unexplained weight loss, anemia, and gastrointestinal bleeding are alarm features that should prompt more aggressive evaluation. Symptoms of heartburn or regurgitation suggest gastroesophageal reflux disease as the underlying etiology, while significant weight loss, anorexia, dysphagia, unexplained iron deficiency, or vomiting may suggest an underlying upper GI malignancy. Biliary colic is suggested by the occurrence of severe episodic epigastric or right upper quadrant pain. Radiation of pain to the back may suggest a pancreatic etiology. Abdominal wall pain is suggested by the presence of localized tenderness during contraction of the abdominal wall muscles (Carnett sign).

Diagnostic investigation

Patients younger than age 45 without weight loss, bleeding, dysphagia, iron deficiency, or recurrent vomiting rarely harbor malignancy. In this population, peptic ulcer disease, gastroesophageal reflux disease, and functional dyspepsia are the most common etiologies of dyspepsia. Initial laboratory testing including complete blood counts, liver chemistries, calcium, and creatinine should be performed. Younger patients with uninvestigated dyspepsia who lack alarm findings may be initially managed using empiric medical therapy (Figure 21.1). Some guidelines suggest that patients in the United States who are younger than age 60 without alarm symptoms may be safely managed with initial empiric therapy due to the low risk of malignancy in this population. The age at which to pursue initial endoscopy likely needs to be individualized based on symptoms, age, nationality, and background risk of gastric cancer.

If there is a high background prevalence of *Helicobacter pylori*, testing for this organism with by stool antigen or urea breath testing is appropriate. If testing is positive, *H. pylori* should be treated. After appropriate therapy, urea breath or stool antigen testing should be used to confirm *H. pylori* eradication. If *H. pylori* is not present, empiric acid-reducing drugs can be administered. Initial empiric acid-suppressive therapy with proton pump inhibitors or histamine-2 (H2) receptor antagonists may be more appropriate if there is a low background prevalence of *H. pylori* or in patients with coexisting reflux-type symptoms.

Initial upper gastrointestinal endoscopy is recommended for patients older than age 50–60 years, for those with long-standing or recurrent symptoms, and for those with "alarm symptoms" including weight loss, gastrointestinal bleeding,

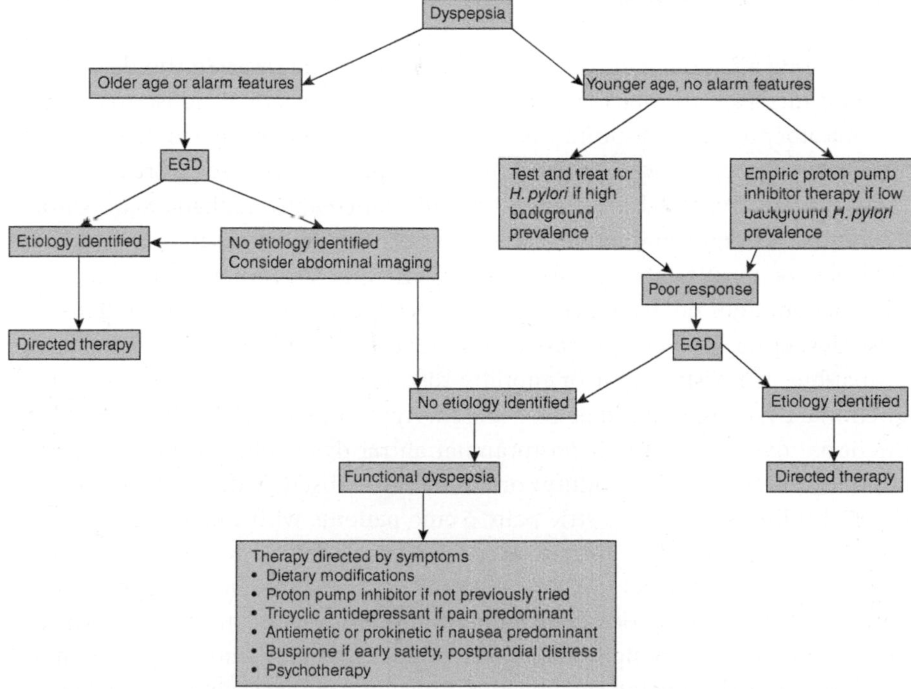

Figure 21.1 Diagnosis and management of uninvestigated dyspepsia. EGD, esophagogastroduodenoscopy.

anemia, or dysphagia to assess for the presence of upper gastrointestinal malignancy. Gastric biopsies should be obtained for histopathology and *H. pylori* testing. In most patients, endoscopy will not reveal a culprit lesion. Whether further testing is needed, for example abdominal ultrasound, CT, or gastric emptying study, will depend upon symptom severity and degree of suspicion for an underlying organic process.

Essentials of diagnosis and potential pitfalls

Decision analyses have been conducted to determine the most cost-effective approach to patients with dyspepsia but no particular diagnostic approach is consistently favored. Young patients without alarm symptoms do not necessarily need endoscopy, and empiric medical therapy is often appropriate. If there is a high background prevalence of *H. pylori*, noninvasive testing for and treatment for this organism if positive are appropriate. Patients at low risk of *H. pylori* may be better managed with a trial of acid suppression. The decision to begin with investigation versus empiric therapy (and if the latter, which therapy to initiate first) depends largely on the prevalence of *H. pylori* in the population and the costs of diagnostic testing. Older patients or those with alarm symptoms should undergo upper endoscopy.

Differential diagnosis

In evaluating a patient with unexplained dyspepsia, the clinician should consider stopping medications that may produce dyspepsia, including nonsteroidal anti-inflammatory agents or aspirin, iron, potassium, and erythromycin. Organic conditions that can present with dyspepsia include peptic ulcer disease, gastroesophageal reflux disease, hepatobiliary disease, chronic pancreatitis, malignancies, chronic mesenteric ischemia, infiltrative diseases (e.g. Crohn's disease, sarcoidosis, eosinophilic gastroenteritis, tuberculosis, and syphilis), and abdominal wall pain.

If a patient does not have evidence of structural disease or infection that could cause dyspepsia, disorders of gastric motility can be considered if symptoms are compatible. If no structural or motility disturbances are noted, a diagnosis of functional dyspepsia should be considered. Approximately 40% of patients with functional dyspepsia exhibit postprandial antral dysmotility or delayed gastric emptying; altered gastric motility correlates more closely with symptoms of postprandial fullness than epigastric pain. Some patients with functional dyspepsia have an impaired gastric fundus accommodation reflex, which may underlie symptoms of early satiety. Many patients with functional dyspepsia exhibit reduced tolerance to balloon distension of the stomach and duodenum, which is not accompanied by changes in wall compliance and may underlie symptoms of epigastric pain. This finding suggests that functional dyspepsia in these individuals stems from visceral hypersensitivity.

Management and prevention

Medical therapy for functional dyspepsia

Once a diagnosis of functional dyspepsia is made, confident reassurance by the clinician is essential to manage patients with functional dyspepsia and may obviate the need for medication therapy in many patients. Patients should avoid aggravating medications and foods if possible. Postprandial symptoms may be reduced by eating low-fat meals or more frequent but smaller meals throughout the day.

Eradicating *H. pylori* has limited benefits and results in symptom resolution in less than 10% of patients with functional dyspepsia. Initial acid suppressive therapy may include H2-receptor antagonists or proton pump inhibitors, which may be more effective in patients with epigastric pain syndrome than with postprandial distress syndrome. Both proton pump inhibitors and H2-receptor antagonists are only moderately effective in relieving dyspeptic symptoms, and data comparing the two medication classes for this indication are sparse. There does not appear to be significant benefit with bismuth, sucralfate, or antacids.

If patients do not benefit from *H. pylori* eradication or acid suppression, tricyclic antidepressant drugs such as amitriptyline or desipramine may provide some benefit by modulating underlying visceral hypersensitivity. However, these agents have prominent side effects including sedation, constipation, dry mouth, and urinary retention. Patients may be able to tolerate these medications if initiated at a low dose with gradual dose titration. In general, doses higher than 75–100 mg are not more effective than lower doses for this indication. Data to support use of selective serotonin reuptake inhibitors for functional dyspepsia are limited. Although widely used, evidence for any benefit from complementary or alternative therapies including probiotics for functional dyspepsia is also limited, and their use is not currently recommended.

Prokinetic drugs such as metoclopramide can be used in patients who do not respond adequately to tricyclic antidepressants. However, their use may also be limited by potential for side effects including dystonia, parkinsonian symptoms, anxiety and, long-term, tardive dyskinesia. Limited data suggests that buspirone may induce relaxation of the gastric fundus, and may be helpful in patients with symptoms of early satiety and postprandial fullness. Complementary and alternative therapies, although commonly used, have limited data to support their effectiveness.

Psychological therapies

Small trials have shown the benefits of cognitive behavioral and hypnotherapy in functional dyspepsia. However, studies of psychological treatment have been heterogeneous and at high risk of bias, and comparisons with drug therapy have not been performed.

Essentials of treatment

There is no universally effective medication for treating functional dyspepsia. Empiric trials of acid suppression, tricyclic antidepressants, and prokinetic agents may be needed. *H. pylori* testing followed by eradication in those testing positive inconsistently improves symptoms. Psychological interventions may be helpful in a subset of patients, particularly those with high levels of depression or anxiety.

Key practice points

- Functional dyspepsia can be diagnosed using Rome IV criteria, and be sub-classified as an epigastric pain, postprandial distress, or overlap syndrome.
- The etiology of functional dyspepsia may vary between patients, and can be attributed to infection or inflammation (such as *H. pylori* infection), or motility disturbances and visceral hypersensitivity. These pathogenic factors can interact with psychological factors to worsen symptom severity and cause patients to seek health care.
- Initial management of dyspepsia may be empiric with either acid suppression (proton pump inhibitors or H2-receptor antagonists) or *H. pylori* testing (with eradication treatment if positive). Initial *H. pylori* testing may be more appropriate in regions with a high background prevalence of this infection. Investigation with upper endoscopy should be reserved for patients presenting with alarm features, patients with new symptoms over the age of 50–60 years of age, or those with persistent or recurrent symptoms after empiric medical therapy.
- No universally effective therapy for functional dyspepsia is available. Patients who do not respond to acid suppression or *H. pylori* eradication can be offered neuromodulators such as tricyclic antidepressants, prokinetic agents, or psychological therapies. There is limited data to suggest use of selective serotonin reuptake inhibitors, buspirone, or complementary and alternative therapies.

Further reading

ASGE Standards of Practice Committee (2015). The role of endoscopy in dyspepsia. *Gastrointest. Endosc.* 82: 227–232.

Moayyedi, P.M., Lacy, B.E., Andrews, C.N. et al. (2017). ACG and CAG clinical guideline: management of dyspepsia. *Am. J. Gastroenterol.* 112: 988–1013.

Yang, Y.X., Brill, J., Krishnan, P. et al. (2015). American Gastroenterological Association Institute guideline on the role of upper gastrointestinal biopsy to evaluate dyspepsia in the adult patient in the absence of visible mucosal lesions. *Gastroenterol.* 149: 1082–1087.

CHAPTER 22
Gastric Neoplasia

A majority of tumors that occur in the stomach are gastric adenocarcinomas, which is the second most common cause of cancer-related mortality worldwide. Other less common gastric tumors include lymphoma, mesenchymal tumors, and endocrine tumors.

Adenocarcinoma

Clinical presentation

Patients with early gastric cancer generally are asymptomatic. Rather, most individuals present at an advanced stage, usually with nonspecific symptoms such as epigastric pain, early satiety, bloating, nausea, vomiting, and weight loss. Gastrointestinal hemorrhage and gastric outlet obstruction are rarely the initial manifestations of a gastric tumor. The results of the physical examination may be normal or evaluation may reveal occult or gross gastrointestinal blood loss, lymphadenopathy, or hepatomegaly with disease dissemination. A Virchow node indicates metastasis to the left supraclavicular lymph node, whereas a periumbilical nodule (Sister Mary Joseph node) may indicate tumor spread along peritoneal surfaces. An ovarian mass (Krukenberg tumor) or a mass in the cul-de-sac (Blumer shelf) may also be present. Paraneoplastic syndromes, such as acanthosis nigricans, membranous glomerulonephritis, microangiopathic hemolytic anemia, arterial, and venous thrombi (Trousseau syndrome), seborrheic dermatitis (Leser–Trélat sign), or dermatomyositis, may also be present.

Diagnostic investigation

Upper gastrointestinal endoscopy

Suggestive symptoms or findings on physical examination require further evaluation by upper gastrointestinal endoscopy or double-contrast upper

Yamada's Handbook of Gastroenterology, Fourth Edition. John M. Inadomi, Renuka Bhattacharya, Joo Ha Hwang, and Cynthia Ko.

gastrointestinal barium radiography. Upper gastrointestinal endoscopy may provide evidence that strongly suggests a neoplasm but endoscopic biopsy is necessary to confirm the diagnosis. The overall sensitivity and specificity of upper gastrointestinal endoscopy with biopsy are 95 and 99%, respectively. Multiple biopsies are necessary to achieve this accuracy. Further, the combined application of brush cytology and forceps biopsy may improve sensitivity. Biopsy specimens of ulcers are best obtained from the base and the four quadrants of the edge of the ulcer. Because of sampling error, any suggestion of malignancy in the appearance of a gastric ulcer warrants re-evaluation by upper gastrointestinal endoscopy after therapy to confirm healing, and biopsy specimens should be taken of any persistent mucosal defect.

Tumors that appear as thickened gastric folds with normal overlying mucosa are caused by infiltration of the tumor into the submucosa. These cancers can be diagnosed with cautious use of a snare to obtain a biopsy specimen from the submucosa. Light-induced fluorescence endoscopy is an emerging diagnostic technique that relies on the naturally occurring fluorescence (autofluorescence) of tissue after irradiation with blue or violet light to distinguish neoplastic from normal tissue.

Radiographic studies

When performed by an experienced radiologist, upper gastrointestinal radiography detects more than 90% of gastric adenocarcinomas. Characteristic radiographic findings include an asymmetrical ulcer crater, distorted, or nodular folds radiating from an ulcer, a lack of distensibility of the stomach, or a polypoid mass. However, radiography does not have the capability of obtaining histological samples and has been largely replaced by endoscopy for diagnosing gastric malignancy.

Staging evaluation

Endoscopic ultrasound (EUS) is ideally suited to the TNM classification for staging gastric cancer because it can accurately assess the depth of tumor penetration. Note, however, that EUS has limited ability to differentiate inflammatory from malignant adenopathy. Computed tomographic (CT) scanning is required to evaluate the M stage because EUS cannot detect the majority of distant metastases. Magnetic resonance imaging (MRI) shows promise as a tool for excluding metastases, but it is not superior to CT for staging. Positron emission tomography (PET) appears to be sensitive in detecting gastric neoplasia but poor differentiation between primary and metastatic lesions precludes its use in staging.

Histopathology

The Borrmann classification of gastric adenocarcinoma contains four distinct morphological subgroups, including polypoid, fungating, ulcerated, and

Table 22.1 TNM staging of gastric carcinoma

Stage	T Stage	N Stage	M Stage	5-year survival (%)
IA	T1	N0	M0	91
IB	T1	N1	M0	82
	T2	N0	M0	
II	T1	N2	M0	65
	T2	N1	M0	
	T3	N0	M0	
IIIA	T2	N2	M0	49
	T3	N1	M0	
	T4	N0	M0	
IIIB	T3	N2	M0	28
	T4	N1	M0	
IV	T4	N2	M0	5
	Any T	Any N	M1	

diffusely infiltrating or linitis plastica. Early gastric cancer is a term that applies to tumors limited to the mucosa and submucosa. It is most commonly diagnosed during screening of asymptomatic high-risk populations and carries a favorable prognosis. The two best predictors of survival are depth of invasion (T stage) and metastases to lymph nodes (N stage) or distant sites (M stage). A TNM staging system categorizes gastric tumors into four stages that correlate with long-term survival (Table 22.1). Young patients, patients with linitis plastica, and patients with proximal tumors have poor prognoses.

Histologically, gastric cancer can be divided into an intestinal type, characterized by epithelial cells that form glandular structures, and a diffuse type, in which undifferentiated cells proliferate in sheets. The intestinal type is more common in countries where gastric cancer is endemic, whereas the diffuse type is more common in low-risk populations, such as in the United States. The intestinal type is more likely to be associated with intestinal metaplasia and atrophic gastritis and has a more favorable prognosis than the diffuse type. Gastric malignancies rarely exhibit adenomatous and squamous features. The adenosquamous variant has a poor prognosis.

Management and course

Table 22.2 outlines the general principles of medical and surgical management of gastric adenocarcinoma.

Surgical therapy

Complete surgical resection is the only therapy that offers a potential cure for gastric adenocarcinoma, but the advanced stage at which more than half of patients present precludes curative surgery. The importance of surgical resection

Table 22.2 Treatment recommendations for gastric adenocarcinoma

	N0	N1	N2	N3
T1 (mucosa)	EMR or modified gastrectomy	Modified or standard gastrectomy	Standard gastrectomy	
T1 (submucosa)	Modified gastrectomy			
T2	Standard gastrectomy	Standard gastrectomy Adjuvant chemotherapy		Extended or palliative gastrectomy or chemotherapy or radiation or palliative care
T3	Standard gastrectomy Adjuvant chemotherapy			
T4	Extended gastrectomy Adjuvant chemotherapy Radiation		Extended or palliative gastrectomy Chemotherapy or radiation or palliative care	
M1 Recurrent	Extended or palliative gastrectomy Chemotherapy or radiation or palliative care			

is reflected in the five-year survival rate of 35–45% of patients with resectable tumors, compared with the five-year survival rate of less than 5% of patients who undergo palliative resection.

Although surgery is recognized as the best treatment option for gastric cancer, there is little consensus on the optimal curative surgical procedure for gastric adenocarcinoma, especially concerning the extent of lymph node dissection. Adenocarcinomas of the proximal fundus are treated by proximal gastric resection. Tumors of the gastroesophageal junction require *en bloc* resection of the distal esophagus and proximal stomach, often by a combined thoracic and abdominal approach. Splenectomy usually is performed if tumors are located along the greater curvature. The role of resection of isolated hepatic metastases at the time of gastrectomy has not been determined in controlled clinical trials. Palliative surgery may be indicated for obstruction, perforation, or bleeding. Bypass procedures provide significantly shorter periods of palliation compared to resection.

Endoscopic procedures

Endoscopic submucosal dissection (ESD) has been shown to cure early gastric cancer with only mucosal involvement or very superficial submucosal invasion (<500 μm). Palliative endoscopic therapy may consist of stent placement or Nd:YAG laser tumor ablation, both of which may be used to treat obstruction. Gastrointestinal hemorrhage may be controlled by Nd:YAG laser coagulation necrosis or hemospray.

Medical therapy

The role of chemotherapy and radiation therapy in treating gastric adenocarcinoma is evolving. Agents shown to decrease tumor mass include 5-fluorouracil, mitomycin C, doxorubicin, cisplatin, and hydroxyurea but there is no evidence of improved survival. Postoperative radiotherapy has likewise not been shown to increase survival.

Key practice points: gastric cancer

- A Virchow node indicates metastasis to the left supraclavicular lymph node.
- A periumbilical nodule (Sister Mary Joseph node) may indicate tumor spread along peritoneal surfaces.
- Gastric cancers are associated with paraneoplastic syndromes, such as acanthosis nigricans, membranous glomerulonephritis, microangiopathic hemolytic anemia, arterial, and venous thrombi (Trousseau syndrome), seborrheic dermatitis (Leser–Trélat sign), or dermatomyositis.
- Esophagogastroduodenoscopy (EGD) with biopsy is necessary to confirm the diagnosis.
- EUS provides accurate local and regional staging (T and N stages) but CT scan should be performed to assess for metastatic disease.
- The two best predictors of survival are depth of invasion (T stage) and metastases to lymph nodes (N stage) or distant sites (M stage).
- ESD can be performed for curative resection of early gastric cancer.

Gastric Lymphoma

Clinical presentation

The presentation of gastric lymphoma is similar to that of gastric adenocarcinoma. Nonspecific symptoms include epigastric pain, weight loss, nausea, vomiting, early satiety, and anorexia. Gastrointestinal hemorrhage and perforation from extensive ulceration are less common manifestations. Physical examination may reveal an abdominal mass or peripheral adenopathy.

Diagnostic investigation

Upper gastrointestinal endoscopy and upper gastrointestinal barium radiography are the primary means for detecting gastric lymphoma; however, the ability to obtain biopsy specimens makes upper gastrointestinal endoscopy the procedure of choice. CT scans are required to determine extragastric involvement. Occasionally, lymphoma appears as a thickened fold on endoscopy and biopsy reveals a submucosal mass with normal overlying mucosa. In this setting, EUS can delineate which layers of the gastric wall are involved, and cytology or biopsy may confirm the diagnosis. Laparotomy may be necessary to define the extent of disease.

Table 22.3 Ann Arbor staging system for gastric lymphoma

Stage	Extent of disease	Relative incidence (%)
I	Limited to stomach	26–38
II	Involvement of abdominal lymph nodes	43–49
III	Involvement of lymph nodes above the diaphragm	13–31
IV	Disseminated disease	–

Management and course

Gastric lymphoma has a favorable prognosis compared with gastric adenocarcinoma. The five-year survival rate is 50%. The Ann Arbor staging system for gastric lymphoma is based on the extent of disease that, once established, determines the appropriate course of management (Table 22.3). Patients with stage I tumors limited to the stomach have cure rates higher than 80% and should undergo total gastrectomy or limited gastrectomy with adequate margins. Postoperative chemotherapy and radiation therapy may improve survival of patients with this early-stage disease. Patients with stage II–IV disease are best treated with combination chemotherapy but if bulky transmural stomach tumors are present, prophylactic gastrectomy is often performed to prevent treatment-related perforation. Patients with disseminated non-Hodgkin lymphoma rarely survive for two years. Most mucosa-associated lymphoid tissue (MALT) lymphomas are stage I. Early mucosal tumors may respond to antibiotic therapy to eradicate *Helicobacter pylori*, whereas more advanced MALT lymphomas require systemic chemotherapy. MALT lymphomas, in particular, have relatively favorable outcomes.

Key practice points: gastric lymphoma

- EGD should be performed to obtain biopsies to establish the diagnosis of gastric lymphoma. If gastric lymphoma is suspected, a biopsy sample should be sent for flow cytometry analysis.
- CT scans are required to determine extragastric involvement.
- Gastric lymphoma has a favorable prognosis compared with gastric adenocarcinoma.
- Early MALT lymphomas may respond to antibiotic therapy to eradicate *H. pylori*.

Gastrointestinal Stromal Cell Tumors

Gastrointestinal stromal cell tumors (GISTs) are mesenchymal neoplasms that are thought to originate from the interstitial cells of Cajal, which is an innervated network of intestinal pacemaker cells. GISTs are composed of a heterogeneous group of neoplasms with predominantly myogenic, neural, or mixed features. Seventy percent of GIST tumors occur in the stomach. The peak incidence occurs in the fifth and sixth decades with equal gender distribution. Symptoms are similar to those of other gastric cancers, although bleeding due to ulceration is more common. Surgical resection is the treatment of choice in patients with tumors >2 cm without evidence of metastasis. High-risk features of GISTs include size >10 cm, any size tumor with >10 mitoses per 50 high-power fields (HPF), tumor >5 cm with a mitosis count >5/50 HPF, or tumor rupture into the peritoneal cavity. Chemotherapy with imatinib should be considered in patients diagnosed with GISTs with high-risk features. No effective therapy exists for advanced metastatic disease. The five-year survival rate is 28–65% in patients with metastatic GIST.

Metastatic tumors

Malignant neoplasms from distant sites may metastasize to the stomach. Common sources include melanoma, ovarian, colon, lung, and breast cancer. Tumors may be mucosal or submucosal with associated ulceration. Patients may experience epigastric pain, vomiting, and gastrointestinal hemorrhage.

Miscellaneous Benign and Malignant Gastric Tumors

Gastric polyps

Most gastric polyps are hyperplastic with no malignant potential. They usually are less than 1 cm in diameter and rarely produce symptoms. Some patients with Ménétrier disease (i.e. hypertrophic gastropathy) may have large numbers of fundic hyperplastic polyps. Adenomatous polyps account for 10% of gastric polyps. Their malignant potential dictates removal, followed by a program of endoscopic surveillance to detect recurrence. Patients with familial adenomatous polyposis (FAP) may have fundic gland polyposis. These polyps usually are hamartomatous, although some are adenomatous. Gastric adenomas in patients with FAP have the potential for malignant degeneration, necessitating excision and endoscopic surveillance.

Gastric carcinoids

Only 3% of all carcinoid tumors are located in the stomach. There are three types of gastric carcinoids. The most common is type 1, which is characterized by generally small multiple tumors localized to the fundus and body. Type 1 gastric carcinoids have the lowest metastatic rate of the three types (9–23%). Associated findings include chronic atrophic gastritis, achlorhydria, and pernicious anemia. Type 2 is associated with multiple endocrine neoplasia type I (MENI) and has an intermediate risk of metastasis. Type 3 is the least common but the most aggressive and most prone to metastasis. Type 3 gastric carcinoids are not associated with a hypergastrinemic state. The tumors are sporadic and generally solitary and large.

Gastric carcinoids are endocrine tumors that produce multiple bioactive substances, including serotonin, histamines, somatostatin, and kinins, but they rarely produce the carcinoid syndrome, which is characterized by flushing, diarrhea, and cardiopulmonary symptoms. Carcinoids usually are submucosal lesions, although they can cause ulceration of the overlying mucosa. Metastatic tumors may require systemic chemotherapy to control tumor bulk. The somatostatin analog octreotide improves symptoms in many patients with the carcinoid syndrome.

Leiomyoma and leiomyosarcoma

Leiomyomas are benign gastric subepithelial masses. They usually cause no symptoms and are often detected incidentally during upper gastrointestinal endoscopy. Leiomyomas rarely undergo malignant transformation to leiomyosarcomas, which account for less than 1% of gastric malignancies. A leiomyosarcoma is a highly vascular tumor that often manifests with massive gastrointestinal hemorrhage. The differentiation of a leiomyoma from a leiomyosarcoma is often problematic and is based on the number of mitotic figures and invasiveness seen on histological examination. The five-year survival rate of patients is about 50% after resection of a leiomyosarcoma.

Key practice points: miscellaneous gastric tumors

- GISTs are neoplasms with variable malignant potential. High-risk features of GISTs include size >10 cm, any size tumor with >10 mitoses per 50 HPF, tumor >5 cm with a mitosis count >5/50 HPF, or tumor rupture into the peritoneal cavity.
- Malignant neoplasms from distant sites may metastasize to the stomach, including melanoma, ovarian, colon, lung, and breast cancer.
- Gastric adenomas in patients with FAP have the potential for malignant degeneration, necessitating excision and endoscopic surveillance.

Case studies

Case 1

A 67-year-old man presents to his gastroenterologist with complaints of early satiety and 15 lb. unintentional weight loss over the past three months. Physical exam demonstrates an enlarged left supraclavicular lymph node and mild epigastric tenderness to palpation. Labs are notable for a hematocrit of 32%.

Endoscopy demonstrates diffusely abnormal gastric mucosa and the lumen does not expand to air insufflation. When taking biopsies, the mucosa is noted to be friable and firm. Stacked biopsies are obtained due to the suspicion of linitis plastica, as these tumors are known to infiltrate the submucosa and mucosal biopsies can be falsely negative. Histology confirms the diagnosis of gastric carcinoma with poorly differentiated, diffuse type histology. A CT scan is performed that shows evidence of metastatic disease to multiple lymph nodes and to the liver. The patient is diagnosed with stage IV gastric cancer and is referred to an oncologist for consideration of palliative chemotherapy.

Case 2

A 55-year-old man is referred for EGD to evaluate new-onset symptoms of epigastric pain. The patient reports a two-month history of epigastric pain that has increased in severity over the last two weeks. He denies any unintentional weight loss, fevers, night sweats, nausea, or vomiting. Physical examination is unremarkable. EGD is performed demonstrating a 3 cm diameter area of mucosal nodularity in the gastric body. Biopsies is obtained for histology and flow cytometry. Histology is consistent with a lymphoma of MALT type. *H. pylori* organisms are also identified in the gastric mucosal biopsy specimens. Flow cytometry demonstrates a clonal B-cell population consistent with extranodal marginal zone B-cell lymphoma MALT type. EUS demonstrates the mucosal nodularity to be limited to the mucosal layer without evidence of extension into the submucosa. There are no abnormal perigastric lymph nodes identified. It is determined that the patient has early-stage MALT type lymphoma and he is treated for *H. pylori* eradication. Urea breath test is performed four weeks following therapy, which confirms eradication. Repeat EGD is performed at two months following eradication therapy demonstrating a decrease in the mucosal nodularity. Repeat biopsies demonstrate residual MALT lymphoma. EGD is repeated at two month intervals and eventually demonstrates no evidence of lymphoma at eight months following eradication therapy.

CHAPTER 23
Celiac Disease

Celiac disease, also known as *celiac sprue* and *gluten-sensitive enteropathy*, is characterized by intestinal mucosal damage and malabsorption from dietary intake of gluten proteins in wheat, rye, or barley. Symptoms may appear with the introduction of cereal into the diet in the first three years of life. A second peak in symptomatic disease occurs in adults during the third or fourth decade, although disease onset as late as the eighth decade has been reported. Epidemiologic studies demonstrate a prevalence of approximately 1% in the United States and Europe. Celiac disease occurs primarily in whites of northern European background, but may occur in other populations with an appropriate genetic background.

Celiac disease results from an interplay of environmental factors, genetic predisposition, and immunological interactions. It is believed that gluten-derived peptides are able to cross into the intestinal submucosa where they undergo deamidation and bind to the antigen-binding groove of human leukocyte antigen (HLA) DQ-2 or DQ8, triggering T-cell activation. Some studies also implicate activation of innate and humoral immune responses within the intestinal epithelium. The vast majority of patients with celiac disease carry the HLA DQ-2 or DQ-8 gene, as the gliadin peptides can bind with high affinity these molecules but not to other HLA sub-types. Symptomatic or asymptomatic celiac disease can occur in 10% of first-degree relatives of patients with defined celiac sprue. Because of this, screening of first-degree relatives using serologic testing is frequently recommended. Three-quarters of identical twins are concordant for the disorder.

Clinical presentation

Classically, celiac disease has presented with symptoms of malabsorption and malnutrition, with clinical improvement upon gluten withdrawal. Celiac disease runs a wide clinical spectrum. In children, celiac disease produces failure to

Yamada's Handbook of Gastroenterology, Fourth Edition. John M. Inadomi, Renuka Bhattacharya, Joo Ha Hwang, and Cynthia Ko.

thrive, pallor, developmental delay, and short stature, in addition to variable abdominal symptoms. Children with celiac disease typically present in the first to third years of life. Adult patients with celiac disease often, but not always, have gastrointestinal symptoms, fatigue, weight loss, or pallor when diagnosed. Gastrointestinal symptoms may include loose stools or diarrhea, bloating, and flatulence, loud borborygmi, and abdominal discomfort. The magnitude of weight loss depends on the extent and severity of the intestinal lesion, and the degree to which the patient increases dietary intake. Rare cases of celiac disease present with intestinal pseudo-obstruction. With more widespread awareness and screening for this disorder, patients are more likely to present with milder symptoms, including nonspecific gastrointestinal complaints, anemia, infertility, osteoporosis, abnormal liver chemistries, and infertility.

Patients with potential celiac disease have abnormal celiac serologic testing but normal duodenal biopsy findings or only increased intraepithelial lymphocytes. These patients have no symptoms or signs of malabsorption but are at risk for future development of overt celiac disease. Patients with refractory celiac disease have ongoing symptoms despite strict gluten avoidance. This condition is rare, but enteropathy-associated T-cell lymphoma or collagenous sprue must be ruled out. Other conditions that can present with villous atrophy such as common variable immunodeficiency or autoimmune enteropathy must also be excluded.

Other regions of the gastrointestinal tract may exhibit inflammatory changes in patients with celiac disease. Ten percent of patients also have lymphocytic gastritis. Microscopic colitis represents a cause of unexplained watery diarrhea and is diagnosed on colonic biopsy. Depending on whether a thickened subepithelial collagen band is demonstrated, microscopic colitis may be subclassified as collagenous or lymphocytic colitis. When this is diagnosed, coexistent celiac disease should be entertained.

Patients with celiac disease can also present with extraintestinal manifestations (Table 23.1). Anemia may be secondary to iron or folate malabsorption or, in the case of severe ileal disease, vitamin B_{12} deficiency. Osteopenic bone disease results from calcium and vitamin D malabsorption. Hypocalcemia (and hypomagnesemia) may be associated with tetany and may lead to secondary hyperparathyroidism. Cutaneous bleeding, epistaxis, hematuria, and gastrointestinal hemorrhage may result from vitamin K malabsorption. Neurological manifestations include peripheral sensory neuropathy, patchy demyelination of the spinal cord, epilepsy, and cerebellar atrophy with ataxia. Psychiatric findings include mood changes, irritability, and depression. The cause of the neurological and psychiatric manifestations is unknown; furthermore, these symptoms may not resolve by excluding gluten from the diet. Muscle weakness may result from a proximal myopathy. Vitamin A deficiency may lead to night blindness. Idiopathic dilated cardiomyopathy has also been reported in association with celiac disease. Women may experience amenorrhea, delayed menarche,

Table 23.1 Clinical associations with celiac disease

Chronic diarrhea with and without malabsorption
Irritable bowel syndrome
Unexplained weight loss
Iron deficiency anemia
Folate deficiency
Vitamin E or K deficiency
Unexplained osteoporosis
Hypocalcemia, vitamin D deficiency, secondary hyperparathyroidism
Unexplained elevation of liver transaminases
Dermatitis herpetiformis
First-degree relative of patients with celiac disease
Down or Turner syndrome
Unexplained peripheral neuropathy, epilepsy, and ataxia
Unexplained infertility

infertility, preterm delivery, and low birth weight. Men may report impotence and infertility. It is also common for liver transaminases to be elevated. Some patients exhibit hyposplenism, which may increase the risk of bacterial infection. There is also a strong association between Down syndrome and celiac disease.

A number of immunological conditions are associated with celiac disease (Table 23.1). The main cutaneous complication is dermatitis herpetiformis, a skin disease with intensely pruritic papulovesicular lesions on the elbows, knees, buttocks, sacrum, face, scalp, neck, and trunk. Approximately 5% of patients with celiac disease report symptomatic dermatitis herpetiformis. Most patients who present initially with dermatitis herpetiformis exhibit celiac sprue-like findings on intestinal biopsy specimens and may respond slowly to a gluten-free diet, although this is not universal. In most patients, a granular or speckled pattern of IgA deposits is noted at the epidermal-dermal junction of uninvolved skin; a linear pattern is less common. Other skin diseases found in patients with celiac sprue include psoriasis, eczema, pustular dermatitis, cutaneous amyloid, cutaneous vasculitis, nodular prurigo, and mycosis fungoides.

Celiac disease exhibits clinical associations with other autoimmune diseases such as insulin-dependent diabetes mellitus, thyroid disease, selective IgA deficiency, Sjögren syndrome, systemic lupus erythematosus, mixed cryoglobulinemia, vasculitis, pulmonary disease, pericarditis, neurological disorders, ocular abnormalities, IgA mesangial nephropathy, primary sclerosing cholangitis, and primary biliary cirrhosis.

Physical findings depend on disease severity. Patients with mild disease exhibit no abnormal physical symptoms. In more severe disease, emaciation, clubbed nails, dependent edema, ascites, ecchymoses, pallor, cheilosis, glossitis, decreased peripheral sensation, and a positive Chvostek or Trousseau sign related to nutritional deficiencies and malabsorption may be detected. Hyperkeratosis follicularis may result from vitamin A deficiency.

Diagnostic investigation

Blood tests in patients with celiac disease may detect anemia (microcytic resulting from iron deficiency or macrocytic resulting from folate or vitamin B_{12} deficiency), hypocalcemia, hypophosphatemia, hypomagnesemia, metabolic acidosis, hypoalbuminemia, hypoglobulinemia, low serum vitamin A levels, prolonged prothrombin time, and an elevated serum alkaline phosphatase level. Fecal fat levels may be increased on qualitative (i.e. Sudan stain) or quantitative assessment.

Antibody testing

If celiac disease is a diagnostic consideration, serological antibody tests are useful initial tests but do not replace the need for small intestinal biopsy. Because of their low sensitivity and specificity, anti-gliadin IgA antibodies are not currently recommended for celiac disease diagnosis and screening. More recently developed antibody tests provide more reliable screening for celiac disease. Anti-endomysial, anti-tissue transglutaminase (tTG), and anti-deamidated gliadin peptide (DGP) IgA antibodies all have a sensitivity and specificity for disease detection of over 90%. Up to 5% of patients with celiac disease have selective IgA deficiency, which may produce false-negative celiac antibody tests. Some clinicians obtain IgG titers of the same antibodies or measure serum IgA levels to exclude this possibility. If patients are already on a gluten-free diet, antibody levels may decline or return to normal. Therefore, serological testing should ideally be performed with patients on a gluten-containing diet. If testing is negative on a gluten-free diet, testing for the presence of HLA DQ-2 or DQ-8 can be obtained. If HLA testing is negative, celiac disease is effectively excluded. A suggested algorithm for the evaluation of suspected celiac disease is shown in Figure 23.1.

Histology of the small intestine

To confirm the diagnosis of celiac disease in those with positive serologic testing or in those with a high suspicion of this disorder regardless of serologic results, biopsy of the small intestinal mucosa is required. If patients are on a gluten-free diet, intestinal histology may gradually revert toward normal. Therefore, biopsies should ideally be obtained when patients are ingesting dietary gluten. With active disease, the endoscopic appearance of the duodenal mucosa is a loss of intestinal villi with scalloping of the folds.

Different grades of enteropathy can be graded histologically using the Marsh classification. Grade 0, or preinfiltrative, histology appears normal but is associated with abnormal serologic testing. It is found in some cases of dermatitis herpetiformis and characterizes potential celiac disease. Grade 1 is an infiltrative lesion with increased intraepithelial lymphocytes but no villous atrophy; patients with grade 1 histology may not have gastrointestinal symptoms. Grade 2 is

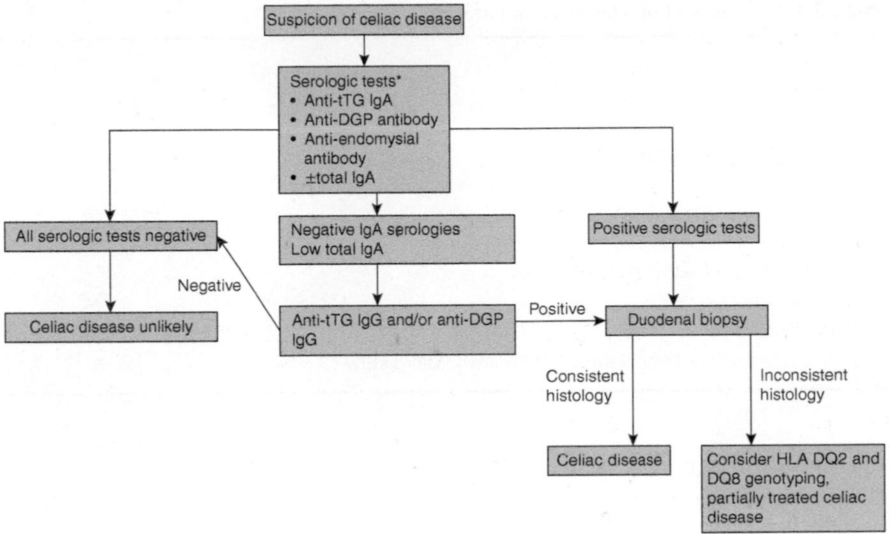

Figure 23.1 Algorithm for the evaluation of a patient for celiac disease. DGP, deamidated gliadin peptide; HLA, human leukocyte antigen; IgA/G, immunoglobulin A/G; tTG, tissue transglutaminase.
*If high suspicion of celiac disease proceeding directly to duodenal biopsy is reasonable. All tests should ideally be performed while patient is on a gluten-containing diet

similar to grade 1 but with crypt hyperplasia and normal villous architecture. Grade 3 is characterized by the typical villous atrophy of untreated celiac disease and is subclassified by the degree of villous atrophy (grades 3a, 3b, and 3c). With this finding, the total thickness of the mucosa is increased by crypt hyperplasia and lamina propria infiltration by plasma cells and lymphocytes. Subtotal villous atrophy may be observed in milder disease or in disease that has been partially treated with a gluten-free diet.

Other infectious or inflammatory diseases produce histological findings similar to celiac disease, including giardiasis, tropical sprue, collagenous sprue, HIV enteropathy, tuberculosis, radiation enteritis, Whipple disease, lymphoma, and Crohn's disease (Table 23.2). Thus, a presumptive diagnosis of celiac disease should be supported by serologic testing and the histologic and clinical response to a gluten-free diet.

Radiologic studies

In 85% of celiac disease patients, barium radiography of the small intestine exhibits the loss of the fine, feathery mucosal pattern with thin mucosal folds. Additional findings in some individuals include straightening of the valvulae conniventes, thickened mucosal folds, luminal dilation, and flocculation of contrast. Such radiographic exams are most important in excluding ulcerative and neoplastic complications of celiac disease. Abdominal computed tomography and magnetic resonance imaging may detect hyposplenism and abdominal lymphadenopathy in some patients. Bone densitometry should be obtained at

Table 23.2 Etiologies of duodenal villous atrophy

Celiac disease
Tropical sprue
Autoimmune enteropathy
Small intestinal bacterial overgrowth
Crohn's disease
Infectious enteritis, e.g. Giardia
Whipple's disease
Drug-induced enteropathy, e.g. olmesartan
Eosinophilic enteritis
Intestinal lymphoma
Acquired immunodeficiency syndrome-associated enteropathy

time of diagnosis to asses for osteopenia or osteoporosis; if abnormal, it should be repeated after one year.

Management

The mainstay for treating celiac sprue is lifelong adherence to a gluten-free diet, which requires completely eliminating wheat (including triticale, spelt, and semolina), rye, and barley products from the diet. As the gluten-free diet is complex, consultation with an experienced nutritionist is essential. Corn, rice, sorghum, buckwheat, potatoes, and soy do not activate the disease. While oats have traditionally been excluded from a gluten-free diet, multiple studies have demonstrated that most patients with celiac disease tolerate oats; in particular pure oat flour is tolerated by many with celiac disease. Gluten is not present in distilled liquor so whisky and other spirits are well tolerated. However, barley-containing beer and ale should be avoided. Because of the loss of brush border lactase activity, dairy products should initially be avoided but these substances can be reintroduced after symptoms improve on a gluten-restricted diet. Symptomatic improvement may be reported as soon as 48 hours after these dietary modifications are initiated. Recovery of normal intestinal histological features often takes much longer (i.e. months), and abnormalities persist in 50% of patients despite strict adherence to the diet. The distal intestinal mucosa heals more rapidly than the proximal mucosa.

Supplemental iron or folate (and rarely vitamin B_{12}) may be needed to treat anemia early in therapy. Vitamin K may be required to treat a coagulation deficit. Osteopenic bone disease is treated with calcium and vitamin D replacement or bisphosphonate therapy. Periodic monitoring with serologic testing and nutritional labs including iron studies and vitamin D is recommended, as is periodic reassessment of dietary adherence. Pneumococcal vaccination is recommended due to the association with hyposplenism. With gluten restriction, antibody levels should gradually decline; if they remain elevated, patients may have ongoing inadvertent or intentional gluten ingestion. The role of repeating the small bowel biopsy in patients with symptomatic improvement is debated.

A subset of patients with celiac disease do not respond to a gluten-free diet and have ongoing gastrointestinal symptoms. In these patients, adherence to the gluten-free diet should be reassessed, as ongoing gluten exposure is the most common cause of nonresponse. Repeat endoscopy with small intestinal biopsies is important to assess the degree of mucosal damage. Other etiologies of diarrhea such as microscopic colitis, lactose intolerance, pancreatic insufficiency, irritable bowel syndrome, inflammatory bowel disease, and small intestinal bacterial overgrowth should be excluded.

Patients with persistent villous atrophy despite strict adherence to a gluten-free diet and in whom other causes of villous atrophy have been excluded have refractory celiac disease. In these patients, small intestinal biopsies should be taken to assess for the presence of clonal lymphocyte populations. Patients with refractory sprue but without clonal lymphocyte populations have type I refractory disease, which is associated with a more favorable prognosis. The presence of clonal lymphocyte populations in small intestinal biopsies indicates type II disease, which may progress to enteropathy-associated T-cell lymphoma. Anti-inflammatory agents such as mesalamine or corticosteroids are sometimes used in patients with refractory sprue. Azathioprine, cyclosporine, methotrexate, and anti-tumor necrosis factor antibodies can be used as steroid-sparing agents, if needed.

The prognosis for type II refractory sprue is particularly poor with development of malnutrition, infection, ulcerative jejunoileitis, or enteropathy-associated T-cell lymphomas. Enteropathy-associated T-cell lymphoma is often multifocal and diffuse and may be difficult to diagnose. Chronic ulcerative jejunoileitis is characterized by multiple ulcers and strictures of the small intestine and presents with anemia, hemorrhage, perforation, or stricture. Patients with celiac disease who have this complication often are refractory to gluten restriction and are further predisposed to developing lymphoma. Carcinoma of the upper gastrointestinal tract and small intestine is more common in patients with celiac disease than in a healthy population, as is lymphoma. Evidence strongly suggests that adherence to a gluten-free diet reduces the subsequent incidence of malignancy.

Essentials of diagnosis of celiac disease

- Maintain a high index of suspicion for celiac disease.
- Serological testing can assess levels of anti-tTG, anti-endomysial, and/or anti-DGP antibodies. The sensitivity and specificity of these antibodies are all greater than 90%. In some patients, total IgA levels may be helpful due to the higher prevalence of selective IgA deficiency. Anti-gliadin antibodies have low sensitivity and specificity, and should not be used to screen for celiac disease.

- The sensitivity and specificity of diagnostic testing is higher if patients are on a gluten-containing diet. Both serological tests and small intestinal histology can improve with initiation of a gluten-free diet, potentially leading to false-negative results.
- HLA genotyping may be helpful in patients with equivocal results on serological or histological testing, or in those on a gluten-restricted diet.
- Biopsy of the small intestine is the gold standard for the diagnosis of celiac disease. However, villous atrophy and intraepithelial lymphocytosis are not specific for celiac disease. Other causes include giardiasis, tropical sprue, eosinophilic gastroenterology, HIV enteropathy, radiation enteritis, and Crohn's disease.

Case Studies

Case 1

A 23-year-old man is referred for iron deficiency anemia. He describes minor symptoms of intermittent loose stool that he has attributed to lactose intolerance, but otherwise has no abdominal pain, nausea, or vomiting. His body-mass index is 23 and his physical examination is normal without rashes or neurological deficits. His white blood count is normal but his hemoglobin is 8.2 mg/dl with a hematocrit of 24% and an MCV of 72. His ferritin is 2 and iron saturation is 5%. His deaminated anti-gliadin and tTG antibodies are abnormally elevated and you perform an upper gastrointestinal endoscopy that is notable for subtle scalloping of the duodenal mucosa. Pathology of duodenal biopsies reveals villous atrophy with crypt hyperplasia and lamina propria infiltration by plasma cells and lymphocytes. You place him on oral iron therapy and refer him to a nutritionist for a gluten-free diet to treat celiac disease.

He returns two months later with no symptoms, but persistent microcytic anemia. He states he has been adherent to a gluten-free diet; however, after careful questioning he admits consumption of one to two beers daily. Further counseling including avoidance of barley-derived alcohol is conducted and on follow up three months later his anemia has resolved and he remains asymptomatic.

Discussion

The presentation of celiac disease ranges from symptomatic disease with abdominal pain, diarrhea, and steatorrhea with weight loss, to an absence of symptoms with subtle signs or biochemical abnormalities including anemia. Positive serologies may be sufficient to provide a diagnosis, although histopathological confirmation is useful for documentation of celiac disease because it requires lifelong lifestyle changes to adhere to a gluten-free diet. The most common reason for nonresponse to dietary prescription is nonadherence, often inadvertent because gluten can be present in numerous foods, drinks, or other ingestible products including beer. Gluten is not present in distilled liquor, which may be an acceptable alternative.

Further reading

Hill, I.D., Fasano, A., Guandalini, S. et al. (2016). NASPGHAN clinical report on the diagnosis and treatment of gluten-related disorders. *J. Pediatr. Gastroenterol. Nutr.* 64: 156–165.

Rubio-Tapia, A., Hill, I.D., Kelly, C.P. et al. (2013). Diagnosis and management of celiac disease. *Am. J. Gastroenterol.* 108: 656–676.

US Preventive Services Task Force (2017). Screening for celiac disease. *J. Am. Med. Assoc.* 317: 1252–1257.

Further reading

CHAPTER 24
Short Bowel Syndrome

Short bowel syndrome is a condition resulting from surgical resection, congenital defect or disease-associated loss of absorption from a substantial portion of small or large intestine. Less than 200 cm of remaining small intestine is often used for the clinical diagnosis: however, a more meaningful criteria for short bowel associated intestinal failure is absorption <1.4 kg/day of wet weight or <84% of energy needs.

Clinical presentation

The symptoms and signs associated with short bowel syndrome include chronic diarrhea, dehydration, steatorrhea, fluid and electrolyte abnormalities (hyponatremia, hypokalemia, hypocalcemia, hypomagnesemia), with nutrient deficiencies. The consequences of small bowel resection are variable but in general relate to the extent of resection, the site of resection, and subsequent adaptive processes. The proximal jejunum is the primary site for carbohydrate, protein and water-soluble vitamin absorption. Active transport of sodium chloride in the ileum allows greater fluid resorption to occur compared with the jejunum. The ileum is also the primary site of bile salt and vitamin B12 absorption, and the source of gut-derived hormones (glucagon-like peptides 1 and 2 and peptide YY) that modulate intestinal motility. Fat absorption occurs over the length of the small intestine. The primary function of the colon is fluid and electrolyte reabsorption; however, bacterial fermentation of malabsorbed carbohydrates to short chain fatty acids allows salvage of energy in short bowel syndrome.

Diarrhea results from a reduction in the absorptive surface area, decreased transit time, increased osmolality of the lumenal contents (as a result of carbohydrate malabsorption), bacterial overgrowth, and fluid hypersecretion from the stomach, small and large intestine. After surgery, fluid losses may exceed 5 l/day, especially with concomitant colectomy. Gastric hypergastrinemia and

Yamada's Handbook of Gastroenterology, Fourth Edition. John M. Inadomi, Renuka Bhattacharya, Joo Ha Hwang, and Cynthia Ko.

hypersecretion cause intestinal mucosal damage, impaired micelle formation, and inhibition of pancreatic enzyme function. Nutritional deficiencies produce weight loss, weakness, fatigue, and growth retardation (in children). Consequences of fatty acid malabsorption include tetany, osteomalacia, and osteoporosis secondary to hypocalcemia and hypomagnesemia. Removal of <100 cm of terminal ileum reduces bile acid absorption and may lead to bile salt-induced secretory diarrhea. Conversely, steatorrhea results from loss of longer ileal segments. Proteins also are metabolized by colonic flora and contribute to osmotic diarrhea to a lesser degree. Zinc deficiency, which may impair intestinal adaptation, is common, as is fat-soluble vitamin deficiency and vitamin B_{12} deficiency. However, other water-soluble vitamins and trace metals are generally well absorbed even if the resection is extensive.

There is a gradual improvement in the absorption of fat, nitrogen, and carbohydrate after extensive resection of the small intestine. The colon also undergoes adaptive dilation, lengthening, and mucosal proliferation and acquires the ability to absorb glucose and amino acids to a limited degree. Enteral nutrients elicit intestinal adaptation by direct effects on epithelial cells and by stimulating trophic gastrointestinal and pancreaticobiliary hormone secretion. Disaccharides are more potent stimulants of adaptation than monosaccharides, and highly saturated fats are more effective stimulants than less saturated fats. Hormones that may have relevant trophic effects include gastrin, cholecystokinin, enteroglucagon, and neurotensin. Growth factors such as epithelial growth factor and insulin-like growth factor 1, prostaglandins, glutamine, arginine, short-chain fatty acids, and polyamines. Conversely, intestinal hypoplasia may result from complete reliance on parenteral nutrition.

Potential pitfalls

Short bowel syndrome presents with a variety of symptoms that may require individualized therapy. Diarrhea is universal and multifactorial. Fat malabsorption (steatorrhea) and carbohydrate malabsorption induce an osmotic diarrhea, while hypersecretion of gastric fluid secondary to hypergastrinemia contributes to a secretory diarrhea. Mineral deficiencies often complicate short bowel syndrome, and vitamin B_{12} is especially common after ileal resection; however, other water-soluble vitamins are absorbed throughout the small intestine and deficiencies are not typical. Similarly, protein absorption is generally preserved.

Diagnostic investigation

Laboratory testing

Laboratory abnormalities relate to the severity of nutrient, vitamin, and mineral deficiencies. Electrolyte determinations may reveal hyponatremia, hypokalemia, hypocalcemia, and hypomagnesemia, whereas a complete blood count may

Table 24.1 Causes of short bowel syndrome

Adult causes	Pediatric causes
Mesenteric ischemia	Necrotizing enterocolitis
Postoperative complications	Intestinal atresia
Crohn's disease	Midgut volvulus
Radiation enteritis	Gastroschisis
Malignancy	Malignancy
Trauma	Trauma

show anemia caused by vitamin B_{12} deficiency or, less commonly, folate and iron deficiencies. Fat-soluble vitamin deficiencies (i.e. A, D, E, and rarely K) may be evident. Urine oxalate levels may be elevated in patients predisposed to oxalate calculi. Stool studies may reveal steatorrhea. Bacterial overgrowth may be detected through hydrogen breath testing.

Radiographic studies

Small intestinal barium radiography can be performed if the length of residual bowel is uncertain. Bone radiography and bone densitometry can be used to assess for osteomalacia and osteoporosis in a patient with calcium and vitamin D malabsorption. Ultrasound may be of value in detecting gallstones. Computed tomography, intravenous pyelography, or renal ultrasound may detect renal calculi.

Differential diagnosis

Causes of short bowel syndrome

The most common disorders in adults that lead to massive resection of the small intestine are vascular insults and Crohn's disease (Table 24.1). Risk factors for vascular disease include advanced age, congestive heart failure, atherosclerotic and valvular heart disease, chronic diuretic use, hypercoagulable states, and oral contraceptive use.

Management and prevention

Nutritional therapy

During the initial postoperative phase, intravenous fluids, electrolytes and total parenteral nutrition are required to prevent dehydration and complications from electrolyte losses. Parenteral nutrition requirements in short bowel syndrome are not specific to the disease and general recommendations should be followed. Energy requirements may be greater than other patients depending on the underlying disease state. Lipids should not exceed 1 g/kg/day, and 1–1.5 g/kg/day of protein should be administered. Over time, many patients can be slowly weaned from intravenous feedings. The length of remaining small intestine, preservation of the colon, and ileocolonic anastomosis predict the ability to wean from intravenous hyperalimentation. Patients who receive long-term parenteral nutrition at home require a permanent intravenous catheter that must be placed surgically.

Limited data suggest that a high-carbohydrate, low-fat diet increases wet weight and mineral absorption, and reduces oxalate absorption, especially among patients who have an intact colon. Caloric goals should be formally calculated; however, short bowel patients absorb only half to two-thirds of ingested energy and therefore require an appropriate increase in energy consumption. Complex carbohydrates are preferred over simple sugars owing to lower osmotic load and enhanced adaptive effects on intestinal mucosa. Sodium supplementation is necessary due to intestinal losses. Dietary protein usually does not need to be increased because nitrogen absorption is preserved. Oral calcium or cholestyramine may reduce dietary oxalate absorption and the risk of oxalate kidney stones. Medium-chain triglycerides can be used as nutritional supplements because they are absorbed directly from the proximal intestine into the portal circulation in the absence of bile salts. However, medium-chain triglycerides are unpalatable, may induce osmotic diarrhea, and do not provide essential fatty acids. Soluble fiber supplementation enhances adaption, slows gastric emptying and provides salvage energy source through bacterial fermentation to short-chain fatty acids. Multivitamin preparations that contain 2–5 times the recommended dietary allowances are advocated. Patients with ileal resections of more than 90 cm should receive intramuscular vitamin B_{12}. Serum retinol, calcium, 25-hydroxyvitamin D, and urinary calcium are monitored to assess the adequacy of vitamin A and D supplementation. Calcium intake of 1000–1500 mg/day is encouraged. Hypomagnesemia may require intravenous magnesium replacement because oral magnesium supplements worsen diarrhea. Iron and zinc deficiency can develop, requiring specific supplementation.

Medical therapy

Reducing diarrhea and correcting malnutrition are the major goals of managing patients with short bowel syndrome. Loperamide (up to 16 tablets daily) or diphenoxylate with atropine may be effective to delay intestinal transit, but many patients require codeine or tincture of opium to control symptoms. In patients with limited ileal resection, cholestyramine may be effective for treating bile salt diarrhea; however, this may worsen steatorrhea in patients with more extensive resection. Subcutaneous octreotide reduces fluid and electrolyte losses in some patients with short bowel syndrome as a result of retarded propulsion, decreased digestive juice secretion, and altered mucosal fluid and electrolyte transport. Oral broad-spectrum antibiotics are warranted if intestinal bacterial overgrowth is detected. There is no evidence to demonstrate benefit from pancreatic enzyme supplementation.

Emerging therapies focus on trophic factors. Glucagon-like peptide-2 (GLP-2) induces epithelial proliferation in the stomach, small bowel and colon by stimulating crypt cell proliferation and inhibiting enterocyte apoptosis. Clinical trials have demonstrated increase in energy absorption, decrease in fecal wet weight, and slowing of gastric emptying. Teduglutide, a recombinant GLP-2 analogue that is FDA approved for short bowel syndrome demonstrated the ability to reduce parenteral nutrition requirements in clinical trials. Side effects include abdominal pain and distention, nausea, stomal changes and peripheral edema. Recombinant-human growth hormone has been approved by the FDA for patients with short bowel syndrome on parenteral nutrition; however, the clinical trials are conflicting with regards to benefit in nutrient and wet weight absorption. Newer therapies may include GLP-1 receptor agonists, epidermal growth factor (EGF), and peptide YY analogues.

Key practice points

Nutritional management of short bowel syndrome evolves over the course of the disease state. One of four long-term outcomes will emerge, depending on the length of intestinal resection and the degree of postsurgical adaptation:

- Maintenance of a balanced nutritional status using an oral diet (normal or modified)
- Requirement for defined enteral formula diet
- Requirement for parenteral electrolyte and fluid supplementation
- Necessity of total or partial parenteral nutritional supplemented by variable amounts of enteral intake

Surgical therapy

A variety of surgical procedures may benefit selected patients with short bowel syndrome. Surgical introduction of antiperistaltic segments that slow intestinal transit can increase water, fat, and nitrogen absorption. Longitudinal intestinal lengthening by tapering enteroplasty (Bianchi procedure) or serial transverse enteroplasty divide the small intestine longitudinally and construct serial anastomoses to lengthen the bowel.

Small intestinal transplantation is indicated if severe complications of parenteral nutrition such as end-stage intestinal failure-associated liver disease, loss of venous access for administration of parenteral nutrition, or recurrent catheter sepsis occur. Five-year survival rates are 75% in some centers. Infection is the primary cause of death after intestinal transplantation, with other causes including lymphoproliferative disease, nontransplant organ failure, thrombosis, ischemia, bleeding, and graft rejection.

Table 24.2 Complications of short bowel syndrome

Complications of central venous catheters (infection, occlusion, thrombosis)
Parenteral nutrition (hepatic, biliary)
Diarrhea
Malnutrition
Fluid and electrolyte abnormalities
Micronutrient deficiency
Essential fatty acid deficiency
Small bowel bacterial overgrowth
D-lactic acidosis
Oxalate nephropathy
Renal dysfunction
Metabolic bone disease
Acid peptic disease
Anastomotic ulceration or stricture

Complications and their management

Short bowel syndrome has significant systemic sequelae. Calcium oxalate renal calculi develop because of increased colonic absorption of dietary oxalate, decreased urinary concentrations of phosphate and citrate, and reduced urinary volume. The incidence of gallstones is increased twofold to threefold by ileal resection. This may be due to bile salt malabsorption, which leads to cholesterol supersaturation of gallbladder bile. However, calcium-containing cholesterol stones and pigment stones are also prevalent after small bowel resection, indicating that other mechanisms are involved.

Intrahepatic steatosis and hepatic dysfunction occur secondary to parenteral nutrition and sepsis, and may lead to liver failure, especially in children. Other complications of short bowel syndrome are indicated in Table 24.2.

Case Studies

Case 1

A 34 year-old woman presenting to the emergency department with abdominal pain is diagnosed to have mesenteric ischemia. Her only identifiable risk factor is use of contraceptive hormones. Unfortunately her course worsens with hypotension and sepsis, and she undergoes resection of the necrotic segment, leaving her with 100 cm of small intestine. She recovers slowly from her surgery and requires total parenteral nutrition for her fluid and nutritional needs. Protein is provided at a dose of 1 g/kg/day and lipids are limited to 1 g/kg/day, with the remainder of caloric administered as dextrose. Vitamins and mineral levels are monitored and replaced appropriately.

Upon resuming oral intake, she has 10–14 loose to watery bowel movements daily despite treatment with 32 mg loperamide daily. Subcutaneous octreotide is administered and her bowel movements reduce to 5–6 per day, but she remains dependent on parenteral nutrition. Teduglutide (0.05 mg/kg subcutaneous daily) is initiated after a colonoscopy is performed that demonstrates no polyps. While she remains dependent on parenteral nutrition, her requirements are reduced and she is able to maintain nutritional balance using parenteral nutrition four days/week.

Discussion

Mesenteric ischemia and necrosis is a common etiology of short bowel syndrome. Remnant intestinal length of <150 cm is an indication for home total parenteral nutrition. Oral intake should consist of a high-carbohydrate, low-fat diet consisting of complex carbohydrates. While caloric needs are routinely increased to account for malabsorption, protein does not need to be increased because nitrogen absorption is preserved. Vitamins and mineral should be routinely checked and replaced.

Loperamide may not be sufficient to control diarrhea and octreotide has been demonstrated to reduce bowel movements in refractory cases. Teduglutide is a GLP-2 agonist that increases the surface area of remaining small intestine and increases fluid and nutrient absorption. Parenteral nutrition requirements were reduced in clinical trials using teduglutide, although continued need for parenteral support is common.

Small intestinal transplantation is indicated if patients with short bowel syndrome develop liver cirrhosis due to parenteral nutrition, experience recurrent line sepsis, or lose venous access for parenteral nutrition as a result of complications of the intravenous line.

CHAPTER 25
Small Intestinal Neoplasia

Tumors of the small intestine account for less than 2% of all gastrointestinal malignancies. Primary cancers of the small intestine include adenocarcinomas, carcinoids, lymphomas, sarcomas, and leiomyosarcomas; however, benign neoplasms such as adenomas, leiomyomas, lipomas, and hamartomas are more common (Table 25.1).

Adenocarcinoma

Clinical presentation

Eighty-five percent of patients with small intestinal adenocarcinomas present after age 50. Symptoms may include abdominal pain, nausea, vomiting, and weight loss. Occult blood loss with anemia may be present. Ileal tumors may cause intussusception, and periampullary tumors (i.e. tumors of the ampulla of Vater) may cause gastric outlet obstruction, biliary obstruction with jaundice, or pancreatitis. Patients with celiac sprue may present with new-onset weight loss and abdominal pain after years of quiescent disease. Similarly, patients with Crohn's disease exhibit symptoms of obstruction that may mistakenly be attributed to a flare of their underlying disease.

The physical examination of patients with adenomas and adenocarcinomas of the small intestine is often normal. A minority of patients have abdominal distension, abdominal masses, gastric outlet obstructions, or evidence of fecal occult blood loss.

Diagnostic investigation

Upper gastrointestinal endoscopy using both forward-viewing and side-viewing endoscopes may be necessary to diagnose small intestinal adenocarcinoma. Most adenomas in patients with familial adenomatous polyposis (FAP) are located in the proximal duodenum and periampullary region, whereas up to half of

Yamada's Handbook of Gastroenterology, Fourth Edition. John M. Inadomi, Renuka Bhattacharya, Joo Ha Hwang, and Cynthia Ko.

Table 25.1 Classification of tumors of the small intestine

Benign epithelial tumors
Adenoma
Hamartomas (Peutz–Jeghers syndrome [PJS], Cronkite–Canada syndrome, juvenile polyposis, Cowden disease, Bannayan–Riley–Ruvalcaba syndrome)
Malignant epithelial tumors
Primary adenocarcinoma
Metastatic carcinoma
Carcinoid tumors
Lymphoproliferative disorders
B-cell
Diffuse large cell lymphoma
Small, noncleaved cell lymphoma
Mucosa-associated lymphoid tissue (MALT) lymphoma
Mantle cell lymphoma (multiple lymphomatous polyposis)
Immunoproliferative small intestinal disease (IPSID)
T-cell
Enteropathy-associated T-cell lymphoma
Mesenchymal tumors
Gastrointestinal stromal cell tumors (GISTs)
Fatty tumors (lipoma, liposarcoma)
Neural tumors (schwannomas, neurofibromas, ganglioneuromas)
Paragangliomas
Smooth muscle tumors (leiomyoma, leiomyosarcoma)
Vascular tumors (hemangioma, angiosarcoma, lymphangioma, Kaposi sarcoma)

Table 25.2 Distribution of malignant tumors of the small intestine

Tumor	Duodenum (%)	Jejunum (%)	Ileum (%)
Primary adenocarcinoma	40	38	22
Malignant carcinoid	18	4	78
Primary lymphoma	6	36	58
Leiomyosarcoma	3	53	44

sporadic carcinomas occur in the jejunum and ileum (Table 25.2). Lesions in the proximal or middle jejunum can be identified and biopsy specimens obtained with enteroscopy. Wireless capsule endoscopy of the small intestine may be useful for visualizing tumors that are too small to detect by radiographic techniques if clinical suspicion remains elevated despite normal radiographic studies. Computed tomographic (CT) scans are helpful in staging tumors of the small intestine by identifying lymph node and hepatic metastases.

Management

Surgical resection is the treatment of choice for adenocarcinoma of the small intestine. Tumors in the jejunum and proximal ileum are treated with segmental resection. A right hemicolectomy is required to treat adenocarcinoma of the distal ileum. Adenocarcinoma involving the ampulla of Vater requires pancreaticoduodenectomy (i.e. the Whipple procedure). The long-term survival for primary small bowel adenocarcinoma is 47.6% (local disease), 33% (regional disease), and 3.9% (distal disease). Neither chemotherapy nor radiation therapy is effective for small bowel adenocarcinoma.

Key practice point: small bowel adenocarcinoma

Most adenomas in patients with FAP are located in the proximal duodenum and periampullary region, whereas up to half of sporadic carcinomas occur in the jejunum and ileum.

Carcinoids

Clinical presentation

The most common clinical presentation of a symptomatic carcinoid tumor of the small intestine is intermittent abdominal pain. Additional complications include intestinal ischemia, intussusception, and gastrointestinal hemorrhage.

The carcinoid syndrome affects 10–18% of patients with small bowel carcinoids. Although localized foregut carcinoids may produce the carcinoid syndrome, carcinoids of the small intestine cause this syndrome only after hepatic metastasis. The characteristic symptoms of the carcinoid syndrome are flushing of the face and neck and intermittent watery diarrhea. Less common symptoms include bronchospasm and right-sided heart failure. Patients with carcinoid syndrome may experience a hypotensive crisis during the induction of general anesthesia.

Diagnostic investigation

Laboratory testing

Measuring the urinary excretion of 5-hydroxyindoleacetic acid (5-HIAA), the major metabolite of serotonin, is a sensitive and specific test for the carcinoid syndrome, but it is less accurate for detecting localized carcinoids. Excretion of more than 30 mg of 5-HIAA in a 24-hour urine sample after provocative testing is diagnostic of the carcinoid syndrome. False-positive tests may be caused by celiac disease, Whipple disease, tropical sprue, and ingesting food rich in serotonin (e.g. walnuts, bananas, and avocados). Elevation of chromogranin A can also be used for diagnosing carcinoid tumors as well as for monitoring treatment response or recurrence. The measurement of neuron-specific enolase levels has also been used, but it is a less accurate diagnostic test for carcinoid tumors than the measurement of chromogranin A.

Imaging studies

Because most carcinoids occur in the ileum, upper gastrointestinal endoscopy and colonoscopy have limited roles in identifying these tumors. Most symptomatic lesions are visible in barium radiographs of the small intestine or CT/MR enterography. The desmoplastic distortion of the mesentery may be evident as kinking and tethering of the intestine. A CT or MR scan is the procedure of choice for documenting hepatic metastases. Scintigraphy with iodine-123 (^{123}I) or ^{131}I-labeled metaiodobenzylguanidine (I-MIBG), indium-labeled pentetreotide, or octreotide may identify primary and metastatic carcinoids not detected by conventional imaging techniques. Positron emission tomography (PET) can also be used to identify metastatic carcinoids.

Management

Localized carcinoids of the small intestine should be completely resected, either endoscopically or surgically. Asymptomatic lesions smaller than 1 cm in diameter may be treated with local excision, but lesions larger than 1 cm require a wide surgical excision. Duodenal lesions require a Whipple procedure, whereas distal ileal lesions require ileocecectomy and lesions in the jejunum and proximal ileum require segmental resection with 10 cm margins. When localized disease is resected, the overall five-year survival is 75%, compared with 20–40% for metastatic disease.

Tumors with regional spread require wide surgical resection. Five-year survival after resection and nodal dissection for regional disease is 65–71%, compared to 38% for patients who do not have surgery.

Patients with metastatic disease and the carcinoid syndrome may benefit from debulking surgery. The somatostatin analog octreotide inhibits serotonin release and reduces flushing in more than 70% and reduces diarrhea in more than 60% of patients with carcinoid syndrome. Initial doses range from 50 to 250 mcg subcutaneously two to three times daily, but as the disease progresses, larger doses may be necessary.

Key practice points: small bowel carcinoid tumors

- The carcinoid syndrome affects 10–18% of patients with small bowel carcinoids.
- Measuring the urinary excretion of 5-HIAA, the major metabolite of serotonin, is a sensitive and specific test for the carcinoid syndrome, but it is less accurate for detecting localized carcinoids.
- Most carcinoids occur in the ileum.
- Most symptomatic small bowel lesions are visible in barium radiographs of the small intestine.
- Localized carcinoids of the small intestine should be completely resected, either endoscopically or surgically. When localized disease is resected, the overall five-year survival is 75%, compared with 20–40% for metastatic disease.

Mesenchymal Tumors

Clinical presentation and diagnostic investigation

Most small gastrointestinal stromal tumors (GISTs) are discovered incidentally and are asymptomatic. Larger tumors may be associated with symptoms of abdominal pain, nausea, vomiting, weight loss, or gastrointestinal hemorrhage. In some series, up to 40% of patients with ileal GISTs present with intussusception.

Small bowel radiography, CT scan, and angiography are useful in diagnosing GISTs. Because the lesions are submucosal, endoscopic diagnosis is often difficult unless ulceration is present. Biopsy specimens or resected tissue should be stained for CD117 to confirm the diagnosis of a GIST.

Management

The treatment of choice for small bowel GISTs is segmental intestinal resection. Despite complete resection with negative margins, recurrence rates approach 50–80% for GISTs with high-risk features (see Chapter 22). Patients found to have GISTs with high risk features should be evaluated by an oncologist for consideration of chemotherapy with imatinib.

Key practice points: small bowel GISTs

- Small bowel GISTs should be surgically resected as long as there is no evidence of metastatic disease or if the lesion is causing a bowel obstruction.
- Patients found to have GISTs with high-risk features should be evaluated by an oncologist for consideration of imatinib therapy.

Lymphoma

Clinical presentation

A discrete mass lesion characterizes primary small bowel lymphoma (PSBL). Intermittent abdominal pain caused by obstruction is the most common complaint. Weight loss is often marked, and a small percentage of patients presents with perforations. Lymphoma should be suspected in patients with celiac sprue who complain of abdominal pain and weight loss after years or decades of quiescent disease. Misinterpreting these symptoms as a flare of celiac sprue may delay diagnosis.

Patients with immunoproliferative small intestinal disease (IPSID) present earlier than those with PSBL. Patients report profuse diarrhea and weight loss in addition to symptoms of obstruction. Many patients have associated clubbing of the digits. Unlike PSBL, a palpable abdominal mass is uncommon.

Diagnostic investigation

Barium radiography of the small intestine is the primary means of detecting small bowel lymphomas. Because most PSBLs occur in the ileum, upper gastrointestinal endoscopy may not visualize the lesion. Tumors within the distal 5–10 cm of the terminal ileum are accessible to colonoscopic biopsy. Double balloon enteroscopy may also identify the lesion. CT scans may be able to stage the tumor based on detecting malignant intra-abdominal and intrathoracic lymph nodes. Because of the diffuse nature of IPSID, a laparotomy may be required to establish the diagnosis. There are no specific laboratory features of PSBL but serum protein electrophoresis demonstrates an α-heavy chain paraprotein in 20–70% of patients with IPSID.

Management

Staging lymphomas of the small intestine is similar to that of gastric lymphomas. Patients with PSBL should be treated with surgical resection with lymph node sampling. Even if curative resection is not possible, palliative resection will prevent perforation resulting from chemotherapy-induced tumor necrosis. Combination chemotherapy is indicated for disease that is incompletely resected or unresectable but the role of adjuvant therapy after curative resection is undefined. Patients with IPSID may respond to antibiotic therapy in the prelymphomatous stage (tetracycline or metronidazole for 6–12 months). Nonresponders or patients in the lymphomatous stage have responded to anthracycline-based chemotherapy. The five-year survival rate after curative resection for PSBL is 44–65%, whereas the corresponding survival rate for unresectable disease is only 20%. A poor prognosis is associated with IPSID, enteropathy-associated T-cell lymphoma, and mantle cell lymphoma.

Key practice points: small bowel lymphomas

- Most PSBLs occur in the ileum.
- Because of the diffuse nature of IPSID, a laparotomy may be required to establish the diagnosis.
- Patients with PSBLs should be treated with surgical resection with lymph node sampling.
- Patients with IPSID may respond to antibiotic therapy in the prelymphomatous stage (tetracycline or metronidazole for 6–12 months).

Case studies

Case 1

A 45-year-old woman with Peutz–Jeghers syndrome (PJS) presents to the gastrointestinal clinic for an annual clinic visit. She states that she feels well overall; however, she reports occasional episodes of severe crampy mid-abdominal pain associated with abdominal fullness, nausea, and vomiting. The episodes typically last for only a few hours and always resolve spontaneously. She denies any weight loss. The patient has already had a colectomy due to multiple adenomatous polyps. She undergoes annual surveillance of her upper GI tract due to extensive polyposis in her stomach and multiple adenomas that have been resected and/or ablated in her duodenum. Physical exam is notable for mucocutaneous pigmentation involving the lips and buccal mucosa. Otherwise, her abdomen is benign with no palpable masses. A barium radiograph of the small bowel demonstrates a 3 cm polyp in the mid-jejunum. A double balloon enteroscopy is then performed and the polyp is endoscopically removed. Histology demonstrates the polyp to be hamartomatous.

Discussion

PJS is an autosomal dominant disorder. Gastrointestinal polyps in patients with PJS are common. Polyps are typically hamartomatous and can occur in the stomach, small bowel, and colon. Obstruction of the small bowel is a common presenting symptom and is due to intussusceptions or obstruction of the lumen by the polyp.

Diagnosis of PJS should be suspected in a patient found to have a hamartomatous polyp. The diagnosis is established clinically if two of the three following criteria are present:

- family history of PJS
- mucocutaneous hyperpigmentation
- small bowel polyps.

In addition, genetic testing should be considered. Patients with PJS are at increased risk for GI (colorectal, stomach, small bowel, and pancreas) and non-GI (lung, breast, uterus, and ovary) cancers.

Case 2

A 64-year-old woman presents to her primary care provider with complaints of intermittent crampy right lower quadrant abdominal pain. She denies any blood in her stool and does not report any change in her bowel habits. The patient had a normal screening colonoscopy one year prior. Physical exam is unremarkable. A CT scan is performed and a 3 cm tumor in the ileum is identified. No other lesions are identified. The patient has the tumor surgically resected and histology demonstrates the tumor to be a carcinoid with extension through the muscularis propria without penetration of the overlying serosa. There is also evidence of nodal metastasis. The patient is staged as stage IIIB (T3N1M0). Six months following resection the patient is found to have a normal urinary 5-HIAA and no evidence of recurrence on CT scan.

Discussion

Small bowel carcinoids are typically found in the ileum. They often are found incidentally or present with nonspecific symptoms of vague abdominal pain. Small bowel carcinoids can metastasize irrespective of size. They often present with multiple lesions. Carcinoid syndrome is usually present only with hepatic metastasis. Following surgical resection of nonmetastatic carcinoid tumors, the patient should be followed clinically to monitor for evidence of recurrence, typically with urinary 5-HIAA measurements and CT scans.

Further reading

National Comprehensive Cancer Network (NCCN) guidelines for neuroendocrine tumors are available at www.nccn.org.

CHAPTER 26
Diverticular Disease of the Colon

A diverticulum (plural: diverticula) is a sac-like protrusion of the wall of the colon. Diverticulosis is an acquired condition. Typical colonic diverticula herniate through defects in the muscle layer where arteries (vasa recta) pass on either side of the mesenteric taenia and on the mesenteric aspect of the antimesenteric taeniae. Because they do not possess muscular layers, they are false or pulsion diverticula. In industrialized nations, 33–50% of individuals over 50 years of age have colonic diverticula and the prevalence steadily increases with age. Diverticula are less common outside the Western hemisphere. Ninety-five percent of patients with diverticulosis have diverticula in the sigmoid colon. Twenty-four percent of patients have diverticula in other regions in addition to the sigmoid colon; 7% have pancolic involvement. Rectal diverticula are rare because of the presence of the circumferential longitudinal muscle layer. Sigmoid diverticulosis is accompanied by thickening of the circular muscle, shortening of the taenia coli, and narrowing of the lumen. Most diverticula are less than 1 cm in diameter.

Development of diverticulosis depends on the strength of the colon wall and the pressure difference between the lumen of the colon and the peritoneal cavity. Muscle thickening in the sigmoid colon is likely to represent a prediverticular condition resulting from high intraluminal pressures in an area of small diameter, with no corresponding increase in wall strength. The elasticity and tensile strength of the colon decrease with age, an effect that is most marked in the sigmoid colon. Deterioration in colonic structural proteins in Ehlers–Danlos and Marfan syndromes may explain the premature development of diverticula in these conditions. The role of primary colonic motor disorders in the pathogenesis of diverticulosis is undefined, and the relationship of diverticulosis and irritable bowel syndrome is controversial.

Identification of risk factors for diverticular disease is an area of active investigation. Cohort studies have implicated low dietary fiber, high intake of

Yamada's Handbook of Gastroenterology, Fourth Edition. John M. Inadomi, Renuka Bhattacharya, Joo Ha Hwang, and Cynthia Ko.

red meat, physical inactivity, high body mass index, and smoking with higher risk of diverticulitis. Although commonly believed, dietary intake of nuts, seeds, and popcorn is not associated with an increased risk of diverticulitis or diverticular bleeding. Medications that may predispose to diverticulitis or diverticular bleeding include nonsteroidal anti-inflammatory drugs (NSAIDs), steroids, and opiates.

Clinical spectrum of diverticulosis and diverticular disease

Diverticulosis implies the presence of diverticula, which may be asymptomatic or symptomatic. Diverticular disease implies symptoms such as diverticulitis, diverticular hemorrhage, segmental colitis associated with diverticulosis, or symptomatic uncomplicated diverticular disease. Seventy percent of persons with diverticulosis never develop significant symptoms, and do not require specific medical intervention. Some patients have mild, intermittent abdominal pain, bloating, flatulence, and altered defecation, although the causal relationship of these symptoms with the diverticula is debated. Three-quarters of the remaining patients develop diverticulitis and one-quarter report diverticular hemorrhage.

Symptomatic uncomplicated diverticular disease

Clinical presentation

Patients with otherwise uncomplicated diverticular disease may present with symptoms such as abdominal pain or altered bowel habits without overt colitis or diverticulitis. However, whether the relationship between symptoms and the presence of diverticulosis is causal remains a matter of debate. In these patients, altered colonic motility or visceral hypersensitivity may play a role in symptom development.

Diagnostic investigation

On barium enema radiography, diverticula appear as contrast-filled colonic protrusions that may persist after evacuation. The presence of diverticula reduces the accuracy of barium enema radiography in detecting coexisting colonic neoplasia. Colonoscopy may reveal diverticular orifices, sigmoid tortuosity, and thickened folds consistent with prior diverticulitis.

Management and prevention

Therapy for symptomatic but uncomplicated diverticular disease relies on increased intake of dietary fiber or the use of fiber supplements. However, lack of vigorous physical activity is associated with diverticulosis, and obesity is associated with an increased risk of complications. Therefore, exercise and weight loss for overweight individuals are recommended.

Segmental colitis associated with diverticulosis

Clinical presentation

Patients may present with symptomatic colitis and evidence of colitis on colonoscopy and mucosal biopsies. Typical symptoms include left lower quadrant abdominal pain, chronic diarrhea, and intermittent hematochezia. Severity of colitis can range from mild inflammation to chronic symptoms similar to inflammatory bowel disease. Symptoms may include chronic diarrhea, abdominal pain, and intermittent rectal bleeding. This entity is relatively rare, estimated to occur in about 1% of patients with diverticulosis. The differential diagnosis for this entity includes inflammatory bowel disease, infectious colitis, radiation colitis, and medication-associated colitis.

Diagnostic investigation

This entity is most commonly diagnosed at the time of colonoscopy. Endoscopic findings may range from patchy erythema in an area of diverticulosis to florid chronic colitis with edema, erythema, and ulcerations. Biopsies can show findings of chronic inflammatory changes. On CT imaging, findings can include colonic wall thickening and pericolic fat stranding.

Management

The management of segmental colitis associated with diverticulosis is not well understood, as there are few long-term prospective studies. Proposed therapies have included antibiotics such as ciprofloxacin and metronidazole, mesalamine, and prednisone. Segmental resection can be offered to patients with steroid-dependent or steroid-refractory disease.

Diverticulitis

Diverticulitis is symptomatic inflammation of a diverticulum and begins as peri-diverticulitis caused by a microperforation of the colon. The incidence of diverticulitis increases with age. Most cases of diverticulitis in Westernized countries are left-sided but inflammation of diverticula at other sites may occur.

Clinical presentation

Early manifestations of diverticulitis include pain over the site of inflammation (usually in the lower abdomen or pelvis), fever, nausea and vomiting, and frequently constipation. On physical examination, abdominal tenderness over the site of inflammation can be detected. There may be a palpable abdominal mass

Table 26.1 Hinchey classification of acute diverticulitis

Grade I	Localized pericolic or mesenteric abscess
Grade II	Pelvic abscess
Grade III	Purulent peritonitis
Grade IV	Feculent peritonitis

or signs of localized peritonitis such as guarding, rigidity, or rebound tenderness. Hemodynamic instability is rare and usually caused by free perforation and peritonitis.

Diverticulitis can be classified as simple or complicated in presentation. The majority of patients have mild, uncomplicated diverticulitis. Complicated diverticulitis is defined the presence of concomitant abscesses, fistulae, strictures, or obstruction. Microperforations can be walled off by the pericolic mesentery and fat, leading to localized abscess or fistulization to adjacent organs. An acute complication, most frequently abscess formation, occurs in approximately 25%. This should be suspected in patients without clinical improvement despite medical therapy. In more severe cases, free perforation and peritonitis can develop. Complicated diverticulitis with abscesses or peritonitis often characterized by the Hinchey classification system (Table 26.1), which can help guide the aggressiveness of surgical management.

Partial colonic obstruction can occur in the acute setting. However, high-grade obstruction is rare and increases risk for future development of a stricture. Fistulas most commonly occur to the bladder, where they may cause symptoms of pneumaturia or dysuria. Vaginal passage of feces or gas should raise suspicion of a colovaginal fistula.

Diagnostic investigation

Mild diverticulitis is often diagnosed clinically, but imaging studies are required to confirm the diagnosis. Computed tomography (CT) scanning is indicated if the diagnosis is uncertain, complications are suspected, medical therapy has failed, or the patient is immunocompromised. CT scans may reveal thickening of the colon wall, pericolic inflammation with fat stranding, fistulae, sinuses, abscesses, and obstruction. Intraperitoneal air implies free perforation and peritonitis. Ultrasound is occasionally useful for detecting and draining pericolonic fluid collections. Barium enema radiography is not recommended during the acute attack. Colonoscopy is generally contraindicated in cases of acute diverticulitis because of the risk of complications, including perforation.

Differential diagnosis

The differential diagnosis of acute diverticulitis is broad and needs to be considered prior to embarking on therapy specific to diverticulitis. Acute appendicitis, inflammatory bowel disease, ischemic colitis, peptic ulcer disease, and infectious colitis can all present with symptoms similar to acute diverticulitis. Ectopic pregnancy and ovarian cysts, torsion or abscess should be suspected in female patients. Neoplasia, especially colorectal carcinoma, should also be considered, particularly in older patients with weight loss or gastrointestinal bleeding.

Management and prevention

Traditionally, the initial management of uncomplicated diverticulitis has included fluid replacement, and oral antibiotics such as quinolones, metronidazole, trimethoprim-sulfamethoxazole, or amoxicillin/clavulanate for 7–10 days (Figure 26.1). Recently, the role of antibiotics for uncomplicated diverticulitis has come into question, and some now advocate supportive care as antibiotic therapy may not accelerate recovery or prevent the development of complications. Nevertheless, standard of care continues to be antibiotic therapy. Repeat imaging is not needed if patients demonstrate clinical improvement. NSAIDs should be avoided because they are associated with increased risk of diverticulitis.

Inpatient treatment may be needed for patients with severe uncomplicated diverticulitis or risk factors for poor treatment response such as immunosuppression or significant comorbidity. Those with complicated diverticulitis always require inpatient management. Patients who do not respond to initial outpatient management may also require hospitalization for more intensive management.

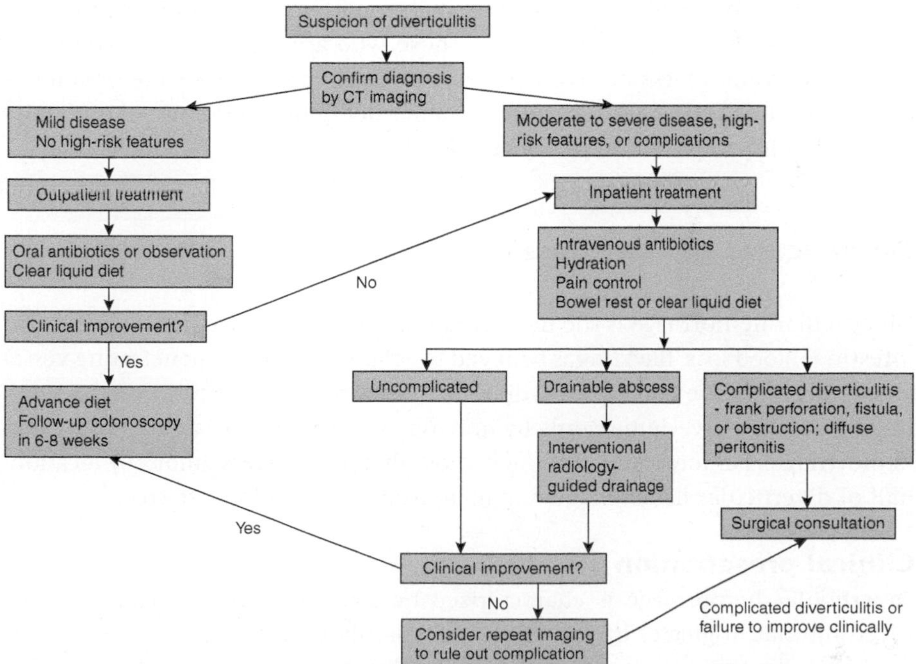

Figure 26.1 Suggested management of acute diverticulitis. CT, computed tomography.

Broad-spectrum antibiotics should be directed at anaerobes, Gram-negative organisms, and Gram-positive coliforms. Nasogastric suction may be needed for ileus or obstruction. Pericolic abscesses less than 2 cm in size usually resolve without further intervention. Percutaneous CT-guided abscess drainage may benefit patients with larger abscesses who are stable and without signs of sepsis. Indications for surgery in the acute setting include frank perforation and peritonitis (e.g. Hinchey class III or IV) and abscesses not responding to conservative therapy or percutaneous drainage. In the case of urgent surgery, primary anastomosis is not attempted because anastomotic breakdown is possible.

Indications for surgery outside the acute setting include the presence of fistula or obstruction. Although surgery was previously recommended for recurrent diverticulitis, evolving standards suggest that it is not indicated for patients with recurrent uncomplicated diverticulitis, as these patients will generally not progress to more complicated disease. If a colonoscopy has not been performed recently, it is indicated after an episode of acute diverticulitis to exclude other causes of symptoms, particularly malignancy or inflammatory bowel disease.

No further therapy is needed if patients recover fully from an attack of acute uncomplicated diverticulitis. Elective colectomy should be offered to patients with episodes of complicated diverticulitis, particularly if recurrent, and should be considered for patients who are immunosuppressed. Patients with recurrent episodes of uncomplicated diverticulitis generally do not benefit from colectomy, but surgery may be offered to patients with symptoms that can be confidently attributed to recurrent diverticulitis or those who are at high risk of complications. Recurrent attacks of diverticulitis are usually not more severe or complicated than the initial attack. Current evidence does not support use of probiotics or mesalamine to prevent recurrences.

Diverticular hemorrhage

Diverticular hemorrhage is the most common cause of acute overt lower gastrointestinal blood loss. Bleeding is believed to originate from the penetrating vessel where it enters the dome of the diverticulum. The vessel at this point is separated from the bowel lumen only by mucosa, predisposing to vascular injury and hemorrhage. Paradoxically, although most diverticula are sigmoid in location, half of diverticular hemorrhages emanate from a right colonic source.

Clinical presentation

Diverticular hemorrhage is characterized by sudden, painless rectal bleeding. Bleeding that originates in the left colon typically presents with hematochezia, while bleeding that originates in the right colon may be appear dark or maroon colored. Rarely, bleeding from the right colon can present as melena. Severe hemorrhage may be associated with hypotension, tachycardia, or syncope.

Bleeding stops spontaneously in 80% of patients. Complications of diverticular hemorrhage are related to hypovolemia and involve the heart, brain, kidneys, and lungs. Diverticulitis and diverticular bleeding rarely coexist, and abdominal pain and fevers are rare in patients with diverticular bleeding.

Diagnostic investigation

It is important to bear in mind that hematochezia may result from a variety of lower gastrointestinal sources as well as from massive upper gastrointestinal hemorrhage. In patients with severe gastrointestinal bleeding, an upper gastrointestinal source should be considered and ruled out by nasogastric lavage or upper endoscopy. This topic is discussed in more detail in Chapter 3.

Management and prevention

The initial management of suspected diverticular hemorrhage, as for other types of gastrointestinal hemorrhage, requires obtaining intravenous access, aggressive fluid resuscitation and blood transfusions if needed. The patient's hemodynamic status must be stabilized, the airway protected, and ventilatory support established, as needed.

The sequence of further evaluation depends upon the severity of the patient's bleeding and hemodynamic status. If an upper gastrointestinal source of bleeding has been excluded, patients with ongoing large-volume blood loss should undergo conventional or CT angiography to attempt to identify the bleeding source. In some centers, scintigraphy with technetium-99m (^{99m}Tc) sulfur colloid or ^{99m}Tc-tagged erythrocytes may be used prior to angiography to identify patients whose bleeding is brisk enough to be detected by angiography. The rate of bleeding must be 0.04 ml/minute or more for scintigraphy to reveal the source. Mesenteric angiography may show extravasation of the contrast agent if the bleeding rate is higher than 0.5 ml/minute. If a site of bleeding is identified, angiographic therapy such as embolization can be utilized. However, patients must be actively bleeding for a site to be identified and treated.

Patients with severe bleeding but who can be adequately resuscitated should undergo bowel preparation and colonoscopy within 24 hours of presentation, as urgent colonoscopy is more likely to identify a site of bleeding. Patients with mild bleeding may undergo more elective colonoscopy. Endoscopically, diverticular bleeding can be treated with electrocautery, banding of the diverticulum, or endoscopic clip placement. Even though endoscopic therapy to stop diverticular hemorrhage may fail, localization of the bleeding site may allow directed evaluation and therapy to the appropriate colonic segment.

Surgery is rarely required for patients with diverticular hemorrhage due to improvements in colonoscopic and radiographic techniques. However, some patients with recurrent, severe hemorrhage may require colectomy for control. Ideally, either endoscopic or radiographic techniques will localize the segment of colon that is involved to allow segmental colectomy. If the site of bleeding cannot be localized, total abdominal colectomy may be required.

Further reading

ASGE Standards of Practice Committee (2014). The role of endoscopy in the patient with lower GI bleeding. *Gastrointest. Endosc.* 79: 875–885.

Feingold, D., Steele, S.R., Lee, S. et al. (2014). Practice parameters for the treatment of sigmoid diverticulitis. *Dis. Colon Rectum* 57: 284–294.

Stollman, N., Smalley, W., Hirano, I. et al. (2015). American Gastroenterological Association Institute guideline on the management of acute diverticulitis. *Gastroenterology* 149: 1944–1949.

Strate, L.L. and Gralnek, I.M. (2016). ACG clinical guidelines: management of patients with acute lower gastrointestinal bleeding. *Am. J. Gastroenterol.* 111: 459–474.

CHAPTER 27
Irritable Bowel Syndrome

Irritable bowel syndrome (IBS) is a disorder characterized by abdominal pain or discomfort with altered bowel habits in the absence of organic disease. It is estimated to affect 10–15% of adults in North America, although the majority of people with symptoms of IBS do not seek medical care. The most widely accepted definition of IBS is provided by the Rome IV criteria: recurrent abdominal pain or discomfort occurring at least one day/week in the past three months associated with two or more of the following: (i) related to defecation, (ii) onset associated with a change in the frequency of stool, and (iii) associated with change in stool form or appearance. IBS can be further subclassified based on the stool pattern as constipation-predominant, diarrhea-predominant, or mixed (Table 27.1).

IBS is associated with decreased health-related quality of life and increased health care costs and is responsible for up to 50% of referrals for gastroenterology consultation. The overall prevalence is two to four times higher in women than in men. IBS is associated with fibromyalgia, chronic fatigue, and functional dyspepsia, and with depression and anxiety. Most affected individuals report disease onset before age 45, although the condition is recognized in both adolescents and the elderly. However, only 25% of people with symptoms of IBS seek medical attention, often because of symptom severity, anxiety, or depression.

Clinical presentation

The intensity, location, and timing of abdominal discomfort or pain in patients with IBS are highly variable. By definition, abdominal pain in IBS is accompanied by change in stool character and is most often described as crampy or achy. The pain may be so intense as to interfere with daily activities. Abdominal pain in IBS commonly is exacerbated by ingesting a meal or by stress and is relieved by defecation or passage of flatus. Despite this, the pain rarely leads to significant

Yamada's Handbook of Gastroenterology, Fourth Edition. John M. Inadomi, Renuka Bhattacharya, Joo Ha Hwang, and Cynthia Ko.

Table 27.1 Rome IV diagnostic criteria[a] for irritable bowel syndrome (IBS)

IBS: Recurrent abdominal pain or discomfort at least one day/week in the last three months, associated with two or more of the following three criteria: 1. Related to defecation 2. Associated with a change in the frequency of stool 3. Associated with a change in the form or appearance
Irritable bowel syndrome with predominant constipation (IBS-C) More than 25% of bowel movements with Bristol stool form[b] types 1 or 2 and less than 25% with Bristol stool form types 6 or 7
Irritable bowel syndrome with predominant diarrhea (IBS-D) More than 25% of bowel movements with Bristol stool form types 6 or 7 and less than 25% with Bristol stool form types 1 or 2
Irritable bowel syndrome with mixed bowel habits (IBS-M) More than 25% of bowel movements with Bristol stool form types 1 or 2 and more than 25% with Bristol stool form types 6 or 7
Irritable bowel syndrome unclassified (IBS-U) Patients who meet diagnostic criteria for IBS but whose bowel habits cannot be accurately categorized into one of the three groups above

[a] Criteria should be fulfilled for the last three months with symptom onset at least six months prior to diagnosis.

[b] Bristol stool form: type 1- separate hard lumps; type 2 – sausage-shaped but lumpy; type 3 – sausage-shaped with cracks on the surface; type 4 – sausage-shaped, smooth, and soft; type 5 – soft blobs with clear-cut edges; type 6 – fluffy pieces with ragged edges, mushy; type 7 – watery without solid pieces.

weight loss or malnutrition and infrequently interrupts sleep. Discomfort may be accompanied by significant complaints of bloating, with or without visible abdominal distension.

Different bowel habit disturbances characterize distinct IBS subsets (Table 27.1). Patients with constipation-predominant symptoms (IBS-C) report stools that are hard or pellet-like, are difficult to pass, and are associated with a sensation of incomplete fecal evacuation. Patients with diarrhea-predominant symptoms (IBS-D) pass soft or loose stools of normal daily volume, and defecation may occur after eating or during stress. Many individuals exhibit a mixed pattern of diarrhea alternating with constipation and report characteristics of each sub-type (IBS-M). Passage of fecal mucus is reported by 50% of patients. Rectal bleeding, nocturnal diarrhea, malabsorption, and weight loss are uncommon in patients with IBS and warrant an evaluation for organic disease.

Patients with IBS frequently report symptoms referable to other organs. Large subsets have associated heartburn, early satiety, nausea, vomiting, and dyspepsia, with many meeting diagnostic criteria for other functional gastrointestinal disorders. A high prevalence of genitourinary dysfunction (dysmenorrhea, dyspareunia, impotence, urinary frequency, and incomplete urinary evacuation), fibromyalgia, low back pain, headaches, fatigue, insomnia, depression, anxiety, and somatization have also been observed in individuals with IBS.

Physical examination of the person with IBS usually is unremarkable. Diffuse tenderness or a palpable bowel loop may be evident on abdominal examination. Organomegaly, adenopathy, or occult fecal blood is not consistent with a diagnosis of IBS and necessitate a search for organic disease.

Diagnostic investigation

Diagnosing IBS confidently involves a directed evaluation to confirm that organic disease is not present. The sensitivity and specificity of the Rome IV criteria are quite high, and the diagnosis of IBS can be made confidently in patients who fulfill these criteria. In these patients, it is reasonable to screen patients for alarm features, but to forego further diagnostic studies if the screening is negative. Otherwise, the extent of the diagnostic investigation depends on patient age, evaluation of any alarm features, and the predominant symptoms.

Laboratory studies

Screening for organic disease can be accomplished with a complete blood count and a sedimentation rate or C-reactive protein. Normal values of these laboratory tests help to confirm a diagnosis of IBS. In contrast, anemia, leukocytosis, leukopenia, or elevations of the sedimentation rate or C-reactive protein suggest organic disease. Thyroid function tests can be performed in some cases of diarrhea-predominant or constipation-predominant disease to exclude hyperthyroidism or hypothyroidism, respectively. Celiac disease serologies, including anti-endomysial, tissue transglutaminase, and/or deamidated gliadin peptide antibodies, can be obtained in individuals with a family history of celiac disease or predominant diarrhea. Stool samples may be obtained to exclude gastrointestinal infections in some patients with diarrhea-predominant disease.

Structural studies

Structural testing is recommended for many patients with suspected IBS. In younger patients with symptoms compatible with IBS who do not have alarm features, the likelihood of organic disease is quite low, and structural studies are not needed. In patients older than age 45–50 years, colonoscopy is recommended to screen for colorectal cancer. Sigmoidoscopy or colonoscopy may be performed in younger individuals, if alarm features are present, the diagnosis is uncertain, or diarrheal symptoms predominate. Biopsy of the colon during lower endoscopy is indicated in some patients with prominent diarrhea to rule out microscopic colitis as a cause of symptoms. Upper endoscopy may be performed for reflux or dyspeptic symptoms. Endoscopic small intestinal biopsy is also indicated if there is clinical suspicion of celiac disease or celiac serologies are suggestive.

Other testing

Other tests occasionally are indicated to evaluate for alternative diagnostic possibilities in patients with IBS symptoms. Hydrogen breath testing often is used to exclude lactase deficiency or small intestinal bacterial overgrowth in patients with bloating and diarrheal symptoms. Patients with constipation refractory to medical management may undergo colonic transit testing using radio-opaque markers or a wireless motility capsule, anorectal manometry, and/or defecography to test for slow transit constipation, pelvic floor dyssynergia, and anatomic pelvic floor abnormalities, respectively. Individuals with severe diarrhea may be evaluated for secretory or malabsorptive processes. Screening for laxative use should be considered because laxative abuse is common in patients with unexplained diarrhea. Liver chemistry studies and ultrasound are performed for suspected biliary tract disease. Computed tomography is obtained if malignancy is a concern in a patient with prominent pain, whereas gastric emptying scintigraphy may be indicated for a patient with prominent nausea, vomiting, or early satiety. In very rare instances, screening for porphyria or heavy metal intoxication is performed.

Differential diagnosis

While the diagnosis of IBS is based upon identifying symptoms that are consistent with the condition, many other conditions may present in a similar manner and need to be excluded in a cost-effective manner. Patients with inflammatory bowel disease, microscopic colitis, celiac disease, thyroid dysfunction, colorectal neoplasia, and infectious diarrhea can have symptoms that mimic IBS. The presence of "alarm features" such as weight loss or gastrointestinal bleeding, refractory diarrhea or a family history of colorectal cancer should be used to help direct the evaluation. In the absence of "alarm features," the Rome criteria for diagnosing IBS are very specific, and many patients can confidently be given a diagnosis of IBS based on their clinical features without extensive additional testing.

Management

After a confident diagnosis of IBS, the clinician should provide reassurance and education to the patient and impart awareness that IBS is a functional disorder without long-term health risks. However, it is important to acknowledge the effect of IBS on patients' quality of life and functional status. Development of a therapeutic physician-patient relationship is important to improve patient outcomes. Many patients appreciate understanding that IBS is a chronic disease with well-defined diagnostic criteria. IBS is not solely a diagnosis of exclusion, and compatible clinical features are sufficient to confirm this diagnosis. In some individuals, particularly those with mild symptoms that do not impact significantly on quality of life, patient education, dietary advice, and lifestyle modification will be sufficient.

IBS usually is characterized by periods of waxing and waning. Despite this, the quality of life for patients with IBS can be improved by appropriate intervention; patients can cope with their symptoms and experience an improved sense of well-being. Patients likely to report good outcomes include those who are male, have a brief history of symptoms, exhibit predominant constipation, and do not have significant psychiatric comorbidities. In some patients, education and dietary modifications are insufficient, and medications may be indicated to reduce symptoms and improve quality of life. Some affected persons will be refractory to drug treatment and are considered for behavioral or psychological therapies. The severity of symptoms and associated distress are often correlated with the presence of concomitant anxiety or depression. Many patients with IBS have a history of physical, emotional, or sexual abuse, which may require separate psychiatric intervention.

Dietary recommendations

Dietary modifications can be recommended for selected patients with IBS. The role of food allergy testing in this setting is limited. Reducing fat content may decrease abdominal discomfort evoked by lipid-stimulated motor activity. Increasing soluble fiber content in the diet or consuming a fiber supplement (psyllium, polycarbophil, or methylcellulose) may improve bowel function in patients with IBS-C. Fiber supplements may take several weeks to produce satisfactory results and can produce bloating in some patients, particularly at initiation of therapy. Some patients may respond to eliminating lactose and/or gas-producing foods, caffeine, and alcohol from their diet.

More recently, a diet low in fermentable oligo-, di-, and monosaccharides, and polyols (the low fermentable oligo-/di-/mono-saccharides and polyol [FODMAP] diet) has shown some efficacy in patients with IBS. These short-chain carbohydrates are osmotically active and fermented in the intestine, producing symptoms of abdominal pain and bloating. Nutritionist education should be provided on implementing this diet. Recommendations are usually to eliminate foods high in FODMAPs from the diet for six to eight weeks, followed by gradually reintroducing foods as tolerated. Nevertheless, this diet is complex and restrictive, and long-term adherence may be difficult. Some patients with IBS but without diagnosed celiac disease may have nonceliac gluten sensitivity. Although there are not strict diagnostic criteria for this entity, many patients with IBS will try a gluten-free diet empirically. Evidence to support gluten avoidance in IBS is mixed.

Medical therapy

Medication regimens should be customized to treat each individual's predominant symptoms. Although many agents have been used for patients with IBS, the evidence for many agents such as fiber is sparse. Randomized controlled trials are needed to prove effectiveness in this syndrome because of high placebo response rates.

Individuals with IBS-C who do not respond to fiber supplements may experience relief with osmotic laxatives such as polyethylene glycol. Although poorly absorbed sugars such as lactulose or sorbitol are often used in this situation, they may worsen symptoms of gas or bloating. Polyethylene glycol may relieve constipation but has less effect in relieving abdominal pain. In patients refractory to osmotic laxatives, chloride channel activators such as lubiprostone or guanylate cyclase inhibitors such as linaclotide or plecanatide may be used.

Opiate agents (e.g. loperamide, diphenoxylate with atropine) are the most useful initial agents for treating IBS-D. Bile acid binders such as cholestyramine or colestipol can be used as second-line therapy for patients who do not respond to these antidiarrheal agents. Eluxadoline is a newer agent with combined mu-opioid receptor agonist and delta-opioid receptor antagonist activity, with efficacy in improving stool consistency and decreasing abdominal pain. This agent should not be used in patients who have undergone cholecystectomy due to a high incidence of acute pancreatitis. The 5-HT_3 receptor antagonist alosetron is a potent treatment for refractory diarrhea-predominant IBS. Because it has not been adequately studied in men, it is only approved for women with severe diarrhea-predominant IBS. It has been associated with severe constipation and ischemic colitis, and therefore is only available through a restricted prescribing program.

Antispasmodic anticholinergic agents such as dicyclomine or hyoscyamine can be used to reduce cramping and pain in IBS. These drugs also blunt the gastrocolonic response and may also be useful in preventing postprandial diarrhea. Oral antibiotics provide benefit to some individuals with IBS and associated bacterial overgrowth. Rifaximin, a minimally absorbed antibiotic, has demonstrated efficacy for improving global IBS symptoms and bloating.

Patients with symptoms refractory to these medications may benefit from antidepressants such as the tricyclic antidepressants. Tricyclic antidepressants exhibit significant potency in patients with significant pain. Tricyclics may also reduce symptoms in those with prominent diarrhea through their anticholinergic effects. Conversely, this class of drugs can exacerbate constipation. Treatment should be started at low dose with dose adjustments based on response and tolerance. Limited evidence suggests that selective serotonin reuptake inhibitors or serotonin-norepinephrine reuptake inhibitors may be useful for modulating symptoms in patients with pain and diarrhea. Antidepressants may also be useful in patients with coexisting depression.

Over-the-counter and alternative therapies are sometimes used for treating IBS. Antigas products, such as simethicone, activated charcoal, and bacterial α-galactosidase, have been proposed for patients with bloating, but controlled trials of these agents have not been performed. Selected herbal remedies reportedly provide benefits to some patients. Although they are frequently used, probiotics are limited by inter-individual variability in response and robust studies to demonstrate their efficacy are lacking.

Psychological and behavioral therapies

Recent research has demonstrated that mindfulness-based stress reduction training, typically in a group setting, can result in improvements in bowel symptom severity and quality of life, while reducing distress among IBS patients. Biofeedback and relaxation training may also reduce symptoms. Hypnosis has been effective in selected patients with medically refractory symptoms. Psychotherapy including cognitive-behavioral therapy can lead to reductions in abdominal pain, diarrhea, and somatic symptoms as well as anxiety, hypervigilance, and catastrophizing. These behavioral and psychologic interventions can be used alone or in combination with medical therapy, and may be particularly helpful in patients with concomitant depression or anxiety.

Complications and their management

Long-term studies show that more than 75% of patients have symptoms persisting beyond five years, despite appropriate therapy. Symptoms often follow a waxing and waning course, and there is significant overlap with other functional gastrointestinal disorders such as dyspepsia. IBS has a significant impact upon the quality of life of affected individuals, and some have considerable limitation of functioning. As no one intervention is consistently effective across individuals, treatment must be individualized, and frequently combinations of diet, medical, and behavioral interventions are used in patients with severe symptoms. Counseling, reassurance and education, along with judicious use of medication and a therapeutic patient-physician relationship, can promote successful outcomes in many patients with IBS.

Key practice points

- IBS may be diagnosed based on clinical presentation without extensive testing. In addition to symptom criteria, limited evaluation to rule out inflammatory bowel disease, celiac disease and chronic infection should be sufficient.
- Management of IBS focuses on reassurance and education, providing insight to the patient to understand the pathogenesis and chronic, waxing and waning nature of this disorder. Depending on the sub-type, additional treatment may include loperamide, tricyclic antidepressants or rifaximin (diarrhea predominant), lubiprostone or linaclotide (constipation predominant).
- Alternatives or adjuncts to medications for management of IBS include mindfulness-based stress reduction therapy, hypnotherapy or cognitive behavioral therapy.

Case Studies

Case 1

A 22-year-old woman is referred to your clinic for symptoms of lower abdominal cramping pain and constipation. The pain is often triggered by eating pizza, hamburgers or ice cream, and is relieved after a bowel movement. She describes having one bowel movement every three to four days consisting of a small amount of hard, pebbly stool. These symptoms do not occur at night and she has not lost weight. She has no hematochezia or melena, and denies a family history of colorectal cancer or colonic polyps.

Her complete blood count, electrolytes and liver tests are normal including an albumin of 4.3. Her thyroid stimulating hormone is normal and a pregnancy test is negative.

You provide counseling about her diagnosis of IBS and advise her to increase her fluid intake and dietary fiber, and give her a list of high FODMAP foods that she should avoid. You also prescribe miralax 17 g once to twice daily with water and titrate to produce one bowel movement every one to two days.

Discussion

The diagnosis of IBS-C does not require structural evaluation – in the absence of warning signs of gastrointestinal bleeding, weight loss, or anemia a positive diagnosis can be made on the basis of Rome IV criteria. The management of IBS-C focuses on dietary counseling, increasing fiber and adding cathartic therapy as needed to reduce symptoms. The low FODMAP diet has been shown to reduce symptoms in many individuals with IBS presumably due to direct dietary effects as well as potential benefit from changes in the metabolic products of intestinal bacteria (the microbiome) that occur as a result of changes in the substrate available to the bacteria.

Case 2

Your patient from Case 1 returns to clinic with a reduction in abdominal cramping and constipation. She describes achieving a bowel movement daily; however, this is associated with increased bloating and an uncomfortable sensation of incomplete evacuation with bowel movements. She states she is avoiding a variety of food high in FODMAPs, in particular dairy, fructans (wheat, onions, garlic), and galactans (beans, lentils, and soybeans), which seem to have triggered her symptoms. You obtain an anorectal manometry, which is notable for her inability to expel a 50 cc rectal balloon. You diagnose pelvic floor dyssynergia and she responds to anorectal biofeedback.

Discussion

Overlap between IBS and other functional gastrointestinal disorders is common. The diagnosis of pelvic floor dyssynergia or other outlet disorders should be considered in any case of constipation, but a history of incomplete evacuation should prompt an anorectal manometry. Dyssynergic motility can be detected with manometry, but the most specific test is the inability to expel a rectal balloon within one minute. The response to biofeedback is excellent.

Further reading

Ford, A.C., Moayyedi, P., Chey, W.D. et al. (2018). American College of Gastroenterology monograph on management of irritable bowel syndrome. *Am. J. Gastroenterology* 113: 1–18.

Weinberg, D.S., Smalley, W., Heidelbaugh, J.J. et al. (2014). American Gastroenterological Association Institute guideline on the pharmacological management of irritable bowel syndrome. *Gastroenterology* 147: 1146–1148.

CHAPTER 28

Inflammatory Bowel Disease

Chronic inflammatory bowel diseases (IBDs) include ulcerative colitis, a disorder in which inflammation affects the mucosa and submucosa of the colon, and Crohn's disease, in which inflammation is transmural and may involve any or all segments of the gastrointestinal tract.

Clinical presentation

Ulcerative colitis

Ulcerative colitis is limited to the rectum in approximately 30% of patients (ulcerative proctitis) and extends proximally to the splenic flexure in 40% (left-sided or distal colitis) or involves the entire colon in 30% (pan-colitis). The dominant symptom in ulcerative colitis is diarrhea, which is often bloody. Bowel movements may be frequent but of low volume as a result of rectal inflammation. Abdominal pain (usually lower quadrant or rectal), fever, malaise, and weight loss may also be reported. Ulcerative proctitis can present with hematochezia and either diarrhea or constipation with associated symptoms of urgency, tenesmus, pain, and incontinence.

Diarrhea and rectal bleeding may the sole complaints of mild disease, which is often associated with a normal physical examination. Most patients with ulcerative proctitis have mild disease. Moderate disease, which occurs in 27% of patients, is characterized by five or six bloody stools per day, abdominal pain, abdominal tenderness, low-grade fever, and fatigue. Nineteen percent of patients exhibit severe ulcerative colitis, which is characterized by frequent episodes of bloody diarrhea (>6 stools/day), profound weakness, weight loss, fever, tachycardia, postural hypotension, significant abdominal tenderness, hypoactive bowel sounds, and anemia and hypoalbuminemia on laboratory investigation.

Severe ulcerative colitis can cause life-threatening complications including toxic megacolon that occurs if inflammation extends into the muscularis

Yamada's Handbook of Gastroenterology, Fourth Edition. John M. Inadomi, Renuka Bhattacharya, Joo Ha Hwang, and Cynthia Ko.

propria, causing dilation of the colonic lumen. Clinical criteria suggestive of toxic megacolon include dehydration, mental status changes, abdominal distension, hypoactive or absent bowel sounds, tenderness, a temperature higher than 38.6 °C, heart rate greater than 120 bpm, hypotension, a neutrophil count of more than 10 500 cells/μl, and electrolyte disturbances. Medications that impair colonic motor function may initiate or exacerbate megacolon including narcotics. Perforation of the colon may complicate toxic megacolon or may occur in cases of severe ulcerative colitis without megacolon.

Crohn's disease

Crohn's disease most commonly affects the terminal ileum and colon, but can involve any portion of the gastrointestinal tract. The main patterns of disease distribution include: involvement of the small and large intestine (40% of patients); disease confined to the small intestine (30%); or disease of only the colon (25%), which is pan-colonic in two-thirds and segmental in one-third. Less commonly, the disease affects the proximal gastrointestinal tract (5%). In addition, approximately 25% of patients develop perianal disease including fissures, fistulae, ulceration and strictures.

Predominant symptoms in Crohn's disease include diarrhea, abdominal pain, and weight loss. Diarrhea may be of small volume with urgency and tenesmus if disease is limited to the colon and rectum; alternatively, larger stool volumes with steatorrhea may be present if disease is extensive and involves the small intestine. Diarrhea due to small intestinal disease occurs via several mechanisms: loss of mucosal absorptive surface area leading to osmotic diarrhea, bile salt malabsorption leading to secretory diarrhea; bacterial overgrowth resulting from strictures or enteroenteric or enterocolonic fistulae. Pain may result from serosal inflammation or intermittent partial bowel obstruction. Weight loss occurs in most patients because of malabsorption and reduced oral intake. Gastroduodenal involvement in Crohn's disease produces epigastric pain, nausea, and vomiting secondary to stricture or obstruction, while esophageal disease can provoke dysphagia or odynophagia. Fatigue, malaise, fever, and chills are constitutional symptoms that contribute to the morbidity of Crohn's disease. The Crohn's Disease Activity Index assigns numerical scores to stool frequency, abdominal pain, sense of well-being, systemic manifestations, the use of antidiarrheal agents, abdominal mass, hematocrit, and body weight, and has been used as a quantitative measure of disease activity in clinical studies.

Crohn's disease often is associated with gastrointestinal complications including abscesses, fistulae, strictures and perianal disease. Abscesses most commonly arise from the terminal ileum but they may occur in iliopsoas, retroperitoneal, hepatic, and splenic regions, and at anastomotic sites. Abscesses present with fever, localized tenderness, and a palpable mass. Infection usually is polymicrobial (e.g. *Escherichia coli, Bacteroides fragilis, Enterococcus,* and α-hemolytic *Streptococcus* species). Twenty to 40% of patients with Crohn's disease have fistulous disease. Fistulae may be enteroenteric, enterocutaneous, enterovesical, or enterovaginal or perianal. They develop when disease is active but may persist after remission if intestinal strictures obstruct the bowel lumen. Large enteroenteric fistulae produce diarrhea, malabsorption, and weight loss. Rectovaginal fistulae lead to foul-smelling vaginal discharge, and enterovesical fistulae produce pneumaturia and recurrent urinary infection. Fistulae drain serous or mucous material, whereas perianal abscesses cause fever, redness, induration, and pain that is exacerbated by defecation, sitting, and walking. Strictures, especially of the small intestine, are a common complication caused by mucosal thickening, muscular hyperplasia and scarring from chronic inflammation or adhesions. Perianal disease, including anal ulcers, abscesses, and fistulae, can also affect the groin, vulva, or scrotum and is a complication that often is difficult to treat.

Extraintestinal features

Extraintestinal manifestations of IBD are more common among individuals with ulcerative colitis and Crohn's colitis than among those with ileal Crohn's disease. Peripheral arthritis is a migratory arthritis commonly affecting the wrists, knees, ankles, proximal interphalangeal and metatarsophalangeal joints that usually lasts a few weeks, rarely produces joint deformity, and usually responds to treatment of bowel inflammation. In contrast, axial arthritidies including sacroiliitis and ankylosing spondylitis may occur in the absence of active bowel disease and may not respond to therapy for intestinal inflammation. The prevalence of ankylosing spondylitis, which is characterized by morning stiffness, low back pain, and stooped posture, increases 30-fold with ulcerative colitis and is associated with the HLA-B27 phenotype. Unlike peripheral arthritis, ankylosing spondylitis can be relentlessly progressive and unresponsive to medications.

Hepatobiliary manifestations of IBD include cholelithiasis, pericholangitis, steatosis, chronic active hepatitis, cirrhosis, and primary sclerosing cholangitis (PSC). PSC is a chronic cholestatic disease characterized by fibrosing inflammation of the intrahepatic and extrahepatic bile ducts; it occurs in 2% of patients with ulcerative colitis and in a smaller proportion of patients with Crohn's disease (0.4%). Conversely, the majority of patients with sclerosing cholangitis have IBD. Cholangiocarcinoma develops in 10–15% of patients with IBD who have long-standing sclerosing cholangitis. Cholesterol gallstones develop in patients with Crohn's disease because of the bile salt depletion that occurs with ileal disease or resection.

Skin lesions include erythema nodosum (painful, raised red nodules usually on the lower extremities), pyoderma gangrenosum (sterile, ulcerated skin lesions), oral aphthous lesions, Sweet syndrome (acute febrile neutrophilic dermatosis appearing as red, painful lesions on the upper extremities, trunk, and face), and pyostomatitis vegetans (oral lesion characterized by pustules and ulcerations along the lips, buccal mucosa, and gingiva).

Ocular complications of IBD include uveitis and episcleritis. Uveitis is inflammation of the anterior chamber and manifests with blurred vision, eye pain, photophobia, and conjunctival inflammation. Slit lamp examination will reveal perilimbic edema and cells in the anterior chamber. Episcleritis causes scleral inflammation and presents with burning pain of the eyes.

The most common renal complication of Crohn's disease is nephrolithiasis that occurs in 20% of patients. Oxalate stones form due to excessive oxalate absorption in the colon caused by unabsorbed free fatty acids binding with calcium that would otherwise bind oxalate and inhibit its absorption.

Thromboembolic complications such as deep vein thrombosis and pulmonary emboli occur in 1–2% of IBD patients.

Diagnostic investigation

Laboratory studies

Laboratory studies that reflect disease activity in ulcerative colitis are hemoglobin level, leukocyte count, electrolytes, serum albumin, erythrocyte sedimentation rate (ESR), and C-reactive protein (CRP). Anemia, hypoalbuminemia, hypokalemia, and metabolic alkalosis may be prominent in severe disease. Granulocyte-derived fecal markers, including calprotectin and lactoferrin, represent noninvasive tests for monitoring intestinal mucosal inflammation. Stool should be inspected for leukocytes and cultures should be obtained to rule out infectious etiologies of diarrhea, including *Campylobacter, Shigella, Salmonella, Yersinia, Giardia lamblia,* and *Clostridium difficile* toxin even in the absence of recent antibiotic use.

Laboratory findings in Crohn's disease are nonspecific. Anemia may be multifactorial, resulting from chronic disease, blood loss, and iron, folate, and vitamin B_{12} deficiency as well as bone marrow suppression from medication. Active Crohn's disease elevates leukocyte counts, CRP, and ESR, but marked increases suggest abscess formation. Hypoalbuminemia may indicate severe disease, malnutrition, or protein-losing enteropathy. Vitamin D may be low due to dietary and absorptive deficiency, or reduced production due to inflammation. Stool testing for infection is indicated to detect identical pathogens found in ulcerative colitis. Increased fecal fat is suggestive of ileal disease.

Complications and extraintestinal manifestations of IBD can be suggested by selected laboratory studies. Profound leukocytosis with a neutrophil predominance in ulcerative colitis is worrisome for perforation or toxic megacolon or *C. difficile* infection. Pericholangitis and sclerosing cholangitis produce elevations of alkaline phosphatase. Pyuria in a patient with Crohn's disease suggests a possible enterovesical fistula, whereas hematuria raises concern for renal stones.

Diagnostic pitfalls

Serological markers have been promoted to diagnose and differentiate ulcerative colitis from Crohn's disease. Perinuclear antineutrophil cytoplasmic antibodies (pANCA) are found in 50–80% of ulcerative colitis patients, but also 31% of individuals with Crohn's disease. Anti-*Saccharomyces cerevisiae* antibodies (ASCA) are found in 60% of Crohn's disease patients, and in 20% of individuals with ulcerative colitis. Because of this broad overlap, these tests cannot reliably differentiate between ulcerative colitis and Crohn's in patients with indeterminant colitis, which represents the group that could have benefited most from this test.

Endoscopy

Colonoscopy at the initial presentation of a patient with suspected IBD can establish the diagnosis and define the extent of disease. With severe disease, sigmoidoscopy may provide enough information to initiate therapy without the risks of perforation associated with colonoscopy in this setting.

In ulcerative colitis, the inflammation begins in the rectum and extends proximally to the point where visible disease ends without skipping any areas (Table 28.1). Mild disease is characterized by loss of vascularity, granularity,

Table 28.1 Colonoscopic findings in inflammatory bowel disease (IBD)

Feature	Ulcerative colitis	Crohn's disease
Inflammation		
Location		
Colon		
Contiguous	+ + +	+
Symmetrical	+ + +	+
Rectum	+ + +	+
Friability	+ + +	+
Topography		
Granularity	+ + +	+
Cobblestoned	+	+ + +
Ulceration		
Location		
Colitis	+ + +	+
Ileum	0	+ + + +
Discrete lesion	+	+ + +
Features		
Size >1 cm	+	+ + +
Deep	+	+ +
Linear	+	+ + +
Aphthoid	0	+ + + +
Bridging	+	+ +

Specificity index range: 0 (not seen) to + + + + (diagnostic).

superficial erosions, and exudation. In severe disease, large ulcers and denuded mucosa may dominate. With chronic disease, the mucosa flattens and inflammatory polyps (pseudo-polyps) develop. Pseudo-polyps are not premalignant and do not need to be resected.

Crohn's colitis exhibits a different appearance in many but not all cases. Aphthous ulcers predominate in early or mild disease, whereas severe disease is characterized by cobblestoning and large, deep, linear or serpiginous ulcers. With gastroduodenal Crohn's disease, antral aphthous and linear ulcers may be seen on upper endoscopy. Unlike ulcerative colitis, mucosal involvement in Crohn's disease is not always contiguous; patches of colon are often relatively disease free (areas skipped), and the rectum may or may not be involved. Ileal disease is common in Crohn's disease.

Strictures are more common with Crohn's disease, as is perianal involvement. Strictures and mass lesions in patients with long-standing IBD (>10 years) suggest malignancy. In addition to its diagnostic capability, colonoscopy has therapeutic potential for dilation of colonic strictures.

Capsule endoscopy has been used in some cases to exclude subtle small intestinal Crohn's disease in patients without obstruction.

Specialized endoscopy can help assess the extraintestinal manifestations of IBD. Magnetic resonance cholangiography can diagnose sclerosing cholangitis; however, endoscopic retrograde cholangiopancreatography (ERCP) with biliary brush cytology and biopsy for histopathology may be necessary to differentiate sclerosing cholangitis from cholangiocarcinoma and can be used to dilate or stent biliary strictures to treat obstructive jaundice.

Radiography

Findings of radiographic evaluation complement those of endoscopy in patients with IBD. Plain abdominal radiography may be normal or show colonic dilation in toxic megacolon, air–fluid levels from intestinal obstruction in Crohn's disease, or pneumoperitoneum with perforation. Computed tomography (CT) may also characterize malignant and benign obstruction in Crohn's disease and is superior to endoscopy for detecting fistulae and strictures. CT detects abscesses and may assist in their percutaneous drainage. Magnetic resonance imaging may be more sensitive than CT in detecting intestinal and extraintestinal Crohn's disease. Scintigraphic scans have been used to localize and characterize areas of intestinal inflammation or abscess.

Imaging studies are useful in characterizing complications and extraintestinal manifestations of IBD. Spine radiography shows squaring of the vertebrae, straightening of the spine, and lateral and anterior syndesmophytes in ankylosing spondylitis, whereas pelvic radiographs of the pelvis in sacroiliitis reveal blurring of the margins of the sacroiliac joints, with patchy sclerosis. Ultrasound is performed on patients with suspected biliary colic or cholecystitis secondary to gallstones in Crohn's disease. Magnetic resonance cholangiopancreatography and percutaneous transhepatic cholangiography are used in some cases to screen for sclerosing cholangitis or cholangiocarcinoma. Intravenous pyelography or CT may demonstrate enterovesical fistulae or renal stones.

Pathology

Histological evaluation of colonic biopsy specimens is usually able to distinguish ulcerative colitis from Crohn's disease, and acute colitis. Distortion of the crypt architectural structure and acute and chronic inflammation of the lamina propria are more common with ulcerative colitis than with acute, self-limited colitis. The presence of granulomas is the best histological distinction of Crohn's disease. In one series, granulomas were found in 60% of Crohn's disease patients versus 6% of patients with ulcerative colitis. Crypt atrophy, neutrophilic infiltration, and surface erosions are more common in ulcerative colitis than in Crohn's disease. Despite these variations, histological discrimination between the two forms of chronic IBD cannot be made in 15–25% of cases.

Ulcerative colitis and Crohn's disease exhibit characteristic findings on gross surgical specimens. Findings in ulcerative colitis are generally limited to the mucosa and submucosa; the muscularis propria is involved only in fulminant disease. Conversely, in Crohn's disease the bowel wall is thickened and stiff and the mesentery is thickened, edematous, and contracted because of transmural involvement. Adipose tissue creeps over the serosal surface, and intestinal loops may be matted together. Lymphoid aggregates may be observed involving the submucosa and occasionally the muscularis propria. Granulomas are found in many surgically resected intestinal, lymph node, mesentery, peritoneal, and liver specimens in Crohn's disease.

Management and prevention

Preventive health maintenance in IBD

Adult patients with IBD should receive pneumococcal vaccination (PCV13 and PPSV23), measles, mumps, rubella, varicella, hepatitis A and B (if not immune), human papilloma virus (HPV), meningococcus, diphtheria, pertussis, herpes zoster, and annual vaccination against influenza. Screening for melanoma is advised, while those on immunomodulators should also undergo screening for nonmelanoma skin cancer. Screening for osteoporosis with bone mineral density testing should be conducted at the time of IBD diagnosis and periodically thereafter. Patients with Crohn's disease should be counseled to quit smoking.

Nutritional management

In most cases, the only nutritional therapy required is a well-balanced diet. Some patients with small intestinal Crohn's disease have secondary lactase deficiency and should restrict lactose intake or use supplemental lactase. Patients with strictures should avoid high-residue foods. Oral or parenteral iron supplements may be indicated for significant blood loss. Specific calcium, magnesium, zinc, vitamin B_{12}, vitamin D, or vitamin K supplements may be required to counter clinical or biochemical evidence of deficiency caused by Crohn's enteritis. Ileal resection may induce bile salt diarrhea that can be treated with the bile salt-binding resin cholestyramine. More extensive terminal ileal disease or resections (>100 cm) cause vitamin B_{12} and fat malabsorption. Treatment includes a low-fat diet; in addition, substitution of dietary fat with medium-chain triglycerides can reduce steatorrhea because they do not require bile salts for absorption in the proximal intestine.

When oral intake is inadequate, enteral feedings may be provided through nasogastric, gastrostomy, or jejunostomy tubes. The use of elemental feedings that consist of amino acids, monosaccharides, vitamins, minerals, and essential fatty acids is controversial due to mixed outcomes from controlled trials. Severe IBD exacerbations or extensive small intestinal resections with Crohn's disease may warrant initiating total parenteral nutrition. Parenteral nutrition also is helpful in improving the nutritional status of patients prior to colectomy or other surgery.

Medication therapy

5-Aminosalicylate preparations

5-aminosalicylates (5-ASA) have been shown to effectively treat mild-to-moderate ulcerative colitis. However, the majority of evidence does not support the efficacy of aminosalicylates in the acute or chronic treatment of Crohn's disease. Sulfasalazine is started at low doses and is gradually increased to 4 g/day, as tolerated, in mild-to-moderate ulcerative colitis. After remission is achieved, doses can be tapered to 2 g/day for long-term maintenance therapy. Dose-related side effects of sulfasalazine include nausea, vomiting, headache, dyspepsia, abdominal discomfort, and hemolysis. Hypersensitive dose-independent reactions include rash, fever, aplastic anemia, agranulocytosis, and autoimmune hemolysis. Other side effects of sulfasalazine include reduced sperm counts (which recover three months after stopping the drug), folate deficiency (caused by inhibition of intestinal folate conjugase), and, rarely, bloody diarrhea (caused by the 5-ASA component).

Other 5-ASA preparations are commonly prescribed in selected groups of patients with ulcerative colitis. Enemas that contain 5-ASA are effective for treating distal ulcerative colitis and induce remission in 93% of patients. 5-ASA suppositories are useful in ulcerative proctitis. 5-ASA have a potential nephrotoxicity; thus caution should be exercised when using these drugs in patients with renal dysfunction, and routine monitoring of renal function should be performed in all patients on aminosalicylate therapy.

Corticosteroids

Corticosteroids are effective in inducing remission in ulcerative colitis and Crohn's disease, but are not advocated for maintaining remission. Oral prednisone is effective in moderate ulcerative colitis and Crohn's disease and produces improvement within three weeks. Intravenous methylprednisolone is useful for inpatients with more severe disease. Steroid enemas are effective in treating left-sided ulcerative colitis reliably up to the level of the mid-descending colon. Systemic absorption of steroid enemas is significant and increases the risks of long-term use. Maintenance steroid therapy is ineffective in preventing recurrences in ulcerative colitis and Crohn's disease.

The side effects of corticosteroids limit their long-term use in IBD. Prednisone at a dose of 10 mg or more taken for longer than three weeks may suppress the hypothalamic–pituitary–adrenal axis for one year after therapy is discontinued. Individuals thus treated should receive supplemental steroids for surgery or severe illness. Common side effects of steroid therapy include increased appetite, centripetal obesity, moon facies, acne, insomnia, depression, psychosis, increased infections, hypertension, glucose intolerance, cataracts, irreversible glaucoma, and growth retardation (in children). Avascular necrosis of the femoral head can produce permanent disability. Osteoporosis is a devastating side effect that can occur with prednisone doses as low as 8–10 mg/day. Patients on long-term steroid therapy should receive supplemental calcium and vitamin D and should undergo periodic bone densitometry studies. More aggressive therapies including bisphosphonates, calcitonin, and hormonal treatments may be indicated in some cases.

Budesonide is a steroid whose systemic toxicity is diminished by rapid first-pass metabolism in the liver. The drug is useful for inducing remission of ileal Crohn's disease and a colonic formulation (MMX) can induce remission in ulcerative colitis. A budesonide foam preparation can treat proctitis. Although observed less frequently than with prednisone, budesonide does suppress plasma cortisol levels so its safety for long-term remission is undefined.

Immunomodulators

Azathioprine (AZA), 6-mercaptopurine (6-MP), and methotrexate (MTX) are effective in inducing remission in ulcerative colitis and Crohn's disease; however, a clinical response may not be observed for three to four months after initiating therapy. For this reason immunomodulators are generally used to maintain remission as steroid-sparing agents, and may be beneficial in healing fistulae in Crohn's disease. Blood counts are monitored frequently because of the bone marrow-suppressive effects of these agents (especially leukopenia). Liver chemistry levels also are monitored to detect possible hepatotoxicity. Other side effects of azathioprine and 6-MP include pancreatitis, infections, and allergic reactions. The therapeutic efficacy and toxicity of these drugs relate to their metabolites. These drugs are metabolized by thiopurine methyltransferase (TPMT) to the inactive metabolite, 6-methylmercaptopurine (6-MMP). Low TPMT activity increases 6-thioguanine (6-TG) production due to less drug inactivation. The therapeutic efficacy and hematological toxicity of 6-MP and azathioprine relate to serum 6-TG levels, whereas elevated 6-MMP levels correlate with hepatotoxicity. TPMT genotyping can identify individuals predisposed to drug toxicity. There is a risk of lymphoma associated with thiopurines; in particular, hepatosplenic T-cell lymphoma has been reported mainly in young male Crohn's disease patients receiving combination anti-tumor necrosis factor (TNF) and immunomodulator therapy for greater than one year.

Methotrexate is considered an effective alternative to 6-MP and azathioprine for induction and maintenance of remission in Crohn's disease. Prominent side effects of methotrexate include nausea, bone marrow suppression, elevated liver chemistry levels, and a long-term risk for development of cirrhosis.

Intravenous cyclosporine is effective for severe ulcerative colitis refractory to intravenous steroid therapy. It is unclear if this approach prevents the ultimate need for colectomy in many patients; however, it may defer surgery to a time when the procedure can be elective. Oral cyclosporine has not shown convincing efficacy in Crohn's disease. In addition to an increase in serious and opportunistic infections, side effects of cyclosporine include renal insufficiency, hypertension, paresthesias, tremor, and headache.

Antibiotics

Broad-spectrum antibiotics are important in treating suppurative complications of Crohn's disease, including abscesses and perianal disease as well as small intestinal bacterial overgrowth from stasis proximal to a stricture. Ciprofloxacin and metronidazole have efficacy for perianal Crohn's disease and may reduce disease activity in Crohn's colitis. Side effects of metronidazole include peripheral neuropathy, dysgeusia, and disulfiram-like reactions. Rifaximin has mixed outcomes in clinical trials. High quality data do not exist to support antibiotics to treat ulcerative colitis, with the exception of ciprofloxacin and metronidazole to treat pouchitis after colectomy with ileal-pouch anal anastomosis.

Biological and small molecule therapy

Infliximab is an intravenously administered mouse-human chimeric monoclonal IgG antibody directed against TNF-α. The drug has demonstrated efficacy in treating refractory flares of Crohn's disease and ulcerative colitis and is intravenously administered (5 mg/kg) at weeks 0, 2, and 6 for induction, followed by every eight weeks thereafter at doses of 5–10 mg/kg. Infliximab also is useful for closing fistulae secondary to Crohn's disease and is increasingly used as maintenance therapy for patients with IBD. Responses; however, may diminish with time secondary to development of antidrug antibodies.

Other anti-TNF drugs include adalimumab and certolizumab. Adalimumab differs from infliximab in that it is a fully humanized IgG antibody administered subcutaneously. Certolizumab pegol is a pegylated Fab fragment targeted against TNF. Both adalimumab and certolizumab pegol are administered subcutaneously and have proven efficacy in patients with Crohn's disease or ulcerative colitis who previously responded to infliximab but discontinued therapy due to loss of response or intolerance.

Adverse events associated with biologicals include hypersensitivity reactions (rash, fever, myalgias, and arthralgias) and infectious complications (varicella zoster virus, *Candida* esophagitis, tuberculosis). Patients must be screened prior to initiating biological therapy to ensure they are not infected with tuberculosis. Vaccination to prevent hepatitis A and B should be performed unless the patient is determined to be immune. Anti-TNF therapy should also not be used in patients with demyelinating disease, severe heart failure or neoplasia. It should be noted that the combination of biological agents in conjunction with 6-MP or azathioprine has been associated with hepatosplenic T-cell lymphoma, a very rare and aggressive lymphoma seen primarily in young male patients.

Vedolizumab is an α-4 β-7 integrin inhibitor that reduces leukocyte migration and has proven efficacy to achieve and maintain remission in Crohn's disease and ulcerative colitis. Natalizumab is a humanized monoclonal antibody that binds to α-4 integrin; however, it has been associated with fatal progressive multifocal leukoencephalopathy (PML) and currently this drug is limited to patients with Crohn's disease who have failed other therapies. Because PML is linked to JC virus, frequent screening should be undertaken and natalizumab discontinued if JC virus is detected.

Ustekinumab is an anti- IL-12 and IL-23 monoclonal antibody that has been demonstrated to be effective in treating Crohn's disease and ulcerative colitis. Tofacitinib is a janus kinase (JAK) 1 and 3 inhibitor. It is a small molecule that is administered orally and is not a biologic agent. Tofacitinib has been approved for treatment of ulcerative colitis, but as of the time of this printing has not been approved for use in Crohn's disease.

Therapeutic drug monitoring in IBD

In adult patients being started on thiopurines, routine TPMT testing (enzymatic activity or genotype) is suggested to guide therapeutic dosing. A target 6-thioguanine (6-TGN) cutoff between 230–450 pmol/8×10^8 red blood cells (RBCs) is recommended for monotherapy, while no specific target has been identified for thiopurines when combined with biologic therapy.

In adult patients with active IBD treated with biologic drugs, it is suggested that reactive therapeutic drug monitoring be used to guide treatment changes.

Medical management of ulcerative colitis

The medical management of ulcerative colitis depends on the extent and severity of disease that is gauged on the risk for colectomy. Patients at low risk for colectomy have limited anatomic extent of colitis and mild endoscopic disease, whereas those harboring extensive colitis, deep ulcers, high CRP and ESR, steroid-requiring disease, history of hospitalization for IBD, *C difficile* infection, cytomegalovirus infection, or age <40 years are at high risk for colectomy.

For outpatients at low-risk for colectomy, induction of remission may be achieved using oral 5-ASA, rectal 5-ASA, oral budesonide, oral prednisone (up to 40 mg orally daily), or any combination of these drugs. Rectal disease may be treated with rectal 5-ASA (first line) or rectal steroids. If patients achieve remission they should taper steroids if taken and continue oral and/or rectal 5-ASA. If remission is not achieved, or if relapse occurs after initial remission, patients should be treated similarly to patients initially deemed at high risk for colectomy.

Outpatients at high risk for colectomy should receive induction therapy that consists of either a short course of steroids simultaneous with initiation of thiopurine; or biologic therapy (anti-TNF, vedolizumab, ustekinumab). Data suggest that induction and maintenance of remission are best achieved with the combination of biologic with an immunomodulator. If remission is achieved, maintenance with the drug used to achieve remission, with the exception of tapering steroids over 60 days.

Failure to maintain steroid-free remission on thiopurine could be due to subtherapeutic 6TGN (<230 pmol 6-TGN/8×10^8 RBCs) in which case the dose of thiopurine should be increased. If the level is therapeutic, however, the best option is to switch to biologic therapy. Similarly, if a patient initially responds to anti-TNF but relapses, this could be due to subtherapeutic drug levels. If drug levels are low, antibodies to anti-TNF should be measured; if drug antibodies are low or absent, the dose of anti-TNF should be increased and/or the interval between administrations shortened and an immunomodulator added if not already administered. If there is a high level of anti-TNF antibodies, switching within the anti-TNF class may be beneficial. Conversely, if the drug level of anti-TNF is therapeutic, management should be switched to another drug class such as vedolizumab, ustekinumab, or tofacitinib.

The mainstays for inpatient treatment of severe ulcerative colitis are intravenous steroids (methylprednisolone 40–60 mg; hydrocortisone 200–300 mg), hydration, and parenteral antibiotics for signs of infection. Prophylaxis against venous thrombosis should be given (heparin 5000 IU three times daily or enoxaprin 40 mg subcutaneously daily). Total parenteral nutrition is provided if oral nutrition is to be withheld for a prolonged period. If there is no response within three to five days, infliximab or intravenous cyclosporine should be considered, in addition to surgical consultation for consideration of colectomy.

The drug necessary to induce remission is usually the drug that is required for maintenance of remission, with the exception of corticosteroids. Steroid weaning may be achieved with the addition of immunomodulators such as azathioprine, 6-MP or methotrexate. For severe or refractory disease, maintenance biological or small molecule therapy has been shown to be effective.

Medical management of Crohn's disease

5-ASA drugs have scant data to support efficacy in Crohn's disease; however, they are often used in mild disease flares and are safe to maintain remission.

Nonsteroidal anti-inflammatory drugs may exacerbate disease activity and should be avoided. Smoking also worsens disease and should be discontinued.

Oral prednisone (40mg daily) may be used to induce remission of moderate-to-severe Crohn's disease. Oral budesonide is an alternative, and has fewer systemic side effects due to its high first-pass hepatic metabolism. Patients who have persistent symptoms despite steroids, who relapse after having achieved remission with steroids, or who relapse after steroids are reduced are candidates for biologic therapy. Fistulae and perianal disease are treated with immunosuppressants or biological therapy. Steroids are not indicated to maintain remission in IBD.

The American Gastroenterological Association (AGA) clinical practice guidelines suggest (weak recommendation) the use of anti-TNF-α drugs in combination with thiopurines over monotherapy (with either anti-TNF-α drugs or thiopurines alone) to induce remission in patients with moderately severe Crohn's disease. Once remission is achieved, combination therapy may be continued, or monotherapy with biological therapy, thiopurines, or methotrexate may be used. Immunological therapy with azathioprine, 6-MP or methotrexate are best used for maintenance due to the prolonged time to effect.

Severe flares of Crohn's disease requiring hospitalization should be treated with intravenous steroids. Anti-TNF therapy may be administered but is usually indicated for patients who fail to respond to intravenous steroids. If anti-TNF drugs are also not effective in achieving remission, other biologic drugs including vedolizumab or ustekinumab may be used. Note that tofacitinib and cyclosporine have not been demonstrated to be effective in Crohn's disease.

CT scans can identify abscesses that require radiolographically guided or surgical drainage, and obstruction or fistulae can be evaluated using CT or magnetic resonance enterography. Fistulae are treated with antibiotics (imidazoles), immunomodulators (azathioprine or 6-mercaptopurine), or biologics; refractory disease should be managed surgically.

Surgical management of IBD

Urgent indications for colectomy in ulcerative colitis include perforation, toxic megacolon, refractory fulminant colitis in the absence of dilation, and severe hemorrhage. Nonurgent indications include failure of medical therapy, dysplasia, carcinoma, and severe drug side effects that prevent adequate medication regimens. For ulcerative colitis, colectomy cures the colonic disease and many but not all of the extraintestinal manifestations. Uveitis, pyoderma gangrenosum, and colitic arthritis usually respond to colectomy, whereas ankylosing spondylitis and sclerosing cholangitis do not.

A colectomy, mucosal proctectomy, with ileal pouch–anal canal anastomosis is the procedure of choice for most patients with uncomplicated ulcerative colitis who undergo colectomy, because it preserves normal continence. In this operation, the colon is completely removed, and the mucosa and submucosa are dissected and removed from the rectum. A pouch is constructed from the distal

30 cm of ileum and sewn to the dentate line. Complications include incontinence, intractable diarrhea, infection, or anastomotic breakdown. In severely ill patients an ileostomy may be performed with proctocolectomy in a one-stage or two-stage (colectomy and ileostomy followed by proctectomy) procedure. Complications of an ileostomy include stomal prolapse, retraction, herniation, and stenosis.

In contrast to ulcerative colitis, surgery does not cure Crohn's disease. Thus, the extent and frequency of resections should be minimized. Indications for surgery in Crohn's disease include failure of medical therapy, obstruction, fistulae, and abscess formation. Stricturoplasty represents an alternative to resection for Crohn's strictures. For extensive colitis with rectal involvement, total proctocolectomy with an ileostomy is the procedure of choice. Subtotal colectomy with ileoproctostomy is only for patients with absolutely normal rectums.

Imidazole antibiotics (metronidazole or ornidazole) 1–2 g/day can be used after small intestinal resection to reduce recurrence. Thiopurines may be used to prevent recurrence after surgery. In high risk patients, anti-TNF agents should be started within four weeks of surgery to prevent postoperative Crohn's disease recurrence.

Complications and their treatment

Toxic megacolon refers to the condition in which colonic dilation (>6 cm diameter) and colitis are accompanied by at least three of the following four signs of systemic compromise are present: fever >38.6 °C; tachycardia >120 bpm; leukocytosis >10 500 cell/mm^3; or anemia. Medical therapy consists of nasogastric suction, intravenous steroids and broad-spectrum antibiotics. Fluid and electrolyte replacement should be aggressive because electrolyte disturbances may contribute to impaired colonic motor function. Narcotics and anticholinergic drugs should be discontinued. A successful medical response is defined by improvement within 24–48 hours in signs of toxicity and reduction in colonic diameter on abdominal radiography. If there is no improvement within 48 hours, colectomy should be performed because of the high risk of perforation.

Broad-spectrum antibiotics with percutaneous or surgical drainage are indicated for abscesses in Crohn's disease. After the abscess has been drained and the inflammation subsides, resection of the affected bowel usually is required. Strictures are a common complication of Crohn's disease, which can be managed by endoscopic dilation or surgery. Surgical excision also is required for fistulae that are proximal to strictures.

Specific therapies are indicated for selected extraintestinal manifestations of IBD. Colitic arthritis usually responds to corticosteroid therapy. Pruritus secondary to sclerosing cholangitis may respond to cholestyramine. Ursodeoxycholic acid decreases liver chemistry abnormalities in sclerosing cholangitis but does not alter the the natural history, which may require liver transplantation.

Surveillance for colonic neoplasia

Patients with ulcerative colitis or extensive Crohn's colitis have an increased likelihood of developing colon cancer. Risk factors for colon cancer in ulcerative colitis include younger age at diagnosis, increased duration and extent of disease, sclerosing cholangitis, and a family history of colon cancer. In contrast to the normal population, development of colon cancer in ulcerative colitis does not follow the standard progression of adenoma to carcinoma. Thus, surveillance programs are designed to detect premalignant dysplasia in mucosal areas that may appear no different from surrounding regions; however, high-definition colonoscopy with chromoendoscopy has demonstrated that many regions harboring dysplasia are nodular, raised or ulcerated. The usual approach to surveillance among patients with pan-colitis or left-sided ulcerative colitis, or Crohn's disease with pan-colitis is colonoscopy every 1–2 years beginning 8–10 years after diagnosis and taking four biopsy specimens every 10 cm of colon. If high-grade dysplasia is found and confirmed by an experienced pathologist, colectomy should be performed. The approach to low-grade dysplasia is more controversial, and an informed discussion should be undertaken with the patient about the risks and benefits of continued surveillance every six months versus colectomy. The risk of cancer in patients with ulcerative proctitis or proctosigmoiditis is not elevated so the screening recommendations are the same as in the general population.

Key practice points

- Treatment of IBD depends on the location, extent, and severity of disease.
- Ulcerative colitis presenting with mild to moderate disease may be treated with topical or systemic 5-ASA drugs; however, Crohn's disease does not typically respond to aminosalicylates.
- Topical and systemic steroids can induce remission in patients who do not respond to 5-ASA drugs, or who present with moderate-to-severe disease. Once in remission, patients should be transitioned to immunomodulators or biologic or small molecule for maintenance therapy. The adverse effects of steroids require that their chronic use be minimized.
- Combination biologic plus immunomodulator therapy achieves higher rates of remission and lower rates of relapse than monotherapy with either biologic or immunomodulator alone in moderate to severe Crohn's disease and ulcerative colitis. The decision to remain on combination therapy should weigh these benefits with the rare adverse effects of malignancy.
- Intravenous cyclosporine is effective in inducing remission in severe ulcerative colitis but has no role in the treatment of Crohn's disease
- Tofacitinib (JAK 1 and 3 inhibitor) is a small molecule indicated for the treatment of ulcerative colitis, but at the time of this review is not indicated for the treatment of Crohn's disease.

Case studies

Case 1

A 19-year-old woman with Crohn's disease involving the terminal ileum and proximal colon is referred to you for recurrent symptoms. She had been treated by her referring physician with oral mesalamine for several years with few symptoms; however, she has had three episodes of right lower quadrant abdominal pain and bloody diarrhea requiring courses of oral steroids over the past year. Her current flare has not responded to two weeks of oral prednisone (40 mg daily) and she is losing weight and is unable to maintain hydration. You admit her to the hospital, rule out infection with *C. difficile,* and obtain cross sectional imaging that confirms contrast-enhancing, thickened mucosa of the terminal ileum and proximal colon. Despite three days of intravenous steroids her symptoms do not abate and you order infliximab to be administered intravenously (5 mg/kg). Over the next three days her pain resolves and she has one to two nonbloody bowel movements per day.

She is discharged from the hospital on a tapering course of prednisone, 6 mercaptopurine 1 mg/kg daily, and infliximab infusions every eight weeks. She achieves remission and during a clinic visit six months after discharge expresses concern over the risk of lymphoma and skin cancer with dual immunosuppression therapy. You check her trough concentration of infliximab, which is 9 mcg/ml, and agree to discontinue the mercaptopurine (Table 28.2).

Discussion

Crohn's disease often involves the terminal ileum and proximal colon. 5-ASA drugs have not been demonstrated to be effective in inducing remission in patients Crohn's disease, although they are frequently used. Multiple courses of steroids should have prompted escalation of therapy to combination biologic plus immunomodulator, which has been demonstrated to achieve higher rates of remission than either drug alone. Combination therapy has been associated with increased incidence of lymphoma and nonmelanoma skin cancer, with the majority of evidence pointing to the azathioprine / mercaptopurine as the etiology of elevated risk. While current guidelines recommend continuation of combination biologic plus immunomodulator to maintain remission, there is indirect evidence to support discontinuation of the immunomodulator if the trough level of biologic is high enough to suppress antibiologic antibody production.

Table 28.2 Suggested target trough concentrations

Drug	Trough Concentration (micrograms/ml)
Infliximab	≥5
Adalimumab	≥7.5
Certolizumab Pegol	≥20
Golimumab	unknown

Case 2

A 22-year-old man with ulcerative pan-colitis is treated with CT-P13 monotherapy (biosimilar to infliximab). Three weeks after initiating therapy he is admitted to the hospital after experiencing one week of bloody diarrhea, five to eight times daily associated with left lower quadrant abdominal pain, fever and anorexia. An unprepped colonoscopy confirms active ulcerative colitis and after three days of intravenous prednisolone and intravenous hydration fail to induce remission he is treated with infliximab 15 mg/kg. However, after three days he still has abdominal pain and 10 daily bowel movements and you prescribe cyclosporine intravenously (4 mg/kg/day). It takes three days to achieve and maintain therapeutic levels, after which the patient improves. You discharge him on oral tofacitinib (10 mg twice daily), and he achieves remission.

Discussion

A biosimilar is a biological product that is approved based on a showing that it is highly similar to an US Food and Drug Administration (FDA)-approved biological product, known as a *reference product*, and has no clinically meaningful differences in terms of safety and effectiveness from the reference product. Several biosimilars based on anti-TNF biologic originator drugs are FDA approved. There is some concern about switching between biosimilar and originator biologic agents, although current evidence does not demonstrate antibody formation or reduction in effectiveness with switching. Cyclosporine administered intravenously can induce remission in patients with severe ulcerative colitis; however, this is not an effective therapy for Crohn's disease. Tofacitinib is a JAK inhibitor that is FDA approved for treatment of moderately to severely active ulcerative colitis. Tofacitinib is not a biologic but rather a small molecule and is not approved for the treatment of Crohn's disease.

Further reading

Farraye, F.A., Melmed, G.Y., Lichtenstein, G.R., and Kane, S.V. (2017). ACG clinical guideline: preventive care in inflammatory bowel disease. *Am. J. Gastroenterol.* 112: 241–258.

Feuerstein, J.D., Nguyen, G.C., Kupfer, S.S. et al. (2017). American Gastroenterological Association Institute guideline on therapeutic drug monitoring in inflammatory bowel disease. *Gastroenterology* 153: 827–834.

Ko, C.W., Singh, S., Feuerstein, J.D. et al. (2019). AGA clinical practice guidelines on the management of mild-to-moderate ulcerative colitis. *Gastroenterology* 156: 748–764; PMID 30576644.

Lichtenstein, G.R., Loftus, E.V., Isaacs, K.L. et al. (2018). ACG clinical guideline: management of Crohn's disease in adults. *Am. J. Gastroenterol.* 113: 481–517.

Terdiman, J.P., Gruss, C.B., Heidelbaugh, J.J. et al. (2013). American Gastroenterological Association Institute guideline on the use of thiopurines, methotrexate, and anti-TNFα biologic drugs for the induction and maintenance of remission of inflammatory Crohn's disease. *Gastroenterology* 145: 1459–1463.

CHAPTER 29
Colonic Neoplasia

Colorectal cancer (CRC) is the second leading cause of cancer death in the United States. Screening with fecal occult blood testing (FOBT) or flexible sigmoidoscopy has been proven to reduce CRC incidence and mortality. Most CRCs arise from neoplastic polyps, and colonoscopic removal of these polyps reduces CRC incidence and mortality. Although several histopathological types of colonic polyps exist, more than 90% are adenomatous or hyperplastic. Several colonic polyposis syndromes have been defined, the most common of which are familial adenomatous polyposis (FAP) and Lynch syndrome (Table 29.1).

Colorectal polyps

Clinical presentation

Colorectal polyps are common and have varying malignant potential depending on the underlying histology. The vast majority of polyps are generally asymptomatic and are detected during screening examinations or during evaluation for symptoms unrelated to the polyps. When symptomatic, the most common manifestations include rectal bleeding (overt and occult), change in bowel habits, and abdominal pain. Digital rectal examination may detect polyps in the distal rectum.

Diagnostic investigation

Laboratory studies

Intermittent bleeding from large polyps may produce a positive result on FOBT or fecal immunochemical test (FIT) or may lead to iron deficiency anemia.

Radiographic studies

Computed tomography colonography (CTC) has 90% sensitivity and 86% specificity for polyps 1 cm in size or larger. The sensitivity for sessile polyps

Yamada's Handbook of Gastroenterology, Fourth Edition. John M. Inadomi, Renuka Bhattacharya, Joo Ha Hwang, and Cynthia Ko.

Table 29.1 Polyposis syndromes

Syndrome	Gene mutation	Risk for colorectal cancer (CRC)	Histology and pathologic features	Distribution	Extraintestinal features
Familial adenomatous polyposis (FAP)	*APC* (regulator of Wnt signaling)	100%	Adenomatous polyps	Stomach, small intestine, colon	Epidermoid cysts, fibromas Gardner syndrome – desmoid tumors, osteomas, dental abnormalities Turcot syndrome – central nervous system malignancies including medulloblastomas, astrocytomas, and ependymomas
Lynch syndrome	*MLH1, MSH2, MSH6, PMS2* (DNA mismatch repair [MMR] genes); *EPCAM*	Depends on genetic mutation; up to 45–50%	Adenomatous polyps, microsatellite instability (MSI)	Colorectal, gastric	Pancreatic, endometrial, renal, central nervous system malignancies
Serrated polyposis syndrome	Unknown	Undefined	Sessile serrated polyps	Colorectal	Undefined
MUTYH-associated polyposis	*MUTYH* (base excision repair gene)	45–50% by age 60 years	Adenomatous, some have hyperplastic and sessile serrated polyps	Gastric, duodenal, colorectal	Ovarian, bladder, thyroid, and skin malignancies
Peutz–Jeghers syndrome	*STK11* (*LKB1*) (regulator of apoptosis through p53)	39%	Hamartomatous	Stomach, small intestine, colon	Orocutaneous melanin pigment, other malignancies (pancreatic, breast, ovarian, uterine, lung)
Juvenile polyposis	*SMAD4* (*DPC4*), *BMPR1A* (regulators of transforming growth factor [TGF]-β signaling)	9–68%	Hamartomatous	Stomach, small intestine, colon	Macrocephaly, hypertelorism
Cowden syndrome	*PTEN* (regulator of cell cycling, translation, and apoptosis)	Minimal	Juvenile, lipoma, inflammatory, ganglioneuroma, lymphoid hyperplasia	Esophagus, stomach, small intestine, colon	Facial trichilemmomas, oral papillomas, multinodular goiter, fibrocystic breast, other malignancies (thyroid, breast, uterine)
Hereditary mixed polyposis syndrome	Chromosome 6	Unknown	Atypical juvenile, adenomatous, hyperplastic	Colon	None

(e.g. those with a flat gross morphology) is lower. However, to optimize performance of CTC, experienced radiologists and state-of-the-art software and hardware are needed. Barium enema (BE) is seldom used for polyp detection since the advent of CTC. Colonoscopy is required when either BE or CTC demonstrates a polyp large enough to require removal.

Endoscopy

Colonoscopy is the procedure of choice for suspected colonic polyps because it has the highest sensitivity and specificity of any modality and allows for biopsy and polypectomy. However, colonoscopy may miss up to 25% of small adenomas. Although flexible sigmoidoscopy allows inspection of the distal colorectum, proximal neoplasia may be missed by this modality.

Histology

Adenomas are the most common premalignant colorectal polyps and are classified by their dominant histology. Tubular adenomas are the most common (85%); tubulovillous adenomas (10%) and villous adenomas (5%) account for the remainder. Although adenomas are premalignant lesions, only a small minority undergo malignant transformation. The risk of high-grade dysplasia or invasive adenocarcinoma correlates with the size of the polyp and the degree of villous architecture. Both the rate of growth and the malignant potential of individual adenomas vary substantially, and many polyps remain stable or even regress. For adenomas that do progress, the mean time from polyp initiation to malignant transformation is estimated to be at least 7–10 years. Adenomas are characterized genetically by the presence of chromosomal or microsatellite instability (MSI).

Serrated polyps are the other major histologic sub-type of polyps. Serrated polyps include hyperplastic polyps, sessile serrated polyps, traditional serrated polyps, and mixed hyperplastic/adenomatous polyps (also known as *sessile serrated polyps with cytological or adenoma-like dysplasia*). Hyperplastic polyps account for more than 80% of serrated polyps, and are quite common, generally <5 mm, most frequently found in the distal colorectum, and believed not to harbor malignant potential. Sessile serrated polyps tend to be more common in the proximal colon. They often have a flat morphology with indistinct borders and are easily missed during colonoscopy due to their subtle appearance. They are distinguished from hyperplastic polyps by the presence of dilated crypts in the deep mucosa, horizontal bending of the crypts, and crypt branching and budding. They develop through genetic pathways characterized by mutation of the BRAF oncogene and/or CpG island hypermethylation. These polyps can undergo malignant transformation and may be a source of interval CRCs. Traditional serrated adenomas and mixed hyperplastic/adenomatous polyps are much less common, but also believed to harbor malignant potential.

Hamartomatous polyps such as juvenile or Peutz–Jeghers polyps may also be seen, but are generally uncommon. Inflammatory polyps may be seen with several different inflammatory conditions, including inflammatory bowel disease and chronic ischemia. Pseudo-polyps may be seen in areas of prior inflammation that have subsequently healed.

Diagnostic pitfalls

Colonoscopy has long been considered the "gold standard" for the evaluation of neoplasia in the colon, but often misses small or flat polyps and occasionally large polyps or cancer. While colonoscopy reduces the risk of cancer for up to 10 years, the protection is not absolute, particularly for right-sided CRC. This may result from a variety of factors, including technical issues (e.g. failure to reach the cecum or to identify and remove polyps completely) or biological factors (e.g. fast-progressing polyps).

Management

Endoscopy and surgery

Most premalignant colorectal polyps can be removed completely by endoscopic polypectomy, although large broad-based polyps may require advanced endoscopic techniques. If endoscopic polypectomy is not possible, surgical resection may be necessary. Colonoscopy complications such as hemorrhage, perforation, and postpolypectomy syndrome occur in <2%.

Patients with adenomatous or sessile serrated polyps usually enter a colonoscopic surveillance program to detect and remove any new polyps before they undergo malignant transformation. The recommended surveillance interval depends upon the number, size, and histology of polyps detected.

Malignant polyps

When malignant cells penetrate the muscularis mucosae, the polyp is considered an invasive carcinoma. Colonoscopic polypectomy is curative if malignant cells have not penetrated this layer. In this case, the decision to perform colonoscopic resection only or surgical resection is based on the characteristics of the malignant polyp. Surgical resection is recommended if at least one poor prognostic feature such as incomplete endoscopic resection, poorly differentiated histology, carcinoma within 2 mm of the polypectomy margin, lymphovascular invasion, sessile morphology, or extension beyond the base of the polyp stalk is present. Pedunculated polyps that can be completely resected and without high-risk features may be treated with polypectomy alone.

Familial Adenomatous Polyposis

FAP and its variants are autosomal dominant diseases characterized by the early onset of hundreds or thousands of intestinal polyps with an extremely high risk of CRC (Table 29.1).

Clinical presentation

Patients with FAP usually develop adenomatous polyps in adolescence or young adulthood, but colonic adenomas have been reported to develop as early as age 4 and as late as age 40. Polyps often carpet the colon, but they rarely produce symptoms until late in the course of disease. CRC is diagnosed at a mean age of 39, and most develop cancer by age 50. Patients with attenuated FAP often have fewer polyps, with development of cancer delayed by 10 years, on average.

Gastric polyps are present in 23–100% of patients with FAP. If present, they usually are numerous, asymptomatic, located in the proximal fundus or body, and have a hamartomatous (nonneoplastic, fundic gland) histology. Adenomatous polyps of the stomach occur in 10% of patients with FAP, usually in the antrum but occasionally in the body or fundus. Duodenal polyps occur in 50–90% of patients with FAP and usually are adenomatous. These polyps tend to be multiple and often develop in the periampullary region. The lifetime risk of developing cancer from duodenal adenomas is 3–5%. Adenomas may also develop in the jejunum (50%) and ileum (20%), but malignant transformation is rare.

Screening and surveillance

Genetic testing may be performed to confirm a suspected FAP diagnosis, to identify the mutation in a patient with known FAP, and to screen relatives of a proband with established FAP. Children with known mutations should be screened by endoscopy every 1–2 years beginning at age 10–12. Because polyps are distributed throughout the colon, flexible sigmoidoscopy is considered an adequate screening procedure. If adenomas are detected, a full colonoscopy should be performed to guide subsequent management. If genetic testing is unsuccessful or unavailable, all relatives should be screened by endoscopy. Patients with established FAP also should be screened by upper endoscopy every one to three years for upper gastrointestinal polyps.

Relatives of a proband with attenuated FAP require colonoscopic screening because this syndrome produces fewer polyps that may be more proximal in the colon. Screening for these persons should be initiated at an age 10 years younger than the earliest age of colon cancer diagnosis within the family.

Endoscopic surveillance for gastric and duodenal polyps should begin at the age of 25–30 or at the onset of colonic polyposis. Surveillance intervals depend on the number and size of duodenal polyps detected.

Management and prevention

Because of the high risk of CRC, elective colectomy is recommended. Indications for colectomy include documented malignancy, multiple large or dysplastic adenomas, or inability to adequately survey the colon due to extensive polyposis. Surgical options for FAP include total proctocolectomy with ileostomy, total colectomy with ileal pouch–anal anastomosis, and subtotal colectomy with ileorectal anastomosis. In the last procedure, the rectal stump remains at risk of developing adenomatous polyps and cancer, and surveillance sigmoidoscopy is required every three to six months. Even after colectomy, ongoing surveillance of the pouch is needed due to risk of malignancy arising from the rectal cuff.

Progression of duodenal adenomas to adenocarcinoma, particularly periampullary cancer, occurs in 3–5% of patients with FAP, at a mean age of 45–50 years. The optimal treatment for adenomatous duodenal polyps is undefined, though endoscopic approaches are appropriate for selected individuals.

Lynch syndrome

Lynch syndrome is the most common cause of inherited colon cancer and is caused by mutation or loss of expression of one of the DNA mismatch repair (MMR) genes, which leads to DNA MSI (Table 29.1). Patients with Lynch syndrome are also at risk of gastric, small bowel, pancreatic, hepatobiliary, endometrial, renal and ureteral malignancies, among others. Colorectal malignancies in these patients tend to be located in the proximal colon, and to progress from adenomas to carcinomas more rapidly. However, overall survival after CRC diagnosis is high.

Because Lynch syndrome is common, all patients with newly diagnosed CRC should have a detailed family history performed looking for Lynch syndrome-associated cancers. Families meeting either Amsterdam II criteria or the revised Bethesda criteria should be referred for genetic counseling (Table 29.2). Testing for MSI or loss of expression of MMR proteins in tumor tissue from newly diagnosed CRCs is also advocated, even in the absence of Lynch syndrome features. Positive results on these tests requires follow-up germline mutation testing to confirm the diagnosis, as some sporadic tumors also have MSI.

Patients with Lynch syndrome should undergo colonoscopic surveillance every 1–2 years, starting at age 20–25 or 2–5 years prior to the earliest age of CRC diagnosis in the family. Colonoscopy should occur annually after age 40. If CRC is found, subtotal colectomy with ileorectal anastomosis is the appropriate therapy, followed by annual surveillance of the rectal stump. Women with Lynch syndrome should undergo annual screening for endometrial and ovarian cancer and may consider prophylactic hysterectomy and bilateral salpingo-oophorectomy at the end of childbearing. Screening for urinary tract, gastric or pancreatic cancers is recommended by some, although the utility and intervals for screening are controversial.

Colorectal adenocarcinoma

Clinical presentation

CRC is the second leading cause of death from cancer in the United States. Most CRCs are diagnosed in patients older than age 50, but the incidence of CRC, and in particular rectal cancer, is increasing in younger individuals. Symptoms or

Table 29.2 Criteria for the diagnosis of Lynch syndrome

Amsterdam criteria

1. Three or more relatives with histologically verified Lynch syndrome-associated cancer[a] (colorectal, endometrial, small bowel, ureter, or renal pelvis), one of whom is a first-degree relative of the other two; familial adenomatous polyposis (FAP) should be excluded.
2. Lynch syndrome-associated cancer involving at least two successive generations.
3. One or more cancer cases diagnosed before the age of 50.

Revised Bethesda criteria for microsatellite instability (MSI) testing of colorectal cancers (CRCs)

1. CRC diagnosed in a patient less than 50 years of age.
2. Presence of synchronous or metachronous colorectal, or other Lynch syndrome-associated tumors, regardless of age.[a]
3. CRC with the MSI-H[b] histology[c] diagnosed in a patient less than 60 years of age.
4. CRC diagnosed in one or more first-degree relatives with a Lynch syndrome-related tumor, with one of the cancers being diagnosed under age 50 years.
5. CRC diagnosed in two or more first- or second-degree relatives with Lynch syndrome-related tumors, regardless of age

[a] Colorectal, endometrial, stomach, small bowel, ovarian, pancreas, ureter and renal pelvis, biliary tract, and brain (usually glioblastoma) cancers, and sebaceous gland neoplasms (carcinomas, adenomas) and keratoacanthomas.

[b] MSI-H, microsatellite instability-high; tumors with changes in two or more of the five National Cancer Institute-recommended panels of microsatellite markers.

[c] Presence of tumor-infiltrating lymphocytes, Crohn's-like lymphocytic reaction, mucinous/signet ring differentiation, or medullary growth pattern.

signs of CRC arise from complications of obstruction, hemorrhage, local invasion, or cancer cachexia. Approximately 15% of patients present with acute complications including obstruction, perforation, and bleeding.

CRC often causes occult gastrointestinal bleeding, but hematochezia may occur from tumor friability and ulceration. Patients with tumors in the distal colon are more likely to have hematochezia or a positive FOBT as the presenting feature, whereas patients with right-sided colonic lesions are more likely to present with iron deficiency anemia.

Diagnostic investigation of symptomatic patients

Colonoscopy is the procedure of choice in patients with symptoms suggestive of CRC. The sensitivity of colonoscopy for detecting malignancies exceeds 90% for neoplasms larger than 1 cm. Baseline complete blood counts, liver function tests, and carcinoembryonic antigen (CEA) levels should be obtained in patients with newly diagnosed CRC.

CTC, or rarely BE, may be used in patients who are at high risk for colonoscopy, but colonoscopy with biopsy or polypectomy is usually required at some point for tissue sampling. When CRC is diagnosed, a CT of the chest, abdomen, and pelvis is recommended for cancer staging. Transrectal endoscopic ultrasound or magnetic resonance imaging can be used to evaluate rectal neoplasms to determine if neoadjuvant chemoradiation is needed and to guide surgical decision-making.

Management

The prognosis in CRC corresponds to tumor stage, with the five-year survival rates of 93, 74–85, 44–83, and 8% for stages I, II, III, and IV, respectively. Poorly differentiated or mucinous histology is also associated with a poorer progosis. Tumors with MSI typically have with better prognosis, despite often higher stage at diagnosis. Tumor size is not a proven independent predictor of survival.

Except for colonoscopic removal of malignant polyps with favorable prognostic features, the only reliable method for curing colorectal adenocarcinoma is surgical resection. Chemotherapy is indicated for patients with stage III colon cancer and may benefit selected patients with stage II disease with high-risk features. Neoadjuvant chemoradiotherapy is commonly used for patients with locally advanced rectal cancer. Chemotherapy is generally indicated for distant metastatic disease, but palliative resection may be considered for patients with metastatic disease to alleviate symptoms of bleeding or obstruction.

Solitary hepatic metastases or a small number of lesions localized to one hepatic lobe may also be surgically treated. Aggressive surgical resection of hepatic metastases can result in a 25–35% five-year disease-free survival rate. Hepatic metastases that are not amenable to surgical resection may be treated with ablative therapy, such as intra-arterial chemoembolization or radiofrequency ablation.

Post-treatment surveillance

Patients who survive curative therapy for CRC should undergo periodic colonoscopic surveillance. If complete colonoscopy was not performed prior to surgery, it should be performed within three to six months postoperatively. Otherwise, surveillance is recommended at 12 months after diagnosis. Subsequently, the surveillance program depends upon the colonoscopic findings.

Screening for CRC in Asymptomatic individuals

Screening for CRC in average-risk individuals is widely recommended, and the most common approaches in the United States are annual FOBT/FIT or colonoscopy (Table 29.3). Annual FOBT reduces the mortality from CRC by about 33%. Prospective trials have shown that screening flexible sigmoidoscopy reduces CRC mortality by 26–31% and CRC incidence by 21–23%. Observational studies suggest that screening colonoscopy reduces CRC incidence by 50–90% and mortality by about 60%. These studies estimate that the protective effect of endoscopic procedures lasts up to 10 years, but may be less in the proximal colon. Large-scale randomized controlled studies comparing colonoscopy to FIT are now in progress.

Other available screening tests include the multi-target stool DNA test, which can detect some of the DNA mutations associated with colorectal neoplasia in stool. This is performed in conjunction with FIT, and has high sensitivity for cancer; however, the specificity of this test is lower than FIT, leading to more

Table 29.3 Current colorectal cancer (CRC) screening guideline recommendations

	US Preventive Services Task Force[a]	American Cancer Society[b]	US Multi-Society Task Force on Colorectal Cancer (CRC)[c]
Age to initiate screening in average risk individuals	50 years	45 years (qualified recommendation) or 50 years (strong recommendation)	50 years
Age to discontinue routine screening	• 75 years • Individualize decisions for patients age 76–85 years • No routine screening if age >85 years	• 75 years • Individualize decisions for patients age 76–85 years • Discourage routine screening if age >85 years	• 75 years • Individualize decisions for patients age 76–85 years • No routine screening if age >85 years
Preferred test	No preferred or rank order	High sensitivity stool test (e.g. fecal immunochemical test [FIT], high sensitivity fecal occult blood testing [FOBT], multi-target stool DNA test) OR structural exam (e.g. colonoscopy, flexible sigmoidoscopy, computed tomography [CT] colonography)	Tier 1 Colonoscopy every 10 years Annual FIT Tier 2 CT colonography every five years FIT-fecal DNA every three years Flexible sigmoidoscopy every 5–10 years Tier 3 Colon capsule every five years

[a] Rex et al. (2017).
[b] Wolf et al. (2018).
[c] US Preventive Services Task Force (2016).

false-positive results. CT colonography is performed in some centers as a noninvasive screening test, but detection of sessile lesions is low; in addition there are risks of cumulative radiation exposure with screening at recommended intervals and extracolonic lesions are common, leading to possible unnecessary diagnostic evaluation. A blood test for methylated septin9 DNA is FDA approved for CRC screening in individuals at average risk for cancer who refuse other forms of screening, although the sensitivity for cancer is lower than other screening tests.

Recommendations for screening average-risk asymptomatic populations

Most guidelines recommend beginning screening in average risk individuals (i.e. those without a family history of CRC, a colonic polypsis syndrome, or a history of inflammatory bowel disease) at the age of 50, although the American Cancer Society conditionally recommends screening initiation at age 45 due to the increasing incidence of CRC in younger populations. Patients with positive screening results obtained through noncolonoscopic strategies should be further evaluated by colonoscopy to diagnose neoplasia and perform polypectomy. A diagnosis of adenomatous or sessile serrated polyps typically necessitates periodic colonoscopic surveillance.

Surveillance for patients with a family history of CRC

Patients with a family history of CRC in a single first-degree relative, but without a defined polyposis syndrome, have a 75–80% increased risk of cancer, compared to patients with no family history of CRC. Persons with multiple first-degree relatives or with one first-degree relative diagnosed with CRC at age 60 or less are at higher risk and should be considered for surveillance colonoscopy 10 years earlier than the earliest age of CRC diagnosis in the family or at age 40, whichever comes first. Subsequent surveillance procedures and intervals are then tailored according to the specifics of the family history.

Key practice points

- Colorectal neoplasia is common and usually asymptomatic. The majority of polyps never progress to cancer.
- CRC is the second leading cause of cancer death. CRC screening is appropriate for average-risk individuals aged 50–75 years, although recent guidelines advocate initiating screening at age 45 years. The best screening modality continues to be a matter for debate.
- Colonoscopy is the procedure of choice for the investigation of symptoms of suspected neoplasia.
- Individuals with a positive CRC screening test (e.g. FOBT/FIT, sigmoidoscopy) should undergo evaluation with colonoscopy.

Further reading

Lieberman, D.A., Rex, D.K., Winawer, S.J. et al. (2017). Guidelines for colonoscopy surveillance after and polypectomy: a consensus update by the U.S. multi-society task force on colorectal cancer. *Gastroenterology* 143: 844–857.

Rex, D.K., Boland, C.R., Dominitz, J.A. et al. (2017). Colorectal cancer screening: recommendations for physicians and patients from the U.S. multi-society task force on colorectal cancer. *Gastroenterology* 153: 307–323.

Rubenstein, J.H., Ens, R.E., Heidelbaugh, J. et al. (2015). American Gastroenterological Association Institute guideline on the diagnosis and management of lynch syndrome. *Gastroenterology* 149: 777–782.

US Preventive Services Task Force (2016). Screening for colorectal cancer: U.S. preventive services task force recommendation statement. *JAMA* 315: 2564–2575.

Wolf, A.M.D., Fontham, E.T.H., and Church, T.R. (2018). Colorectal cancer screening for average-risk adults: 2018 guideline update from the American Cancer Society. *CA Cancer J Clin* 68: 250–281.

CHAPTER 30
Anorectal Diseases

Anorectal disorders are common among patients presenting to gastroenterologists and can be challenging to manage. Often, co-management by gastroenterologists and surgeons is required.

Hemorrhoids

Hemorrhoids result from dilation of the superior and inferior hemorrhoidal veins that form the physiological hemorrhoidal cushion. Internal hemorrhoids arise above the dentate line in three locations and are covered by columnar epithelium. External hemorrhoids arise below the dentate line and are covered by squamous epithelium. Skin tags are redundant folds of skin arising from the anal verge. They may be residua of resolved, thrombosed, external hemorrhoids. Although it is widely believed that constipation is an important risk factor for hemorrhoids, recent studies suggest a more prominent role for diarrheal disorders.

Patients with internal hemorrhoids may exhibit gross but not occult bleeding (rarely requiring transfusion), discomfort, pruritus ani, fecal soiling, and prolapse. First-degree hemorrhoids do not protrude from the anus. Second-degree hemorrhoids prolapse with defecation but spontaneously reduce. Third-degree hemorrhoids prolapse and require manual reduction, and fourth-degree hemorrhoids cannot be reduced and are at risk of strangulation.

Most patients with new-onset rectal bleeding should be evaluated endoscopically to confirm the source of hemorrhage, even if hemorrhoids are noted on physical examination or anoscopy. Laboratory testing is not routinely recommended. Hemorrhoids should initially be managed medically with a high-fiber diet, adequate fluid intake, good anal hygiene, and avoidance of prolonged sitting or straining with bowel movements. The role of suppositories, ointments, and witch hazel is relatively limited. Most first-degree and second-degree hemorrhoids can be managed with these conservative measures. Patients with

Yamada's Handbook of Gastroenterology, Fourth Edition. John M. Inadomi, Renuka Bhattacharya, Joo Ha Hwang, and Cynthia Ko.

symptomatic, bothersome grade 1 or grade 2 hemorrhoids who do not respond to conservative measures may need more definitive therapy, such as rubber band ligation. Surgical hemorrhoidectomy is the treatment of choice for large third-degree hemorrhoids, all fourth-degree hemorrhoids, and other hemorrhoids refractory to nonsurgical therapy.

Thrombosis of an external hemorrhoid can produce severe pain and bleeding. Most thrombosed external hemorrhoids can be managed with sitz baths, bulking agents, stool softeners, and topical anesthetics; resolution occurs after 48–72 hours. If surgical evacuation or excision is required, it should be performed within 48 hours of symptom onset. Symptoms of skin tags include sensation of a growth and difficulty with anal hygiene. Treatment is conservative and surgical resection is rarely needed.

Anal fissure

An anal fissure is a painful linear ulcer in the anal canal. Idiopathic anal fissures are usually located in the posterior (90%) or anterior midline. Nonmidline fissures suggest a predisposing illness such as Crohn's disease, malignancy, or infection. Fissures are caused by traumatic tearing of the anal canal during passage of hard stool. They may become chronic from high resting anal sphincter tone, which promotes a relative ischemia that prevents fissure healing. Reflex anal contraction after defecation contributes to spasm and pain.

Severe pain, often worse with bowel movements, with scant red bleeding is the hallmark of an anal fissure. The fissure is best identified by simple physical examination. Anoscopy is usually not necessary and is poorly tolerated due to pain. An acute anal fissure is a small, linear tear perpendicular to the dentate line. Chronic anal fissures appear as the triad of a fissure, a proximal hypertrophic papilla, and a sentinel pile at the anal verge. Patients with acute fissures usually respond to a high-fiber diet, topical anesthetics, and warm sitz baths. Topical vasodilators such as nifedipine or nitroglycerine are helpful, but topical corticosteroids have a limited role. Patients with chronic fissures should be treated with topical vasodilators. If patients do not respond to topical agents, intramuscular injection of botulinum toxin may promote fissure healing. Surgical internal anal sphincterotomy may be necessary for some patients with chronic fissures who do not respond to more conservative measures.

Anorectal abscess and fistula

An anorectal abscess usually originates from an obstructed anal crypt gland due to trauma, diarrhea, hard stools, or foreign bodies. Anorectal fistulae are abnormal communications between the anorectal canal and the perianal skin that are often the result of chronic infection. Abscess and fistula formation may occur without primary glandular infection in patients with Crohn's disease, anorectal malignancy, tuberculosis, actinomycosis, lymphogranuloma venereum, radiation proctitis, leukemia, and lymphoma. Abscesses are classified by site of origin and potential pathways of extension. Fistulae are divided into intersphincteric, trans-sphincteric, suprasphincteric, and extrasphincteric types.

Acute pain and swelling, exacerbated by sitting, movement, and defecation, are the main symptoms of an anorectal abscess. Malaise and fever are common. A purulent discharge suggests that the abscess is spontaneously draining through the primary anal orifice. Examination reveals erythema and fluctuance, although deeper abscesses may not produce any external findings with the abscess only palpable on rectal exam. Anal ultrasound, computed tomography (CT) or magnetic resonance (MR) imaging can determine the location of an abscess relative to the sphincters. Anorectal abscesses require surgical drainage to prevent development of systemic infection. Superficial abscesses may be drained under local anesthesia but other abscesses require surgical drainage. Antibiotics usually are not necessary and may mask signs of underlying suppurative infection. Broad-spectrum antibiotics are indicated for patients with signs of systemic infection, diabetes, immunosuppression, valvular heart disease, or extensive soft tissue infection. Warm sitz baths, stool-softening agents, and analgesics can minimize disease recurrence postoperatively.

Anorectal fistulae produce chronic, purulent drainage, pain on defecation, and pruritus ani. Examination may reveal a red, granular papule that exudes pus. Multiple perineal openings suggest the possibility of Crohn's disease or hidradenitis suppurativa. Anoscopy and endoscopy are performed to locate the primary orifice at the level of the dentate line and to exclude proctitis. MRI may help guide management of complex fistulas. Simple primary anorectal fistulae may be treated by fistulotomy, in which the primary orifice is opened with conservation of the external sphincter. Postoperative care is the same as that for anorectal abscesses.

Patients with pre-existing fecal incontinence, Crohn's disease or other complex chronic fistulae may benefit from placement of a seton through the fistula, and generally should not undergo fistulotomy due to risk for nonhealing.

Rectal prolapse

Rectal prolapse is protrusion of the rectum through the anus. The prolapse may be complete (all layers visibly descend), partial (protrusion of distal rectal tissue but not the entire circumference), or occult (internal intussusception without visible protrusion). In adults, the condition is associated with older age, female gender, pelvic floor weakness or dysfunction, chronic constipation or diarrhea, and neurological disease.

Patients report prolapse of tissue as well as defecatory straining, incomplete evacuation, tenesmus, and incontinence. On examination, the prolapse may be obvious with straining. Endoscopy or barium enema radiography excludes malignancy but may reveal a concomitant solitary rectal ulcer. Defecography, either with barium or MRI, may identify occult prolapse and other pelvic floor anatomic abnormalities. Persistently prolapsed tissue must be promptly reduced manually to avoid strangulation, ulceration, bleeding, or perforation. Surgical repair such as rectopexy should be offered to those who are surgical candidates. Perineal strengthening exercises can be suggested to patients who refuse or who cannot undergo surgery. Perineal repair may be offered to patients who are poor operative candidates. Occult prolapse is treated surgically if incontinence or solitary rectal ulcer is present; otherwise, conservative therapy is recommended.

Fecal incontinence

Fecal incontinence affects women, elderly individuals, and institutionalized persons most commonly. Patients often will not voluntarily disclose incontinence, and direct questioning may be needed. Traumatic obstetric and surgical injuries, rectal or hemorrhoidal prolapse, and neuropathic disease may impair anal sphincter function and lead to incontinence (Table 30.1). Other factors that

Table 30.1 Causes of fecal incontinence

Causes
Diarrhea
Fecal impaction
Constipation with overflow incontinence
Irritable bowel syndrome
Anal diseases
Anal carcinoma
Congenital abnormalities
Protruding internal hemorrhoids
Rectal prolapse
Perianal infections
Fistulae
Injury (e.g. surgical, obstetric, accidental)
Sphincteric weakness
Rectal diseases
Rectal carcinoma
Rectal ischemia
Proctitis (e.g. inflammatory bowel disease, radiation therapy, infection)
Neurological diseases
Central nervous system (e.g. cerebrovascular accident, dementia, toxic or metabolic disorders, spinal cord injury or tumors, multiple sclerosis, tabes dorsalis)
Peripheral nervous system (e.g. diabetes, cauda equina lesions)

predispose to fecal incontinence include loss of anal or rectal sensation secondary to neuropathy; poor rectal distension with ulcerative proctitis, radiation proctitis, or ischemia; and overwhelming diarrhea. Hypersensitivity to distension and abnormal rectal motility probably account for the incontinence often seen in patients with irritable bowel syndrome.

Partial incontinence is defined as minor soiling and poor flatus control. The elderly and those with internal anal sphincter deficiency, fecal impaction, and rectal prolapse are prone to partial incontinence. Some patients have near normal sphincter pressures and experience soiling secondary to hemorrhoids or fissures. Major incontinence is the frequent loss of large amounts of stool. It is caused by neurological disease, traumatic injury, and surgical damage. Examination may reveal anal deformity, tumors, infections, fistulae, prolapsing hemorrhoids, loss of anal tone, and absence of the anal wink.

Several different examinations may be needed for evaluation of fecal incontinence. Physical examination can assess the anorectal angle and puborectalis function with simulated squeeze and defecation as well as look for evidence of fistulae, prolapse, and hemorrhoids. Endoscopy excludes malignancy and proctitis. Anorectal manometry defines resting and maximal anal pressures, rectal compliance, and rectal sensitivity to distension, and can determine the efficiency of evacuation by simulated expulsion of an inflated balloon. MR defecography, allows evaluation of the pelvic floor and anorectal anatomy and allows dynamic assessment of the pelvic floor anatomy and function. Anorectal ultrasound and endoanal MRI measure sphincter muscle thickness and detect muscle defects from trauma or surgical injury. Electromyography assesses external sphincter and puborectalis muscle activity in patients with a suspected neurogenic cause of incontinence.

Adequate management of fecal incontinence often requires a combination of interventions. Fiber therapy or opiate antidiarrheals are indicated for stool bulking and treating diarrhea. Anticholinergics may blunt the gastrocolonic response and reduce meal-associated incontinence. Fecal impactions are removed with enemas or by manual disimpaction. For individuals who fail conservative measures, pelvic floor physical therapy and biofeedback produces high success rates in appropriate patients. Biofeedback can also be used to improve rectal sensation in patients with underlying neuropathy. Conditions that respond poorly to biofeedback therapy include severe organic disease with reduced rectal sensation, irritable bowel syndrome, anterior rectal resection, and prior anal sphincterotomy. Selected patients may benefit from sacral nerve stimulation.

Surgery is generally reserved for patients with major incontinence. Prior anal injury may be repairable with anal sphincteroplasty. Gracilis muscle transposition with or without electrical stimulation may benefit a patient with severe sphincter dysfunction or a congenital pelvic floor abnormality. Artificial sphincters may be implanted, but complication rates are high. As a last resort, placing a colostomy should be considered.

Pruritus ani

Pruritus ani is an itchy sensation of the anus and perianal skin that may result from perianal disease (fissures, fistulae, hemorrhoids, malignancy) or from residual fecal material (Table 30.2). *Candida albicans* and dermatophyte infections appear as localized erythematous rashes but may also be present on apparently normal skin. Pinworm (*Enterobius vermicularis*) causes nocturnal pruritus ani. Scabies (*Sarcoptes scabiei*) and pubic lice produce pruritus ani that may be associated with genital itching. Sexually transmitted diseases associated with the condition include herpes simplex, gonorrhea, syphilis, condyloma acuminatum, and molluscum contagiosum. Generalized skin conditions (e.g. psoriasis, atopic dermatitis) as well as local irritants, allergens, and chemicals may produce perianal itching. Clinical experience suggests that certain dietary products such as coffee, cola, beer, tomatoes, chocolate, tea, and citrus fruits may be causative. Idiopathic pruritus ani results from a combination of perianal fecal contamination and trauma.

Most cases of pruritus ani can be successfully managed. If identified, the underlying disorder should receive specific treatment. A diagnosis of pinworms can be confirmed by detecting eggs on adhesive cellophane tape applied to the perianal skin early in the morning. Foods that predispose to diarrhea or pruritus

Table 30.2 Causes of pruritus ani

Causes of pruritus ani
Anorectal diseases
Diarrhea
Fecal incontinence
Hemorrhoids
Anal fissures
Fistulae
Rectal prolapse
Anal malignancy
Infections
Fungal (e.g. candidiasis, dermatophytes)
Parasitic (e.g. pinworms, scabies)
Bacterial (e.g. *Staphylococcus aureus*)
Sexually transmitted (e.g. herpes, gonorrhea, syphilis, condyloma acuminatum)
Local irritants
Moisture, obesity, perspiration
Soaps, hygiene products
Anal creams and suppositories
Dietary (e.g. coffee, beer, acidic foods)
Medications (e.g. mineral oil, ascorbic acid, quinidine, colchicine)
Dermatological diseases
Psoriasis
Atopic dermatitis
Seborrheic dermatitis

should be eliminated. The key to management in most cases rests on keeping the anal area clean and dry while minimizing trauma induced by wiping and scratching. The perianal skin should be cleansed with a moistened pad after defecation. The area should be dried with a blow dryer or with a soft towel using a blotting motion. Thin cotton pledgets may be needed for those with fecal discharge. Excess perspiration can be controlled with talcum powder and loose cotton clothing. In some patients, a barrier cream such as zinc oxide can be used. Nocturnal pruritus may benefit from oral antihistamines (e.g. diphenhydramine). Topical capsaicin may be beneficial if these conservative measures fail.

Proctalgia fugax and levator ani syndrome

Proctalgia fugax is characterized by sudden, brief episodes of severe rectal pain and is associated with irritable bowel syndrome and psychogenic disorders. In most cases, the cause is unknown. Attacks of proctalgia fugax are described as intense stabbing or aching midline pain above the anus, lasting seconds to minutes. Frequently, no clear precipitating cause is identified. Patients are asymptomatic between episodes. Other causes of rectal pain should be excluded by physical examination and endoscopy. Unproven local therapies include rectal massage, firm perineal pressure, and warm soaks or baths. Anecdotal reports claim that topical nitroglycerin, pudendal nerve block, or botulinum toxin injections into the anal sphincter may reduce symptoms.

The levator ani syndrome refers to aching rectal pain due to tenderness and spasm of the levator ani muscle group. The pain of the levator ani syndrome is more chronic, aching, and pressure-like than that of proctalgia fugax. Defecation and prolonged sitting precipitate the pain. On examination, palpable tenderness and spasm of the levator muscles may be elicited. Pelvic floor physical therapy with biofeedback training is the preferred method of treatment. Other therapies that have been tested include electrical stimulation of the pelvic floor muscles, levator ani massage, sitz baths, and botulinum toxin injections.

Miscellaneous conditions

Coccygodynia is a sharp or aching pain in the coccyx that may radiate to the rectal region or buttocks and can be caused by traumatic arthritis, dislocation or fracture, difficult childbirth, or prolonged sitting. Manipulating the coccyx on examination reproduces the pain. Therapies include warm soaks, analgesics, local corticosteroid injection, and, rarely, coccygectomy.

Pilonidal disease is an acquired condition of the midline coccygeal skin in which small skin pits precede development of a draining sinus or abscess. In contrast to anorectal fistula or hidradenitis suppurativa, there is no communication with the anorectum. Patients, usually young men, present with a painful swelling and drainage. Definitive treatment usually is surgical. Squamous cell carcinoma may complicate the course of pilonidal disease.

Hidradenitis suppurativa is a suppurative condition of apocrine glands in the axilla and inguinoperineal regions that manifests in adolescence and young adulthood. It can present as recurrent inflamed nodules, abscesses, or draining sinus tracts. Risk factors include obesity, acne, perspiration, and mechanical trauma. Repeated inflammation and healing produce fibrosis and draining sinus tracts, including anal and rectal fistulae. Avoidance of skin trauma and weight management are important first steps for management. Topical and/or systemic antibiotics can be used for mild-to-moderate disease. Surgery may be needed for treatment of severe or recurrent disease.

Key practice points

- Symptomatic hemorrhoids can often be managed conservatively with stool bulking and lifestyle modifications.
- Those with symptomatic first-, second-, or third-degree internal hemorrhoids in whom conservative management fails should be treated with band ligation. Fourth-degree internal hemorrhoids often require surgical management.
- Chronic anal fissure should be initially treated with topical nitrate or calcium channel blocker, or botulinum toxin injection. Lateral internal sphincterotomy is indicated for patients with chronic anal fissure in whom these measures fail.
- Fecal incontinence has multiple potential etiologies. Anorectal manometry may help define function and sensation of the pelvic floor muscles. Pelvic floor physical therapy with biofeedback can be helpful.

Further reading

American Society for Gastrointestinal Endoscopy (2010). The role of endoscopy in patients with anorectal disorder. *Gastrointest. Endosc.* 72: 1117–1123.

Davis, B.R., Lee-Kong, S.A., Migaly, J. et al. (2018). The American society of colon and rectal surgeons clinical practice guidelines for the management of hemorrhoids. *Dis. Colon Rectum* 61: 284–292.

Stewart, D.B., Gaertner, W., Glasgow, S. et al. (2017). Clinical practice guidelines for the management of anal fissures. *Dis. Colon Rectum* 60: 7–14.

Wald, A., Bharucha, A.E., Cosman, B.C., and Whitehead, W.E. (2014). ACG clinical guideline: management of benign anorectal disorders. *Am. J. Gastroenterol.* 109: 1141–1157.

CHAPTER 31
Pancreatitis

Acute Pancreatitis

Clinical presentation

Acute pancreatitis is a clinical syndrome of sudden-onset abdominal pain and elevations in the levels of serum pancreatic enzymes caused by an acute necro-inflammatory response in the pancreas. The differential diagnosis for the etiology of acute pancreatitis is provided in Table 31.1. In the United States, more than 80% of acute pancreatitis cases are caused by ethanol or biliary stones.

The initial symptom of acute pancreatitis is almost always abdominal pain, which is described as a deep, visceral pain that develops over several hours in the epigastric and umbilical region. Pain persists for hours to days and may radiate to the middle to lower back. Patients often are restless. Increased pain when supine prompts many patients to sit leaning forward in an effort to minimize discomfort. However, 5% of patients with acute pancreatitis present without abdominal pain.

Nausea and vomiting are present in most patients. Low-grade fever is commonly observed in uncomplicated pancreatitis but high fever and rigors suggest coexisting infection. In some cases of severe pancreatitis, the diagnosis is overlooked because of the patient's inability to report pain because of delirium, hemodynamic instability, or extreme respiratory distress.

Physical examination

Physical examination of a patient with pancreatitis may reveal several findings. Abdominal tenderness with guarding is common and usually most pronounced in the epigastric region. Bowel sounds are diminished as a result of superimposed ileus. Tachycardia may be secondary to severe pain but hypovolemia is common, and severe cases may be complicated by hypotension from extravasation of fluids or hemorrhage in the retroperitoneum. Rare patients present with periumbilical (Cullen sign) or flank (Grey Turner sign) ecchymoses.

Yamada's Handbook of Gastroenterology, Fourth Edition. John M. Inadomi, Renuka Bhattacharya, Joo Ha Hwang, and Cynthia Ko.

Table 31.1 Differential diagnosis of acute pancreatitis

Ethanol
Gallstones
Choledocholithiasis
Biliary sludge
Microlithiasis
Mechanical/structural injury
Sphincter of Oddi dysfunction
Pancreas divisum
Trauma
Following endoscopic retrograde cholangiopancreatography (ERCP)
Pancreatic malignancy
Peptic ulcer disease
Inflammatory bowel disease
Medications
Azathioprine/6-mercaptopurine
Dideoxyinosine
Pentamidine
Sulfonamides
L-Asparaginase
Thiazide diuretics
Metabolic
Hyperlipidemia
Hypercalcemia
Infectious
Viral
Bacterial
Parasitic
Vascular
Vasculitis
Atherosclerosis
Genetic mutations
Cationic trypsinogen (hereditary) (serine protease-1, PRSS1)
Serine protease inhibitor, Kazal-type 1 (SPINK1)
Cystic fibrosis transmembrane conductance regulator (CFTR)
Miscellaneous
Scorpion bite
Idiopathic pancreatitis
Cystic fibrosis
Coronary bypass
Tropical pancreatitis

Ethanol-induced pancreatitis is occasionally accompanied by signs or symptoms of alcoholic liver disease, including jaundice, hepatomegaly, ascites, and encephalopathy. Gallstone pancreatitis may be accompanied by jaundice caused by a retained common bile duct stone, although any severe cause of pancreatitis may be associated with jaundice that is caused by biliary obstruction from an edematous pancreas or associated fluid collection.

Diagnostic investigation

Laboratory studies

Elevated serum amylase and lipase levels are the most common abnormalities seen in laboratory studies of patients with acute pancreatitis and result from increased release and decreased renal clearance of the enzymes. Elevations greater than fivefold are virtually diagnostic of pancreatitis but disease severity does not correlate with the degree of enzyme elevation. Total serum amylase is composed of pancreatic and salivary isoforms. Salivary amylase levels increase with salivary gland disease, chronic alcoholism without pancreatitis, cigarette smoking, anorexia nervosa, esophageal perforation, and several malignancies. The pancreatic amylase isoform may also be elevated in cholecystitis, intestinal perforation, renal failure, and intestinal ischemia. Five to 10% of episodes of acute pancreatitis produce no increases in serum amylase and lipase levels, which are most common in underlying chronic alcoholic pancreatitis, long-term glandular destruction, and fibrosis with loss of functional acinar tissue.

Serum lipase is reportedly a more specific marker of pancreatitis but mild elevations are observed in other conditions (e.g. renal failure and intestinal perforation). In pancreatitis, lipase levels may remain elevated for several days after amylase levels have normalized. Therefore, if the diagnosis is delayed, hyperlipasemia may be the only abnormal laboratory finding. A lipase-to-amylase ratio higher than two is reportedly specific for alcoholic pancreatitis; however, this should not replace the history and physical examination as the primary means for discerning the cause of pancreatitis.

Patients often have other laboratory abnormalities. Leukocytosis can result from inflammation or infection. An increased hematocrit (HCT) may signal decreased plasma volume caused by extravasation of fluid; a decreased HCT may be caused by retroperitoneal hemorrhage. Pancreatic necrosis develops in about half of the patients whose HCT is higher than 44% when admitted to the hospital or if the HCT fails to decrease 24 hours after admission. Electrolyte disorders are common, particularly hypocalcemia, which in part is caused by sequestration of calcium salts as saponified fats in the peripancreatic bed. Patients with underlying liver disease or choledocholithiasis may have abnormal liver chemistry levels. Bilirubin levels higher than 3 mg/dl suggest a biliary cause of pancreatitis.

Imaging studies

Ultrasound is the most sensitive noninvasive means for detecting gallstones, biliary tract dilation, and gallbladder sludge. Intralumenal gas may obscure images of the pancreas in 30–40% of patients, making ultrasound an insensitive technique for detecting the changes associated with pancreatitis. Computed tomographic (CT) scanning is superior to ultrasound for imaging the peripancreatic bed. In mild cases, the pancreas may appear edematous or enlarged. More severe inflammation may extend into surrounding fat planes, producing a pattern of peripancreatic fat stranding. CT scanning also is optimal for defining inhomogeneous pancreatic phlegmons with ill-defined margins or well-defined pseudo-cysts. A dynamic arterial phase CT scan can identify areas of tissue necrosis, which are at risk of subsequent infection. The magnitude of pancreatic necrosis predicts the prognosis. Given its high cost and the limited yield in evaluating mild disease, CT scanning should be reserved for patients where the diagnosis is unclear or have not improved clinically within 48–72 hours. Once pancreatitis has resolved, CT scanning may have a role in excluding pancreatic cancer as a cause of pancreatitis in older patients. Magnetic resonance (MR) cholangiopancreatography, which is considerably more expensive than ultrasound or CT scanning, has a sensitivity higher than 90% for detecting bile duct stones. Endoscopic ultrasound (EUS) is a sensitive test for detecting persistent biliary stones and can be used to distinguish patients who may benefit from treatment with endoscopic retrograde cholangiopancreatography (ERCP). EUS also is useful for detecting small pancreatic or ampullary tumors, pancreas divisum, and chronic pancreatitis.

ERCP is primarily a therapeutic tool in acute biliary pancreatitis; it has no role in diagnosing acute pancreatitis. The primary role of ERCP in the setting of acute pancreatitis is to remove stones from the bile duct in the setting of acute cholangitis. Otherwise, ERCP can be performed to removed bile duct stones after the episode of acute pancreatitis has resolved.

Differential Diagnosis

See Table 31.1.

Management

Prognosis

The most common prognostic criteria used to assess acute pancreatitis are the Ranson criteria, which are observations made at admission and at 48 hours after admission, and the simplified Glasgow criteria, which are variables measured at any time during the first 48 hours after admission (Table 31.2). The prognostic accuracy of the two scales is similar. Although the Ranson criteria were developed to assess alcoholic pancreatitis, they are frequently applied to pancreatitis from other causes. If two signs or fewer are present, mortality is less than 1%; three to five signs predict a mortality rate of 5%; and six or more signs increase the mortality rate to 20%. Other factors associated with a poor prognosis include obesity and extensive pancreatic necrosis. A CT-based scoring system, measurement of serum levels of the trypsinogen activation peptide, and the APACHE II score have also been used to assess the severity of acute pancreatic damage.

Complications

Patients with severe pancreatitis may develop peripancreatic fluid collections or pancreatic necrosis; either can become infected. The role of prophylactic antibiotics in patients with severe pancreatitis is controversial. Current American

Table 31.2 Prognostic criteria for acute pancreatitis

Ranson criteria	Simplified Glasgow criteria
At admission	**Within 48 h of admission**
Age > 55	Age > 55
Leukocyte count >16,000/μl	Leukocyte count >15,000/μl
Lactate dehydrogenase >350 IU/l	Lactate dehydrogenase >600 IU/l
Glucose >200 mg/dl	Glucose >180 mg/dl
Aspartate aminotransferase >250 IU/l	Albumin <3.2 g/dl
	Calcium <8 mg/dl
	Arterial PO_2 < 60 mmHg
	Serum urea nitrogen >45 mg/dl
48 h after admission	
Hematocrit (HCT) decrease >10%	
Serum urea nitrogen increase >5 mg/dl	
Calcium <8 mg/dl	
Arterial PO_2 < 60 mmHg	
Base deficit >4 meq/l	
Estimated fluid sequestration >6 l	

Source: adapted from Agarwal et al. (1990) and Marshall (1993).

Gastroenterological Association guidelines suggest against the administration of prophylactic antibiotics to prevent infection of peripancreatic fluid collections or necrosis. Infections of peripancreatic fluid collections or pancreatic necrosis are characterized by florid symptoms. More indolent courses are characteristic of pancreatic abscesses, which can arise several weeks after a bout of pancreatitis in well-defined pseudo-cysts or areas of resolving pancreatic necrosis. Infected necrotic tissue and pancreatic abscesses require immediate debridement, which can be performed either surgically or endoscopically. Infected fluid collections may be drained percutaneously or endoscopically. Sterile pancreatic necrosis should be managed with supportive medical care unless symptomatic or if significant clinical deterioration occurs.

Pseudo-cysts develop in 10% of patients with acute pancreatitis, most commonly in those with alcoholic pancreatitis. Pseudo-cysts can persist for several weeks, causing pain, compressing adjacent organs, and eroding into the mediastinum. Cysts more than 5–6 cm in diameter have a 30–50% risk of complications, including rupture, hemorrhage, and infection. Although most pseudo-cysts spontaneously resolve or decrease in size, persistent (>6 weeks) large cysts or rapidly expanding cysts should be drained using surgical, endoscopic, or percutaneous procedures. Percutaneous drainage may be complicated by formation of a pancreaticocutaneous fistula. Endoscopic drainage may be achieved by transpapillary stent placement or transgastric placement of a cystenterostomy. The use of EUS in endoscopic drainage can decrease the risk of hemorrhage and free perforation. Rarely, pseudo-cysts may erode into the splenic artery and present as hemosuccus pancreaticus, a life-threatening event.

Pancreatitis may be complicated by several pulmonary processes. Mild hypoxemia is present in most patients with pancreatitis. Chest radiography may demonstrate increased interstitial markings or pleural effusions, which usually are left-sided and small but occasionally are large enough to compromise respiration. The interstitial edema occurs in the setting of normal cardiac function; the etiology is unclear. Severe adult respiratory distress syndrome requires artificial respiratory support. Multisystem organ failure develops in about 50% of patients with pancreatic necrosis and is an independent predictor of mortality.

Other systemic complications of severe pancreatitis include stress gastritis, renal failure, coagulopathy, hypocalcemia, delirium, and disseminated fat necrosis (involving bones, joints, and skin). Extension of the inflammatory process into the peripancreatic bed may produce splenic vein thrombosis, which may be complicated by development of splenomegaly, gastric varices, and gastrointestinal hemorrhage.

Therapy

Therapy for most cases of acute pancreatitis is supportive, although severe cases may require massive volume repletion. Goal-directed therapy (based on hemodynamics, urine output, blood urea nitrogen [BUN], and HCT) should be used for fluid management. Early enteral feeding within 24 hours is recommended in patients with severe acute pancreatitis; compared to parenteral nutrition, it is less expensive and decreases infectious complications. For patients with persistent nausea, vomiting, and pain nasoenteric feeding is recommended. Total parenteral nutrition should be considered for patients with pronounced ileus who fail enteral nutrition trials. Nasogastric suction is useful primarily for intractable vomiting but it is not needed in most cases. There is no evidence to support the routine use of antibiotics or somatostatin. The decision to reinitiate feeding should not be based on serum enzyme levels but rather on the clinical status of the patient. Resolution of pain and emergence of hunger reliably indicate that the patient is ready to eat in patients with mild acute pancreatitis.

For patients with biliary pancreatitis, urgent ERCP with sphincterotomy and stone extraction is only recommended in patients with cholangitis. Patients with mild gallstone pancreatitis should be treated conservatively; ERCP is performed after recovery to assess for retained bile duct stones. The risk of recurrent gallstone pancreatitis is up to 33%; therefore, all patients should undergo expeditious and definitive surgical therapy. For patients who are poor operative risks, endoscopic sphincterotomy without cholecystectomy is an acceptable therapeutic option.

Key practice points: acute pancreatitis

- Elevations of amylase and/or lipase greater than three times the upper limit of normal are virtually diagnostic of pancreatitis but disease severity *does not* correlate with the degree of enzyme elevation.
- Bilirubin levels higher than 3 mg/dl suggest a biliary cause of pancreatitis.
- Ultrasound is the most sensitive noninvasive means for detecting gallstones, biliary tract dilation, and gallbladder sludge.
- The severity of acute pancreatitis needs to be determined based upon clinical, laboratory, and radiological risk factors as well as the application of a severity grading system (Ranson criteria, APACHE II score, CT severity score, etc.).
- Early enteral feeding within 24 hours should be initiated in patients with severe acute pancreatitis. If oral feeding is not tolerated, then nasoenteric feeding should be initiated. Total parenteral nutrition (TPN) should be reserved for patients who are not able to tolerat nasojejunal feeding due to severe ileus.
- Administration of prophylactic antibiotics is not recommended for patients with acute pancreatitis and peripancreatic fluid collections or necrosis.
- In patients with acute biliary pancreatitis, urgent ERCP is only recommended if there is evidence of cholangitis.
- Patients who present with acute biliary pancreatitis should have cholecystectomy during the initial admission.

Chronic Pancreatitis

Clinical presentation

Chronic pancreatitis implies irreversible morphological and functional damage to the pancreas. In many cases, there are intermittent flares of acute pancreatitis. The clinical distinction between acute recurrent pancreatitis with restoration of normal pancreatic function and structure between attacks, and chronic pancreatitis may be difficult. Ethanol use accounts for most cases of chronic pancreatitis in the United States whereas in Asia and Africa, malnutrition is the major cause (Table 31.3). The prevalence of chronic pancreatitis in autopsy series is 0.04–5.0%, although it may be as high as 45% among alcoholics. Most cases are probably subclinical; only 5–10% of heavy ethanol users develop clinical pancreatitis.

Abdominal pain and malabsorption are the most common clinical features of chronic pancreatitis. Pain, which is present in 85% of patients, is likely to be caused by noxious stimulation of peripancreatic afferent nerves or increased intraductal pressure. Morphological studies show that the pancreatic nerves are larger and more numerous in patients with chronic pancreatitis. Pain typically is felt in the upper quadrants and may radiate to the back. It often is less intense while sitting forward. Patients may report steady, unremitting pain or several days of pain with pain-free intervals. Food ingestion increases the intensity of pain, leading to a fear of eating (sitophobia), which is the main cause of weight loss in early chronic pancreatitis.

Table 31.3 Causes of chronic pancreatitis

Causes
Ethanol (70%)
Idiopathic (including tropical) (20%)
Other (10%)
Hereditary
Hyperparathyroidism
Hypertriglyceridemia
Obstruction
Trauma
Cystic fibrosis
Autoimmune pancreatitis
Pancreas divisum

Malabsorption in late chronic pancreatitis results from inadequate secretion of pancreatic enzymes. Maldigestion is the physiological defect that occurs when the exocrine function is less than 10% of normal. Steatorrhea is the initial manifestation of malabsorption; azotorrhea occurs in more advanced disease. Because the mucosal absorptive capacity is intact, voluminous diarrhea is unusual; most patients complain of bulky or greasy stools. A pattern of steatorrhea and weight loss in the absence of abdominal pain is common in idiopathic chronic pancreatitis.

Most patients eventually develop symptomatic hyperglycemia. Although insulin often is required to control symptoms, most patients are not prone to ketosis. Patients with ethanol-induced chronic pancreatitis may have symptoms of liver disease, including ascites, encephalopathy, variceal bleeding, and jaundice. Jaundice can also result from compression or stricturing of the intrapancreatic portion of the common bile duct.

Physical examination findings may be normal or there may be marked abdominal tenderness. Patients may have stigmata of chronic alcoholism including gonadal atrophy, gynecomastia, and palmar erythema. A midline mass suggests the presence of a pseudo-cyst or complicating neoplasm. Patients rarely have pancreatic ascites. Marked deficiencies of fat-soluble vitamins (A, D, E, and K) are seldom seen.

Diagnostic investigation

Laboratory studies

The findings of laboratory evaluation are often normal in chronic pancreatitis. Patients rarely exhibit hyperbilirubinemia and abnormal liver chemistry levels as a result of concurrent alcoholic liver disease or common bile duct stricture. Acute flares of pancreatitis may be accompanied by leukocytosis. Macrocytic anemia occurs in the rare patient with vitamin B_{12} deficiency. Coagulopathy may result from vitamin K malabsorption or alcoholic liver disease. Because azotorrhea occurs only in advanced disease, serum albumin levels usually are normal despite profound weight loss. Serum amylase and lipase levels may be slightly elevated but marked elevations, as observed in acute pancreatitis, are unusual. If exocrine function is severely impaired, serum lipase levels may be low, whereas serum amylase levels usually are normal in this setting because salivary amylase production is normal.

Assessment of pancreatic exocrine function

Numerous methods for assessing pancreatic enzyme output are available. The simplest tests are those that detect increased fat in the stool, which develops if exocrine secretion is less than 10% of normal. Steatorrhea may be detected by qualitative fecal fat tests (Sudan stain) or quantitative 72-hour fecal fat measurements. In severe cases, the amount of fat excreted in the feces may approach the amount of fat ingested, which is indicative of profound reductions in pancreatic enzyme output. Such high degrees of steatorrhea are rarely observed with mucosal disease of the small intestine.

Pancreatic exocrine function is more accurately assessed by pancreatic stimulation tests after injecting secretin or cholecystokinin (CCK), or after ingesting a high protein meal, with simultaneous collection of pancreatic secretions through a catheter positioned in the distal duodenum. The collected fluid is assayed for bicarbonate (for secretin stimulation) or lipase and trypsin (for CCK stimulation). Chronic pancreatitis is characterized by decreased secretory output in response to these stimulants. Pancreatic stimulation tests may yield false-positive results in diabetes mellitus and cirrhosis, and after Billroth II gastrojejunostomy. Incomplete duodenal recovery of pancreatic juice or gastric acid inactivation of enzymes may lead to underestimation of pancreatic function. The sensitivity of pancreatic function tests for detecting chronic pancreatitis is 70–95%, which includes most patients with only mild-to-moderate pancreatic insufficiency.

The findings from a Schilling test are abnormal in chronic pancreatitis because of impaired cleavage of R protein, which prevents the binding of vitamin B_{12} to intrinsic factor. Expanding this test to include vitamin B_{12} bound to intrinsic factor can differentiate the maldigestion of R protein from the malabsorption of the vitamin B_{12}–intrinsic factor complex. Ingestion of the triglyceride ^{14}C-olein with subsequent measurement of breath $^{14}CO_2$ excretion assesses triglyceride digestion and absorption.

Structural studies

Confirming the diagnosis of chronic pancreatitis usually requires imaging studies of the pancreas. Abdominal radiography demonstrates the diagnostic finding of pancreatic calcifications in 30–40% of patients with chronic pancreatitis. This obviates the need for more expensive imaging procedures. Ultrasound has a sensitivity of 70% and a specificity of 90% for detecting chronic pancreatitis. If abdominal radiography and ultrasound fail to confirm the diagnosis, a CT scan demonstrates the architectural changes of chronic pancreatitis with a sensitivity of 80% and specificity of 90%. Findings may include duct dilation, calcifications, and cystic lesions. CT scans can also be useful in differentiating chronic pancreatitis from pancreatic carcinoma, and can reveal splenomegaly and venous collaterals resulting from splenic vein thrombosis.

EUS is sensitive for diagnosing chronic pancreatitis. Findings on EUS that suggest the diagnosis of chronic pancreatitis include pancreatic duct stones, parenchymal calcifications, visible side branches irregular main pancreatic duct, echogenic main pancreatic duct wall, hyperechoic strands and foci, hypoechoic lobules, and cysts. EUS-guided fine needle aspiration can differentiate chronic pancreatitis from malignancy.

Advances in MR imaging and MR cholangiopancreatography allow detailed examination of the pancreatic and biliary ducts without exposure to radiation or the use of oral or intravenous contrast agents. These techniques also can be used to direct endoscopic therapy.

Management and course

Medical therapy

Medical therapy for chronic pancreatitis focuses on relief of pain and repletion of digestive enzymes. If the patient has symptoms of maldigestion, pancreatic enzyme supplements should be taken before all meals. Steatorrhea usually is more difficult to treat than azotorrhea. At least 25,000–30,000 units of lipase per meal are necessary to provide adequate lipolysis; therefore, patients will need to take 2–10 pills with each meal, depending on the preparation.

Analgesics remain the primary means of controlling the pain of chronic pancreatitis. An initial trial of acetaminophen or nonsteroidal anti-inflammatory drugs (NSAIDs) is preferable. Patients should be cautioned about excessive doses of acetaminophen. Severe cases require opiate analgesics and co-management with a chronic pain management specialist.

The somatostatin analog octreotide inhibits pancreatic secretion and has visceral analgesic effects; thus, it might be expected to decrease pain in chronic pancreatitis. Octreotide may also have a role in managing refractory pancreatic fistulae or pseudo-cysts.

Nonmedical therapy

A small percentage of patients are refractory to medical measures and require more invasive procedures to control pain. Although celiac plexus neurolysis has been effective for pain control in patients with pancreatic adenocarcinoma, results in patients with chronic pancreatitis have been disappointing. Most patients experience only transient relief. Endoscopic pancreatic stone extraction, occasionally performed in conjunction with extracorporeal shock wave lithotripsy, reduces pain in 50–80% of cases. Patients with tight strictures may obtain pain relief after endoscopic balloon dilation and stent placement.

For severe debilitating pain unresponsive to medical therapy, surgical therapy is a legitimate means of restoring the quality of life to a patient with chronic pancreatitis. Patients with dilation of the main pancreatic duct are optimal candidates for pancreaticojejunostomy (modified Puestow procedure), a procedure with initial success rates of 80%. Unfortunately, many patients develop recurrent pain several years postoperatively. Patients without significant ductal dilation may require partial or subtotal pancreatectomy according to the extent of parenchymal disease. One-half of patients experience pain relief. Ketosis-prone diabetes invariably complicates subtotal pancreatectomy. Pancreatic islet cell autotransplantation at the time of the operation may prevent postoperative diabetes.

Complications

Patients with chronic pancreatitis who report severe refractory pain or worsening of pain should be evaluated for the development of a pseudo-cyst. Ultrasound detects many pseudo-cysts but a CT scan is the definitive diagnostic procedure. Pseudo-cysts in chronic pancreatitis usually are found in the body of the gland. They may rupture, bleed, or become infected; the risk of these complications is much lower than the corresponding risk of complications from acute pseudo-cysts. Cysts larger than 6 cm rarely resolve and require internal drainage using endoscopic techniques. EUS can be used to direct endoscopic drainage of mature cysts that impinge on the gastric or duodenal walls. Percutaneous CT-guided catheter drainage has proved successful in some cases, although a persistent pancreaticocutaneous fistula may develop.

Key practice points: chronic pancreatitis

- Serum amylase and lipase levels may be slightly elevated but marked elevations, as observed in acute pancreatitis, are unusual.
- The classic triad for diagnosing chronic pancreatitis includes pancreatic calcifications, steatorrhea, and diabetes mellitus but this triad is usually seen only in advanced disease.

Case studies

Case 1

A 45-year-old man presents to the emergency department with a two-day history of severe periumbilical abdominal pain that was rapid in onset and has become progressively worse. The pain radiates to his back. He has developed severe nausea and vomiting. He denies any alcohol consumption. He does report having had intermittent episodes of right upper quadrant abdominal pain for the past year that would often occur after meals but would always resolve. On physical exam his heart rate is 120, blood pressure is 90/50, respiratory rate is 22, and temperature is 38.5 °C. The patient is alert and appears uncomfortable. Eyes show mild scleral icterus. Abdomen is tender to palpation in the periumbilical region and bowel sounds are absent. Labs are notable for a white blood count (WBC) 22,000, HCT 56%, BUN 25 mg/dl, glucose 220 mg/dl creatinine 1.3 mg/dl, aspartate aminotransferase (AST) 330, alanine aminotransferase (ALT) 370, total bilirubin 3.2, amylase 2120, and lipase 1950.

Abdominal ultrasound demonstrates a dilated common bile duct but visualization of the head of the pancreas is obscured by bowel gas. The patient is aggressively hydrated with 4 l of normal saline over a period of eight hours. A diagnosis of severe acute gallstone pancreatitis with cholangitis is made and the patient has urgent ERCP performed, at which time a 1 cm gallstone is found to be impacted at the ampulla of Vatter and is removed after performing a sphincterotomy.

Discussion: gallstone pancreatitis

- Gallstone pancreatitis should be suspected based on history of right upper quadrant abdominal pain, elevated liver function tests (especially bilirubin), and finding of dilated bile duct on ultrasound imaging.
- Urgent intervention with ERCP is indicated in patients with severe acute pancreatitis with evidence of cholangitis.

Case 2

A 55-year-old man presents with four or five loose, oily stools per day and notes a 30-pound weight loss over the past year. He has a long history of heavy alcohol consumption; however, his alcohol consumption has decreased due to worsening abdominal pain. He has chronic mid-epigastric abdominal pain that is worse after meals. He has had a 30-pound unintentional weight loss over the past year that he attributes to decreased oral intake because of abdominal pain. He was also diagnosed with diabetes one year ago. On physical examination he has a scaphoid abdomen and has tenderness to palpation in the mid-epigastric region. Labs are significant for a 24-hour fecal fat collection that weighs 350 g and has 35 g of fat. An abdominal radiograph demonstrates diffuse calcifications of the pancreas (Figure 31.1). The patient is prescribed pancreatic enzyme replacement therapy for his steatorrhea. He achieves some pain relief with pancreatic enzymes but continues to experience significant epigastric pain. He is prescribed amitriptyline 10 mg po before bed, which further controls his pain.

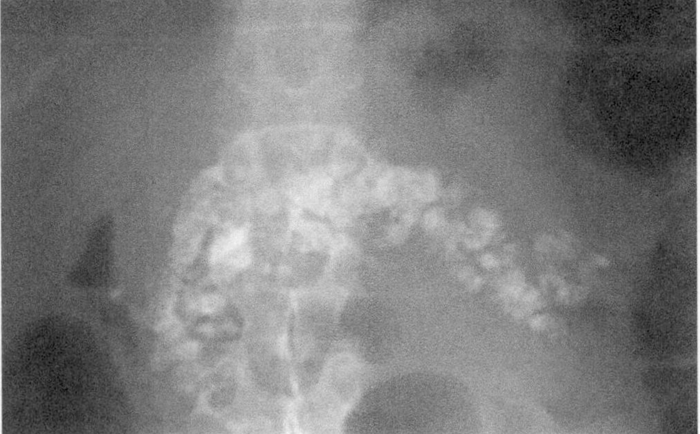

Figure 31.1 Abdominal radiograph demonstrating diffuse calcifications of the pancreas.

Discussion: chronic pancreatitis

- The classic triad to diagnose chronic pancreatitis includes steatorrhea, pancreatic calcifications, and diabetes. This triad of symptoms occurs in advanced chronic pancreatitis where <10% of the gland remains functional.
- Management of chronic pancreatitis is based on symptoms. Steatorrhea can be managed with a low-fat diet and pancreatic enzymes. Pain management can be challenging and should be performed in a stepwise fashion, beginning with pancreatic enzyme therapy, nonopioid analgesics, low-dose tricyclic antidepressants for neuropathic pain modulation, and then opioid analgesics. For patients with severe chronic abdominal pain requiring long-term narcotic use, a chronic pain specialist should be involved in the patient's management.

Further reading

Agarwal, N., Pitchumoni, C.S., and Sivaprasad, A.V. (1990). Evaluating tests for acute pancreatitis. *Am. J. Gastroenterol.* 85: 356.

Crockett, S.D., Wani, S., Gardner, T.B. et al. (2018). American Gastroenterological Association Institute guideline on initial management of acute pancreatitis. *Gastroenterology* 154: 1096–1101.

Marshall, J.B. (1993). Acute pancreatitis: a review with an emphasis on new developments. *Arch. Intern. Med.* 153: 1185.

CHAPTER 32
Pancreatic Neoplasia

Ductal adenocarcinoma

Pancreatic ductal adenocarcinoma is the fourth leading cause of cancer mortality in the United States and has a five-year survival rate of less than 7%. Gastroenterologists play a critical role in the diagnosis and management of patients with this disease.

Clinical presentation

Most patients experience abdominal pain that often radiates to the back. The indolent onset of the pain contrasts with the acute severe pain of acute pancreatitis and cholangitis. Careful questioning of the patient often reveals that pain developed up to three months before the onset of jaundice. The pain of pancreatic cancer results from ductal obstruction or malignant perineural invasion. It usually is poorly localized and constant. Persistent severe pain often reflects unresectability and is associated with perineural invasion. As with other forms of pancreatic pain, the severity may be increased by lying supine and decreased by leaning forward while sitting.

Seventy percent of pancreatic adenocarcinomas occur in the head of the pancreas, and virtually all of these lesions produce obstructive jaundice. Cancers in the body or tail of the gland only rarely cause jaundice because of the anatomical spacing between the tumors and the common bile duct that courses posterior to the head of the pancreas. Jaundice in patients with tumors in the pancreatic body or tail usually results from adenopathy in the porta hepatis or extensive liver metastasis. Pruritus and pale-colored stools are common with jaundice, owing to impaired bile excretion caused by an extrahepatic biliary obstruction.

The loss of more than 10% of body weight almost invariably occurs with pancreatic cancer. Weight loss usually results from anorexia and inadequate caloric intake. Sixty percent of patients with pancreatic adenocarcinoma have delayed gastric emptying, most often in the absence of mechanical

Yamada's Handbook of Gastroenterology, Fourth Edition. John M. Inadomi, Renuka Bhattacharya, Joo Ha Hwang, and Cynthia Ko.

gastroduodenal obstruction. Gastroparesis may be secondary to infiltration of the local splanchnic neural network and disruption of the neurohumoral mechanisms responsible for coordinated gastroduodenal motility. Reduced secretion of pancreatic enzymes with consequent maldigestion can also contribute to weight loss. Maldigestion is particularly prominent with tumors of the pancreatic head because obstruction of the pancreatic duct in this location results in nearly total loss of pancreatic enzyme secretion.

Diabetes mellitus is present in more than 60% of patients with pancreatic adenocarcinoma. Most patients first experience glucose intolerance within two years of the diagnosis of pancreatic cancer, which suggests that the malignancy causes diabetes. Enhanced secretion of islet amyloid peptide from the islets of Langerhans adjacent to the tumor is the purported cause. Elevated serum levels of this peptide produce marked insulin resistance and relative glucose intolerance.

Acute pancreatitis is the initial manifestation in 5–10% of pancreatic tumors. Adenocarcinoma of the pancreas should be considered in any older adult with acute pancreatitis unrelated to gallstones or ethanol. Duodenal obstruction caused by local invasion of the pancreatic mass occurs in 10% of patients. Obstruction is rarely a presenting feature, and it is almost always a preterminal event. Other uncommon complications include gastric variceal hemorrhage resulting from splenic vein thrombosis, major depression, and migratory superficial thrombophlebitis (Trousseau syndrome).

The physical examination of patients with pancreatic adenocarcinoma often reveals jaundice and evidence of significant weight loss. The chest and extremities may have extensive excoriations and lichenification from constant scratching because of the effects of jaundice. Tumors in the body and tail may be detected as palpable masses because they grow to enormous size before causing symptoms. With long-standing biliary obstruction, the gallbladder may become markedly distended and palpable, defining the classic Courvoisier sign.

Diagnostic investigation

Laboratory studies

At the time of clinical presentation, patients often have several laboratory abnormalities but none is specific for the diagnosis of pancreatic adenocarcinoma. Serum amylase and lipase levels may be mildly elevated but this finding is not universal, and normal levels should not preclude further testing. There may be mild elevations of liver chemistry levels and disproportionate increases in alkaline phosphatase levels. Hematological abnormalities include anemia caused by nutritional deficiencies or blood loss and thrombocytopenia caused by splenomegaly associated with splenic vein thrombosis. The tumor markers carcinoembryonic antigen (CEA) and CA19-9 are elevated in 75–85% of patients with pancreatic adenocarcinoma. Assays of these serum markers lack the specificity necessary for a reliable diagnosis and the search for better diagnostic markers is ongoing.

Imaging studies

Ultrasound has a sensitivity of 70% for identifying pancreatic cancer but overlying intralumenal gas and excess adipose tissue often compromise image quality. Even if examination of the pancreas is incomplete, ultrasound may demonstrate ancillary findings of pancreatic cancer, including dilation of the biliary tract and enlargement of the gallbladder. Computed tomography (CT) is superior to ultrasound and provides a sensitivity of 80% for detecting pancreatic masses. CT can define the tumor stage using dynamic contrast-enhanced imaging and can identify unresectable lesions with a positive predictive value of 98%. False-positive results may occur in the presence of focal pancreatitis or if normal anatomical variants are mistaken for tumors.

Endoscopic retrograde cholangiopancreatography (ERCP) has a sensitivity and specificity of 90% in diagnosing pancreatic malignancy. Abrupt obstruction of both a dilated common bile duct and a dilated pancreatic duct is termed the *double-duct sign*. This finding is virtually diagnostic of pancreatic cancer and is usually indicative of an advanced tumor in the pancreatic head. Less advanced lesions and cancers in the body or tail more often produce discrete pancreatic duct strictures. Cytological samples of a pancreatic stricture can be obtained at the time of ERCP but the yield is limited and the sensitivity is only 30–40%.

Endoscopic ultrasound (EUS) has a sensitivity of 90% for detecting pancreatic tumors. It is more sensitive than CT or ultrasound for detecting tumors smaller than 2 cm. EUS-guided fine needle aspiration (FNA) or fine needle biopsy (FNB) is the preferred method for obtaining tissue for diagnostic purposes (cytology, pathology, molecular analysis). If the needle track is confined to the area of surgical resection (duodenum), there is no concern for tumor seeding outside the field of resection.

Management and course

Staging

Curative surgical resection provides the only chance for long-term survival to patients with pancreatic adenocarcinoma. Unfortunately, more than 85% of patients have unresectable disease at presentation. Preoperative staging of pancreatic cancer is essential to establish the prognosis and to plan the optimal treatment strategy. As with many other cancers of the gastrointestinal tract, pancreatic tumors are staged on the basis of the TNM classification system (Table 32.1). The staging system continues to evolve and now allows for attempted curative resection in patients with superior mesenteric and even portal vein invasion (T3). Only those primary tumors involving the celiac axis and superior mesenteric artery (T4) are deemed unresectable. Most tumors involving the major splanchnic vessels cannot be resected for cure. Because splenectomy and hence splenic vein resection are often performed at the time of pancreatic cancer resection, invasion of the splenic vein does not preclude complete excision of the tumor. Although metastasis to regional lymph

Table 32.1 TNM classification of pancreatic cancer

Primary tumor (T)	
T1	Tumor ≤2 cm
T2	Tumor >2 cm and ≤4 cm in greatest dimension
T3	Tumor >4 cm in greatest dimension
T4	Tumor involves the celiac axis, superior mesenteric artery, and/or common hepatic artery, regardless of size
Regional lymph nodes (N)	
N0	No regional lymph node metastasis
N1	Regional lymph node metastasis
Distant metastasis (M)	
M0	No distant metastasis
M1	Distant metastasis

Source: reproduced with permission from Amin et al. (2017).

nodes (N1) does not preclude complete surgical excision, patients with these tumors have an unfavorable prognosis relative to patients without lymph node metastasis.

Several complementary procedures are used to define the stage of pancreatic cancer. Contrast-enhanced CT scanning is the best noninvasive means for detecting liver metastasis. Invasion of the large splanchnic vessels can be detected with a sensitivity of 30–50%. Angiography detects vascular invasion with a sensitivity of 75%. EUS has emerged as the most accurate means of detecting vascular invasion, with a sensitivity and specificity approaching 90%. As with angiography, EUS is not a reliable method for detecting distant metastatic disease so the optimal staging strategy combines CT and EUS studies. Magnetic resonance imaging has been refined to improve the definition of the vascular anatomy of the peripancreatic bed. Ongoing studies will define the staging role of this imaging method.

Surgical therapy

Surgical exploration to perform curative resection should be attempted in all patients who have apparently resectable disease. An initial staging laparoscopy should be part of the planned resection to inspect the peritoneum and liver for evidence of distant metastases not detected on CT scans. Even when all staging procedures, including laparoscopy, indicate a resectable tumor, unresectable disease is found in 10–20% of patients after surgical dissection. Cancers localized to the pancreatic head require a pancreaticoduodenectomy – the Whipple procedure. Lesions in the body or tail can be treated with distal pancreatectomy. Alternative procedures, including total pancreatectomy and the pylorus-sparing Whipple procedure, have no proven advantage relative to standard operations. In the past, operative mortality rates for curative resection averaged 10–20% but specialized centers are reporting mortality rates of 2–5%.

The poor overall prognosis for pancreatic cancer is underscored by five-year survival rates of 10–25% for patients who undergo surgical resection. Neoadjuvant therapy with chemotherapy and/or radiation is often administered prior to surgical resection. The long-term survival of patients with T1 cancers is only 35–40%; most deaths result from recurrent disease. Unfortunately, survival for five years does not guarantee a cure from this disease; 40% of these persons eventually die of recurrent pancreatic adenocarcinoma. Lymph node metastasis, poorly differentiated histology, and tumors larger than 2.5 cm are all associated with a poor prognosis.

Palliative therapy

Because most patients with pancreatic cancer have unresectable disease at presentation and have an expected survival of six months, palliation of symptoms is the primary goal. Correction of nutritional deficiencies and control of pain can be achieved with supportive measures. Malabsorptive symptoms can be alleviated with adequate pancreatic enzyme supplementation. Adequate protein and caloric intake may require enteral nutrition, given the high rate of malnutrition in these patients. Nonsteroidal anti-inflammatory drugs (NSAIDs) and acetaminophen may be adequate for pain control, but if pain is severe, narcotics should be administered. Narcotics may have constipating effects, necessitating the concomitant use of osmotic or stimulant laxatives. For relief of tumor-associated refractory pain, surgical or radiologically guided percutaneous injection of alcohol into the celiac ganglion is 90% effective.

Obstructive jaundice and pruritus may be treated by surgical biliary bypass or by endoscopic or percutaneous placement of a biliary stent. Endoscopic stent placement and surgical bypass are more than 90% successful in relieving biliary obstruction but surgical therapy is associated with longer hospitalizations, higher morbidities, and higher periprocedural mortality rates. Percutaneous stent placement for distal common bile duct malignant strictures has higher morbidity and mortality relative to endoscopic stent placement because of the hemorrhage and bile leaks associated with transhepatic puncture. Therefore, endoscopic placement is preferred. Unfortunately, 40% of biliary stents become obstructed with debris and sludge five to six months after placement. As a prophylactic measure, plastic stents often are replaced every three to six months to prevent cholangitis secondary to stent occlusion. Expandable metallic biliary stents have shown lower occlusion rates, and should be considered in patients who are not candidates for surgical resection.

In contrast to biliary obstruction, symptomatic duodenal obstruction is best managed surgically. This complication occurs in 10% of patients with pancreatic cancer. Gastrojejunostomy is the procedure of choice. Unfortunately, duodenal obstruction is often preterminal, and surgical intervention may be contraindicated because of the overall poor clinical status of the patient.

The role of chemotherapy and radiation therapy for patients with pancreatic cancer is limited. Combined radiation and chemotherapy may prolong survival by two to four months but there is often significant therapeutically induced toxicity. The chemotherapeutic agent gemcitabine slightly improves survival, reduces pain, and improves the quality of life.

Key practice points: Pancreatic cancer

- Pancreatic cancer often presents as advanced disease due to lack of symptoms in early disease. Symptoms include abdominal pain radiating to the back, unintentional weight loss, and jaundice.
- CT scan should be performed for staging to evaluate for metastatic disease.
- EUS-guided FNA is the optimal modality for obtaining tissue diagnosis if indicated.
- Placement of a metal biliary stent should be considered for patients with unresectable tumors causing biliary obstruction.

Other malignant and premalignant diseases of the pancreas

Cystic neoplasms

Cystic neoplasms of the pancreas may be benign or malignant. These lesions must be differentiated from the pseudo-cysts that often complicate the course of acute and chronic pancreatitis. Differentiation of cysts can be difficult based on appearance on imaging and management of pancreatic cystic lesions is highly controversial due to extremely high incidence of pancreatic cystic lesions incidentally identified on cross-sectional imaging and the relatively low rate of progression to malignancy for a majority of pancreatic cysts. However, the risk of progression to malignancy is significant for certain types of cystic neoplasms. Cystic neoplasms (excluding pseudo-cysts) can be categorized as follows: serous cystadenomas, mucinous cystadenomas, intraductal papillary mucinous neoplasms (IPMNs), and cystic neuroendocrine tumors.

Serous cystadenomas

Serous cystadenomas have extremely low malignant potential and often have a characteristic appearance of a central calcification on CT imaging and multiple microcystic cavities on EUS imaging.

Mucinous cystic neoplasms

Mucinous cystic neoplasims have a 10–20% rate of progression on to adenocarcinoma and are characterized by the presence of ovarian stroma, occurring almost exclusively in women. Due to their high risk of malignant transformation, surgical resection is recommended, especially for cysts greater than 3 cm.

Despite these characteristic anatomical features, distinguishing the two neoplasms on the basis of imaging alone is difficult. CEA levels and K-RAS mutations are useful in establishing the diagnosis of mucinous cystic neoplasms but they are unable to identify presence of malignancy or risk for malignant progression. Asymptomatic serous lesions require no further therapy but all mucinous lesions should be referred for consideration of surgical resection or monitored closely. In comparison with the poor survival rate of ductal adenocarcinoma, patients with adenocarcinoma associated with a mucinous cystic neoplasm have a five-year survival rate higher than 50% after surgical resection.

Intraductal papillary mucinous neoplasms

IPMNs are premalignant ecstatic/cystic lesions involving the pancreatic duct. They are typically classified as either main duct or side branch type. Main duct IPMN often is associated with significant dilation of the main pancreatic duct upstream of the lesion. The risk of malignancy in main duct IPMN is approximately 40% whereas the risk of malignancy in side branch IPMN is approximately 15–20%. Patients present with abdominal pain, weight loss, and steatorrhea. By endoscopic examination, the ampulla of Vater may be seen to release copious amounts of viscous mucus into the duodenum and have a characteristic "fish mouth" appearance. Papillary projections of dysplastic mucosa and intraductal collections of mucinous debris often produce diffuse filling defects on ERCP. At presentation, patients may have coexisting adenocarcinoma. Surgical excision is curative if the lesion is detected before carcinoma develops.

Solid pseudo-papillary neoplasms

Solid pseudo-papillary neoplasms arise from the epithelium of ductules, usually in the tail of the pancreas. Most patients are adolescent girls or women in their early 20s. Tumors are often larger than adenocarcinomas and frequently exhibit a cystic appearance on CT or ultrasound studies as a result of liquefaction necrosis. Despite their large size, many tumors remain localized. Resection is associated with long-term survival.

Key practice points: Pancreatic cysts

- Cysts and IPMNs are often asymptomatic at presentation and are often identified incidentally.
- Mucinous cyst adenomas and IPMNs have risk of malignancy.
- Main duct IPMN has a 40% risk of malignancy and should be surgically resected.

Case studies

Case 1

A 65-year-old woman presents to her physician with new-onset jaundice. She denies any abdominal pain. She does report a 10lb. unintentional weight loss over the past three months. She denies any nausea, vomiting, or fevers. Physical examination is unremarkable. Labs are notable for a total bilirubin 6.0mg/dl, aspartate aminotransferase (AST) 230U/l, alanine aminotransferase (ALT) 180U/l, white blood count (WBC) 5.0, and hematocrit (HCT) 35%. A CT scan demonstrates a 3cm ill-defined mass in the head of the pancreas, dilated common bile duct and intrahepatic ducts, and a dilated main pancreatic duct. There is no evidence of metastatic disease but the mass appears to be adjacent to the portal vein. EUS FNA is then performed that demonstrates the portal vein to be free from the tumor. FNA of the mass is performed, confirming the diagnosis of pancreatic adenocarcinoma. The patient has an ERCP to place a plastic biliary stent to relieve the biliary obstruction. The patient is later taken to surgery for a Whipple resection.

Discussion: Pancreatic cancer

Pancreatic head masses often present with painless jaundice. CT scan should be performed to evaluate for a pancreatic head mass. EUS FNA is the best method to obtain tissue to confirm the diagnosis of pancreatic cancer. Tissue diagnosis is recommended because benign inflammatory masses from autoimmune pancreatitis may also present as a pancreatic head mass causing biliary obstruction and do not require resection. Finally, resection of a pancreatic head mass requires a Whipple resection (pancreaticoduodenectomy).

Case 2

A 50-year-old woman is involved in a car accident and has a CT scan performed in the emergency department due to complaints of abdominal pain. There is no evidence of abdominal trauma on CT scan, but a 3cm pancreatic cyst is incidentally identified. The patient is then referred for further evaluation with EUS FNA, which demonstrates a 3cm cystic lesion without any septae or associated masses. The pancreatic duct and parenchyma are normal in appearance. FNA is performed on the cyst, revealing a clear, nonviscous fluid. Fluid analysis demonstrates a CEA 252ng/dl, amylase 40U/l, and cytology does not show any atypical cells. The patient is informed that the cyst is likely to be a mucinous cystic neoplasm. Given the size of the lesion, patient is referred for surgical management.

Discussion: Pancreatic cyst

Pancreatic cysts are often incidentally identified on cross-sectional imaging. Certain pancreatic cysts have malignant potential. Evaluation with EUS FNA can be used to obtain high-resolution imaging of the cyst and adjacent tissue to evaluate for a possible mass and to aspirate the fluid from the cyst for biochemical analysis (CEA, amylase, and possibly K-RAS mutation analysis). IPMNs and mucinous cystic neoplasms have malignant potential. Serous cystadenomas are benign.

Further reading

Amin, M.B., Edge, S.B., Greene, F.L. et al. (2017). *AJCC Cancer Staging Manual,* 8e. New York: Springer.

Elta, G.H., Enestvedt, B.K., Sauer, B.G., and Lennon, A.M. (2018 Apr). ACG clinical guideline: diagnosis and management of pancreatic cysts. *Am. J. Gastroenterol.* 113 (4): 464–479. https://doi.org/10.1038/ajg.2018.14. Epub 2018 Feb 27. PubMed PMID: 29485131.

Vege, S.S., Ziring, B., Jain, R. et al. (2015 Apr). American gastroenterological association institute guideline on the diagnosis and management of asymptomatic neoplastic pancreatic cysts. *Gastroenterology* 148 (4): 819–822; quize12-3. doi:10.1053/j.gastro.2015.01.015. PubMed PMID: 25805375.

CHAPTER 33
Biliary Tract Stones and Cysts

Gallstones

Gallstone-related conditions are among the most common gastrointestinal disorders requiring hospitalization. Cholesterol stones account for 75% of gallstones in western countries, whereas pigment or bilirubinate stones predominate in Africa and Asia. Gallstones are more prevalent in females across all age and ethnic groups.

Clinical presentation

Gallbladder stones produce a wide spectrum of clinical presentations, including episodic biliary pain, acute cholecystitis, and chronic cholecystitis. Passage of a gallstone through the common bile duct may lead to acute cholangitis or acute pancreatitis. Despite the high incidence of these complications in the general population, more than two-thirds of patients with gallstones will never develop symptoms.

Biliary colic

Most patients with symptomatic cholelithiasis present with biliary pain. This visceral pain is caused by transient gallstone obstruction of the cystic duct. The pain typically is severe and episodic and lasts 30 minutes to several hours. The common use of the term biliary "colic" is a misnomer because the pain is steady and does not fluctuate in intensity. It is usually epigastric and is often referred to the right shoulder or interscapular region. During attacks, patients are restless and may have associated diaphoresis and vomiting. The interval between attacks is highly variable and may be days to years. There is no convincing evidence that ingesting fatty foods precipitates an attack of biliary colic.

Yamada's Handbook of Gastroenterology, Fourth Edition. John M. Inadomi, Renuka Bhattacharya, Joo Ha Hwang, and Cynthia Ko.

Acute cholecystitis

When a biliary colic attack lasts longer than three hours, or if localized right upper quadrant tenderness and fever develop, the diagnosis of acute cholecystitis should be considered. The pain of acute cholecystitis may wane but the tenderness usually increases. A Murphy sign, the abrupt cessation in inspiration in response to pain on palpation of the right upper quadrant, is a classic finding observed in 60–70% of patients. High fever, hemodynamic instability, and peritoneal signs suggest gallbladder perforation, which is a complication in 10% of patients with acute cholecystitis. Ten to 15% of patients develop jaundice, which is a symptom that may be caused by gallstone obstruction of the common bile duct or by Mirizzi syndrome, which is an obstruction of the common hepatic duct caused by edema and inflammation at the origin of the cystic duct. Most patients with acute cholecystitis have had previous attacks of biliary pain.

Chronic cholecystitis

Patients with chronic cholecystitis usually have gallstones and have had repeated attacks of biliary pain or acute cholecystitis, which results in a thickened and fibrotic gallbladder. It is uncommon for the gallbladder to be palpable during an attack of pain. In fact, patients may have few symptoms referable to the gallbladder itself, presenting instead with complications such as cholangitis and gallstone pancreatitis.

Acalculous cholecystitis

There is no evidence of cholelithiasis in 5–10% of patients with acute cholecystitis. Acalculous cholecystitis is caused by ischemia and occurs in critically ill patients, often with multiorgan failure, extensive burn injuries, major surgery, and trauma. Perforation is more common and the course is more fulminant.

Diagnostic investigation

Laboratory studies

Most patients with acute cholecystitis exhibit leukocytosis. Some may have elevations in aminotransferases, alkaline phosphatase, bilirubin, or amylase caused by choledocholithiasis or cystic duct edema with resulting biliary obstruction. Patients with uncomplicated biliary colic usually have normal biochemical profiles.

Structural studies

Ultrasound is highly sensitive and specific for diagnosing cholelithiasis. In uncomplicated biliary pain, gallstones may be the only finding. Thickening of the gallbladder wall is a nonspecific finding commonly observed in acute and chronic cholecystitis. Pericholecystic fluid and intramural gas are specific ultrasonographic features of acute cholecystitis. Dilation of the intrahepatic or extrahepatic ducts suggests choledocholithiasis; however, ultrasound is insensitive for imaging common bile duct stones. 99mTc-labeled iminodiacetic scintigraphy can confirm a diagnosis of acute cholecystitis. The tracer is injected intravenously and excreted in bile. Failure to image the gallbladder within 90 minutes suggests cystic duct obstruction. The gallbladder cannot be visualized in 85% of patients with acalculous cholecystitis. Computed tomography (CT) may be beneficial in evaluating patients with complicated disease (e.g. perforation or gangrene).

Management and course

Most patients with gallstones remain asymptomatic, but over a 20-year period, 15–25% of these asymptomatic patients develop symptoms. Once symptoms occur, there is a high risk of recurrent attacks of pain and complications such as cholecystitis, pancreatitis, and cholangitis.

Although there are many nonsurgical alternatives, cholecystectomy is the definitive treatment for symptomatic cholelithiasis. Laparoscopic cholecystectomy is favored because there are fewer wound-related complications, shorter hospital stays, and more rapid recoveries. However, the technique results in a 2–3% incidence of bile duct injuries, a higher incidence than with open cholecystectomy. Open cholecystectomy is preferred if acute cholecystitis is evident, if there is extensive scarring from prior abdominal surgery, if exploration of the common bile duct is planned, or if visualization by laparoscopy is inadequate.

Given the overall benefits of surgical therapy, dissolution therapy with chenodeoxycholic acid or ursodeoxycholic acid should be reserved for patients who are at high risk of surgery. Because of its superior side-effect profile, ursodeoxycholic acid is preferred. Small (<1.5 cm diameter) noncalcified stones that float on oral cholecystography are suitable for dissolution. Candidate patients should demonstrate adequate gallbladder filling and emptying by oral cholecystography. Dissolution often requires longer than six months of therapy. Response rates range from 60 to 70%. There are frequent recurrences after therapy is discontinued. Direct-contact dissolution therapy with mono-octanoin and methyl-*tert*-butyl ether is often successful in days to weeks but it has a high rate of complications and thus remains experimental.

Extracorporeal shock wave lithotripsy is 90% successful in achieving stone fragmentation and clearance of solitary, small, radiolucent stones. Most patients also require dissolution therapy. As with dissolution therapy, it may take months of extracorporeal shock wave lithotripsy to clear the gallbladder of stones. About 20% of patients experience biliary pain for several weeks after fragmentation.

Choledocholithiasis

In the United States, most bile duct stones are cholesterol stones that have migrated from the gallbladder. Ten to 15% of patients who undergo cholecystectomy have concomitant bile duct stones, and 1–4% exhibit residual postoperative choledocholithiasis, even after the common bile duct is explored. Conversely, more than

80–90% of patients with choledocholithiasis have gallbladder stones. The incidence of choledocholithiasis increases with age; one-third of octogenarians who undergo cholecystectomy have coexistent bile duct stones. The prevalence of choledocholithiasis and intrahepatic stones is higher in Asian societies. These populations have higher incidences of pigment stones, which usually are formed de novo in the bile ducts.

Clinical presentation

Unlike gallbladder stones, most patients with bile duct stones develop symptoms. Some remain asymptomatic for decades while others present suddenly with potentially life-threatening cholangitis or pancreatitis. Patients with choledocholithiasis often present with biliary pain indistinguishable from the pain of cystic duct obstruction. The pain is steady, lasts for 30 minutes to several hours, and is located in the epigastrium and right upper quadrant.

Cholangitis is the result of superimposed infection in the setting of a biliary obstruction. The Charcot classic triad of right upper quadrant pain, fever, and jaundice may be present in only 50–75% of patients with acute cholangitis. Ten percent of episodes are marked by a fulminant course with hemodynamic instability and encephalopathy. Reynolds pentad refers to the constellation of the Charcot triad plus hypotension and confusion.

Diagnostic investigation

Laboratory studies

Immediately after an attack, levels of serum aminotransferases are often elevated because of hepatocellular injury. Alkaline phosphatase levels are often elevated, mildly in asymptomatic patients, and not more than five times higher than normal in symptomatic patients. Most symptomatic patients have hyperbilirubinemia; the bilirubin level is in the range of 2–14 mg/dl. Higher elevations of alkaline phosphatase or bilirubin levels suggest malignant obstruction of the biliary tree.

Structural studies

In contrast to gallbladder stones, bile duct stones are not readily detected by ultrasound due to gas-filled surrounding structures; the sensitivity is less than 20%. The technological advances of CT and magnetic resonance imaging (MRI) scanning have led to improved accuracy in sensitivity and specificity of 80–85% in detecting bile duct stones. Magnetic resonance cholangiopancreatography (MRCP) is a noninvasive means to confirm suspected choledocholithiasis. MRCP has a sensitivity of 90% for diagnosing choledocholithiasis; however, endoscopic retrograde cholangiography (ERCP) is necessary for therapeutic sphincterotomy and stone extraction. Endoscopic ultrasound (EUS) can detect 95% or more of common bile duct stones but likewise cannot extract stones.

There is no consensus on the optimal evaluation of choledocholithiasis in patients undergoing elective cholecystectomy for gallstone disease. If open cholecystectomy is planned, intraoperative cholangiography and common bile duct palpation can be used. If stones are found, the common bile duct should be explored and stones should be extracted. Several alternative strategies are available to patients undergoing planned laparoscopic cholecystectomy. One strategy involves minimal preoperative assessment, including ultrasound and CT scanning. An intraoperative cholangiogram is performed during the laparoscopic procedure. Those patients with documented intraductal stones undergo stone extraction laparoscopically or by open cholecystectomy. Alternatively, ERCP with endoscopic sphincterotomy may be performed postoperatively. A second strategy identifies patients preoperatively at high or low risk of coexisting cho- ledocholithiasis on the basis of the biochemical profile and the presence or absence of biliary tract dilation on ultrasound. Patients at high risk undergo preoperative endoscopic ultrasonography or ERCP; those with confirmed biliary stones undergo endoscopic stone extraction. When the stones are cleared from the bile duct, the patient then proceeds to laparoscopic cholecystectomy. Patients with a low risk of choledocholithiasis undergo laparoscopic cholecystectomy with intraoperative cholangiography, as previously described. Benefits and risks are associated with each strategy; the approach is largely determined by the resources available at individual institutions.

Management and course

Common bile duct stones, even if asymptomatic, generally require therapy because of the high complication rate (e.g. cholangitis and pancreatitis). Secondary biliary cirrhosis may develop in cases of persistent biliary obstruction (i.e. >five years). In such cases, reversal of portal hypertension and cirrhosis has been reported, suggesting that even late efforts to relieve obstruction are warranted. Definitive therapy involves common bile duct exploration and stone extraction but this procedure increases the operative mortality rate of a cholecystectomy from 0.5 to 3–4%. The perioperative mortality rate for patients younger than age 60 is 1.5%, whereas the risk for patients older than 65 is 5–10%.

Based on this high mortality rate, endoscopic sphincterotomy and stone extraction represent a favorable approach, especially in older patients. The risk of recurrent symptoms is high if patients have intact gallbladders; therefore, cholecystectomy should be performed. In elderly patients with severe comorbid illness, however, the surgical risks may outweigh the risk of recurrent gallstone symptoms. Endoscopic sphincterotomy alone may be an acceptable therapy for these patients. If bile duct stones cannot be extracted endoscopically, long-term internal stenting is also a therapeutic option for this high-risk group.

Young, healthy patients who have minimal operative risk factors may be treated with primary cholecystectomy and common bile duct exploration with stone extraction. Local expertise and resources may determine the choice of endoscopic versus surgical removal of bile duct stones in this group. It is worth noting that even after surgical common bile duct exploration, 1–4% of patients have retained common bile duct stones.

Patients presenting with cholangitis or pancreatitis are treated initially with conservative measures, including parenteral fluid repletion, bowel rest, and parenteral antibiotics (for cholangitis). In patients with severe pancreatitis that progresses or fails to improve within 48 hours and in patients with cholangitis, emergency ERCP with stone extraction reduces morbidity and mortality.

Miscellaneous complications of biliary tract stones

Bile duct strictures

Trauma and the chronic inflammatory response induced by biliary stones can result in benign strictures of the extrahepatic bile ducts. Other common causes of benign strictures include surgical trauma, chronic pancreatitis, parasitic infection, and sclerosing cholangitis. Patients may present with cholangitis, painless jaundice, or asymptomatic elevations of alkaline phosphatase levels. Diagnosis requires direct bile duct visualization by MRCP, ERCP, or EUS. Given the inadequate long-term efficacy of biliary stenting, surgical decompression is the treatment of choice for benign strictures. Failure to relieve the obstruction predisposes the patient to cholangitis, stone formation, and secondary biliary cirrhosis.

Biliary fistula

The most common cause of biliary fistula formation is surgical trauma during cholecystectomy. Hepatobiliary scintigraphy can detect bile leaks and fistulae with more than 90% sensitivity. Most leaks respond to endoscopic therapy using biliary sphincterotomy and/or stenting. Most spontaneous biliary-enteric fistulae are produced by gallstones; alternative causes include malignancy, peptic ulcer disease, and penetrating trauma. Patients with gallstone-induced fistulae can be asymptomatic, or they may present with nonspecific symptoms of anorexia, weight loss, and malabsorption. Gallstone ileus results when a large gallstone (>3 cm) passes into the gut through a cholecystenteric fistula and causes lumenal obstruction in the distal ileum. Biliary fistulae can often be detected on abdominal radiographs or upper gastrointestinal barium radiographs as air or barium in the biliary tree. Treatment requires surgical excision of the fistula, cholecystectomy, and extraction of all bile duct stones.

Hematobilia

Hematobilia, also referred to as hemobilia, refers to hemorrhage from the biliary tract. Common causes include penetrating trauma or iatrogenic trauma from a liver biopsy. In the United States, hepatobiliary tumors and aneurysms are possible causes, whereas parasitic diseases are possible causes in Asian societies. This is a rare complication of gallstones. Diagnosis requires upper gastrointestinal endoscopy to exclude other sources of upper gastrointestinal hemorrhage. Angiography can confirm the site of bleeding. Angiographic embolization is the preferred initial treatment of hepatic causes of hematobilia. Surgical intervention is recommended to treat hemorrhage from the extrahepatic biliary tree.

Recurrent pyogenic cholangitis

In selected regions of South East Asia, the most common presentation of gallstone disease is a syndrome characterized by intrahepatic bile duct stones, ductal dilation and stricturing, and recurrent cholangitis, known as *recurrent pyogenic cholangitis* (RPC) or *oriental cholangiohepatitis*. It occurs primarily in patients older than 50 and is associated with malnutrition and low socioeconomic status. There are inconsistent associations with infections caused by *Clonorchis sinensis* and *Ascaris lumbricoides* but the pathogenetic role of these parasites remains unclear.

The stones in this disease are pigmented calcium bilirubinate stones that preferentially involve the left intrahepatic ducts. Patients typically present with relapsing cholangitis and hepatic abscesses. Ultrasound is of limited value because echogenic material often fills the intrahepatic ducts. The diagnosis relies on cholangiography. The primary treatment is surgical and often requires hepatic resection and extensive biliary reconstruction to relieve any obstruction and clear the ductal system of stones. Most patients require reoperation, although long-term prophylactic antibiotics may reduce the frequency of infectious complications.

Biliary cysts

Biliary cysts can occur throughout the biliary tract, involving the intrahepatic and extrahepatic bile ducts. Biliary cysts can lead to biliary complications, with some cysts having an increased risk of malignancy.

Clinical presentation

Patients with type I choledochal cysts typically present in infancy with jaundice and failure to thrive, although 20% of patients present after age two with intermittent abdominal pain and recurrent jaundice. Patients rarely remain asymptomatic. Cirrhosis and portal hypertension are frequent complications, particularly if the cysts present in infancy. Patients with type II cysts classically present with obstruction of the common bile duct. Seventy-five percent of patients with choledochoceles (type III cysts) present after age 20 with pain and obstructive jaundice. Pancreatitis is a complication in 30–70% of cases of choledochocele. Patients with type IV and type V cysts typically have recurrent cholangitis, liver abscesses, and portal hypertension. Type V, or Caroli disease, may be

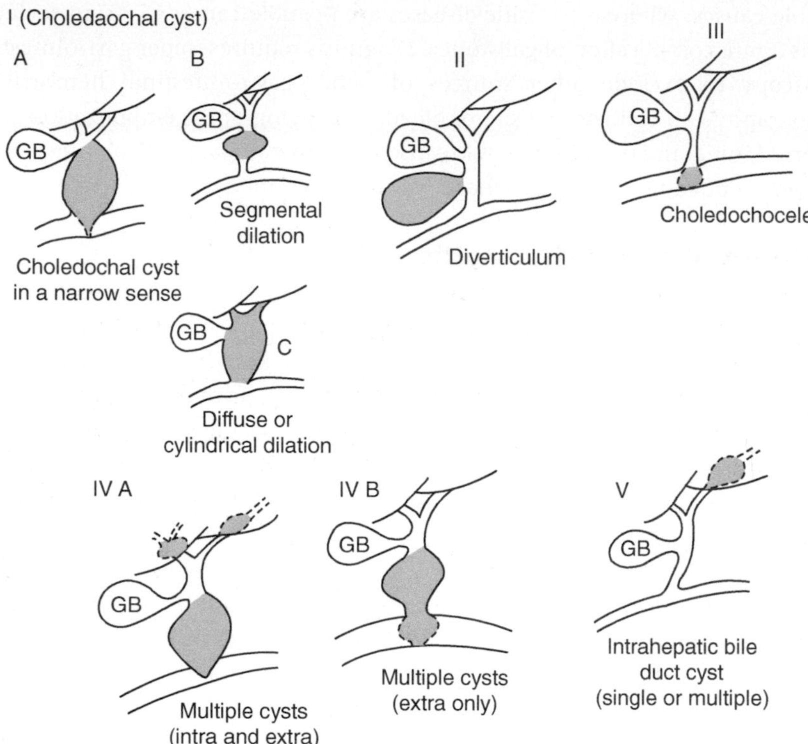

Figure 33.1 Today's classification of biliary cysts based on location. Hatched areas represent cystic dilations. Source: from Yamada et al. (2009).

associated with medullary spongy kidney, which should be distinguished from autosomal dominant polycystic kidney disease. The latter disease is characterized by hepatic cysts, which are pathologically distinct from biliary cysts. Unlike biliary cysts, hepatic cysts do not communicate with the biliary tract. Figure 33.1 diagrams the classification of biliary cysts.

Diagnostic investigation

Imaging with ultrasound or CT may detect biliary cysts. Advances in MRI have made MRCP useful for diagnosis and MRCP has replaced ERCP and percutaneous transhepatic cholangiography (PTC) for initial evaluation of these patients. EUS can provide detailed images of cyst structure, and intraductal ultrasound can evaluate malignant transformation. ERCP and PTC can be used to remove stones or obtain a tissue diagnosis of malignant disease.

Management and course

Small intraduodenal choledochoceles are best treated by endoscopic sphincterotomy but all other biliary cysts may require surgical therapy. For extrahepatic cysts, excision and drainage is preferable to drainage alone because of the risks of recurrent cholangitis and malignant transformation. Resection is the preferred treatment for localized intrahepatic cysts. The patient with diffuse intrahepatic cysts may require hepatic transplantation if hepatic failure or portal hypertension develops. Chronic antibiotic therapy may reduce the risk of recurrent cholangitis, particularly in Caroli's disease.

In addition to cholangitis, pancreatitis (type III), biliary cirrhosis, and liver abscesses may complicate the course of disease in patients with biliary cysts. Cyst rupture during pregnancy or labor has prompted the recommendation that pregnant women with symptomatic cysts deliver by cesarean section. The most feared complication is malignant degeneration. This risk is particularly high for adult patients, as 15% develop carcinoma. Carcinoma may occur throughout the biliary tract and pancreas, including the gallbladder and sites uninvolved by the cysts. The prognosis of these tumors is dismal.

Key Practice Points

- Ultrasound is highly sensitive and specific for diagnosing cholelithiasis.
- Cholecystectomy is the definitive treatment for symptomatic cholelithiasis.
- The Charcot classic triad consists of right upper quadrant pain, fever, and jaundice and is present in 50–75% of patients with acute cholangitis.
- MRCP can diagnose choledocholithiasis, but ERCP is the procedure of choice for sphincterotomy and stone removal.
- Common bile duct stones, even if asymptomatic, require therapy because of the high complication rate (e.g. cholangitis and pancreatitis).
- MRCP is the diagnostic method of choice for imaging suspected choledochal cysts.

Further reading

Yamada, T., Alpers, D.H., Kalloo, A.N. et al. (eds.) (2009). *Textbook of Gastroenterology*, 5e, 2010. Oxford: Blackwell Publishing.

CHAPTER 34
Viral Hepatitis

Hepatitis is a nonspecific clinicopathological term that encompasses all disorders characterized by hepatocellular injury accompanied by histological evidence of a necroinflammatory response. Hepatitis is classified into acute hepatitis, defined as self-limited liver injury of less than six months' duration, and chronic hepatitis, in which the inflammatory response persists after six months. These two fundamental forms of hepatitis can be further subdivided on the basis of the underlying disease process or cause. Viral hepatitis refers to liver injury, either acute or chronic, caused by infection with hepatitis A, B, C, D, and/or E (Table 34.1), among others. Hepatitis B and C may manifest as both acute and chronic hepatitis. Others, such as viral hepatitis A, are strictly acute.

Hepatitis A

Epidemiology

Hepatitis A virus (HAV) causes 200,000 cases of acute hepatitis annually. It is transmitted primarily by fecal–oral routes. Epidemics can be traced to contaminated water or food. HAV is rarely acquired by parenteral exposure. About 30% of the population of the United States has serum IgG antibody to HAV, which suggests prior exposure. Significant racial and ethnic differences in the prevalence of antibody to HAV are likely to reflect both country of origin and socioeconomic status. In developing countries, essentially all children are exposed to the virus, which often produces subclinical illness in this age group. Risk factors for acquiring HAV include male homosexuality, household contact with an infected person, travel to developing countries, and contact with children in day care. Outbreaks have also been associated with the consumption of raw shellfish, frozen strawberries, salads, and raw onions.

Yamada's Handbook of Gastroenterology, Fourth Edition. John M. Inadomi, Renuka Bhattacharya, Joo Ha Hwang, and Cynthia Ko.

Table 34.1 Human hepatitis viruses

Virus	Genome	Genome size (kb)	Envelope	Classification family	Genus
HAV	RNA positive sense, single-stranded, linear	7.5	–	Picornaviridae	Hepatovirus
HBC	DNA partially double-stranded, circular	3.2	+	Hepadnaviridae	
HCV	RNA positive sense, single-stranded, linear	9.6	+	Flaviviridae	Hepacivirus
HDV	RNA positive sense, single-stranded, linear	1.7	+	Unclassified (viroid)	Deltavirus
HEV	RNA positive sense, single-stranded, linear	7.5	–	Unclassified	Togavirus-like and alphavirus-like

Pathogenesis

HAV is an RNA virus that produces hepatocellular injury by mechanisms that remain poorly understood. Both direct cytopathic and immunologically mediated injury seem probable but neither has been proven. After exposure, there is a two to six-week incubation period before symptom onset, although the virus may be detectable in the stool one week before clinically apparent illness. The immune response to HAV begins early and may contribute to hepatocellular injury. Immunological clearance of HAV is the rule and unlike hepatitis viruses B and C, HAV never enters a chronic phase. By the time symptoms are manifest, patients invariably have IgM antibodies to HAV (anti-HAV IgM), which typically persist for three to six months. IgG antibodies to HAV (anti-HAV IgG) then develop and provide life-long immunity against reinfection.

Clinical course

Many patients with HAV infection, in particular 80–90% of children, are asymptomatic. Only 5–10% of patients with serological evidence of prior HAV infection recall an episode of jaundice. Factors that contribute to subclinical versus clinical infection remain unclear.

The syndrome of acute hepatitis caused by HAV is clinically indistinguishable from other viral causes of acute hepatitis. Patients usually present with a nonspecific prodrome of fatigue, anorexia, nausea, headache, myalgias, and arthralgias. This may be followed by jaundice and right upper quadrant pain. Some patients may experience pruritus but this rarely requires treatment. Vomiting is common and may lead to fluid and electrolyte imbalance. Physical signs include icterus and tender hepatomegaly. The spleen is palpable in a minority of patients. A prolonged form of HAV infection is characterized by pruritus, fever, weight loss, serum bilirubin >10 mg/dl and a clinical course lasting a minimum of 12 weeks. It is seen more often in older individuals. A relapsing variant characterized by initial clinical improvement followed by recrudescent symptoms 5–10 weeks after recovery affects 20% of patients, and the clinical course is rarely protracted, lasting no longer than 12 weeks. Resolution of HAV infection with complete recovery, except in the rare cases of fulminant hepatitis (~1%), is the rule.

Diagnostic and serological studies

Elevations in levels of aminotransferases usually occur one to two weeks before the onset of symptoms and persist for up to four to six weeks. The alanine aminotransferase (ALT) level usually is higher than the aspartate aminotransferase (AST) level; absolute values often exceed 1000 IU/l. The level of enzyme elevation does not correlate with disease severity; asymptomatic cases may have serum AST or ALT levels in the thousands. Serum bilirubin levels usually peak one to two weeks after symptoms appear but they rarely exceed 15–20 mg/dl. HAV infection occasionally produces a cholestatic pattern of liver biochemical abnormalities with a disproportionate elevation in the alkaline phosphatase level. Other laboratory abnormalities include relative lymphocytosis with a normal total leukocyte count.

Diagnosis relies on detecting anti-HAV IgM in the serum. Because this IgM component of the humoral immune response lasts only three to six months, its presence implies recent or ongoing infection (Figure 34.1). Liver biopsy is not necessary if the findings from serological testing are positive and is performed only if the diagnosis is in doubt. Although there are no distinguishing features of any form of viral hepatitis, patchy necrosis and lobular lymphocytic infiltrates

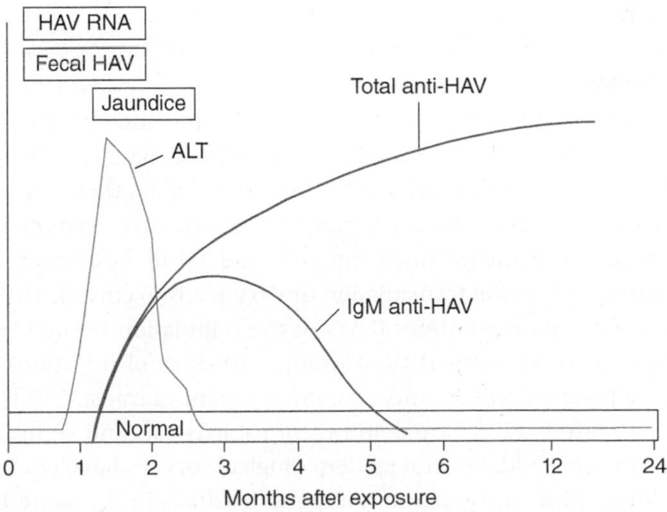

Figure 34.1 Typical serological course of acute hepatitis A virus (HAV) infection. ALT, alanine aminotransferase; IgM, immunoglobin M.

are typical findings. Occasionally, ultrasound scanning may be necessary to exclude biliary obstruction, particularly in patients with the cholestatic variant of HAV infection. This test may confirm hepatomegaly and reveal a heterogeneous liver parenchyma but findings usually are nonspecific.

Management

HAV is self-limited, and symptoms resolve in most cases over the course of two to four weeks. There is no specific treatment, and patients should be encouraged to maintain fluid and nutritional intake. Ten percent of patients require hospitalization for intractable vomiting, worsening laboratory values, or comorbid illnesses. The overall mortality rate for hospitalized patients is less than 1%. Deaths are mainly the result of the rare case of fulminant hepatitis, which is characterized by signs of hepatic failure, including encephalopathy. These patients are typically older and may have coexisting liver disease, and should be referred to liver transplant centers for management and potential transplantation.

Prevention

Infection with HAV can be prevented by either passive or active immunization. Patients exposed to feces of HAV-infected individuals should be given immunoglobulin (0.02 ml/kg) within two weeks of exposure. Travelers to endemic areas may be given immunoglobulin, which provides protection for about three months, or the formalin-inactivated hepatitis A vaccine, which provides long-term immunity to more than 90% of persons, beginning one month after the first dose of the two-dose regimen.

Hepatitis B

Epidemiology

Hepatitis B virus (HBV) is an important cause of acute and chronic hepatitis. In regions of Africa, Asia, and the Mediterranean basin where HBV is endemic, there are high rates of chronic HBV infection. Worldwide, there are 400 million HBV carriers. In the United States during the 1990s, HBV accounted for more than 175,000 cases of acute hepatitis annually, and 5% of these entered a chronic phase. In contrast, perinatal transmission of HBV leads to chronic HBV infection in more than 90% of cases. About 0.3% of the population in the United States suffers chronic infection with HBV. Although 30–50% of infections with HBV have no identifiable source, the most common means of transmission are sexual contact with an infected individual, intravenous drug use, and vertical transmission from mother to child. Several epidemiological surveys have emphasized the importance of contact transmission among individuals in the same household, even in the absence of intimate or sexual contact. The mechanism of this contact-associated transmission remains poorly defined. Blood transfusion is an unlikely source of HBV in western countries with the use of blood bank screening but poses a major risk in developing countries that do not screen blood or blood products for HBV.

Pathogenesis

HBV is a DNA virus that has seven genotypes, A–G, based on differences in sequence. One component of HBV is an envelope that contains a protein called *hepatitis B surface antigen* (HBsAg). Inside the envelope is a nucleocapsid that contains the hepatitis B core antigen (HBcAg), which is not detectable in serum. During viral replication, a third antigen, termed the *hepatitis B e antigen* (HBeAg), and HBV DNA are detectable in the serum. While in the replicative phase, HBV produces hepatocellular injury primarily by activating the cellular immune system in response to viral antigens on the surface of hepatocytes. The vigor of the immune response determines the severity of acute HBV hepatitis and the probability that the infection will enter a chronic phase. An exuberant response can produce fulminant hepatic failure, whereas a lesser response may fail to clear the virus.

After exposure to HBV, there is an incubation period of several weeks to six months before the onset of symptoms. HBsAg appears in the serum, followed shortly by HBeAg late in the incubation period. Detectable levels of HBeAg correlate with active viral replication, as does the quantity of HBV DNA. The first detectable immune response is antibody to HBcAg (anti-HBc), which is usually present by the time symptoms occur. As with HAV, the initial antibody response is primarily IgM, which persists for four to six months and is followed by a life-long IgG response. Antibodies to HBsAg (anti-HBs) develop in more than 90% of adult individuals with acute hepatitis. The appearance of anti-HBs, usually several weeks after the disappearance of HBsAg and resolution of symptoms, signifies recovery. Anti-HBs provides life-long immunity to reinfection, although titers may decrease to undetectable levels over the course of years.

Antibodies to HBeAg (anti-HBe) appear earlier than anti-HBs and usually signify the clearance of HBeAg and cessation of replication. In chronic HBV infection, the virus may be in a replicative phase characterized by the presence of HBsAg, HBeAg, and high levels of HBV DNA, along with an immune-mediated chronic inflammatory response. Alternatively, HBV may enter a nonreplicative state, formerly referred to as the carrier state, in which HBV is maintained by insertion into the host genome. In this phase, HBsAg persists but HBeAg disappears and anti-HBe appears. HBV DNA is present at low levels (fewer than 100,000 copies/ml). The inflammatory response in this nonreplicative state usually is minimal but due to integrated HBV DNA in the hepatocytes, the risk of hepatocellular carcinoma persists

Clinical course

Most acute HBV infections are asymptomatic, especially if acquired at a young age when chronicity is more likely. Thirty percent of infections with HBV in adults result in acute hepatitis, which is indistinguishable from other forms of acute viral hepatitis. The illness usually has a one to six-month incubation period. Hepatitis may be preceded by a serum sickness syndrome characterized by fever, urticaria, arthralgias, and, rarely, arthritis. This syndrome is likely caused by immune complexes of HBV antigens and antibodies, which may also produce glomerulonephritis and vasculitis (including polyarteritis nodosa) in patients with chronic HBV infection. Patients with chronic HBV infection may have a distant history of acute hepatitis but a history of jaundice is unusual. Most patients with chronic HBV infection remain asymptomatic for years. When symptoms develop, they usually are nonspecific, including malaise, fatigue, and anorexia. Some patients exhibit jaundice and complications of portal hypertension, such as ascites, variceal hemorrhage, or encephalopathy. Physical examination in the chronic phase may be normal. Some patients may present with stigmata of cirrhosis and portal hypertension, including ascites, dilated abdominal veins, gynecomastia, and spider angiomata.

Diagnostic and serological studies

Diagnosis of acute hepatitis B is based on a typical serological pattern in acute hepatitis. Serum aminotransferase elevations in the thousands and other liver biochemical abnormalities are indistinguishable from alternative causes of acute viral hepatitis. Acute infection is diagnosed by the presence of IgM antibodies to HBcAg (anti-HBc IgM) and evidence of ongoing infection represented by HBsAg, HBeAg, and HBV DNA. In 5–10% of patients with acute hepatitis, the latter three markers may be cleared before clinical presentation, leaving anti-HBc IgM as the only indicator of recent infection. It is important to measure the anti-HBc IgM because the isolated presence of IgG antibodies to HBcAg (anti-HBc IgG) is the most common serological pattern in resolved HBV infection (Figure 34.2). The timing of HBsAg disappearance is variable but it is absent in 80–90% of cases by four months after infection. Persistence of HBsAg beyond six months indicates chronic infection. Anti-HBs will appear several weeks after the disappearance of HBsAg. This antibody provides life-long immunity but titers may drop to undetectable levels over the course of years. As with acute HAV, liver biopsy for acute HBV is needed only if the diagnosis is not substantiated by serological testing.

Chronic HBV may produce several serological patterns based on the replicative state of the virus. The presence of HBsAg, HBeAg, and HBV DNA and the absence of anti-HBs and anti-HBe are characteristic of active viral replication. The presence of HBsAg and anti-HBe in the absence of HBeAg, along with low levels of HBV DNA, is representative of the nonreplicative or chronic inactive state. All patients with chronic HBV have anti-HBc IgG. A small number of patients may have low titers of anti-HBc IgM, particularly when the virus is transiting from the replicative phase to the nonreplicative phase. In addition, several mutations exist, including precore mutations that result in negative HBeAg in serum and positive anti-HBe but significant HBV DNA as well as pre-S and polymerase mutations. The latter usually arise in response to therapy, such as the YMDD mutation that is associated with lamivudine resistance.

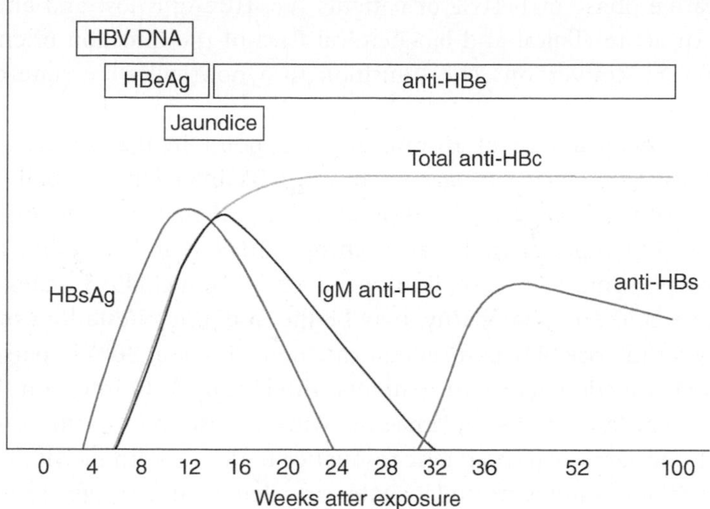

Figure 34.2 Typical serological course of acute hepatitis B virus (HBV) infection. HBeAg, hepatitis Be antigen; HBsAg, hepatitis surface antigen; IgM, immunoglobulin M.

Biochemical variables and symptoms correlate poorly with the histological severity of liver damage. Liver biopsy provides important prognostic information in patients with chronic hepatitis B. Patients with active viral replication demonstrate a variable degree of chronic periportal inflammation. Extension of chronic inflammatory cells into the hepatic lobule is termed *piecemeal necrosis*, whereas inflammation and hepatocellular destruction extending from portal tract to portal tract is termed *bridging necrosis*. Patients in the nonreplicative phase usually have minimal to no inflammation. Variable stages of fibrosis or even cirrhosis can be present in any patient with chronic HBV. Determining the extent of inflammation and fibrosis is often critical in making therapeutic decisions for chronic HBV.

Management

Acute HBV hepatitis usually resolves clinically and biochemically over several weeks to months. As with other forms of acute viral hepatitis, treatment is supportive. One percent of cases follow a fulminant course that results in hepatic failure and encephalopathy. These patients should be referred to transplantation centers.

The risk that HBV infection will become chronic is in large part related to the patient's age at acquisition. Chronicity rates are 90% for infections acquired perinatally. The rate is lower in older children and is about 5% in adults. The mechanism of this variability in the ability of HBV to enter a chronic phase appears related to changes in immune tolerance with aging. Once established, chronic HBV infection is usually life-long. Annually, only up to 1% of chronic HBV carriers lose HBsAg and develop anti-HBs, suggesting complete viral eradication. Each year, the replicative phase of the virus transforms into the nonreplicative phase in 1–10% of patients (i.e. HBeAg is lost and anti-HBe is gained). An acute clinical and biochemical flare of the infection often accompanies this seroconversion. The transition to a nonreplicative state does not indicate complete clearance of HBV. Many patients exhibit reactivation of replication with reappearance of HBeAg at some point in the future. Although cirrhosis may develop at any stage of chronic HBV infection, it usually requires many years of infection. The risk is greatest for patients with bridging necrosis and active viral replication. Because chronic HBV is indolent and produces minimal or no symptoms, complications of cirrhosis, including ascites, variceal hemorrhage, and encephalopathy, may be the initial manifestations of chronic HBV. The lifetime risk of hepatocellular carcinoma is about 20% in persons with chronic HBV infection; therefore, patients with chronic HBV infection should be screened every six months by imaging with ultrasound (or in some cases computed tomography or magnetic resonance imaging) with or without serum α-fetoprotein measurements, to facilitate early detection. The age of the patient, duration of infection, country of origin, and family history determine the age at which screening should begin. The course of acute and chronic HBV infection can also be complicated by superinfection with hepatitis D virus (HDV).

Treatment

Treatment of acute HBV infection is rarely indicated, although it is often pursued for fulminant infection. The goals of antiviral therapy include bringing the HBV DNA down to undetectable levels. The options for treatment of chronic HBV include antiviral or immunomodulatory therapy with nucleoside analogs and interferon-α. Candidates for interferon therapy ideally have higher levels of serum liver enzymes, lower serum levels of HBV DNA, and genotype A disease. They should not have histological evidence of cirrhosis or decompensated liver disease. Interferon therapy consists of standard or pegylated interferon for 12 months. With this therapy, the virus in 30–50% of cases will transition from the active replicative phase to the nonreplicative phase (HBeAg clearance) and up to 15% of patients will experience HBsAg clearance with long-term follow-up. Side effects are substantial; there is an almost universal occurrence of an influenza-like illness with myalgia, fever, chills, and headache. Other adverse reactions include depression, bone marrow suppression, alopecia, and autoimmune thyroiditis. Patients should be selected with this side-effect profile in mind, especially if there are pre-existing psychiatric conditions and cytopenias.

Treatment is typically reserved for patients with chronic active hepatitis B (Figure 34.3). There are currently five oral agents that are approved by the Food and Drug Administration for treatment of chronic hepatitis B in the United States: lamivudine, adefovir, entecavir, telbivudine, and tenofovir. These medications can be used by individuals who are HBeAg positive or negative, including those with decompensated liver disease. Lamivudine has been associated with a

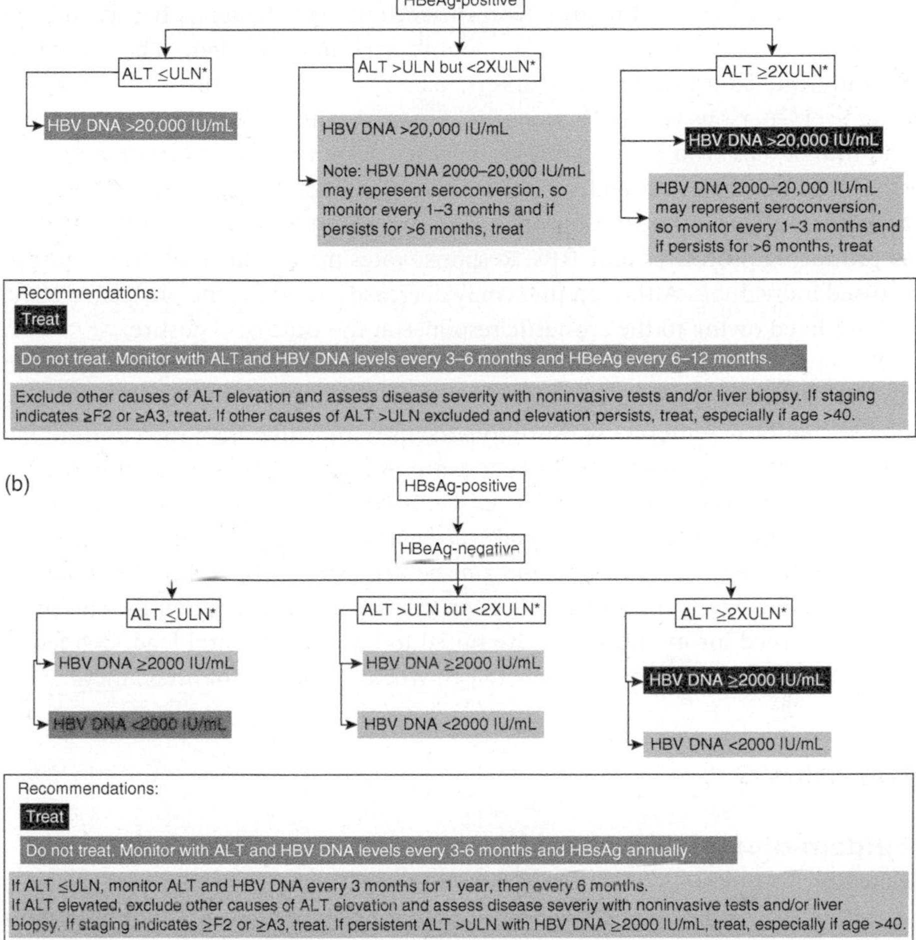

Figure 34.3 Algorithm for management of HBsAg-positive persons without cirrhosis who are HBeAg-positive (a) or HBeAg-negative (b). ALT, alanine aminotransferase; HBeAg, hepatitis Be antigen; HBsAg, hepatitis surface antigen; HBV, hepatitis B virus; ULN, upper limit of normal. Source: Terrault A. et al. 2018.

high rate of viral resistance (50–70% at three years), as has adefovir, although to a lesser degree (11% at three years, 30% at 4.5 years). Resistance to telbivudine is also common after one to two years of monotherapy, with cross-resistance with lamivudine. Currently, entecavir and tenofovir (available as tenofovir disoproxil and tenofovir alafenamide) are first-line agents, with similar and highly effective antiviral efficacy. These agents provide superior rates of biochemical and virological response as well as marked improvements in histology over time, with vanishingly low rates of resistance in treatment-naïve patients.

Prevention

Prevention of HBV has widespread public health implications. A program of universal vaccination of infants with the recombinant hepatitis B vaccine is in place in the United States and other countries around the globe. This vaccine is also indicated for healthcare workers, patients on hemodialysis, intravenous drug users, persons who have household contact with HBV carriers, adolescents and individuals who are sexually active with more than one partner, and travelers who reside in an endemic area longer than six months. The three-dose regimen is given at time 0, 1 month, and 6 months. It is more than 90% effective in producing protective anti-HBs. Response rates may be lower in immunosuppressed individuals. Although titers may decrease over time, the protective effect is long-lived owing to the amnestic response at the time of exposure.

Postexposure prophylaxis requires the use of hepatitis B immune globulin (HBIG) (0.06 mg/kg) in addition to the recombinant vaccine. Those who have had sexual or parenteral exposure to persons with active HBV infection should receive HBIG within two weeks of exposure. All exposed persons should receive the vaccine on the usual dosing schedule. Infants born to mothers with HBsAg should receive HBIG at birth and vaccination should be initiated. Further reduction of perinatal transmission can be achieved by lowering the maternal viral load during the third trimester of pregnancy using oral antivirals. This practice is reserved for mothers who are noted to have a high viral load, defined as ≥200,000 IU/ml when measured between weeks 28 and 32 of pregnancy.

Hepatitis C

Epidemiology

Hepatitis C virus (HCV) is an RNA virus in the Flaviviridae family that has been classified into six genotypes, based on sequence variation. Because most infections with HCV assume a chronic phase, preventing transmission is critical. Along with human immunodeficiency virus (HIV), screening of the blood supply for antibodies to HCV has dramatically reduced the incidence of posttransfusion hepatitis. Most HCV infections in the United States result from intravenous drug use. Given that the main mode of transmission is parenteral, the epidemiology of HCV infection mirrors to some extent that of HBV and HIV infections; however, sexual and perinatal transmission are rare for HCV. The risk of sexual transmission is poorly defined but appears to be 3–5% in long-standing monogamous relationships.

In most regions of the world, the prevalence of HCV antibodies ranges from 0.5 to 2%. In the United States, 70% of HCV infections are caused by genotypes 1a and 1b; the remaining 30% of infections are caused by genotypes 2 and 3. Although parenteral exposure is the primary means of contracting HCV, 10% of cases still have no identifiable source of infection. Groups at high risk of infection with HCV include intravenous drug users and persons who required transfusions or other blood products prior to 1991 or in countries outside the United States. The risk of vertical transmission from mother to fetus is 3–5%. The risk is higher (12–14%) if the mother is seropositive for HIV-1. Nosocomial infections from contaminated instruments or multidose vials, and needlestick injuries account for a small proportion of HCV infections.

Pathogenesis

Based on the observation that HCV infection follows a slightly more aggressive course with immunosuppression secondary to medications or HIV infection, HCV does not appear to rely solely on immune-mediated injury. Dual mechanisms of hepatocellular injury include a direct cytopathic effect of HCV as well as injury from specific and nonspecific T-cell-mediated immunological injury. No protective antibodies to HCV have been demonstrated. In addition, the immune response in HCV infection is responsible for the syndrome of mixed cryoglobulinemia observed in a small fraction of chronic HCV infections. In this disorder, HCV antigens associated with monoclonal IgM and polyclonal IgG antibody complexes are deposited in the end organ and activate complement, producing dependent purpura, glomerulonephritis, arthritis, and vasculitis. The incubation period after exposure is usually 2–12 weeks; the average is six to seven weeks. Similar to HBV infection, antibodies develop against several viral proteins and are detected by the enzyme-linked immunosorbent assay (ELISA) and the immunoblot assay (RIBA). Anti-HCVs may not be detectable for up to two months after the onset of acute hepatitis; however, HCV RNA is detectable within one to three weeks after the onset of acute infection. HCV antibodies are neither neutralizing nor protective, and 70–85% of HCV infections assume a chronic phase.

Clinical course

Most patients infected with HCV never develop a clinical syndrome of acute hepatitis. About 15–20% of patients develop malaise, fever, fatigue, nausea, vomiting, arthralgia, and right upper quadrant pain. Systemic symptoms may be followed by jaundice. Although fulminant HCV has been reported, it is exceedingly rare. After acute infection, 75–85% of adults and 55% of children with HCV infections enter a chronic phase. Spontaneous clearance of chronic HCV is observed, but rare. Many patients remain asymptomatic for years and are detected only during health screening or when donating blood. The most common symptoms of chronic HCV are nonspecific malaise, fatigue, and right upper quadrant abdominal discomfort. Some patients may remain asymptomatic even as the disease progresses to cirrhosis. Chronic HCV leads to cirrhosis in at least 20–25% of immunocompetent patients within 20 years of infection. The factors that influence the rate of progression to cirrhosis include coexisting liver disease and consumption of alcohol.

In recent years, much has been learned about a single nucleotide polymorphism (rs12979860 C/T) 3 kb upstream of the interleukin 28B (IL-28B) gene.

This IL-28B polymorphism has been shown to be associated with the likelihood of spontaneous hepatitis C clearance as well as likelihood of treatment response, and possibly disease severity. The CC genotype is associated with greater spontaneous clearance and superior response rates to interferon-based treatment, with the TT genotype having the least favorable profile.

Diagnostic and serological studies

Patients with acute hepatitis caused by HCV usually have aminotransferase levels lower than 1000 IU/l; less than 10% have levels higher than 2000 IU/l. Serum bilirubin levels rarely exceed 10–15 mg/dl. Severe liver dysfunction with abnormal coagulation variables is uncommon. As with other forms of acute viral hepatitis, the cornerstone of diagnosis is serological testing. The main obstacle to diagnosing acute infection is the variable delay in the appearance of anti-HCV. Only 65% of patients have anti-HCV within two weeks of symptom onset but 90% are seropositive after three months. The remaining 10% usually develops anti-HCV over several months. The presence of virus can be assessed for using polymerase chain reaction (PCR) or branched DNA (bDNA) amplification methods. HCV RNA is detectable within 7–21 days of infection. For patients with established chronic HCV infection, quantitative HCV PCR does not correlate with disease severity or histology. It may help to predict the likelihood of response to antiviral therapy. HCV genotype can be determined using genetic sequence detection techniques. Genotype does not correlate with disease severity but can be associated with the likelihood of treatment success.

Liver biopsy is generally not useful for diagnosing acute HCV infection but can be used for staging of fibrosis in chronic HCV. In chronic HCV, there is a variable degree of periportal chronic inflammation, often with discrete lymphoid aggregates. The severity may vary from a minimal increase in periportal lymphocytes to the confluent destruction of hepatocytes in bridging necrosis. There is also a variable degree of fibrosis, ranging from no fibrosis to cirrhosis. The severity of histological injury correlates poorly with symptoms and elevations in levels of aminotransferases. While liver biopsy remains the gold standard for staging fibrosis in hepatitis C infected patients, newer assays and technology provide less invasive alternatives to biopsy. Testing options include panels of serum markers, and the use of ultrasound technology including transient elastography using a Fibroscan device.

Management

With supportive therapy, most patients with acute HCV experience a gradual resolution of symptoms over weeks to months. The infection is self-limited in 15–30% of cases and the virus is cleared. In the remaining 70–85% of cases, the infection becomes chronic. Consideration should be given to treating all patients with chronic HCV infection, unless the life expectancy of the patient is limited. The goal of treatment is to prevent progression of fibrosis to cirrhosis. Cirrhosis occurs in 20–25% of patients within 20 years of infection. Once a patient develops cirrhosis, careful monitoring for complications of portal hypertension and hepatocellular carcinoma is indicated. Referral for liver transplantation should be considered if a patient experiences decompensation of their liver disease.

There have been many recent advances in the treatment of chronic hepatitis C. Pangenotypic oral agents are now available, offering a high likelihood of cure with 8 to 12 weeks of treatment for most patients. Due to the multiple advances and frequent changes in available medication regimens, it is difficult to identify optimal therapy in this handbook; therefore, it is recommended that one reviews the most current treatment recommendations for hepatitis C that are updated frequently by national and international societies, including the American Association for the Study of Liver Diseases (AASLD) and the Infectious Diseases Society of America (IDSA) at https://www.hcvguidelines.org. Guidelines are tailored for treatment of patients based on genotype, prior therapy, and whether cirrhosis is present. Successful antiviral treatment is defined as an undetectable viral load at 12 and/or 24 weeks after completing treatment, which is labeled a sustained virologic response (SVR). Once achieved, an SVR is associated with long-term clearance of the HCV and can be regarded as a "cure," with positive impact on morbidity and mortality.

Hepatitis D

The HDV, also termed the delta agent, is a defective RNA virus that requires the presence of HBV to replicate. Only patients with acute or chronic HBV infection are susceptible to infection with HDV, occurring as either an acute coinfection or as superinfection. HDV is present worldwide, with high incidences in regions of Africa, South America, and the Mediterranean but a low incidence in the United States. Modes of transmission appear to be both parenteral and sexual. Diagnosis requires a high level of suspicion. Identification of HDV infection has improved as there is now a quantitative HDV RNA assay available, in addition to antibody testing. Infection with HDV in chronic HBV carriers may result in increased severity of hepatitis and clinical decompensation of patients with cirrhosis. Thus far, only interferon-α treatment has been shown to exert significant antiviral activity against HDV and has been linked to improved long-term outcomes. Studies of other medication options are ongoing.

Hepatitis E

The hepatitis E virus (HEV) is an RNA virus epidemiologically and clinically similar to HAV. It is endemic in developing countries, especially Mexico, Africa, central Asia, and southern Asia. Reports in the United States are rare and usually represent infection acquired while traveling in endemic regions. Transmission is mainly by the fecal–oral route. Outbreaks are typically caused by contaminated water or food. The incubation period and clinical syndromes of acute hepatitis E are identical to those for HAV. For reasons that remain poorly defined, HEV infection in the third trimester of pregnancy is associated with a fulminant course in 15–25% of cases and has a high mortality rate. Diagnosis relies on detecting IgM antibodies to HEV. Detection of IgG antibodies to HEV signifies resolved infection and is associated with immunity. Treatment is supportive, and except for the high rate of fulminant hepatitis in pregnancy, full recovery from HEV infection is the rule. An exception to this rule is in the immunosuppressed patient who has undergone solid organ or bone marrow transplantation, as there are multiple published reports of chronic hepatitis E in this population.

Key practice points

- Hepatitis A is an RNA virus spread primarily via fecal–oral contact. The majority of cases have only mild symptoms, although <1% will have a fulminant presentation. There are cases of prolonged cholestatic and relapsing variants, but resolution of disease with complete recovery is the rule. Passive and active immunization is available for disease prevention.
- Hepatitis B is a DNA virus, with the most common modes of transmission including sexual, vertical, and via intravenous drug use. Approximately 95% of adults recover without chronic infection, while >90% of perinatally exposed persons develop chronic infection. There are multiple phases of disease activity, depending on the replicative state of the virus. Treatment is rarely curative but rather aimed at viral suppression. Persons with chronic HBV infection are at increased risk for hepatocellular carcinoma, so screening for HCC is recommended. Effective vaccination is available.
- Hepatitis C is an RNA virus that is transmitted parenterally, largely via intravenous drug use in the United States. Sexual and perinatal transmission is rare. The majority of patients with acute HCV infection are asymptomatic. Seventy to 85% of HCV infections become chronic, and 20–25% of infected patients progress to cirrhosis over 20 years. Patients with HCV-associated cirrhosis require screening for hepatocellular carcinoma. Due to numerous treatment advances in recent years, well-tolerated oral antiviral treatment regimens are available with a high rate of cure of infection.

Further reading

American Association for the Study of Liver Disease (AASLD) and Infectious Diseases Society of America (IDSA) guidance: Recommendations for testing, managing and treating hepatitis C. 2019. www.hcvguidelines.org.

Terrault, A. et al. (2018). Update on prevention, diagnosis, and treatment of chronic hepatitis B: AASLD 2018 hepatitis B guidance. *Hepatology* 67: 1560–1599.

CHAPTER 35
Genetic and Metabolic Diseases of the Liver

While much of the burden of liver disease is caused by viral hepatitis, there are many nonviral etiologies of liver disease that must be considered. These include highly prevalent diseases, such as nonalcoholic fatty liver disease (NAFLD), and rare disorders such as Wilson disease and α1-antitrypsin deficiency. Autoimmune hepatitis, primary biliary cirrhosis, and primary sclerosing cholangitis are discussed in other chapters.

Nonalcoholic steatohepatitis

A form of liver injury histologically indistinguishable from alcoholic hepatitis is often observed in patients who do not have histories of ethanol abuse. This syndrome has been termed *NAFLD*, representing a spectrum of disease from simple steatosis to nonalcoholic steatohepatitis (NASH) (Table 35.1).

Clinical Presentation

NASH is more common in obese patients and in those with hyperlipidemia, diabetes mellitus, or insulin resistance. Most patients do not have symptoms, but a minority may have nonspecific symptoms of fatigue, anorexia, and abdominal discomfort. The prevalence of NAFLD continues to rise, likely due to increasing rates of obesity and diabetes, and NASH is steadily increasing as an indication for liver transplant.

Diagnostic Evaluation

Laboratory testing will reveal mild elevations in levels of serum amino- transferases. The presence of Metabolic Syndrome, the NAFLD Fibrosis Score or FIB-4, or liver stiffness measured by VCTE or magnetic resonance elastography (MRE) may be used for identifying patients who are at risk for steatohepatitis (SH) and/or advanced fibrosis. Liver biopsy should be considered in patients with NAFLD who

Yamada's Handbook of Gastroenterology, Fourth Edition. John M. Inadomi, Renuka Bhattacharya, Joo Ha Hwang, and Cynthia Ko.

Table 35.1 Nonalcoholic fatty liver disease (NAFLD) and related definitions

NAFLD	Encompasses the entire spectrum of fatty liver disease (FLD) in individuals without significant alcohol consumption, ranging from fatty liver to steatohepatitis (SH) to cirrhosis.
NAFL	Presence of ≥5% hepatic steatosis (HS) without evidence of hepatocellular injury in the form of ballooning of the hepatocytes or evidence of fibrosis. The risk of progression to cirrhosis and liver failure is considered minimal.
NASH	Presence of ≥5% HS with inflammation and hepatocyte injury (ballooning) with or without fibrosis. This can progress to cirrhosis, liver failure, and rarely liver cancer.
NASH cirrhosis	Presence of cirrhosis with current or previous histological evidence of steatosis or SH.
Cryptogenic cirrhosis	Presence of cirrhosis with no obvious etiology. Patients with cryptogenic cirrhosis are heavily enriched with metabolic risk factors such as obesity and metabolic syndrome.
NAS	An unweighted composite of steatosis, lobular inflammation, and ballooning scores. NAS is a useful tool to measure changes in liver histology in patients with NAFLD in clinical trials. Fibrosis is scored separately.
SAF score	A semiquantitative score consisting of steatosis amount, activity (lobular inflammation plus ballooning), and fibrosis.

are at increased risk of having SH and/or advanced fibrosis. Histopathologically, NASH is characterized histologically by the presence of steatosis, inflammation, hepatocyte ballooning, Mallory hyaline and pericellular fibrosis.

Management

There are currently only limited treatment options for NASH, although multiple pharmaceutical trials are ongoing. Clinicians advise weight loss for obese patients and aggressive treatment of hyperlipidemia and diabetes. Studies of Pioglitazone and Vitamin E have shown promising results.

Key Practice Points

- Initial evaluation of patients with suspected NAFLD should carefully consider the presence of commonly associated comorbidities such as obesity, dyslipidemia, diabetes, hypothyroidism, polycystic ovary syndrome, and sleep apnea.
- There should be a high index of suspicion for NAFLD and NASH in patients with type 2 diabetes. Clinical decision aids such as NAFLD Fibrosis Score or fibrosis-4 index (FIB-4) or vibration controlled transient elastography (VCTE/Fibroscan) can be used to identify those at low or high risk for advanced fibrosis (bridging fibrosis or cirrhosis).

- Liver biopsy should be considered in patients with NAFLD who are at increased risk of having SH and/or advanced fibrosis.
- Pharmacological treatments aimed primarily at improving liver disease should generally be limited to those with biopsy-proven NASH and fibrosis.
- Weight loss of at least 3–5% of body weight appears necessary to improve steatosis, but a greater weight loss (7–10%) is needed to improve the majority of the histopathological features of NASH, including fibrosis.
- Metformin is not recommended for treating NASH in adult patients.
- Pioglitazone improves liver histology in patients with and without T2DM with biopsy-proven NASH. Therefore, it may be used to treat these patients. Risks and benefits should be discussed with each patient before starting therapy.
- Vitamin E (rrr a-tocopherol) administered at a daily dose of 800IU/day improves liver histology in nondiabetic adults with biopsy-proven NASH and therefore may be considered for this patient population. Risks and benefits should be discussed with each patient before starting therapy. Until further data supporting its effectiveness become available, vitamin E is not recommended to treat NASH in diabetic patients, NAFLD without liver biopsy, NASH cirrhosis, or cryptogenic cirrhosis.
- Foregut bariatric surgery can be considered in otherwise eligible obese individuals with NAFLD or NASH. It is premature to consider foregut bariatric surgery as an established option to specifically treat NASH.
- Patients with NAFLD are at high risk for cardiovascular morbidity and mortality. Thus, aggressive modification of CVD risk factors should be considered in all patients with NAFLD.
- Patients with NAFLD or NASH are not at higher risk for serious liver injury from statins. Thus, statins can be used to treat dyslipidemia in patients with NAFLD and NASH. While statins may be used in patients with NASH cirrhosis, they should be avoided in patients with decompensated cirrhosis.

Wilson Disease

Wilson disease, or hepatolenticular degeneration, is an autosomal recessive disorder caused by mutations in the *ATP7B* gene that lead to excessive accumulation of total body copper. It is a rare disorder with a worldwide incidence of three cases per 100,000 of population. The incidence of heterozygotes is 1 in 90. Abnormal copper metabolism is established from birth. Patients usually are diagnosed in adolescence, although rarely cases manifest after age 50.

The gene for Wilson disease is a copper-transporting P-type ATPase expressed exclusively in the liver. A defective structure or function of the transporter results in impaired biliary excretion and increased hepatic stores of copper. Free copper is also released into the serum and deposited in end organs. Accumulations in the brain, kidneys, bones, and eyes are responsible for the extrahepatic complications of Wilson disease.

Clinical presentation

Patients with Wilson disease almost universally present between ages 5 and 50; the second decade of life is the peak time of onset. Liver disease affects 50% of patients but the proportion who present with hepatic or neuropsychiatric symptoms varies with age. Potential hepatic manifestations include chronic active hepatitis with associated malaise, fatigue, and anorexia. Alternatively, patients present with complications of cirrhosis or a syndrome of fulminant hepatic failure with marked jaundice, encephalopathy, and hemolytic anemia. The diagnosis might be suggested by asymptomatic elevations of serum aminotransferase levels in an adolescent or young adult, often with a very low alkaline phosphatase level. Because the primary metabolic defect is localized in the liver, all symptomatic patients with Wilson disease have some degree of liver disease but 50% of patients present with extrahepatic manifestations. In 40% of patients, neuropsychiatric complications dominate. For unclear reasons, Wilson disease never leads to sensory deficits but spasticity, choreiform movements, dysarthria, ataxia, and intention tremor result from copper accumulation in the lenticular nuclei. Patients also may have subtle behavioral or psychiatric changes. The diagnosis should be suspected in adolescents with marked declines in scholastic or social performance. Patients with neuropsychiatric manifestations universally have Kayser–Fleischer rings, which are deposits of copper in the peripheral cornea. Other extrahepatic manifestations include Fanconi syndrome and proximal renal tubular acidosis, osteoporosis with spontaneous fractures, and copper-induced hemolytic anemia.

Diagnostic investigation

All siblings of Wilson disease patients should undergo diagnostic testing, in addition to young persons with abnormal liver chemistry profiles or clinical symptoms suggestive of Wilson disease. Screening for Wilson disease in a young patient with elevated levels of aminotransferases should include measurement of serum ceruloplasmin, which is decreased in more than 95% of homozygotes. Ceruloplasmin may also be low in 20% of heterozygotes and in patients with malnutrition, protein-losing enteropathy, and other forms of hepatic failure. Therefore, low ceruloplasmin levels should be confirmed by demonstrating 24-hour urinary copper excretion of more than 100 mg. The diagnosis cannot be excluded on the basis of a normal ceruloplasmin level. If Wilson disease is strongly suspected, further diagnostic evaluation with 24-hour urinary copper measurement should be performed with or without penicillamine challenge. Urinary copper also may be elevated in patients with cholestasis from other causes. Detection of Kayser–Fleischer rings may require slit-lamp examination. Although the presence of Kayser–Fleischer rings helps to confirm the diagnosis in the appropriate clinical setting, they may be absent in early Wilson disease. The standard for diagnosis is quantitation of hepatic copper levels in liver biopsy specimens. Histological findings include steatosis, glycogenated nuclei, and variable degrees of periportal mononuclear infiltrates and fibrosis. Genetic testing is challenging because of the large number of mutations described for the *ATP7B* gene.

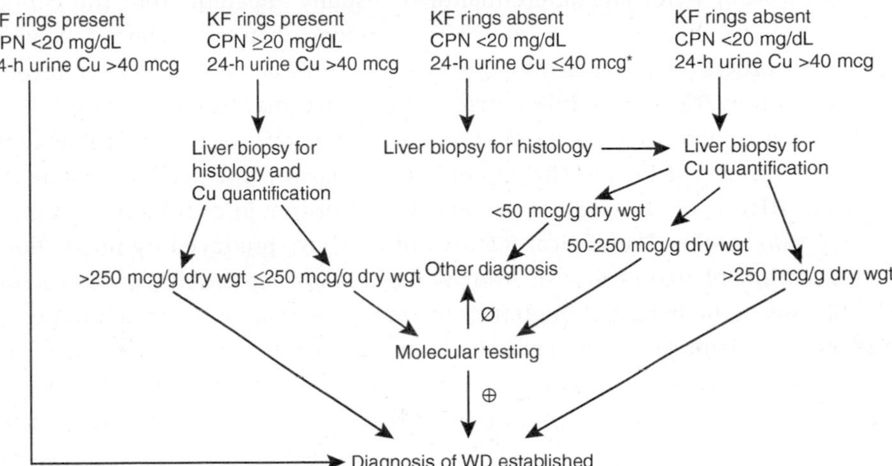

Figure 35.1 AASLD practice guidelines: diagnosis and treatment of Wilson disease (WD).

The American Association for the Study of Liver Diseases (AASLD) practice guidelines for the diagnosis of Wilson disease are shown in Figure 35.1.

Management and course

The critical factor in managing Wilson disease is establishing a definitive diagnosis early in its clinical course. Untreated, the disease is universally fatal. When treated, patients have a normal life expectancy but because treatment is lifelong, the diagnosis should be established with certainty. The cornerstone of treatment has been copper chelation with oral penicillamine or trientine. Zinc inhibits copper absorption in the gut and cannot be used to treat pre-existing copper overload but can be used for maintenance therapy. Although neurological symptoms may not resolve completely, patients with cirrhosis may experience long-term survival if they comply with therapy. Fulminant hepatic failure is not responsive to copper chelation and is universally fatal unless liver transplantation is performed. Transplantation should also be considered in the small fraction of patients with advanced cirrhosis who develop complications of progressive portal hypertension despite therapy.

Hemochromatosis

Hemochromatosis is characterized by pathological accumulation of toxic levels of iron in the cells of various organs and tissues, including the liver. Hemochromatosis may be caused by a genetic disorder of iron homeostasis termed *hereditary hemochromatosis* (HHC), or it may be caused by a secondary disorder, such as transfusional iron overload, sickle cell anemia, or dyserythropoiesis (e.g. thalassemia). The hepatic manifestations of secondary hemochromatosis are similar to those of HHC, but differentiation is usually apparent from the clinical features of the disorders associated with secondary hemochromatosis. Several hepatic disorders including alcoholic liver disease may be associated with uncomplicated iron overload, and differentiation from HHC may be challenging.

HHC is inherited as an autosomal recessive trait, with the responsible gene, designated *HFE*, localized to chromosome 6. The basic pathophysiological mechanism in HHC is increased intestinal absorption of iron in conditions of normal dietary iron intake. The clinical features of HHC are produced by intracellular accumulation of toxic levels of iron, which causes hepatocellular destruction and fibrosis in the liver. Although the mechanism of iron toxicity remains poorly understood, damage to cellular and organelle membranes by increased lipid peroxidation has been proposed as an important factor. Iron deposition in the heart, pituitary, pancreas, skin, and gonads is responsible for the extrahepatic manifestations of HHC.

Clinical presentation

Liver disease is the most common clinical feature of HHC. Most patients remain asymptomatic until complications of cirrhosis develop but many cases of precirrhotic HHC are diagnosed after detection of asymptomatic mild elevations in levels of serum aminotransferases. Advanced liver disease may present with jaundice, weight loss, fatigue, variceal hemorrhage, ascites, and encephalopathy. The most common extrahepatic manifestation is diabetes mellitus, which occurs in more than 50% of patients with HHC. An additional 50% of patients develop other endocrinopathies, including hypogonadism from pituitary and primary gonadal iron overload. Most patients with advanced disease have bronze or slate gray discolorations of exposed skin from increased melanin production and iron deposition in the basal layers. Degenerative arthropathy with a characteristic predilection for the second and third metacarpophalangeal joints occurs in 25% of patients.

Diagnostic investigation

Serum aminotransferase levels rarely exceed 100 IU/l, and they are normal in many cases. Serum measurements of total body iron levels are almost invariably elevated in HHC. The serum ferritin level is usually higher than 500 ng/ml and is often measured in the thousands. However, the serum ferritin level is elevated in any inflammatory disorder or iron overload condition such as alcoholism. Although a transferrin saturation of more than 55% is more specific for HHC, the predictive accuracy is less than 90% and the sensitivity is less than 80%. Therefore, patients with abnormal iron indexes should have their diagnoses confirmed. HHC can be diagnosed by liver biopsy with hepatic iron quantification and determination of the hepatic iron index (HII). The HII is calculated as micromoles of iron per gram of dry liver divided by the patient's age. A HII higher than 1.9 is diagnostic of hemochromatosis, whereas an index less than two essentially excludes HHC. Patients with alcoholic liver disease and those who are heterozygous for HHC often have markedly abnormal serum iron indexes but the HII is always less than 2.0. Histological evaluation with Prussian blue staining usually shows impressive stores of intracellular iron in more than 50% of hepatocytes but this finding may also occur in advanced alcoholic liver disease. Noninvasive magnetic resonance imaging can also document iron overload and quantify the degree of hepatic iron. Increasingly, diagnosis is made by detecting the C282Y mutation in the *HFE* gene, which detects more than 90% of HHC. A second mutation, H63D, is of less clinical import. C282Y/H63D compound heterozygotes can develop liver disease related to iron overload.

Management

The mainstay of HHC treatment is phlebotomy. The usual regimen removes 1 unit (250 mg of iron) every one to two weeks. Patients may require a total of 75–100 sessions over two to three years before iron stores return to normal levels. Once the transferrin saturation falls to less than 45% and the serum ferritin level is below 50 ng/ml, patients can be maintained on regimens of phlebotomy every three to four months. If diagnosed before the onset of cirrhosis or diabetes, patients with HHC compliant with phlebotomy programs can expect normal survival. Although phlebotomy does not reverse cirrhosis, it improves survival and should be considered at all stages of HHC. In patients with dyserythropoiesis or other causes of anemia intolerant of phlebotomy, iron chelation therapy is an alternative.

Up to 30% of patients with HHC develop hepatocellular carcinoma. Screening patients with established cirrhosis by using biannual alphafetoprotein measurement and ultrasound, computed tomography, or magnetic resonance imaging may result in early detection. Patients with advanced cirrhosis should be considered for liver transplantation but the post-transplantation survival of patients with HHC has historically been lower than that of patients with other forms of chronic liver disease, possibly because of a higher incidence of diabetes and cardiac disease.

The current AASLD practice guidelines for the diagnosis and management of hemochromatosis are shown in Figure 35.2.

α1-Antitrypsin Deficiency

Individuals who have inherited the PiZZ phenotype of α1-antitrypsin may manifest various liver disorders as a result of the accumulation of mutant Z α1-antitrypsin in the endoplasmic reticulum of hepatocytes. Patients usually present in infancy with cholestatic hepatitis or cirrhosis but some present in adulthood with chronic hepatitis, cirrhosis, or hepatocellular carcinoma. Only 20% of persons with PiZZ phenotype develop clinical liver disease. The other phenotypes (e.g. PiSS, PiSZ), including those commonly associated with emphysema, are not independently associated with liver disease, although may serve as a cofactor in

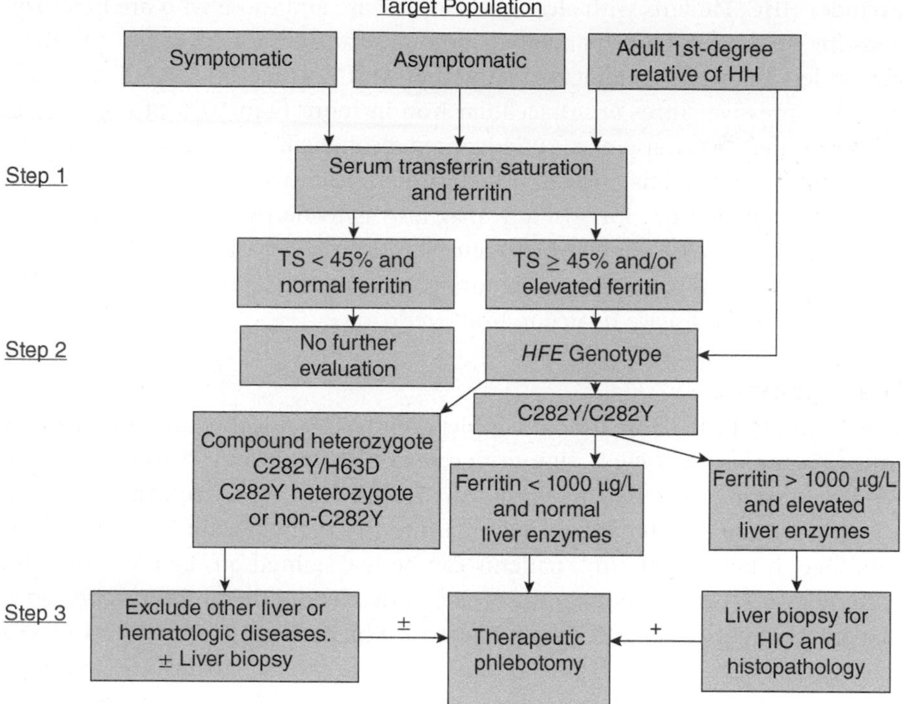

Figure 35.2 AASLD practice guidelines: diagnosis and management of hemochromatosis.

other liver disorders such as alcoholic liver disease. Diagnosis is usually suspected in a patient with liver disease who exhibits decreased levels of the α1 band in serum protein electrophoresis. Determining the specific phenotype of patients can provide more direct evidence for the diagnosis. Liver biopsy specimens can confirm the diagnosis by the presence of intracellular periodic acid–Schiff (PAS)-positive globules.

There is no specific treatment for liver disease due to α1-antitrypsin deficiency, and liver transplantation should be considered in patients with complications of cirrhosis. In addition to treating complications of cirrhosis, transplantation cures the underlying metabolic defect.

Further reading

Bacon et al. (2011). Diagnosis and management of hemochromatosis: 2011 practice guideline by the American Association for the Study of Liver Diseases. *Hepatology* 54: 328–343.

Chalasani et al. (2018). The diagnosis and management of nonalcoholic fatty liver disease: practice guidance from the American Association for the Study of Liver Disease. *Hepatology* 67: 328–357.

Roberts and Schilsky (2008). AASLD practice guidelines: diagnosis and treatment of Wilson disease: an update. *Hepatology* 47: 2089–2111.

CHAPTER 36
Cholestatic Liver Diseases

Cholestasis is a defect in bile excretion. It can be classified as intrahepatic or extrahepatic based on the anatomical site of the disturbance. Extrahepatic cholestasis is caused by diseases that structurally impair bile secretion and flow in the large bile ducts. Intrahepatic cholestasis is caused by a functional defect in bile formation and excretion at the level of the hepatocyte and terminal bile ducts. This chapter reviews the most common causes of intrahepatic cholestasis outlined in Table 36.1.

Primary biliary cholangitis

Primary biliary cholangitis (PBC) is a chronic, progressive, cholestatic disease that affects mainly middle-aged women. Patients may present as early as age 30 or as late as age 90, with a median age between 40 and 55 at presentation. PBC has been observed in all races but is more common in whites. Although several disease associations and well-characterized disturbances in immune regulation suggest that PBC is an immune-mediated disease, the etiology remains unknown. Associated immunological abnormalities include antimitochondrial autoantibodies, increased IgM levels, multiple antinuclear antibodies (ANAs) (~30%), circulating immune complexes, and other associated autoimmune phenomena. Autoimmune diseases associated with PBC include Sjögren syndrome, CREST syndrome, autoimmune thyroiditis, and, possibly, rheumatoid arthritis. PBC has also been linked to the HLA-DR8 antigen, which suggests that the disease may have a genetic component. Liver injury results from the nonsuppurative destruction of small bile ducts in the lobule. Reduced biliary excretion leads to cholestasis and toxic hepatocyte injury from the accumulation of bile acids and copper.

Yamada's Handbook of Gastroenterology, Fourth Edition. John M. Inadomi, Renuka Bhattacharya, Joo Ha Hwang, and Cynthia Ko.

Table 36.1 Differential diagnosis of intrahepatic cholestasis

Primary biliary cholangitis
Sclerosing cholangitis
Hepatocellular disease
Viral hepatitis
Alcoholic hepatitis
Medications
Intrahepatic cholestasis of pregnancy
Systemic infection
Total parenteral nutrition-associated cholestasis
Postoperative cholestasis

Clinical presentation

Forty to 50% of persons with PBC are asymptomatic at presentation. The disease is detected in most of these individuals from elevated serum alkaline phosphatase or γ-glutamyltransferase levels. About 50–60% of patients have presenting symptoms, usually fatigue and pruritus, and in some, upper right quadrant discomfort. Less than 25% present with jaundice. Pruritus may be severe, and the skin may become excoriated and hyperpigmented from incessant scratching. Other physical findings include hepatomegaly, splenomegaly, palmar erythema, spider angiomata, xantho- mas, and xanthelasma. The last finding correlates with the hypercholesterolemia (particularly of high-density lipoprotein) that is observed in PBC. The defect in bile acid secretion leads to impaired fat digestion with resultant steatorrhea, weight loss, and fat-soluble vitamin deficiencies. Long-standing cholestasis can also result in bone resorption and osteoporosis, which often lead to vertebral compression fractures and long bone fractures. A rare patient may have hepatic failure or a complication of portal hypertension (e.g. variceal bleeding) as the initial manifestation of PBC.

Most patients with PBC have associated autoimmune diseases. These diseases are usually mild, and survival is dictated by the severity of hepatic dysfunction. Autoimmune thyroiditis with hypothyroidism and CREST syndrome also often occur with PBC and may predate the diagnosis of liver disease. Other diseases associated with PBC include rheumatoid arthritis, gallstones, decreased pulmonary diffusion capacity, psoriasis, Raynaud phenomenon, and distal renal tubular acidosis (Table 36.2).

Diagnostic investigation

Laboratory studies

Patients with PBC typically have elevated serum alkaline phosphatase levels. Similar elevations in levels of 5′-nucleotidase and γ-glutamyltransferase help confirm the hepatic origin of the elevated alkaline phosphatase level. Serum bilirubin levels usually are normal at diagnosis. As the disease progresses, more than 50% of patients develop hyperbilirubinemia, a poor prognostic indicator.

Table 36.2 Extrahepatic manifestations of primary biliary cholangitis (PBC)

Extrahepatic disease	Prevalence (%)
Sjögren syndrome	30–58
Gallstones	30–50
Decreased pulmonary diffusion capacity	40–50
Renal tubular acidosis	20–33
Osteoporosis	15–40
Bacteriuria	11–35
Arthropathy	4–38
Rheumatoid arthritis	3–26
Hypothyroidism	11–32
Raynaud phenomenon	7–14
CREST[a] syndrome	3–6
Autoimmune thyroiditis	3–6
Autoimmune anemias	1–2
Psoriasis	1–13
Lichen planus	0.5–6
Ulcerative colitis	0.5–1

[a] CREST: syndrome of calcinosis, Raynaud phenomenon, esophageal dysmotility, sclerodactyly, and telangiectasias.

As with other cholestatic syndromes, levels of aminotransferases usually are only slightly elevated. Other nonspecific surrogate markers of cholestasis include increased levels of serum bile acids, cholesterol, triglycerides, elevated serum and hepatic copper levels, and decreased levels of fat-soluble vitamins A, D, E, and K.

Serological testing

The immunological abnormalities observed in PBC provide useful diagnostic information. Antimitochondrial antibodies (AMAs) are present in 90–95% of patients with PBC. Although other autoantibodies are present in a large number of cholestatic syndromes, elevated titers of AMAs rarely occur in other diseases and therefore are quite specific for PBC. Similarly, the finding of elevated IgM levels on serum protein electrophoresis, often in the absence of hyperglobulinemia, has high predictive value for PBC. Other serological abnormalities include increased titers of ANAs in 25–70% of patients and other autoantibodies but these findings are not specific to PBC and are of limited diagnostic value.

Liver biopsy

The diagnosis of PBC can be confirmed with a percutaneous liver biopsy. The pathognomonic lesion is characterized by patchy destruction of interlobular bile ducts with a mononuclear inflammatory infiltrate. Granulomas may be present in some portal tracts but their presence is not required to confirm a diagnosis of PBC.

The disease evolves through four histologically described stages. In stage I, chronic inflammatory cells and noncaseating granulomas adjacent to the damaged bile ducts, including the classic "florid duct lesion", expand the portal tracts. Stage II is characterized by expansion of the inflammatory infiltrate into the hepatic parenchyma and proliferation of the bile ductules. In stage III, interlobular fibrous septa and ductopenia are present. Stage IV represents cirrhosis.

Structural studies

Several imaging procedures may be used in the evaluation of PBC. These procedures are used primarily to exclude extrahepatic causes of cholestasis. Ultrasound generally demonstrates bile ducts of normal size. Gallstones are revealed in more than 30% of cases. Computed tomographic scanning also helps to exclude bile duct dilation and may demonstrate portosystemic collaterals that suggest portal hypertension. In patients lacking the serological markers of PBC, endoscopic retrograde cholangiopancreatography (ERCP) may be necessary to exclude large bile duct disease. Although the terminal intrahepatic ducts may be irregular, the larger ducts appear to be normal in size and contour on ERCP.

Management

PBC is an invariably progressive disease but the rate of progression varies. About half of the patients with PBC are asymptomatic at presentation but many become symptomatic within two to four years. As the disease progresses from the asymptomatic to symptomatic stages, serum alkaline phosphatase and globulin levels often dramatically increase and subsequently reach a plateau. Once symptoms appear, there is an indolent worsening of fatigue and pruritus, usually over the course of years. Patients eventually develop muscle wasting, progressive jaundice, and hepatic dysfunction. Once jaundice develops, life expectancy declines markedly, with mean survival times of four years if bilirubin levels are higher than 2 mg/dl and two years if higher than 6 mg/dl. The final stage of PBC is marked by complications of portal hypertension, including ascites, variceal hemorrhage, and encephalopathy.

The chronic inflammatory response and immune dysfunction observed in PBC have prompted clinical trials of several immunosuppressive regimens. Corticosteroids fail to alter the biochemical, histological, and clinical progression observed in PBC. Azathioprine, cyclosporine, colchicine, and D-penicillamine may result in biochemical improvements but none of these agents alters disease progression or survival. Some clinical trials of weekly regimens of methotrexate have shown improvement in biochemical and histological abnormalities. Given the potential for toxicity and the lack of clear benefit, the use of methotrexate is not recommended.

The synthetic bile acid ursodeoxycholic acid (ursodiol, UDCA) is the standard therapy for PBC. Given at a daily dose of 13–15 mg/kg, ursodiol may stabilize hepatocyte membranes, decrease the rate of biliary epithelial apoptosis, and decrease the production of more toxic bile acids. Most patients experience biochemical improvement but effects on histological improvement have been inconsistent in short-term trials. Long-term studies of ursodiol treatment have shown improved survival and delay in time to transplantation but meta-analysis has not confirmed these results, perhaps due to the short duration of the placebo phase before the cross-over to ursodiol in several large trials. Obeticholic acid (OCA), a farnesoid X receptor (FXR) agonist, is approved to be used in combination with UDCA in patients with PBC who have an inadequate biochemical response to at least one year of treatment with UDCA, or as monotherapy for those patients who are intolerant to UDCA. OCA has been shown to result in a significant reduction in alkaline phosphatase levels, although studies examining the effect of OCA on survival of patients with PBC are still ongoing. Pruritus, at times severe, is the most common adverse event reported with OCA use and can result in drug discontinuation.

The control of pruritus is the goal of symptomatic treatment of PBC. Oral antihistamines are occasionally of benefit in cholestasis-associated pruritus. Cholestyramine and colestipol are effective in a majority of patients but they often cause profound constipation and bloating. These ionic resins bind intraluminal bile acids and other pruritogens, thus preventing the absorption of these substances. Cholestyramine and other resins also interfere with the absorption of medications such as digoxin, thyroxine, and penicillins. Steatorrhea and fat-soluble vitamin deficiencies can be exacerbated. Patients intolerant of cholestyramine may respond to phenobarbital or rifampin. Refractory pruritus may respond to naloxone or other opioid antagonists, ondansetron, or therapy with ultraviolet B light, but data are limited.

Hypercholesterolemia rarely leads to cardiac disease except in the presence of other cardiac risks or unfavorable lipid profiles. Osteoporosis can be severe so monitoring the vitamin D level and supplementation of vitamin D as well as additional pharmacotherapies are useful in preventing bone loss.

Prediction of survival is critical in enabling the clinician to select optimal candidates for liver transplantation. Transplantation should be considered for patients with complications of portal hypertension, severe symptomatic osteodystrophy, or a predicted survival of less than two years. In properly selected candidates, liver transplantation is highly successful in treating PBC, with outcomes similar to transplant for other indications.

Primary Sclerosing Cholangitis

Primary sclerosing cholangitis (PSC) is a disorder of the bile ducts involving chronic inflammation leading to structuring of bile ducts and liver fibrosis. The majority of patients with PSC have ulcerative colitis (up to 90%). PSC may lead to end-stage liver disease.

Clinical presentation

The onset of PSC is insidious, and it can be diagnosed when asymptomatic elevations in serum liver biochemistry values are detected. Alternatively, symptomatic patients may have progressive fatigue, pruritus, weight loss, and jaundice for an average of two years before a diagnosis is made. Patients with associated inflammatory bowel disease are more likely to have both intrahepatic and extrahepatic ductal disease. Isolated involvement of the extrahepatic ducts is more common in patients without inflammatory bowel disease (38%) than in patients with inflammatory bowel disease (7%). A small percentage of patients with PSC have other associated immune disorders (e.g. Sjögren syndrome, hereditary acquired immunodeficiency syndromes, or the antiphospholipid antibody syndrome). PSC should be differentiated from other causes of chronic cholestasis, including primary biliary cirrhosis and recurrent pyogenic cholangitis.

Diagnostic investigation

Most patients have at least a twofold elevation of alkaline phosphatase levels, often out of proportion to the elevations of serum bilirubin levels. Aminotransferase levels are only mildly increased. Magnetic resonance imaging is often used in the initial evaluation of patients with suspected PSC and can reveal characteristic cholangiographic features including multifocal strictures, usually in the intrahepatic and extrahepatic ducts, with intervening normal or dilated ductal segments that produce a "string of beads" pattern. However, this pattern is not specific for PSC and may be seen in patients with metastatic cancer to the liver, allograft ischemic injury, and the diffuse form of cholangiocarcinoma. Differentiating cholangiocarcinoma from PSC can be difficult, especially because bile duct cancer is a potential complication of PSC. Liver biopsy can be helpful with diagnosis and staging of the disease, but biopsy information can be nondiagnostic due to the heterogeneous nature of the disease.

Management

PSC usually follows a slow, progressive course. A small subset of patients has stable disease for decades, but over years, most patients with PSC progress to portal hypertension and death caused by liver failure. The five-year survival rate is 60–70%. Patients who present with symptomatic disease have significantly worse prognoses. Cholangiocarcinoma complicates the course of disease in 7–15% of patients with PSC; it can be difficult to diagnose in view of the cholangiographic abnormalities observed in PSC. The mean age at diagnosis of cholangiocarcinoma in these patients is 42, compared with the mean age of 66 for the general population.

The treatment of PSC patients is primarily supportive. Orthotopic liver transplantation is reserved for patients with end-stage disease, recurrent cholangitis despite medical therapy, or uncontrolled peristomal variceal bleeding. No immunosuppressive regimen has been demonstrated to slow the progression of the disease. Although UDCA (ursodiol) may relieve pruritus and improve biochemical profiles, it fails to halt disease progression. Prophylactic colectomy in patients with ulcerative colitis does not alter the natural course of PSC nor does it prevent the complication of cholangiocarcinoma. Dominant symptomatic biliary strictures may be treated with ERCP and endoscopic balloon dilation and stenting. Surgical resection and biliary reconstruction may be necessary for selected patients with refractory strictures or for those who may have bile duct carcinoma.

Hepatocellular Diseases

Several liver diseases that characteristically produce hepatocellular injury may demonstrate biochemical and clinical features more consistent with cholestasis. Alcoholic hepatitis may produce profound increases in levels of serum bilirubin and alkaline phosphatase with normal to minimally elevated levels of aminotransferases, a pattern that often correlates with severe hepatocellular injury. Atypical variant forms of acute viral hepatitis A, B, and E include a syndrome of prolonged cholestasis. Although patients with hepatitis C typically manifest acute hepatitis, liver allograft recipients with recurrent infection from hepatitis C virus may rarely develop recurrent cholestatic hepatitis C, which is characterized by pericholangitis and cholestasis with minimal inflammation, rapid graft failure, requiring urgent antiviral therapy.

Cholestasis of Pregnancy

Pregnancy may be associated with abnormal liver chemistry values attributable to numerous physiological alterations and disease processes. Perhaps the most common finding is a mild increase in the serum alkaline phosphatase level from placental release of this enzyme. Women may also have coincident liver diseases unrelated to their pregnancy, for example, alcohol-, viral-, and immune- mediated liver diseases. The impact of pregnancy on the natural history of these disorders remains unclear. Pregnancy may be complicated by several disorders unique to pregnancy, for example, HELLP syndrome with pre-eclampsia, and the rare but devastating syndrome of acute fatty liver of pregnancy. These two disorders present in the third trimester, often with cholestasis and systemic complications such as disseminated intravascular coagulation and renal and hepatic failure. Acute fatty liver and pre-eclampsia-related liver injury require prompt delivery of the fetus. Unless diagnosed early, these disorders have high maternal mortality rates.

The most common liver disease unique to pregnancy is intrahepatic cholestasis of pregnancy. It occurs in less than 1% of all pregnancies in the United States and accounts for 30–50% of all causes of jaundice in pregnancy. It is distinguished from the other disorders by its benign course. The syndrome is similar to the cholestasis associated with estrogen supplements. Moreover, women with a prior history of intrahepatic cholestasis of pregnancy often manifest cholestasis when challenged with oral contraceptives in the nonpregnant state. The etiology remains unknown but familial clustering suggests the presence of a genetically acquired sensitivity to the cholestatic effects of estrogens. Patients usually present with pruritus and mild jaundice in the third trimester. Liver chemistry values demonstrate a cholestatic pattern. A biopsy specimen from the liver reveals bland cholestasis with no inflammatory reaction. A biopsy is occasionally needed to differentiate the syndrome from acute fatty liver of pregnancy or other more morbid disorders. Supportive treatment with ursodiol and cholestyramine may relieve the pruritus; cholestasis and pruritus resolve within 24–48 hours of delivery.

Systemic Infection

Systemic gram-negative bacterial infections are often accompanied by cholestasis. Endotoxemia decreases bile flow and may result in conjugated hyperbilirubinemia, with bilirubin levels in the range of 5–10 mg/dl. Levels of aminotransferases are usually near normal, and the alkaline phosphatase level is variably elevated. Clinical manifestations are dominated by the underlying infection. Cholestasis improves with successful treatment of the responsible micro-organisms.

Cholestasis Associated with Total Parenteral Nutrition

Patients who receive long-term total parenteral nutrition (TPN) may manifest any of several distinct patterns of hepatic dysfunction, including cholestasis. TPN-induced intrahepatic cholestasis is common in premature newborn infants. The mechanism is undefined but probably results from alterations in serum bile acid pools caused by changes in intestinal bacteria. Patients who receive TPN are often subjected to bowel rest; the resulting bile stasis promotes biliary sludge and stone formation. Therefore, extrahepatic cholestasis also should be considered when evaluating patients on long-term TPN.

Postoperative Cholestasis

The postoperative state may be complicated by jaundice caused by cholestasis and impaired bile formation or alterations in the production or excretion of bilirubin. Increased bilirubin production, which may exceed the excretory capacity of the liver, can be caused by several factors in a patient undergoing surgery. Hemolysis caused by systemic infections, transfusion reactions, mechanical trauma caused by artificial valves or a circulatory bypass, or pre-existing red blood cell defects and hemoglobinopathies increase the production of bilirubin. Similarly, massive transfusions and resorption of large hematomas may overwhelm the liver's ability to excrete bilirubin. Increased bilirubin loads lead to predominantly unconjugated hyperbilirubinemia. Patients with Gilbert syndrome, a common autosomal dominant defect of bilirubin conjugation, often develop unconjugated hyperbilirubinemia from physiological stress and fasting in the perioperative period.

Hepatocellular injury also may cause jaundice in postoperative patients. Hypoxia and hypotension in the perioperative period can produce ischemic hepatitis. Drug-induced hepatotoxicity, especially from anesthetic agents, can cause jaundice. Rarely, viral hepatitis acquired from transfusions results in jaundice, weeks after an operation. All of these insults usually produce a marked increase in levels of aminotransferases in addition to hyperbilirubinemia.

Cholestasis in the postoperative state can be extrahepatic or intrahepatic in origin. Patients undergoing biliary surgery are prone to extrahepatic cholestasis if there are retained bile duct stones and bile duct injuries. Systemic infection, medications, and TPN can produce intrahepatic cholestasis. When all other causes of postoperative jaundice and cholestasis have been excluded, the probable diagnosis is benign postoperative intrahepatic cholestasis. This transient syndrome of unknown etiology usually causes conjugated hyperbilirubinemia and elevated serum alkaline phosphatase levels by the third postoperative day. It typically gradually resolves over one to two weeks.

Key practice points

- Cholestasis is a defect in bile excretion. It can be classified as intrahepatic or extrahepatic based on the anatomical site of the disturbance.
- PBC results in intrahepatic cholestasis due to destruction of small bile ducts. It is characterized by a positive antimitochondrial antibody, and the recommended first-line treatment is ursodiol.
- Cholestatic liver diseases can result in jaundice, pruritus, fat-soluble vitamin deficiency, hypercholesterolemia, and reduced bone density.
- Treatment of pruritus in cholestatic liver disease can include antihistamines, cholestyramine, rifampin, naloxone, and ultraviolet light therapy.

CHAPTER 37
Alcoholic Liver Disease

Alcohol-related liver disease is among the most common liver diseases in the United States. The amount of alcohol that can be safely consumed is unknown, but it is estimated to be 20 g/day (two drinks) for men and 10 g/day (one drink) for women. The risk of alcoholic cirrhosis increases with daily alcohol consumption of 60–80 g/day (men) or 20 g/day (women).

Metabolism of ethanol

Most ethanol is metabolized by hepatic alcohol dehydrogenase (ADH) to acetaldehyde, which is subsequently converted by acetaldehyde dehydrogenase (ALDH) to acetate. ADH is the rate-limiting enzyme. Its activity is decreased by fasting, protein malnutrition, and chronic liver disease. A smaller portion of ethanol is oxidized by the cytochrome CYP2E1. This enzyme is inducible by chronic ethanol ingestion and may contribute to the increased rate of ethanol elimination in alcoholics. Because CYP2E1 is responsible for metabolizing other drugs, ethanol can increase or decrease the rate of elimination of some medications

Clinical presentation

The clinical manifestations of alcoholic liver disease (ALD) can be divided into three disease processes: steatosis, alcoholic hepatitis, and alcoholic cirrhosis. Steatosis is generally benign, asymptomatic, and reversible with abstinence. Patients with alcohol-related steatosis may be asymptomatic or have mild hepatomegaly.

Although a rare patient may be asymptomatic, patients with alcoholic hepatitis generally experience fever, anorexia, malaise, and abdominal pain. Physical examination findings of icterus, tender hepatomegaly, or tachycardia are common. Severe alcoholic hepatitis manifests portal hypertension, including splenomegaly, enlarged collateral abdominal veins, ascites in 40–70% of cases,

Yamada's Handbook of Gastroenterology, Fourth Edition. John M. Inadomi, Renuka Bhattacharya, Joo Ha Hwang, and Cynthia Ko.

encephalopathy in 20%, and upper gastrointestinal bleeding in 30%. Portal hypertension may be present in the absence of histological evidence of cirrhosis. The mortality rate of acute alcoholic hepatitis is high.

Eighty to 90% of patients with alcoholic cirrhosis have nonspecific complaints of weight loss, malaise, failure to thrive, or complications of portal hypertension (e.g. ascites, spontaneous bacterial peritonitis, variceal hemorrhage, and hepatic encephalopathy). Patients with alcoholic cirrhosis often have classic stigmata on physical examination, including palmar erythema, Dupuytren contracture, testicular atrophy, gynecomastia, and feminization in male patients.

Diagnostic evalution

Laboratory abnormalities in alcoholic fatty liver are typically mild. Bilirubin may be elevated but less than 5 mg/dl. As with all stages of ALD, serum aspartate aminotransferase (AST) and alanine aminotransferase (ALT) levels are usually less than 300 IU/l. The AST is usually higher than the ALT, with AST/ALT ratio ≥2 in the vast majority of cases.

Bilirubin is increased, whereas albumin is decreased and prothrombin time is typically prolonged. Electrolyte abnormalities are common, including hyponatremia, hyperchloremia, hypokalemia, and hypophosphatemia.

Liver biopsy

The classification of ALD into fatty liver, alcoholic hepatitis, and cirrhosis is based on clinical and pathological correlations; therefore, confirmation of these abnormalities and exclusion of alternative causes of liver disease may require liver biopsy. For patients with coagulopathy, tense ascites, or thrombocytopenia, the risk of biopsy may outweigh the benefit of obtaining pathological confirmation.

Fatty liver or steatosis is characterized histologically by large intracytoplasmic fat droplets often concentrated in the pericentral zone or zone 3. By definition, simple steatosis is not accompanied by significant inflammation or necrosis but pericentral fibrosis, a network of collagen surrounding the central vein, may be present. In addition to alcohol, other causes of fatty liver should be considered (Table 37.1).

In contrast, inflammation and hepatocellular necrosis are hallmarks of alcoholic hepatitis. The inflammatory infiltrate is primarily neutrophilic, and necrosis may range from ballooning degeneration of isolated hepatocytes to confluent centrilobular necrosis. Mallory hyaline and pericellular and perisinusoidal fibrosis, which has a characteristic "chicken wire" appearance, are common.

Cirrhosis, the final stage of ALD, requires documenting the presence of bands of fibrosis extending between the portal tracts and the central veins and the presence of regenerative nodules. Alcoholic cirrhosis may be confused with primary hemochromatosis because of the high levels of hepatic iron. These two disorders can be distinguished by calculating the hepatic iron index:

Table 37.1 Potential causes of fatty liver

Macrovesicular fat
Alcoholic steatohepatitis
Nonalcoholic steatohepatitis
Hepatitis C
Toxins and drugs: methotrexate, halogenated hydrocarbons, niacin, human immunodeficiency virus (HIV) protease inhibitors, glucocorticoids, heavy alcohol use
Nutritional disorders: obesity, diabetes, choline deficiency, systemic carnitine deficiency, celiac disease, kwashiorkor, parenteral nutrition
Lipodystrophy
Wilson disease
Aβ-lipoproteinemia
Inflammatory bowel disease
Weber–Christian disease
Q fever
Microvesicular fat[a]
Reye syndrome
Parenteral alimentation
Yellow fever
Heat stroke
Toxins and drugs: valproic acid, intravenous tetracycline, toxic shock syndromes, salicylate overdosage in children, Jamaican vomiting disease, fialuridine (FIAU), nucleoside reverse transcriptase inhibitors, mycotoxins
Metabolic diseases: cholesterol ester storage disease, galactosemia, Wolman disease, long-chain 3-hydroxyacyl-conenzyme A (CoA) dehydrogenase deficiency, medium-chain acyl-CoA deficiency
Complications of pregnancy: acute fatty liver of pregnancy, eclampsia, HELLP syndrome

[a] Microvesicular fatty liver is usually the result of mitochondrial damage and defects in lipid oxidation pathways; however, there is significant overlap with many disorders occasionally producing microvesicular fatty liver.

the micromoles of iron per gram of dry liver divided by the patient's age. In hemochromatosis, the iron index is higher than 1.9 μmol/g and in alcoholic cirrhosis without hemochromatosis, it is less than 1.9.

There is no pathognomonic histological feature of ALD. Mallory bodies are aggregates of perinuclear eosinophilic material once considered diagnostic of alcohol-induced injury. They are present in at least 30% of patients with alcoholic hepatitis or cirrhosis but they are also present in other liver disorders, including Wilson disease, cholestatic liver disease, nonalcoholic steatohepatitis, drug-induced and total parenteral nutrition-induced liver disease.

Management

The prognosis for ALD is determined mainly by the pathological stage at presentation and the patient's ability to abstain from ethanol consumption. The single most important therapeutic intervention is complete avoidance of ethanol consumption. This often requires a multidisciplinary approach, involving social workers, psychiatrists, primary care physicians, hepatologists, and social support groups. No therapy for ALD has benefit if heavy drinking continues.

Alcoholic fatty liver is generally benign and resolves completely after three to six weeks of abstinence. The major clinical importance of this condition is its representation of significant alcohol-related end-organ damage, for which patients should be counseled to abstain before more severe or irreversible damage develops.

Alcoholic hepatitis carries a far worse prognosis, with a high associated mortality. Early (two month) mortality rates range from 19 to 78%. Patients with encephalopathy, renal failure, ascites, and variceal bleeding have higher mortalities. Several methods of predicting disease severity and survival have incorporated clinical and laboratory findings but the most accurate and widely used is the Maddrey discriminant function (DF): serum bilirubin (mg/dl) + [4.6 × (patient's prothrombin time − control prothrombin time)]. A DF of more than 32 identifies patients with severe alcoholic hepatitis who have a 30-day mortality rate higher than 50%.

Corticosteroids have been used to reduce the inflammatory response of alcoholic hepatitis. Several studies have demonstrated improved survival of patients with a DF of more than 32 or with spontaneous encephalopathy. Studies have used prednisone, prednisolone, or 5-methylprednisolone in doses of 35–80 mg/day for four to six weeks. The American College of Gastroenterology (Table 37.2) has recommended the use of prednisolone 40 mg daily for four weeks, followed by a taper, in patients with severe alcoholic hepatitis (DF > 32) with hepatic encephalopathy. Treatment should exclude patients with active infection, renal failure, pancreatitis, or gastrointestinal hemorrhage. The mortality rate in this selected group is reduced by 25%. If a patient fails to respond to steroids after one week, consideration should be given to discontinuing steroids. Failure to respond can be measured by the Lille Score, with a score of >0.45 on day seven of treatment suggesting that a patient is not responding to glucocorticoid therapy.

The possible contribution of protein and calorie malnutrition to alcohol toxicity has led to several trials of enteral and parenteral nutritional supplementation for treating patients with alcoholic hepatitis. These supplements result in accelerated biochemical improvement, and some studies have demonstrated improved survival. Patients with alcoholic hepatitis should have their caloric intake monitored and supplemented if deficient. Aggressive enteral supplementation may be warranted if oral intake is inadequate.

Pentoxifylline, which has anti-tumor necrosis factor-α properties, has been shown to reduce the risk of hepatorenal syndrome in a large study of patients with severe alcoholic hepatitis. Pentoxifylline, given at a dose of 400 mg three times daily, reduced mortality by 40%, due in large part to a reduction in renal failure. Subsequent studies have been unable to reproduce these findings, and the routine use of Pentoxifylline is not typically recommended. Numerous additional medications have been studied for the management of alcoholic hepatitis, including anabolic steroids (oxandrolone), propylthiouracil (PTU),

Table 37.2 American College of Gastroenterology clinical guideline: alcoholic liver disease (ALD)

Environmental and genetic determinants

1. Patients with obesity or chrome hepatitis C virus (HCV) should avoid consumption of alcohol. (Conditional recommendation, very low level of evidence)
2. Patients with ALD should be advised to abstain from cigarettes. (Conditional recommendation, very low level of evidence)

Diagnosis of alcoholic use disorder

3. Patients who have heavy alcohol use (>three drinks per day in men and >two drinks in women for >fiveyears) should be counseled that they are at increased risk for ALD. (Strong recommendation, low level of evidence)

Management of ALD

Management of alcohol use disorder

4. In patients with ALD, baclofen is effective in preventing alcohol relapse. (Conditional recommendation, low level of evidence)
5. In patients with ALD, brief motivational interventions arc effective in reducing alcohol relapse compared with no intervention. (Conditional recommendation, very low level of evidence)

Alcoholic hepatitis

Treatment of alcoholic hepatitis

6. Patients with alcoholic hepatitis should be considered for nutritional supplementation to ensure adequate caloric intake and to correct specific deficits, yet its effects on patient survival has not been proven. (Conditional recommendation, very low level of evidence)
7. Patients with severe alcoholic hepatitis should be treated with corticosteroids if there are no contraindications for their use. (Strong recommendation, moderate level of evidence)
8. The existing evidence does not support the use of pentoxifylline tor patients with severe alcoholic hepatitis. (Conditional recommendation, low level of evidence)

Liver transplantation in alcoholic fever disease

9. Liver transplantation may be considered for highly selected patients with severe alcoholic hepatitis. (Strong recommendation, moderate level of evidence)

infliximab, colchicine, and vitamin E, without convincing evidence of benefit and some with potential risk.

As with all forms of ALD, long-term survival of patients with alcoholic cirrhosis is directly related to the stage of the disease and the patient's ability to abstain from ethanol consumption. Liver transplantation should be considered for patients who have abstained from alcohol but continue to suffer from complications of portal hypertension and are in Child class B or C. The period of abstinence and other patient characteristics to select candidates who will have low rates of recidivism is controversial. A six month period of abstinence allows for potential improvement in liver function to a condition that may not warrant transplantation. Patients may be referred to a transplant center before completing this prolonged period of abstinence. Although guidelines for pretransplant and post-transplant treatment vary from center to center, survival post-transplant has been excellent. With appropriate patient selection, only 10–30% of patients return to drinking. Alcohol-related liver disease accounts for over 25% of adult liver transplants in the United States.

Key practice points

- ALD is highly prevalent, affecting men more than women (3/1), typically at the ages of 40–55.
- The histological findings in alcoholic fatty liver disease include steatosis in a zone 3 distribution, neutrophilic inflammation, Mallory hyaline, and pericentral fibrosis.
- ALD can be divided into three disease processes: steatosis, alcoholic hepatitis, and alcoholic cirrhosis, and all three can coexist.
- Alcoholic hepatitis carries a poor prognosis. Multiple models exist to measure disease severity, most notably Maddrey's DF.
- Treatment options for severe alcoholic hepatitis (DF >32 ± encephalopathy) include the use of corticosteroids and nutritional supplementation.
- Ultimately, prognosis of ALD depends on abstinence from alcohol.
- For those who do not recover liver function despite alcohol abstinence, the criteria for selection of patients for liver transplant is challenging, and the recommendation for a prolonged period of abstinence is controversial.

Further reading

Singal, Bataller, R., Ahn, J. et al. (2018). ACG clinical guideline: alcoholic liver disease. *Am. J. Gastroenterol.* 113: 175–194.

CHAPTER 38

Autoimmune Hepatitis

Autoimmune hepatitis (AIH) can affect patients of all ages and races, and women are affected four times more often than men. The disease prevalence in the European population is approximately 1.9 per 100,000. The etiology of AIH remains poorly defined but current evidence suggests that a genetic predisposition to aberrant immunological responses is the fundamental pathogenic mechanism. Associations of HLA-DRB*301 and DRB*401 with type 1 AIH and DRB1*07, DRB1*15, and DQB1*06 with type 2 AIH suggest potential genetic components of AIH relating to immune dysregulation. AIH has been reported to be precipitated by acute viral infection, the use of interferon for hepatitis C treatment, and the use of certain drugs, such as minocycline and nitrofurantoin. The autoantibodies typically associated with AIH, antinuclear antibody (ANA) and anti-smooth muscle antibody (ASMA), are not thought to be pathogenic and are not infrequently noted in other nonautoimmune liver diseases. Perhaps the most convincing evidence in favor of the role of the immune system in the pathogenesis of AIH is the nearly complete resolution of the inflammatory response with immunosuppressive therapy.

Classification

AIH is classified into type 1 (anti-actin) and type 2 (anti-liver and kidney microsomal [LKM]). Type 1 AIH is the most common form of disease in North America, and occurs in young and older women. It is associated with a high frequency of positive ANA and ASMA. Type 2 is more common in the European population, and typically affects children and adolescents. It is associated with positive anti-LKM, and only rarely with ANA and ASMA. Progression to cirrhosis occurs in three years in 82% of patients with type 2 disease, compared to 43% with type 1 disease. Type 3 (anti-SLA) AIH is rare, and follows a clinical

Yamada's Handbook of Gastroenterology, Fourth Edition. John M. Inadomi, Renuka Bhattacharya, Joo Ha Hwang, and Cynthia Ko.

and epidemiological pattern similar to that of type 1, except that serum tests are reliably positive only for anti-soluble liver antigen (SLA), and ANAs and SMAs may be negative.

Clinical presentation

The initial symptoms of AIH can be mild and nonspecific, with fatigue, malaise, right upper quadrant abdominal pain, pruritis and arthralgias. Patients can present with secondary amenorrhea or delayed menarche. Some patients are entirely asymptomatic, and are diagnosed upon further evaluation of abnormal liver tests. The majority of patients will present with markedly abnormal liver tests, and patients may be jaundiced at the time of diagnosis. Occasionally, patients will present with fulminant liver disease and hepatic decompensation. There may be a personal or family history of other autoimmune diseases. Physical examination can reveal a spectrum of findings, from a normal exam to the presence of jaundice, ascites, and encephalopathy.

Diagnostic investigation

Patients with AIH will have elevated serum aminotransferase levels. Typically, aminotransferase levels are threefold to 10fold above normal but occasionally, levels higher than 1000 IU/l are encountered. Patients with advanced disease may present with varying degrees of hyperbilirubinemia or with symptoms of fulminant or subfulminant hepatitis. Similarly, prolongation of prothrombin time, hypoalbuminemia, thrombocyto- penia, leukopenia, and anemia may be present in patients with cirrhosis or portal hypertension. Viral testing for hepatitis A, B, and C should be performed to rule out viral infection, and serological testing for alternative causes of liver disease, such as Wilson disease, should be completed.

The key to diagnosing AIH is documenting the presence of circulating autoantibodies. Testing for ANA, ASMA, anti-LKM, SLA, and IgG levels should be performed. Patients with AIH may have other autoantibodies, including asialoglycoprotein receptor, anti-liver cytosol I, anti-actin, antineutrophil cytoplasmic antibodies, and low titers of antimitochondrial antibodies. Conversely, other chronic liver diseases may have low titers of ANA and ASMA, but titers higher than 1:320 and higher than 1:40, respectively, are unusual outside of AIH. A small group of patients with the typical clinical features of AIH have no detectable viral serological features or autoantibodies.

Liver histology

The role of liver biopsy is important in confirming the diagnosis of AIH, even though histological findings are not entirely specific. Viral hepatitis and drug-induced hepatitis may have indistinguishable histological findings. The typical histological findings in AIH include an interface hepatitis consisting of lymphoplasmacytic chronic inflammatory cells. The intrahepatic bile ducts generally appear normal. Staining for α1-antitrypsin and excess iron should be negative. In patients with a more severe presentation, bridging necrosis may be seen. It is not uncommon to find advanced histological injury, including cirrhosis, at the time of initial diagnosis and biopsy.

Diagnostic scoring systems

Several scoring systems have been proposed to aid the accurate diagnosis of AIH. The initial scoring system published in 1993 was subse- quently modified in 1999, and more recently a simplified version has been proposed. This scoring system uses results of autoantibody and immunoglobulin testing as well as liver histology to allow for a diagnosis of probable or definite AIH (Table 38.1).

Management

Patients with AIH may progress to liver failure, so AIH patients with elevated aminotransferase levels and inflammation in biopsy specimens should be treated. Immunosuppressive therapy is successful in more than 80% of patients. Therapeutic trials have shown significant survival benefit from the use of corticosteroids, with or without azathioprine. Therapy may be divided into an induction phase and a maintenance or withdrawal phase. Therapy is initiated with prednisone alone or in combination with azathioprine. Azathioprine alone is not effective for induction but can be used alone for maintenance.

Table 38.1 Diagnostic criteria for autoimmune hepatitis (AIH)

Variable	Cutoff	Points
Antinuclear antibody (ANA) or smooth muscle antibody (SMA)	≥1 : 40	1
ANA or SMA	≥1 : 80	
or liver and kidney microsomal antibody (LKM)	≥1 : 40	2[a]
or soluble liver antigen (SLA)	Positive	
IgG	>Upper normal limit	1
	>1.10 times upper normal limit	2
Liver histology (evidence of hepatitis is a necessary condition)	Compatible with AIH	1
	Typical AIH	2
Absence of viral hepatitis	Yes	2
		≥6: probable AIH
		≥7: definite AIH

Source: from Hennes et al. (2008).

[a] Addition of points achieved for all autoantibodies (maximum, two points).

Table 38.2 Suggested therapy for autoimmune hepatitis (AIH)

Initial therapy Prednisone 30–40 mg/day monotherapy or prednisone 30 mg/day and azathioprine 50–100 mg/day combined therapy
Dose reduction Slowly reduce prednisone (2.5–5 mg every 1–3 months) if alanine aminotransferase (ALT) in normal range
Maintenance Minimum-dose prednisone or azathioprine to maintain ALT in normal range
Stop therapy If ALT and immunoglobulin G (IgG) normal for 1–2 years; liver biopsy indicates inactivity
Treatment of relapse Reintroduce therapy as for initial treatment
Failure to respond To above, use either high-dose prednisone 40–60 mg/day or another immunosuppressant, or consider liver transplant if appropriate

Source: from Yamada et al. (2009).

Once remission is achieved, steroids should be tapered and discontinued if possible. Patients who do not tolerate azathioprine can try an alternative immunosuppressive agent such as mycophenolate mofetil or a calcineurin inhibitor. For patients with excessive systemic side effects related to prednisone, the use of budesonide has been shown to be effective in AIH. There is no consensus on the need to repeat a liver biopsy to establish histological improvement. Patients occasionally can be tapered completely off immunosuppressants but a significant proportion will relapse in the first few months after stopping therapy. For any patient, the risks of life-long therapy must be weighed against the risk of disease recurrence. A proposed treatment algorithm is outlined in Table 38.2.

Key practice points

- The diagnosis of AIH is based on serological and histological findings.
- Type 1 AIH is the most common in the United States, with a high frequency of positive antinuclear and anti-smooth muscle antibodies.
- Type 2 AIH typically affects children and adolescents. It is associated with positive anti-LKM and only rarely with ANA and ASMA. It is associated with a more aggressive disease course.
- Treatment of AIH is indicated for those with abnormal liver tests and significant inflammation on liver biopsy. Treatment is typically initiated with prednisone and azathioprine. For patients who fail or are intolerant to this regimen, alternative agents such as mycophenolate, cyclosporine, or tacrolimus may be used. Most patients require life-long treatment.

Further reading

Hennes, E.M., Zeniya, M., Czaja, A.J. et al. (2008). Simplified criteria for the diagnosis of autoimmune hepatitis. *Hepatology* 48 (1): 169–176.

Yamada, T., Alpers, D.H., Kalloo, A.N. et al. (eds.) (2009). *Textbook of Gastroenterology*, 5e. Oxford: Blackwell.

CHAPTER 39
Complications of Cirrhosis

Cirrhosis represents the final common pathway of many hepatic disorders characterized by chronic cellular destruction. An intervening stage of increased fibrosis is followed by the formation of parenchymal regenerative nodules. The nodular distortion of the lobules and vascular network defines cirrhosis and ultimately plays a critical role in the development of portal hypertension. A clinically relevant method of classifying cirrhosis is based on the primary disease processes responsible for hepatocellular injury (Table 39.1). In the United States, most cases of cirrhosis are related to alcoholic liver disease and chronic viral hepatitis, with a rising incidence of nonalcoholic steatohepatitis (NASH) cirrhosis. Other more common causes of cirrhosis include hereditary hemochromatosis, primary biliary cholangitis, primary sclerosing cholangitis, and autoimmune hepatitis. Several rare disorders that frequently are complicated by cirrhosis should always be considered in the differential diagnosis, including Wilson disease and α1-antitrypsin deficiency. Medications such as nitrofurantoin, amiodarone, and methotrexate may produce chronic hepatitis and cirrhosis. Cirrhosis in childhood can be caused by congenital anomalies (e.g. biliary atresia), metabolic conditions (e.g. tyrosinemia, galactosemia), α1-antitrypsin deficiency, cholestatic liver disease (e.g. total parenteral nutrition, progressive familial intrahepatic cholestasis), Wilson disease, glycogen storage disease, cystic fibrosis, and idiopathic neonatal hepatitis.

When all other causes of cirrhosis are excluded, the diagnosis is idiopathic (cryptogenic) cirrhosis. This disorder may result from an immunological or viral disease process that cannot be detected by serological assays or from "burned-out" nonalcoholic fatty liver disease (NAFLD). Cryptogenic cirrhosis may account for 10–20% of all cases with cirrhosis; it is clinically indistinguishable from other common causes.

Yamada's Handbook of Gastroenterology, Fourth Edition. John M. Inadomi, Renuka Bhattacharya, Joo Ha Hwang, and Cynthia Ko.

Table 39.1 Causes of cirrhosis

Common	Infrequent	Rare
Chronic hepatitis C	Primary biliary cirrhosis	α1-Antitrypsin deficiency
Chronic hepatitis B	Primary sclerosing	Wilson disease
Alcoholic cirrhosis	Autoimmune hepatitis	Sarcoidosis
Nonalcoholic fatty liver disease	Hemochromatosis	Cystic fibrosis

Table 39.2 Classification and differential diagnosis of portal hypertension

Prehepatic causes
Portal vein thrombosis
Splenic vein thrombosis
Arterioportal fistula
Splenomegaly
Intrahepatic causes
Cirrhosis
Fulminant hepatitis
Veno-occlusive disease
Budd–Chiari syndrome
Schitosomiasis
Metastatic malignancy
Posthepatic causes
Right ventricular failure
Constrictive pericarditis
Inferior vena cava web

Portal hypertension

Portal hypertension occurs if there is increased splanchnic flow or increased resistance in the hepatic vasculature. In cirrhosis, both mechanisms contribute to the development of portal hypertension. Nodular regeneration and fibrosis in the space of Disse increase postsinusoidal and sinusoidal resistance, respectively. Cirrhosis is also accompanied by increased splanchnic flow from decreased tone in the splanchnic arterioles. In extrahepatic causes of portal hypertension, such as portal vein thrombosis or massive splenomegaly, either increased resistance or increased flow is the principal mechanism of increased portal pressure. The anatomical site of increased flow or resistance has been used to classify portal hypertension into prehepatic, intrahepatic, and posthepatic portal hypertension (Table 39.2). Intrahepatic causes are often further subdivided into presinusoidal, sinusoidal, and postsinusoidal according to the site of increased resistance.

Clinical presentation

Although patients with early cirrhosis may be asymptomatic, cirrhosis is typified by a general decline in health with nonspecific complaints of anorexia, weight loss, malaise, fatigue, and weakness. More advanced disease may present with one of the complications of portal hypertension.

Endocrine manifestations

Patients with cirrhosis may manifest several endocrine disturbances. The prevalence of diabetes mellitus increases in all forms of cirrhosis but particularly in patients with hemochromatosis, alcoholic liver disease, or hepatitis C. Hypogonadism in males and females is also common in hemochromatosis and alcoholic liver disease, primarily because of the direct gonadal toxicities of iron and alcohol, respectively. In addition, androgenic steroids may bypass metabolism in the liver and subsequently undergo conversion in adipose tissue to the estrogenic steroid estrone. Increased plasma estrogen levels may lead to gynecomastia, telangiectasias, and palmar erythema.

Pulmonary manifestations

End-stage liver disease is often accompanied by pulmonary disorders. Chronic hyperventilation is likely caused by the same central nervous system alterations responsible for hepatic encephalopathy (HE). Patients may have hypoxemia because of mismatches of ventilation and perfusion induced by ascites, which restricts the ventilation of dependent lung spaces. The hepatopulmonary syndrome, a distinct form of right-to-left shunting with impaired gas exchange caused by intrapulmonary vascular dilation, is increasingly recognized. Portopulmonary hypertension, in contrast, is caused by pulmonary vasoconstriction, which produces markedly elevated pulmonary pressure and is a relative contraindication to liver transplantation. Patients with or without ascites may develop a transudative pleural effusion, termed *hepatic hydrothorax,* which may impair respiratory function. Hydrothorax probably develops from ascites traversing pores in the diaphragm. The onset of hepatic hydrothorax often signals rapid clinical deterioration.

Renal manifestations

Numerous disturbances of sodium and water homeostasis are observed in cirrhosis but the most devastating complication is the hepatorenal syndrome. In its most severe form, hepatorenal syndrome type I progresses to oliguric renal failure and prerenal physiology despite adequate filling pressure. It is associated with extreme intrarenal vasoconstriction that leads to sodium retention. Potential precipitants include intravascular volume depletion from hemorrhage, diuretics, or paracentesis. Alternative causes of renal failure include acute tubular necrosis caused by hypovolemia, nephrotoxic drugs, nonsteroidal anti-inflammatory agents, and radiocontrast agents. These disorders can often be distinguished from hepatorenal syndrome based on a normal or elevated urine sodium concentration. Pulmonary artery catheter placement or central venous pressure monitoring should be considered because they facilitate optimal management of volume status. Hepatorenal syndrome type 1 usually is irreversible without transplantation. A milder form, hepatorenal syndrome type 2, affects many cirrhotics and is characterized by a mildly depressed glomerular filtration rate and marked sodium and water retention refractory to diuretics.

Diagnostic investigation

Laboratory results

Coagulation profiles, complete blood counts, electrolytes, and albumin should all be obtained. Patients with pathological evidence of cirrhosis may have normal biochemical profiles; however, those with advanced cirrhosis will have a prolonged prothrombin time and a decrease in serum albumin levels because of impaired hepatic synthetic function. Protein malnutrition and vitamin K deficiency, which are particularly common in alcoholics, may also produce these abnormalities. Patients with portal hypertension may have thrombocytopenia, anemia, or leukopenia on the basis of congestive hypersplenism. Thrombocytopenia from splenic sequestration rarely is less than 30,000/μl; lower levels suggest an alternative diagnosis, such as drug-induced, immune-mediated, or disseminated intravascular coagulation-associated thrombocytopenia. In addition to splenic sequestration, anemia may result from gastrointestinal hemorrhage, nutritional deficiencies (e.g. folate, iron, or vitamin B12), or hemolysis. Hyponatremia, hypokalemia, and renal insufficiency are common complications of the altered renal hemodynamics and sodium and water homeostasis observed in cirrhosis.

An accurate determination of the cause of cirrhosis requires a serological evaluation, whose extent is largely dictated by the clinical setting. The initial screen should include serum assays for antibody to hepatitis C; hepatitis B surface antigen and antibodies to hepatitis B surface antigen and core antigen; antimitochondrial antibodies; antinuclear antibodies; anti-smooth muscle antibodies; ferritin, transferrin, total iron-binding capacity; and serum protein electrophoresis to measure the $\alpha 1$ band and γ-globulins. Patients younger than age 50 and those with a high level of clinical suspicion should be screened for Wilson disease to detect low serum ceruloplasmin. Selected patients may require specialized studies based on the preliminary results above, for example, hepatitis C viral RNA, hepatitis B DNA.

Imaging and endoscopic studies

Imaging procedures are often helpful in providing evidence of cirrhosis or portal hypertension. Ultrasound, computed tomographic (CT), and magnetic resonance imaging (MRI) studies may demonstrate lobular, heterogeneous, hepatic parenchyma or findings attributable to portal hypertension, including ascites, splenomegaly, and portosystemic collaterals. Upper gastrointestinal endoscopy permits detection of varices or portal hypertensive gastropathy but does not allow differentiation of cirrhosis from other causes of portal hypertension. MRI and CT with contrast may help exclude primary vascular causes of portal hypertension, including the hepatic vein thrombosis of Budd–Chiari syndrome and portal vein thrombosis. Patients with suspected secondary biliary cirrhosis caused by primary sclerosing cholangitis should undergo magnetic resonance cholangiopancreatography (MRCP) or endoscopic retrograde cholangiopancreatography (ERCP).

Liver biopsy

Liver biopsy is the gold standard for diagnosing cirrhosis and often provides clues to the underlying cause. Liver biopsy also can be used to quantify iron and copper if hemochromatosis or Wilson disease is in the differential diagnosis. In the setting of coagulopathy, the risk of biopsy-associated hemorrhage may outweigh the benefit of obtaining information from the biopsy specimen. A transjugular biopsy may be performed if histological confirmation is deemed critical.

Portal venous pressure measurement

Although not frequently needed in clinical practice, direct and indirect measurements of portal pressure are the definitive means of diagnosing portal hypertension. The more commonly used indirect method involves angiographic positioning of a balloon occlusion catheter in the hepatic vein and, with the balloon inflated, measuring the hepatic vein wedge pressure. Analogous to pulmonary capillary wedge pressure, the hepatic vein wedge pressure measures sinusoidal pressure and is an estimate of portal pressure. It is inaccurate if the causes of portal hypertension are presinusoidal or prehepatic because the major pressure gradient is upstream from the sinusoids. The difference between the hepatic vein wedge pressure and free hepatic vein pressure, the hepatic venous pressure gradient (HVPG), provides an estimate of the portosystemic gradient, or the pressure drop across the resistance bed of the liver. A portosystemic gradient higher than 5 mmHg is consistent with portal hypertension, and a gradient greater than 12 mmHg identifies patients at risk for variceal hemorrhage. The pressure in the portal circulation can be measured directly by a pressure transducer placed in the portal vein. This can be done through the parenchyma from the hepatic vein, similar to transjugular intrahepatic portosystemic shunt (TIPS) or transhepatic placement.

Clinical management of patients with cirrhosis is focused on control of ascites, varices and HE, and screening of hepatocellular carcinoma. The management of ascites is reviewed separately in Chapter 13, and hepatocellular carcinoma is reviewed in Chapter 40.

Management of variceal hemorrhage

Portal hypertension can lead to the formation of portosystemic collaterals. The major sites of collateral formation are through the umbilical vein, producing abdominal wall collaterals (the caput medusae); through the superior rectal vein to the middle and inferior rectal vein, producing rectal varices; and through the coronary and left gastric veins to the azygos vein, producing gastroesophageal varices. Collaterals may form in numerous other sites within the abdomen but hemorrhage from gastroesophageal varices is the primary cause of morbidity from portosystemic collaterals.

The formation of varices is closely related to portal pressure. Bleeding occurs in 25–30% of patients with varices but variables for identifying patients at high risk are less than perfect. Absolute portal pressures above the threshold of 12 mmHg do not correlate well with the risk of bleeding but the endoscopic size of varices does seem to indicate the patients at highest risk.

Primary prevention of acute variceal hemorrhage includes nonselective β-adrenergic antagonists (e.g. propranolol, nadolol, and carvedilol). β-Blocker therapy in multiple studies reduced the rate of first bleeds as well as rebleeding. These medications should be dose titrated to produce a 25% decrease in resting heart rate. Contraindications include bradycardia, hypotension, congestive heart failure, reactive airway disease, and peripheral vascular disease. For large varices, endoscopic band ligation can be used for primary prophylaxis and reduces the rate of initial variceal bleeding.

Acute variceal hemorrhage from esophageal or gastric varices is a medical emergency. Patients should be managed in intensive care; volume resuscitation and optimizing the hemodynamic status are the first priorities. Nonvariceal hemorrhage may account for up to 50% of gastrointestinal bleeding in patients with known cirrhosis. Therefore, early upper gastrointestinal endoscopy is needed to confirm the source of bleeding. Endoscopic band ligation has replaced sclerotherapy as the first-line treatment for endoscopic management of gastroesophageal varices. Band ligation has superior efficacy with fewer side effects. Injection sclerotherapy of varices is occasionally used for acute variceal bleeding that is difficult to control, particularly if extensive bleeding impairs visualization and makes banding difficult. Complications of sclerotherapy include esophageal ulceration, pneumonia, and bacteremia. Combination therapy with banding and sclerotherapy does not have higher rates of efficacy than either technique alone and has more complications. Continuous infusion of the somatostatin analog octreotide (25–50 mcg/hour for 24–48 hours) reduces splanchnic blood flow by inhibiting the vasodilating hormones (e.g. glucagon) and lowers portal pressure. It does not cause systemic vasoconstriction and thus is safer than vasopressin. If portal hypertensive bleeding is suspected, therapy should be started immediately and continued for 72 hours. Continuous infusion of vasopressin (0.1–0.4 U/minute) may also control acute hemorrhage but 50% of patients fail to respond and side-effects of systemic vasoconstriction, including myocardial and cerebral ischemia, are common. Vasopressin therapy should be limited to less than 24–48 hours.

If bleeding persists despite the above measures, balloon tamponade may be required. Balloon tamponade is 90% effective in stopping variceal hemorrhage but it is only a temporizing measure, usually while awaiting placement of a TIPS. Adverse effects are common and include esophageal rupture and aspiration. Tamponade should never be continued for longer than 24–36 hours and should be limited to inflating the gastric balloon whenever possible. Endotracheal intubation should be performed before balloon insertion to prevent airway compromise. In refractory or recurrent variceal hemorrhage, portosystemic shunting should be considered by using TIPS or a surgically created shunt. Although both procedures are highly effective in controlling hemorrhage, encephalopathy results in 10–20% of patients. The lower morbidity and less invasive nature of TIPS make it the logical choice in this setting. After acute variceal bleeding has been stopped, secondary prophylactic interventions lower the risk of rebleeding. The preferred therapy is endoscopic band ligation. Complete obliteration of varices is the goal, and several sessions separated by approximately two weeks are often required. Pharmacotherapy with the nonselective β-adrenergic antagonists alone also reduces the rate of rebleeding but does not improve survival. Combination therapy with serial banding and β-adrenergic antagonists is the most effective means to prevent recurrent bleeding.

Transjugular intrahepatic portosystemic shunt has added a new dimension to therapies for secondary prophylaxis of variceal bleeding. Although TIPS clearly has a role in patients with hemorrhage refractory to endoscopic therapy, its role in secondary prophylaxis remains to be established. Reports suggest that TIPS improves rebleeding rates compared with endoscopic therapy but risks of encephalopathy have generally limited the applicability of TIPS to failure of endoscopic therapy with rebleeding.

Current American Association for the Study of Liver Diseases (AASLD) guidelines for primary and secondary prophylaxis of variceal bleeding are outlined in Figure 39.1.

Management of Hepatic Encephalopathy

The mechanism for developing HE in severe liver disease remains ill defined. Possible explanations include decreased clearance of gut-derived neurotoxins, including ammonia; disturbances of central neurotransmission resulting from an accumulation of false neurotransmitters that activate γ-aminobutyric acid receptors or catecholamines; and accumulation of glutamate in astrocytes. None of these explanations is satisfactory. Although serum ammonia is often elevated in HE, some patients have normal ammonia levels.

Management of Patients With Moderate/Large Varices That Have Not Bled

Therapy	Recommended Dose	Therapy Goals	Maintenance/Follow-up
Propranolol	• 20-40 mg orally *twice* a day • Adjust every 2-3 days until treatment goal is achieved • Maximal daily dose: ◦ 320 mg/day in patients without ascites ◦ 160 mg/day in patients with ascites	• Resting heart rate of 55-60 beats per minute • Systolic blood pressure should not decrease <90 mmHg	• At every outpatient visit make sure that heart rate is on target • Continue indefinitely • No need for follow-up EGD
Nadolol	• 20-40 mg orally *once* a day • Adjust every 2-3 days until treatment goal is achieved • Maximal daily dose: ◦ 160 mg/day in patients without ascites ◦ 80 mg/day in patients with ascites	• Resting heart rate of 55-60 beats per minute • Systolic blood pressure should not decrease <90 mmHg	• At every outpatient visit make sure that heart rate is on target • Continue indefinitely • No need for follow-up EGD
Carvedilol	• Start with 6.25 mg *once* a day • After 3 days increase to 6.5 mg twice daily • Maximal dose: 12.5 mg/day (except in patients with persistent arterial hypertension)	• Systolic arterial blood pressure should not decrease <90 mmHg	• Continue indefinitely • No need for follow-up EGD
EVL	• Every 2-8 weeks until the eradication of varices	• Variceal eradication (no further ligation possible)	• First EGD performed 3-6 months after eradication and every 6-12 months thereafter

Any of these four therapies can be used, but current data do not support the use of combination therapy.

Treatments for the Prevention of Recurrent Esophageal Variceal Hemorrhage

Therapy	Recommended Dose	Therapy Goals	Maintenance/Follow-up
Propranolol	• 20-40 mg orally *twice* a day • Adjust every 2-3 days until treatment goal is achieved • Maximal daily dose: ◦ 320 mg/day in patients without ascites ◦ 160 mg/day in patients with ascites	• Resting heart rate of 55-60 beats per minute • Systolic blood pressure should not decrease <90 mmHg	• At every outpatient visit make sure that heart rate is on target • Continue indefinitely
Nadolol	• 20-40 mg orally *once* a day • Adjust every 2-3 days until treatment goal is achieved • Maximal daily dose: ◦ 160 mg/day in patients without ascites ◦ 80 mg/day in patients with ascites	• Resting heart rate of 55-60 beats per minute • Systolic blood pressure should not decrease <90 mmHg	• At every outpatient visit make sure that heart rate is on target • Continue indefinitely
EVL	• Every 1-4 weeks until the eradication of varices	• Variceal eradication (no further ligation possible)	• First EGD performed 3-6 months after eradication and every 6-12 months thereafter

The combination of either propranolol or nadolol *plus* EVL is recommended. Carvedilol is not recommended in this setting.

Figure 39.1 AASLD practice guidance. EGD, esophagogastroduodenoscopy. (Source: Garcia Tsao et al. 2017.)

HE is often graded according to the patient's level of consciousness, using indexes such as the West Haven criteria and the Glasgow Coma Scale. *Minimal HE*, previously called *subclinical*, can be measured by Reitan trail testing, neuropsychiatric testing, electroencephalography, or evoked potentials. Imaging of the brain has little diagnostic yield but may be more important to exclude other causes, such as intracranial hemorrhage in an alcoholic patient with coagulopathy.

New-onset HE or acute decompensation of chronic HE should always prompt a search for precipitating causes. Common causes include gastrointestinal hemorrhage, psychotropic medications (in particular benzodiazepines), electrolyte and fluid disturbances, infection, new-onset renal insufficiency, constipation, and medical or dietary noncompliance. In addition to providing specific therapy for HE, the clinician should always attempt to correct the precipitating factors.

Because many of the responsible neurotoxins appear to be produced by intestinal flora, therapy is directed at altering the colonic microenvironment. Lactulose, titrated to produce two to three soft stools per day, is the first-line therapy. It promotes catharsis and lowers intraluminal pH to decrease ammonia absorption. It can cause flatulence and bloating; higher doses cause diarrhea, with possible fluid and electrolyte disturbances. Rifaximin is a minimally absorbed enteric antibiotic that is approved by the Food and Drug Administration for treatment of HE. It has been shown in studies to reduce the risk of overt HE recurrence and may reduce HE-related hospitalizations. The antibiotics metronidazole or neomycin also may be added to treat refractory HE but generally are second-line agents because of side-effects, including nephrotoxicity with neomycin and neuropathy with metronidazole. Other agents being studied include benzoate, L-ornithine-L-aspartate, branched-chain amino acids, levodopa, and bromocriptine.

Severe restriction of dietary protein is no longer recommended as a means of preventing encephalopathy in cirrhotic patients, as long-term nitrogen restriction is potentially harmful. Protein intake of 1–2 g/kg/day is generally recommended.

Orthotopic liver transplantation

The decision to perform orthotopic liver transplantation depends mostly on the expected survival of the patient with end-stage liver disease. Several prognostic indicators have been developed, including the Child–Turcotte–Pugh classification (Table 39.3) and the Model for End-Stage Liver Disease (MELD). MELD is a mathematical model based on log-transformed serum bilirubin, serum creatinine, and the international normalized ratio (INR) for prothrombin time. It predicts three-month mortality more accurately than a Child–Turcotte–Pugh score and is now used to prioritize candidates for transplantation. The benefit of orthotopic liver transplantation for any person must also account for the individual's clinical complications such as spontaneous bacterial peritonitis, intractable ascites, refractory encephalopathy, recurrent variceal bleeding, or debilitating fatigue.

Pretransplant evaluation should include an assessment for contraindications and an evaluation of factors that may complicate the posttransplant period. Absolute contraindications include active ethanol or substance abuse, extrahepatic or metastatic malignancy, untreated sepsis, and severe cardiopulmonary

Table 39.3 Child–Turcotte–Pugh classification system

Prothrombin time	Bilirubin	Albumin	Ascites	Encephalopathy	Score
0–4 sec above control	0–2.0 mg/dl	>3.5 mg/dl	Absent	Absent	1
4–6 sec above control	2.0–3.0 mg/dl	2.8–3.5 mg/dl	Nontense	Grade I–II	2
>6 sec above control	>3.0 mg/dl	0–2.8 mg/dl	Tense	Grade III-IV	3

Class A = 5–6 points; class B = 7–9 points; class C = 10–15 points.

disease. Relative contraindications include previous malignancy and poor social support. Chronological age is not a contraindication but patients significantly older than 70 are acceptable candidates for orthotopic liver transplantation only if there are no other comorbidities. The evaluation usually includes ultrasound with Doppler examination, cardiac stress testing, contrast-enhanced (bubble) echocardiography, serological testing for herpes viruses (e.g. cytomegalovirus, herpes simplex virus, and varicella zoster virus), serum α-fetoprotein, and tuberculosis skin testing. Women require a Papanicolaou smear. Women older than 40 years should undergo mammography, and all patients older than 50 should have screening colonoscopies.

Investigation of a patient's social support system is critical and requires the input of a trained social worker. Psychiatric consultation should be sought for patients with prior substance or alcohol abuse. Dental evaluation may be necessary. The complex decision to approve a patient for orthotopic liver transplantation requires the input of several disciplines. This multidisciplinary approach should consider the medical and social implications of transplantation as well as the limited availability of donor organs and the long pretransplant waiting period.

Key practice points

- Cirrhosis is the common endpoint of multiple liver diseases and is the result of progressive fibrosis leading to nodular distortion of the liver.
- Portal hypertension results from increased splanchnic flow and increased resistance to flow (at the level of the sinusoid and/or pre- or postsinusoidal).
- Numerous complications can develop in patients with cirrhosis and portal hypertension, including variceal bleeding, HE, ascites, and hepatocellular carcinoma. More rare complications include hepatic hydrothorax, hepatopulmonary syndrome, and portopulmonary hypertension.
- Liver transplant should be considered for patients with poor expected survival and no significant contraindications based on multidisciplinary evaluation.

Further reading

Garcia-Tsao, G., Abraldes, J.G., Berzigotti, A., and Bosch, J. (2017). AASLD practice guidance: Portal hypertensive bleeding in cirrhosis. *Hepatology* 65: 310–335.

CHAPTER 40
Primary Hepatic Neoplasms

The liver is a frequent site of metastasic disease from extrahepatic neoplasms, due to its rich blood supply and inflow from the mesenteric vasculature. Primary hepatic neoplasms, arising from hepatocytes (hepatocellular carcinoma [HCC]) and cholangiocytes (cholangiocarcinoma) are also increasingly common tumors.

Hepatocellular Carcinoma

HCC is the fifth most common cancer and the third leading cause of cancer deaths worldwide. While all forms of cirrhosis are associated with an increased risk of HCC, the risk is particularly high in patients with cirrhosis secondary to chronic viral infection, and in hepatitis B-infected patients even in the absence of cirrhosis. In the United States, there has been a well-documented rise in the number of HCC cases over the past decade. This recent increase in incidence has been attributed to chronic hepatitis C infection as well as the rising prevalence of cirrhosis due to nonalcoholic steatohepatitis (NASH).

Clinical presentation

Ninety percent of patients with HCC have superimposed cirrhosis, and many of the presenting signs and symptoms are often mistakenly attributed to coexisting cirrhosis. Nonspecific symptoms of fatigue, anorexia, weight loss, and jaundice are common. Patients may complain of right upper quadrant pain or increasing abdominal girth. HCC may cause well-compensated cirrhosis to become decompensated, with progressive ascites, encephalopathy, jaundice, or hemorrhage. Invasion of the portal and, less commonly, hepatic veins can greatly worsen portal hypertension that leads to refractory ascites or variceal bleeding. HCC should be suspected in all new cases of portal vein thrombosis. Patients can occasionally exhibit paraneoplastic phenomena, such as fever and hypercalcemia. Rarely, patients will present with hemoperitoneum due to tumor rupture, which

Yamada's Handbook of Gastroenterology, Fourth Edition. John M. Inadomi, Renuka Bhattacharya, Joo Ha Hwang, and Cynthia Ko.

requires urgent angiography for embolization. On physical examination, an abdominal mass may be palpable, and a bruit related to arterioportal shunting may be heard.

Diagnostic investigation

Laboratory studies

Aminotransferase levels are often mildly elevated but can be normal. Alkaline phosphatase may be elevated in infiltrative tumor or if there is biliary obstruction due to malignancy. In advanced tumors, serum bilirubin may be markedly elevated. Paraneoplastic hypercalcemia and erythrocytosis have been observed. The tumor marker most often associated with hepatocellular carcinoma is α-fetoprotein (AFP), which is a glycosylated protein expressed in proliferating hepatocytes. Although chronic hepatitis and cirrhosis may be associated with levels in the hundreds, levels higher than 400 ng/ml are likely to be caused by HCC. An AFP level higher than 1000 ng/ml associated with a liver mass is diagnostic of HCC. Unfortunately, AFP is elevated in only 60–70% of patients with HCC and may be only mildly elevated in certain tumors, which compromises the ability of AFP to serve as a screening test for early HCC.

Imaging studies

Imaging studies are the mainstay of screening for HCC, which is recommended for all patients with cirrhosis and many hepatitis B patients without cirrhosis. Screening guidelines proposed by the American Association for the Study of Liver Diseases (AASLD) are outlined in Figure 40.1. The difficulty in imaging the cirrhotic liver is to distinguish macroregenerative nodules, also known as *dysplastic nodules*, from HCC. The distinguishing feature of HCC is increased arterial vascularity, which results in enhancement on the arterial phase of CT or MRI imaging, compared with the surrounding normal liver, and "washout" of contrast from the lesion on the portal venous and delayed phases, unlike the surrounding liver tissue (Figure 40.2). For lesions >2 cm in size, this enhancement pattern is associated with a 98% specificity for the diagnosis of HCC, and liver biopsy is not required.

Management

The safety, tolerability, and outcome of HCC treatment is dependent on the severity of the underlying liver disease, tumor characteristics such as size and vascular invasion, the patient's performance status, and the efficacy of the treatment intervention

Surgical resection

Resection of HCC is limited to patients with Child A cirrhosis with localized disease. Patients with signficant liver dysfunction and/or portal hypertension (hepatic venous pressure gradient >10 mmHg) are unlikely to tolerate a liver

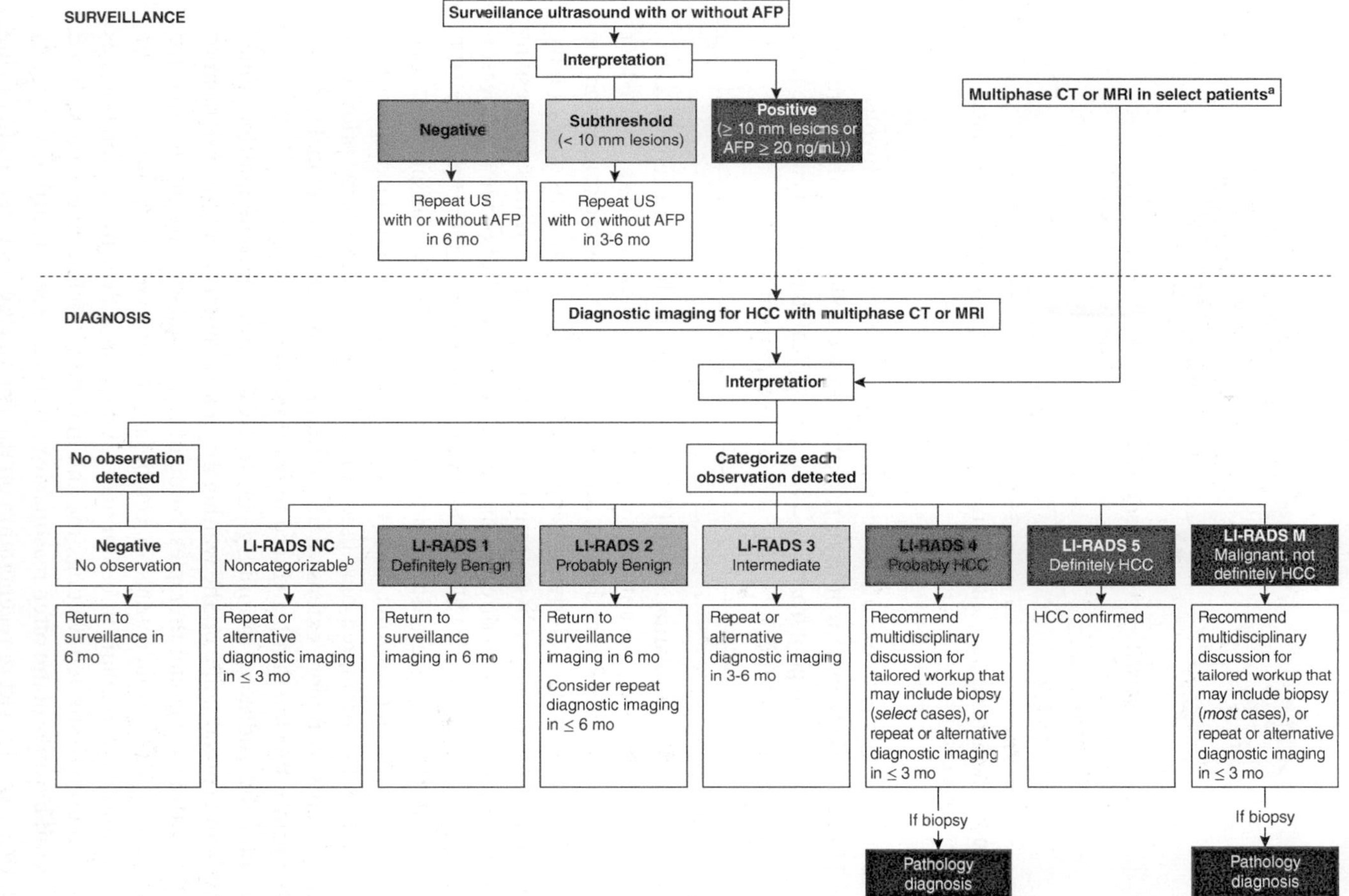

Figure 40.1 AASLD surveillance and diagnostic algorithm. AFP, α-fetoprotein; CT, computed tomography; HCC, hepatocellular carcinoma; MRI, magnetic resonance imaging; US, ultrasound. (Source: Marrero et al. 2018.)

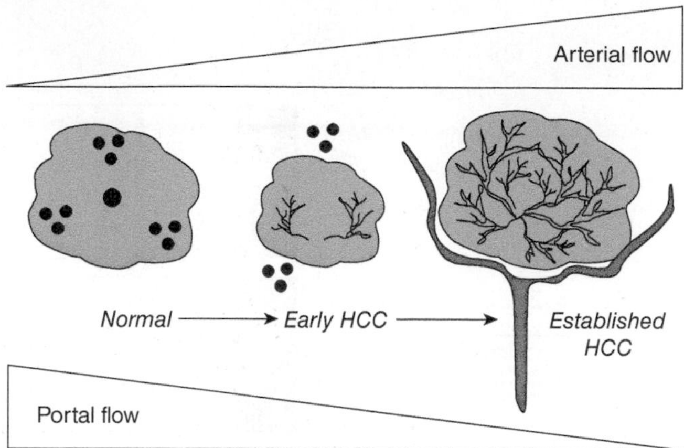

Figure 40.2 Schematic representation of arterialization during hepatocellular carcinoma (HCC) development.

resection. Patients with extrahepatic tumor spread or diffuse liver involvement by HCC are unlikely to benefit from resection. Resectability rates, therefore, are typically very low, ranging from 5 to 20%. The typical five-year recurrence rates after resection are around 50%, due to new or recurrent tumors.

Liver transplant

Orthotopic liver transplantation (OLT) for patients with hepatocellular carcinoma offers significant advantages over partial hepatectomy. It can be used for patients with advanced liver disease, and it removes the existing cancer and the diseased liver with its underlying neoplastic potential. Numerous studies have shown excellent results of liver transplantation for patients with single lesions smaller than 5 cm or up to three lesions, each 3 cm or smaller (stage I–II disease). Patients who meet these "Milan" criteria are given additional priority for OLT. Other studies have suggested that larger tumors can also be transplanted, such as the University of California, San Francisco (UCSF) criteria that extend to 8 cm of HCC. This has prompted new guidelines allowing for transplant priority for select patients with more extensive tumor that responds to locoregional therapy, with a tumor burden that is reduced to within Milan criteria.

Despite the additional priority given to HCC, with the potential for tumor growth and spread while on the waiting list, many centers treat the lesions prior to OLT with locoregional therapies. None of these therapies has been subjected to randomized controlled trials in combination with OLT and, therefore, the optimal approach remains to be defined. Living donor liver transplantation has also been used to shorten waiting time and may be an optimal use of the reduced sized graft because of the often reasonably preserved hepatic function in patients with HCC. The impact of regeneration on the risk of HCC recurrence after living donor liver transplantation remains controversial.

Locoregional therapy

Percutaneous ethanol injection

Percutaneous ethanol injection (PEI) is widely accepted as a form of therapy for small (<3 cm), discrete HCC lesions. The advantage of PEI is its relatively simple technique and low cost. PEI can be performed even for patients with advanced liver disease. Larger lesions may require several rounds of therapy, and the extent of necrosis achieved is dependent on the tumor size. Survival data have been reported but there have been no prospective, randomized controlled trials comparing PEI to other therapies.

Radiofrequency ablation

Radiofrequency ablation (RFA) is emerging as a preferred therapeutic option in the management of HCC. RFA destroys tissue by thermal energy. It is typically performed via the percutaneous approach with ultrasound guidance. RFA can be done via a laparoscopic approach if necessary, due to tumor location or proximity to structures such as diaphragm or colon. Large blood vessels act as a heat sink and thereby reduce the effectiveness of RFA for tumors adjacent to large veins. The accumulating data regarding RFA suggest that it may be equivalent to surgical resection for small tumors.

Transarterial chemoembolization

Transarterial chemoembolization (TACE) is a technique that uses angiography to selectively embolize the arterial supply of an HCC. A cytotoxic agent, such as doxorubicin, is injected into the feeding artery of the tumor, either as a suspension or adhered to drug-eluting beads. This results in both selective ischemic and chemotherapeutic effects on the HCC. The value of TACE as a palliative measure has been established in trials demonstrating survival benefit over untreated controls. The risks of TACE include arterial pseudoaneurysm formation, worsening liver function tests, hepatic abscess, and ischemic cholangiopathy/cholecystitis. The technique cannot be used if there is significant portal venous thrombosis.

Transaterial radioembolization

Transaterial radioembolization (TARE) is similar to TACE, with radiolabeled particles infused via the hepatic artery into the HCC. The embolic load of radioembolization microspheres is small, and therefore does not occlude the vasculature as in TACE. TARE can therefore be administered to patients with portal venous thrombosis. There are risks of radiation injury to the lungs or gastrointestinal tract, therefore a planning angiogram is necessary during which any hepatic artery branches that supply the stomach and duodenum are occluded, and the degree of shunt to the lungs is measured. TARE may provide superiority in downstaging patients to resection, RFA, or transplantation.

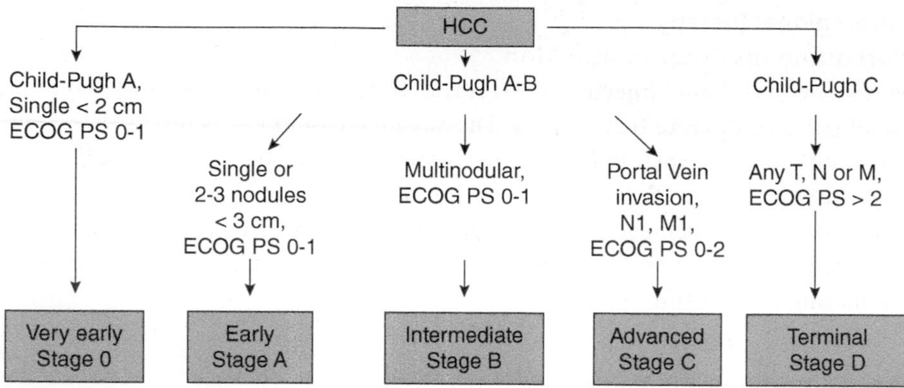

Figure 40.3 Barcelona Clinic Liver Cancer hepatocellular carcinoma staging system. N, nodal metastasis; M, extrahepatic metastasis. (Source: Marrero et al. 2018.)

Systemic therapy

HCC is typically refractory to currently available cytotoxic therapies, with overall response rates <20%. Further, systemic chemotherapy is often poorly tolerated in patients with advanced liver disease. Recent advances in understanding of the molecular pathogenesis of HCC have led to potential treatment targets, including tyrosine kinase signaling pathways and their down- stream proangiogenic pathways mediated by vascular endothelial growth factor (VEGF). The tyrosine kinase inhibitor sorafenib has shown modest survival benefit in patients with advanced HCC. Large studies have been completed in patients with Child–Turcott–Pugh Class A disease, and the safety and tolerability of the drug are being evaluated for those with more advanced liver disease. It is recommended for those with Barcelona Clinic Liver Cancer (BCLC) stage C disease. The BCLC staging and treatment system has become widely accepted into clinic practice (Figure 40.3). There have been more recent advances in systemic treatment options for HCC, including approval by the US Food and Drug Administration (FDA) of lenvatinib, a multiple kinase inhibitor against the VEGFR1, VEGFR2, and VEGFR3 kinases, and the PD1 inhibitors nivolimab and pembrolizumab.

Cholangiocarcinoma

Cholangiocarcinoma is an aggressive malignancy that arises from the epithelial cells of the bile duct. It can involve the intrahepatic or extrahepatic bile ducts and often leads to biliary obstruction.

Clinical presentation

Nonspecific symptoms of anorexia and weight loss are common in patients with cholangiocarcinoma. Jaundice develops if the extrahepatic ducts become obstructed. Pain and cholangitis are not typical symptoms unless the patient has had prior surgery or superimposed choledocholithiasis. Fifty percent of extrahepatic tumors involve the hilum of the right and left hepatic ducts (i.e. Klatskin tumor), and the other 50% involve the common hepatic duct or common bile duct. Ten percent of tumors spread diffusely throughout the biliary tract and may mimic PSC. Bile duct tumors tend to invade locally, and patients generally do not present with widely metastatic disease.

Diagnostic investigation

Initially, ultrasound should be used to evaluate patients suspected of having bile duct tumors. Intrahepatic bile duct dilation with no evidence of extrahepatic dilation suggests an extrahepatic bile duct tumor. A CT scan is more accurate in defining distal common bile duct lesions and is more sensitive than ultrasound in detecting intrahepatic lesions. The definitive imaging procedure is cholangiography by percutaneous transhepatic cholangiography (PTC) or endoscopic retrograde cholangiopancreatography (ERCP). Contrast-enhanced CT, angiography, and magnetic resonance imaging can define vascular invasion.

Histological confirmation of malignancy can be obtained by transhepatic or endoscopic cytological brushings. These tests have sensitivities of only 30–50% but show specificities approaching 100%. Because of this, cytology is useful if results are positive but of little value if negative. The addition of forceps biopsy to cytological testing increases the diagnostic yield to 70%. Many tumors are well differentiated and occur in PSC, making diagnosis very difficult without surgical resection.

Management

Surgical resection is the best option for long-term survival. At diagnosis, 20–30% of proximal duct tumors and 60–70% of distal duct tumors are resectable. Involvement of both the right and left hepatic lobes or invasion of the portal vein or hepatic artery indicates unresectability. The median survival time for patients who successfully undergo resection with tumor-free margins is three years, compared with one year for patients who have unresectable tumors.

Jaundiced patients with unresectable tumors should be considered for palliative biliary-enteric anastomosis. If the patient is a poor operative candidate, placement of a biliary stent during ERCP or PTC usually provides adequate drainage. Radiation therapy may also palliate symptoms and improve survival. Liver transplantation prolongs survival but the high incidence of recurrent disease in these patients suggests that transplantation should be limited to a highly select subset of patients. Liver transplant following an extensive neoadjuvant chemoradiation protocol is now offered at a number of transplant centers for patients meeting strict inclusion criteria.

Key practice points

- HCC is a leading cause of cancer deaths worldwide.
- Primary risk factors are cirrhosis of any cause and hepatitis B even in the absence of cirrhosis.
- The diagnosis depends largely on imaging characteristics that reflect the increased arterial vascularity of the tumor. Liver biopsy is often not required for diagnosis.
- Treatment modalities for HCC include surgical resection, transplantation, various locoregional therapies (TACE, transarterial radioembolization, RFA, PEI) and chemotherapy.
- Cholangiocarcinoma is an aggressive malignancy with limited treatment options. Liver transplant is an option only for a small subset of patients meeting restrictive criteria following a course of chemoradiation.

Further reading

Marrero, J.A., Kulik, L.M., Sirlin, C.B. et al. (2018). Diagnosis, staging, and management of hepatocellular carcinoma: 2018 practice guidance by the American Association for the Study of Liver Diseases. *Hepatology* 68: 723–750.

CHAPTER 41
Infections of the Gastrointestinal Tract

Bacterial and viral infections of the large and small intestine cause disease by direct destruction of intestinal epithelial cells or mediated by toxin production. Ingestion of food or water contaminated with pathogens accounts for most cases. An estimated 76 million cases of food-borne disease occur per year in the United States, accounting for 325,000 hospitalizations and 5000 deaths. The most common bacterial and viral pathogens of the gastrointestinal tract are reviewed below.

Bacterial infections of the gastrointestinal tract

Infection with *Campylobacter* Species

Campylobacter species (*Campylobacter jejuni* and *Campylobacter coli*) are the most common cause of bacterial diarrhea in the United States. The Centers for Disease Control and Prevention estimate that *Campylobacter* is responsible for two million illnesses per year. Seasonal variation of infection exists and the peak incidence is during the summer. The organism is transmitted by ingesting contaminated poultry, unpasteurized milk, or contaminated water, or by exposure to infected pets. Children younger than five years are most susceptible to infections caused by *Campylobacter*.

Clinical presentation

The incubation period of *Campylobacter* is 18 hours to 8 days. A prodrome of fever, headache, malaise, and myalgia may precede symptoms of watery and bloody diarrhea with abdominal pain. Other reported symptoms include nausea, vomiting, and weight loss. Although the disease usually resolves within one week, some patients experience a relapsing course similar to ulcerative colitis. Physical examination may reveal localized tenderness suggestive of appendicitis. Complications of infections with *Campylobacter* species include bacteremia,

Yamada's Handbook of Gastroenterology, Fourth Edition. John M. Inadomi, Renuka Bhattacharya, Joo Ha Hwang, and Cynthia Ko.

hemorrhage, toxic megacolon, Reiter syndrome, erythema nodosum, urticaria, cholecystitis, pancreatitis, abortion, Guillain–Barré syndrome, and hemolytic uremic syndrome.

Diagnostic investigation

Laboratory studies may show evidence of volume depletion and peripheral leukocytosis. Stool examination usually reveals leukocytes and erythrocytes. The diagnosis is confirmed by positive stool cultures. Rapid detection methods that use DNA probes and polymerase chain reaction (PCR) have been developed.

Management

The mainstay of therapy for infections with *Campylobacter* species is fluid and electrolyte replacement. By the time a diagnosis is confirmed, most patients will have experienced a decrease in their symptoms, obviating the need for treatment. For severe dysentery, relapsing symptoms, systemic infection, or immunosuppression, antibiotic therapy can effectively eradicate the organism. Erythromycin (500 mg, twice daily, or 250 mg, four times daily, for five days) is efficacious but there is no evidence that the antibiotics reduce the duration or severity of symptoms. Ciprofloxacin is an alternative choice but quinolone-resistant strains are frequent. Azithromycin (500 mg daily for three days) is effective in areas of quinolone resistance. Adding an aminoglycoside is recommended for cases of systemic infection.

Infection with *Shigella* Species

About 15,000 cases of shigellosis occur annually in the United States. Most infections (69%) occur in children younger than five years. The organism is transmitted by the fecal–oral route, via infected food or water, or in chronic care facilities, day-care centers, and nursing homes. Shigellosis is highly contagious, requiring only small inoculums (180 organisms) to establish infection. Ninety percent of infections occur from *Shigella sonnei* or *Shigella flexneri*, although *Shigella dysenteriae* has been associated with pandemic disease.

Clinical presentation

Shigella infection is characterized by the acute onset of bloody diarrhea with mucus, accompanied by fever and abdominal pain. After a one to three-day incubation period, symptomatic disease generally persists for five to seven days in adults and two to three days in children. The illness may have two phases: an initial small bowel phase of severe watery diarrhea, followed by a dysenteric phase with smaller volumes of blood-tinged mucus or blood clots. Symptoms may be severe in malnourished children or debilitated adults, whereas some healthy individuals may note only mild diarrhea. Physical examination may reveal lower abdominal tenderness with normal or increased bowel sounds. Dehydration may occur in some cases but peritoneal findings are rare and should suggest other diagnoses. The infection most severely affects the rectosigmoid colon but 15% of cases exhibit pan-colitis.

Complications of *Shigella* infection include bacteremia, Reiter syndrome, and the hemolytic uremic syndrome. Bacteremia has a 20% mortality rate as a result of renal failure, hemolysis, thrombocytopenia, gastrointestinal hemorrhage, and shock. Reiter syndrome, a triad of arthritis, urethritis, and conjunctivitis, occurs most commonly in men between ages 20 and 40 and presents two to four weeks after infection with *Shigella* species (or certain strains of *Salmonella*, *Yersinia*, or *Campylobacter*). Eighty percent of patients who develop Reiter syndrome are HLA-B27 positive. The arthritic manifestations, which are distributed asymmetrically, often are chronic and relapsing and require management with nonsteroidal anti-inflammatory drugs (NSAIDs). Although hemolytic uremic syndrome is most often associated with enterohemorrhagic *Escherichia coli* (EHEC) infection, it may complicate infections with *Shigella*. The syndrome is characterized by microangiopathic hemolytic anemia, thrombocytopenia, and renal failure. It has been postulated that hemolytic uremic syndrome results from the systemic effects of Shiga toxin. The syndrome has a mortality rate of less than 10%.

Diagnostic investigation

Examination of stool will identify leukocytes and erythrocytes. The laboratory diagnosis of infection with *Shigella* species is made by identification in stool culture.

Management

Antibiotics reduce the duration and severity of symptoms in shigellosis, shorten the period of fecal excretion of the organism, and are recommended for all patients with diarrhea, except those with mild symptoms. Ciprofloxacin is the drug of choice, or azithromycin in cases of fluoroquinolone resistance. As for other diarrheal illness, oral or intravenous rehydration should be administered. Antidiarrheal agents are contraindicated because they may prolong symptoms and delay clearance of the organism.

Infection with *E. Coli*

Most strains of *E. coli* do not produce gastrointestinal disease. However, four clinically and epidemiologically distinct syndromes are associated with *E. coli*: enterotoxigenic, enteropathogenic, enteroinvasive, and enterohemorrhagic infections. Enterotoxigenic and enteropathogenic *E. coli* infections affect the small intestine, while enteroinvasive and enterohemorrhagic infections primarily affect the colon.

Enterotoxigenic *E. coli*

Enterotoxigenic *Escherichia coli* (ETEC) causes disease by producing a heat-labile toxin and two heat-stable toxins. The heat-labile toxin increases cAMP levels, leading to chloride secretion and secretory diarrhea. One of the heat-stable toxins activates guanylate cyclase. Disease occurs in the absence of invasion or damage to intestinal epithelial cells. ETEC is a major cause of diarrhea in children in developing countries and accounts for most cases of traveler's diarrhea resulting from ingesting food contaminated by human waste.

Patients with ETEC present with watery diarrhea, abdominal cramping or pain, headache, arthralgias, myalgias, vomiting, and low-grade fever. The period of illness is generally two to five days. Less than 10% of patients complain of symptoms for more than one week. Dehydration is severe only in the very young or very old. Fluid and electrolyte replacement are emphasized. Therapy includes trimethoprim-sulfamethoxazole (double strength [DS] twice daily for three days), fluoroquinolone twice daily for three days (ciprofloxacin 500 mg, norfloxacin 400 mg, ofloxacin 300 mg), or ciprofloxacin (one 750 mg dose). Prophylaxis with bismuth subsalicylate, two 262 mg tablets four times daily, is more than 60% effective in preventing illness. Probiotic prophylaxis using *Lactobacillus* species also may be efficacious. Vaccine trials have met with variable success.

Enteropathogenic *E. coli*

Enteropathogenic *Escherichia coli* (EPEC) produces disease as a result of its ability to adhere to the epithelial cell and destroy microvilli. It is an endemic pathogen with fecal–oral transmission and affects primarily infants and children younger than two years. Older children and adults may serve as reservoirs for this illness. Patients with EPEC present with profuse watery diarrhea and associated symptoms of vomiting, fever, failure to thrive, metabolic acidosis, and possibly life-threatening dehydration. The diagnosis is by stool culture with serotyping, documentation of tissue culture adherence, or detecting the adherence factor by DNA probe techniques. Therapy relies on fluid and electrolyte replacement, as the illness is usually self-limited.

Enteroinvasive *E. coli*

Enteroinvasive *Escherichia coli* (EIEC) is a rare cause of traveler's diarrhea. The pathogenesis initiates with attachment and invasion of colonocytes by the organism, which proliferates within cells and finally destroys the host cell. EIEC possesses a virulence plasmid identical to that possessed by *Shigella*. The clinical presentation of EIEC includes fever, malaise, anorexia, abdominal cramps, and watery diarrhea, followed by passage of blood-tinged stool or mucus. Fecal blood and leukocytes are present in many but not all patients. Laboratory confirmation of EIEC in clinical practice requires serotyping *E. coli* O and H antigens. The disease usually is self-limited and uncomplicated.

Treatment should concentrate on fluid and electrolyte replacement. The role of antibiotic therapy in EIEC infection is undefined but it is reasonable to give patients with dysentery a five-day course of either trimethoprim-sulfamethoxazole (160 mg/800 mg, twice daily), ampicillin (500 mg, four times/day), or ciprofloxacin (500 mg, twice daily).

Enterohemorrhagic *E. coli*

Infection with EHEC is caused by the O157:H7 strain, which is transmitted to humans in poorly cooked ground beef, unpasteurized dairy products or fruit juices, and fecally contaminated water. The highest incidence of infection occurs in children younger than five years, although elderly patients are also affected. Outbreaks are clustered in schools, day-care centers, and nursing homes. Factors that enhance EHEC virulence include adhesins that provide attachment to host cells, plasmid-encoded hemolysin, and two Shiga-like toxins that cause damage through thrombus formation and vasculitis leading to ischemia and hemorrhage. After an incubation of three to nine days, EHEC-associated hemorrhagic colitis manifests watery diarrhea and abdominal cramping pain, followed by bloody diarrhea two to five days later. The severity of blood loss ranges from blood-tinged mucus to passage of large clots. Vomiting is present in three-quarters of patients, whereas fever is generally absent.

Complications of infection with EHEC include hemolytic uremic syndrome and intestinal hematoma causing intestinal obstruction, rhabdomyolysis, and pancreatic necrosis with subsequent development of diabetes mellitus. Fecal leukocytes are typically not present. *E. coli* O157:H7 can be identified by culturing on sorbitol-MacConkey medium and agglutination with O157 and H7 antiserum.

The most important goal of treatment is replacement of fluid and electrolytes. Recovery without sequelae is the usual outcome, although patients with hemolytic uremic syndrome may have long-term renal failure or neurological deficits. Antibiotics are not recommended for this infection because they do not diminish the duration of symptoms or prevent complications and may increase the risk of developing hemolytic uremic syndrome. Novel therapies for treating *E. coli* O157:H7 include reagents that bind the Shiga-like toxins to prevent interaction with host cell receptors.

Infection with *Salmonella* Species

Etiology and pathogenesis

Although all *Salmonella* are grouped into a single species, *Salmonella choleraesuis*, there are seven species subgroups, of which subgroup I contains almost all the serotypes that cause human disease. Nontyphoidal *Salmonella* species account for 1.5 million cases of food-borne enteric illness in the United States annually. *Salmonella* may be acquired from infected eggs, poultry, beef, dairy products, pet turtles, carmine red dye, aerosols, marijuana, thermometers, endoscopes, and platelet transfusions. Outbreaks of infection tend to occur during the summer and autumn, likely from picnics and barbecues during which food is not cooked at temperatures necessary to kill the organism (>150 °F for 12 minutes). Person-to-person transfer is important only in institutional settings where fecal contamination is prevalent. Other persons at risk include patients with malignancy, immunosuppression, alcoholism, hypochlorhydria, sickle cell anemia, cardiovascular disease, hemolytic anemia, or schistosomiasis, and those who have recently undergone surgery.

The development of symptomatic infection depends on the volume of organisms ingested and various host factors. Diarrhea develops only if the mucosa of the small intestine is invaded. The pathogenicity is poorly understood but is thought to involve regulatory proteins that control the synthesis of proteins at the level of transcription. Unlike *Shigella* infection, *Salmonella* only rarely causes ulceration, hemorrhage, and microabscesses. Invasion of the bloodstream by nontyphoidal *Salmonella* species is infrequently beyond the mesenteric lymph nodes, and blood cultures are positive in less than 10% of cases.

Clinical presentation, diagnosis, and management

Nontyphoidal *Salmonella* species are associated with a spectrum of disease severity ranging from infrequent loose stools to a cholera-like diarrhea with dehydration. Associated symptoms include fever, abdominal pain, nausea, and vomiting. Symptoms manifest within 48 hours of exposure and persist for 3–7 days. Complications include osteomyelitis, focal abscesses, bacteremia, sepsis, and infection of aortic or iliac aneurysms. Diagnosis is by stool culture and the mainstay of treatment is supportive care.

Antimicrobials are not recommended for mild-to-moderate disease because they may prolong intestinal carriage of the organism and increase the risk of relapse. Antimicrobials do not shorten symptom duration. Indications for antibiotics include extremes of age, immunodeficiency, sepsis, abscess, osteomyelitis, and chronic typhoid carrier states. Multidrug resistance is emerging in the United States, mediated by large complex plasmids. In seriously ill patients, administration of two antimicrobial agents of different classes for 10–14 days orally or parenterally is indicated. Antibiotics with proven efficacy include ampicillin, amoxicillin, trimethoprim-sulfamethoxazole, chloramphenicol, cefotaxime, ceftriaxone, and quinolones. To eradicate the chronic carrier state, six-week regimens of amoxicillin and trimethoprim-sulfamethoxazole and norfloxacin or ciprofloxacin for three weeks have known efficacy.

Salmonella typhi

The pathogenesis of *S. typhi* resides with the Vi antigen, which prevents antibody binding and subsequent phagocytosis by the host. The organism is transmitted by the fecal–oral route and humans are the only known reservoir. Initially, transient bacteremia results from organism release from dying macrophages in Peyer patches. Persistence of *S. typhi* in the circulating macrophages leads to seeding of distant sites and a second phase of bacteremia that coincides with enteric fever.

Clinical presentation, diagnosis, and management

After an incubation period of about 1 week (range 3–60 days), enteric fever (temperature of 39–40 °C) develops and persists for 2–3 weeks. Associated symptoms include headache, malaise, mental confusion, anorexia, abdominal discomfort, bloating, and upper respiratory symptoms. Initially, diarrhea may be short-lived and resolves prior to the onset of fever, only to recur in the late phase of illness. The liver and spleen may be enlarged, and abdominal tenderness may mimic appendicitis. Rose spots – a faint salmon-colored maculopapular rash on the anterior trunk – develop in 30% of patients but last only three to four days. Relative bradycardia (pulse slow for degree of fever) may be seen. Hematological abnormalities include leukopenia and anemia. Complications include hemorrhage, intestinal perforation, pericarditis, orchitis, and splenic or liver abscess.

A combination of cultures from blood, bone marrow, and intestinal secretions will provide the diagnosis in more than 90% of patients, although the sensitivity of blood culture alone is 50–70%. Third-generation cephalosporins and fluoroquinolones are effective in treating typhoid fever and have replaced chloramphenicol as the treatment of choice. Symptom relapse occurs in 3–13% of cases. Oral (live attenuated virus) and parenteral (whole-cell and purified capsular polysaccharide) vaccines are effective in preventing illness.

Infection with *Yersinia* Species

Yersinia species are Gram-negative, nonlactose-fermenting coccobacilli that cause gastrointestinal illness primarily in children. *Yersinia enterocolitica* causes 0.1% of reported food-borne illness in the United States. The organism is transmitted by the fecal–oral route, by animals (e.g. dogs), and by contaminated milk, ice cream, tofu, and water.

Clinical presentation, diagnosis, and management

Y. enterocolitica manifests clinically as a self-limited, febrile, diarrheal illness. Abdominal pain often occurs in the right lower quadrant and may mimic appendicitis. Other symptoms include vomiting, dysentery, arthritis, and pharyngitis. Most cases resolve over two to three days, although diarrhea can persist for months, especially in children. Rare complications of appendicitis, intestinal perforation, ileocolic intussusception, peritonitis, toxic megacolon, or cholangitis have been reported. Sepsis is uncommon but is associated with iron overload states (e.g. hemochromatosis, cirrhosis, and hemolysis). Focal *Yersinia* infections may involve the meninges, joints, bone, sinuses, and pleural spaces. Thyroiditis or glomerulopathy have developed in the postinfectious state.

Moreover, patients who are HLA-B27 positive are susceptible to postinfectious Reiter syndrome, carditis, arthritis, rashes, erythema nodosum, ankylosing spondylitis, and inflammatory bowel disease.

Yersinia is diagnosed by stool examination that shows leukocytes and erythrocytes and by stool cultures using special techniques specific for *Yersinia* species. There is no evidence supporting the general use of antimicrobial therapy because the disease is usually self-limited and antibiotics do not decrease the risk of postinfectious complications. If septicemia occurs, however, therapy may consist of aminoglycosides, tetracycline, chloramphenicol, trimethoprim-sulfamethoxazole, piperacillin, or third-generation cephalosporins.

Infection with *Vibrio Cholerae*

Cholera is caused by *V. cholerae*, a motile, monoflagellated, Gram-negative, curved rod that classically causes voluminous watery diarrhea by elaborating an enterotoxin. Cholera is transmitted mainly via seafood or fecally contaminated water, and the disease primarily affects children (age 2–9) and women of childbearing age who live in crowded conditions with poor water and waste sanitation. Other persons at increased risk of infection include those with hypochlorhydria or impaired immune function. Person-to-person transmission is not considered important.

There are seven *Vibrio* species that are known to cause gastroenteritis. Although the risk of cholera in the United States is small, cases involving sero-groups O1 and O139 have been reported. Cholera toxin consists of an "A" subunit, which is internalized and irreversibly activates mucosal adenylate cyclase, thus producing massive electrolyte and fluid secretion, and a "B" subunit, which binds to specific surface receptors and enables the A subunit to enter into the cell. The inoculum required to produce illness is larger than 10^6 organisms.

Clinical presentation, diagnosis, and management

The clinical presentation of cholera is highly variable, ranging from subclinical gastroenteritis to severe cholera (cholera gravis) that may lead to hypovolemic shock within one hour. After an incubation period of a few hours to seven days, cholera manifests with diarrhea, which is described as having the consistency of rice water. Associated symptoms include vomiting, metabolic acidosis, hyponatremia, hypokalemia, hypoglycemia, lethargy, altered sensorium, and seizures. Paralytic ileus, muscle cramps, weakness, and cardiac arrhythmias may result secondary to electrolyte abnormalities. The diagnosis is based on the characteristic clinical presentation, direct stool examination identifying the "shooting star" motility under dark-field or phase microscopy or stool culturing of *V. cholerae* O1 or *V. cholerae* O139 Bengal.

The mainstay of therapy is prompt initiation of oral rehydration with glucose and electrolyte solutions endorsed by the World Health Organization. Intravenous lactated Ringer solution may be required to treat severe dehydration or concomitant vomiting. Antibiotics reduce the volume and duration of diarrhea and shorten the period of excretion of *V. cholerae*. Tetracycline (250–500 mg, four times daily for three days) and doxycycline are effective, as are streptomycin, chloramphenicol, trimethoprim-sulfamethoxazole, nalidixic acid, ampicillin, and furazolidone. Eradication with a single 1 g dose of ciprofloxacin has been effective. Primary infection with *V. cholerae* confers immunity to subsequent infection for at least three years. Parenteral and oral vaccines have been formulated but they confer only about 50% protection.

Other *Vibrio* Species

Vibrio parahaemolyticus is found in salt water or in its inhabitants and frequently causes food-borne illness in the United States. Reported cases generally involve ingestion of raw or incorrectly stored seafood or contamination of food with sea-water. It elaborates an enterotoxin and produces inflammation in the small intestine. In addition to *V. parahaemolyticus*, a group of vibrios termed *non-O1 cholera vibrios* (they do not agglutinate in antiserum against O-group 1 antigen) can cause gastroenteritis. Infection may result from ingesting oysters, eggs, and potatoes or from exposure to dogs. Other vibrios (e.g. *fluvialis, furnissii, hollisae,* and *mimicus*) may also cause diarrheal illness.

Clinical presentation, diagnosis, and management

V. parahaemolyticus produces a range of illness from mild diarrhea to dysentery after an incubation of longer than 24 hours, with associated nausea, vomiting, headache, and fever. Non-O1 cholera vibrio illness presents with diarrhea, which lasts one to six days and is associated with abdominal cramping, fever, nausea, and vomiting. Most cases of gastroenteritis caused by *V. parahaemolyticus* and non-O1 cholera vibrios are self-limited, and antibiotics do not shorten the duration of symptoms. Severe illness, however, may be effectively treated with tetracycline.

Additional Food-Borne Bacterial Pathogens

Staphylococcus aureus

S. aureus is a Gram-positive coccus that accounts for 1–2% of recognized food-borne illness in the United States. Epidemics often occur during warm weather, reflecting the association of *S. aureus* outbreaks with large gatherings (e.g. picnics). The high sugar or salt content of certain foods (e.g. salads, pastries, and meats) allows selective growth of the organism. The organism produces at least seven enterotoxins and a δ-toxin that can evoke fluid secretion in the intestine. The clinical features of food poisoning with *Staph. aureus* include nausea, vomiting, and diarrhea. These symptoms occur with an attack rate of 80–100% within 8 hours after ingesting preformed enterotoxin. Full recovery usually occurs within 48 hours. The diagnosis is clinical but may be confirmed by culturing the organism from the food or food handler.

Bacillus cereus

B. cereus is an aerobic, motile, spore-forming Gram-positive rod. It accounts for less than 1% of food-borne disease in the United States. The organism produces two types of toxins, depending on the media upon which it grows. Two distinct clinical syndromes are associated with food-borne illness caused by *B. cereus*. Patients with the emetic illness present with vomiting and cramping. Symptoms appear 1–6 hours after ingestion and persist for 2–10 hours. Patients with the diarrheal illness have profuse watery diarrhea, abdominal cramping, and occasional vomiting. The illness has an incubation period of 6–24 hours and lasts for 16–48 hours. The diagnosis is based primarily on clinical information. Both syndromes are self-limited. Prevention of *B. cereus* infection requires proper food handling and storage.

Clostridium botulinum

C. botulinum is a ubiquitous, anaerobic, spore-forming, Gram-positive bacterium that produces a neurotoxin capable of blocking acetylcholine release at the neuromuscular junction. Incorrectly canned food is the usual source of infection. Mild nausea, vomiting, abdominal pain, and diarrhea occur within 12–36 hours after ingestion. Associated neurological symptoms may also be present, including diplopia, ophthalmoplegia, dysarthria, dysphagia, dysphonia, descending weakness, paralysis, postural hypotension, and respiratory muscle paralysis. The latter is the major cause of mortality and occurs in 15% of patients; otherwise, full recovery may take months. The diagnosis is confirmed by detecting botulinum toxin in the stool and vomitus of infected patients or in the contaminated food. Electromyography can be used to differentiate this illness from Guillain–Barré syndrome. Treatment is supportive in addition to administering the antitoxin early in the course of disease.

Clostridium perfringens

C. perfringens is a nonmotile, obligate anaerobe that is responsible for approximately 2% of all food-borne cases reported to the Centers for Disease Control and Prevention (CDC). Spores are heat resistant and grow in temperatures that vary from 15° to 50 °C. The organism produces a heat-labile enterotoxin that binds to mucosal cell surfaces, causing structural damage and leading to loss of electrolytes, fluids, and proteins. Most outbreaks occur in the autumn and winter and result from ingesting incorrectly stored beef, fish, poultry, pasta salads, and dairy products. *C. perfringens* causes watery diarrhea and cramping abdominal pain 8–24 hours after ingestion of contaminated food. The disease is self-limited and full recovery is expected within 24 hours, although dehydration may cause death of elderly patients. *C. perfringens* has also been implicated in antibiotic-associated diarrhea. Other toxins (e.g. α-toxin and β-toxin) can produce necrotizing enterocolitis, ileus, and pneumatosis intestinalis. Definitive diagnosis is made by demonstrating more than 10^5 organisms per gram in contaminated food or more than 10^6 spores per gram in stools of affected individuals, or by detecting *C. perfringens* enterotoxin in assays.

Therapy for infection with *C. perfringens* is supportive, although oral metronidazole (400 mg, three times/day for 7–10 days) may facilitate eradication of the infection.

Listeria monocytogenes

L. monocytogenes is a non-spore-forming, Gram-positive bacillus that is notorious for causing gastrointestinal illness from ingesting unpasteurized milk products, although an association with ingesting contaminated meats, fruits, vegetables, and seafood is also known. It is uncommon and is reported to the CDC in only 0.1% of food-borne outbreaks. Populations at risk include pregnant women, infants, immunosuppressed individuals, the elderly, veterinarians, and laboratory workers. The varied clinical presentation of *Listeria* ranges from mild febrile illness to an overt episode of bacteremia, meningitis, and sepsis. Complications include perinatal listeria septicemia (granulomas and abscesses in multiple organs), cervical adenitis, endocarditis, arthritis, osteomyelitis, brain abscess, peritonitis, and cholecystitis. It is diagnosed by isolating the organism with "tumbling motility." Early treatment with ampicillin and an aminoglycoside is indicated because of the seriousness of the illness. Trimethoprim-sulfamethoxazole, macrolides, and tetracycline have also been advocated; cephalosporins are not effective. The duration of therapy has not been well studied but at least two weeks, and up to six weeks, is recommended.

Aeromonas, Plesiomonas, and *Edwardsiella*

Aeromonas species, *Plesiomonas shigelloides*, and *Edwardsiella tarda* are pathogens responsible for gastroenteritis (including traveler's diarrhea), wound infection, and meningitis. All are water-borne: *Aeromonas* species are commonly identified and isolated from freshwater fish and shrimp, *P. shigelloides* is present in contaminated oysters and seafood, and *E. tarda* is found primarily in water and aquatic animals. All produce illness by elaborating an enterotoxin and by cytotoxic activity.

Enterocolitis induced by *Clostridium Difficile*

C. difficile is the most common cause of nosocomial diarrhea. The major risk factors for symptomatic *C. difficile* infection are exposure to antimicrobials, hospitalization, and host susceptibility. The antibiotics most commonly used for treatment include clindamycin, ampicillin, and cephalosporins. *C. difficile* is prevalent in chronic care facilities, nursing homes, newborn nurseries, and neonatal intensive care units. To reduce transmission of *C. difficile*, hospital personnel should wear disposable gloves when handling stool or linen, and they should wash their hands after patient contact. Incontinent patients with diarrhea caused by *C. difficile* should be placed in isolation. Bleach solutions may be effective against environmental contamination.

C*C. difficile* is a Gram-positive, obligate anaerobic rod. Colonic damage is mediated by the release of two potent toxins, A and B. These toxins inactivate Rho proteins, leading to collapse of the cell cytoskeleton, increased tight junction permeability, and fluid secretion. An intense inflammatory response is initiated by the toxins and mediated by nuclear factor-κB (NF-κB), which in turn increases production of interleukin-8 (IL-8), tumor necrosis factor-α (TNF-α), prostaglandin E_2, and leukotriene B_4.

Clinical presentation

C. difficile is associated with a wide spectrum of disease ranging from, in order of decreasing severity, pseudomembranous colitis, antibiotic-associated colitis withoutpseudomembranes,toantibiotic-associateddiarrhea.Pseudomembranous colitis presents with diarrhea and cramps generally within the first week of antibiotic therapy, although delays in symptom onset of up to six weeks have been reported. Associated symptoms include fever, nausea, vomiting, tenesmus, and dehydration. Physical findings may include abdominal distension and diffuse tenderness. Peripheral leukocytosis usually is present. Occult fecal blood loss is common but hematochezia is rare. Complications of pseudomembranous colitis include toxic megacolon, perforation, and peritonitis. Findings that suggest a fulminant course include fever, tachycardia, localized abdominal tenderness with guarding, ascites, decreased bowel sounds, and signs of toxemia. In these cases of toxic megacolon, striking leukocytosis (white blood cell count of up to 40,000–80,000 cells/μl), and hypoalbuminemia, caused by protein-losing enteropathy, may be present.

Antibiotic-associated colitis without pseudomembranes follows a more benign course, with insidious development of fecal urgency, cramps, watery diarrhea, malaise, fever, and abdominal tenderness. Antibiotic-associated diarrhea without colitis is characterized by the absence of systemic findings and by diarrhea that resolves when antibiotics are stopped. Infection with *C. difficile* can also complicate the course of inflammatory bowel disease. A stool toxin assay is recommended for patients with Crohn's disease or ulcerative colitis who have unexplained relapses, especially after recent exposure to antibiotics.

Diagnostic investigation

Stool examination reveals leukocytes in 50% of patients with pseudomembranous colitis but fecal leukocytes are less common with milder infections caused by *C. difficile*. The gold standard for diagnosing *C. difficile* intestinal infection is a tissue culture assay. If a stool specimen submitted for testing contains toxin, cellular rounding or detachment of cultured human fibroblasts is observed after an incubation of 24–48 hours. The cytotoxin assay is positive in 95–100% of patients with pseudomembranous colitis and in 60–75% of patients with colitis without pseudomembranes. Enzyme-linked immunosorbent assays (ELISAs) that detect *C. difficile* toxins are also widely available and used. Although less sensitive than the cell culture assay, results are available the same day and are highly specific for infection. New panels for stool detection of enteric pathogens use PCR technology to identify multiple organisms including *C. difficile*. Stool cultures do not differentiate asymptomatic carriers from patients with colitis and thus are of limited clinical use.

Sigmoidoscopy is not necessary to diagnose infection with *C. difficile*; however, endoscopic evaluation may be considered for very ill, hospitalized patients for whom reliance on stool toxin assays may delay initiation of appropriate therapy. Endoscopic diagnosis hinges on the presence of pseudomembranes, which appear as yellow-white raised plaques 2–5 mm in diameter. Histological examination of the pseudomembrane reveals a summit lesion, which is composed of fibrin, mucus, and inflammatory cells erupting from an epithelial microulceration.

Management

The initial step in management should be to discontinue the inciting antimicrobial, which effectively resolves symptoms in 15–23% of patients. In patients who do not respond, metronidazole and vancomycin have proven efficacy in eradicating infection. Oral metronidazole (250 mg four times daily, or 500 mg three times daily, for 10 days) is the recommended initial course for treating pseudomembranous colitis. In patients with ileus, intravenous metronidazole (500 mg every six hours) is an alternative therapy. Oral vancomycin (125 mg, four times daily for 10 days) can effectively eradicate *C. difficile* after one week. Opiate antidiarrheals (e.g. loperamide, diphenoxylate with atropine) should be limited or avoided.

Fifteen to 20% of patients with pseudomembranous colitis relapse after successful antibiotic treatment, usually one to two weeks after completing therapy. Possible etiologies for relapse include persistence of spores or vegetative forms of the organism or reinfection from environmental sources. A repeated course of the initial antibiotic regimen is recommended. Strategies for treatment of relapses are presented in Table 41.1. A pulsed regimen of vancomycin is recommended for treatment of a second relapse. Fecal microbiota transplant (FMT) should be considered if relapse occurs after a pulsed regimen of vancomycin.

Table 41.1 Treatment recommendations for first-occurrence *Clostridium difficile*-associated diarrhea and recurrences

	Agent	Adult dose[a]	Duration	Side effects
First-line treatment, first occurrence	Metronidazole	250 mg tid	10 days	Disulfiram-like reaction, nausea, vomiting, metallic taste in mouth, peripheral neuropathy (rare during short-course therapy). Should not be used during pregnancy
	Vancomycin	125 mg po qid	10 days	None
First recurrence (confirm diagnosis with antigen test for all recurrences; consider withholding treatment if symptoms are not severe)	Metronidazole	250 mg tid	14 days	Disulfiram-like reaction, nausea, vomiting, metallic taste in mouth, peripheral neuropathy (rare during short-course therapy). Should not be used during pregnancy
	Vancomycin	250 mg po tid	14 days	None
Second recurrence	Tapering course of vancomycin	125 mg po qid 125 mg po tid 150 mg qd 125 mg qod 125 mg q3days	1 week 1 week 1 week 2 weeks 2 weeks	
	Pulsed course of vancomycin	125 mg qid 125 mg q3days	10 days 10 doses over 30 days	
Third recurrence	Fecal microbiota transplant (FMT)			

[a] Dosage recommendations are for adults and might need adjustment based on body habitus and other factors.

bid, twice a day; po, orally; qd, once a day; qid, four times a day; q3days, every three days; qod, every other day; tid, three times a day.

Viral infections of the gastrointestinal tract

Infection with Rotavirus

Rotavirus is a nonenveloped, spherical, segmented, double-stranded RNA virus that is the single most important cause of severe diarrhea in young children worldwide. Transmission is by fecal–oral transfer, most likely person to person, and children and asymptomatic adults are the major reservoirs. Recurrent infections with differing serotypes are not uncommon. Infection with rotavirus causes loss of mature villus absorptive cells and loss of brush border hydrolases, resulting in fluid loss and osmotic diarrhea. In addition, a nonstructural protein of the virus appears to have enterotoxin-like activity and may augment diarrhea.

Clinical presentation, diagnosis, and management

Most rotavirus infections are not associated with symptomatic disease. Clinical cases present after an incubation period of one to three days with a rapid onset of fever, malaise, vomiting, and watery diarrhea. The illness typically lasts three to eight days. A mild elevation of blood urea nitrogen and metabolic acidosis are common. Stools are watery but devoid of red or white blood cells. A number of diagnostic assays have been developed to detect rotavirus infection. Solid-phase immunoassays have sensitivities and specificities higher than 90%. Nucleic acid hybridization assays are also available, as are reverse transcriptase–PCR assays; however, both are generally more expensive than solid-phase immunoassays. Electrophoretic analysis of stool RNA is both sensitive and inexpensive. Culture of the virus from fecal specimens is also feasible.

Therapy for rotaviral diarrhea is supportive. Oral rehydration therapy is the cornerstone of treatment; no effective antiviral medication is available. Several live, attenuated, rotavirus vaccines are being tested.

Infection with norwalk virus

Norwalk virus is a nonenveloped, round, viral particle that causes epidemic diarrhea in both developed and underdeveloped countries. The virus, named after the 1968 outbreak of gastroenteritis that affected half of the teachers and students of an elementary school in Norwalk, Ohio, was the first evidence of a viral etiology for diarrhea. The settings of Norwalk virus outbreaks include homes, schools, cruise ships, swimming pools, and military facilities. Transmission is primarily through the fecal–oral route, although person-to-person, air-borne, and fomite transmissions have also been implicated. Biopsy specimens of the small intestine show broad and blunted villi, crypt cell hyperplasia, cytoplasmic vacuoles, and infiltration of the lamina propria with polymorphonuclear and mononuclear cells. Brush border enzymes are reduced and gastric emptying may be delayed.

Clinical presentation, diagnosis, and management

The incubation period is 10–50 hours. The most frequently reported symptoms are nausea, abdominal cramps, headache, diarrhea and fever, which last 12–72 hours. There are no commercially available diagnostic tests for Norwalk virus infection. Research centers have diagnosed infection through detection of viral antigen by ELISA, the presence of viral RNA by reverse transcriptase – PCR, or the serological response to infection. Therapy centers on fluid and electrolyte replacement and symptomatic treatment of diarrhea. Prevention should be directed toward hand washing and hygienic food preparation.

Infection with astrovirus

Astrovirus infection mainly affects children but it also occurs in institutionalized elderly patients. Other groups at risk of infection are bone marrow transplant recipients and patients infected with human immunodeficiency virus. Viral aggregates are seen in enterocytes, which appear to cause villus atrophy and crypt cell hyperplasia.

Clinical presentation, diagnosis, and management

After an incubation period of one to four days, symptoms that consist of watery diarrhea with vomiting, fever, and abdominal pain ensue for about two to three days. An ELISA based on monoclonal antibodies to all eight types of human astroviruses is commercially available. Supportive therapy is advocated. Immunoglobulin administered intravenously, orally, or by a combination of routes has been reportedly efficacious, although not yet studied in controlled clinical trials.

Infection with enteric adenovirus

Adenoviruses are DNA viruses, of which serotypes 40 and 41 in particular are known to cause gastroenteritis. The infection affects mainly children younger than age 2. Viral infection appears to vary geographically but does not exhibit seasonal variation. Infection is transmitted from person to person.

Clinical presentation, diagnosis, and management

The presentation of adenovirus is similar to that of other viral agents. The incubation period is about seven days. Symptoms include watery diarrhea and vomiting, in addition to respiratory complaints and fever. An ELISA kit is available for diagnosis. Viral particles can be evaluated directly by electron microscopy and by PCR. The goal of therapy is rehydration and adequate nutritional intake.

Key practice points

- Bacterial infections of the gastrointestinal tract are common and can lead to significant disease. The most common pathogens include *Campylobacter*, *Shigella*, *Salmonella*, *Yersinia*, *E. coli*, and *Vibrio* species.
- *C. difficile* is an increasingly common infection. Retreatment for relapse or reinfection may be necessary.
- Viral infections of the gastrointestinal tract are most commonly due to rotavirus, norovirus (including Norwalk virus), adenovirus, and astrovirus infections.
- Treatment is usually supportive for both bacterial and viral infections of the gastrointestinal tract, although there is a role for antibiotic use for certain infections.

Further reading

Riddle, M.S., HL, D.P., and Connor, B.A. (2016). ACG clinical guideline: Diagnosis, treatment, and prevention of acute diarrheal infections in adults. *Am. J. Gastroenterol.* 111: 602–622.

Surawicz, C.M., Brandt, L.J., Binion, D.G. et al. (2013). Guidelines for diagnosis, treatment, and prevention of *Clostridium difficile* infections. *Am. J. Gastroenterol.* 108: 478–498.

CHAPTER 42
Gastrointestinal Vascular Lesions

A variety of vascular lesions manifest in the gastrointestinal tract. They can be broadly categorized as being intrinsic or extrinsic (Figure 42.1). Intrinsic lesions can be further sub-classified as vascular ectasia, vascular neoplasia, and other vascular lesions (Table 42.1).

Dieulafoy lesion

The Dieulafoy lesion results from an unusually large (1–3 mm) submucosal artery and can be associated with massive gastrointestinal hemorrhage. The majority of Dieulafoy lesions occur in the proximal stomach (75%) with a smaller proportion in the distal stomach and duodenum; however, they can also form in the jejunum, ileum, colon, and rectum.

Clinical presentation

Upper gastrointestinal Dieulafoy lesions usually present with massive upper gastrointestinal bleeding and an absence of associated gastrointestinal symptoms. Hypotension, orthostasis, tachycardia, and prerenal azotemia are common. Lower gastrointestinal lesions manifest as hematochezia with hemodynamic instability.

Diagnostic investigation

Upper gastrointestinal endoscopy is the principal means of diagnosing an upper tract Dieulafoy lesion. There may be a pigmented protuberance, identifying the vessel stump, and an adherent clot with little surrounding edema. No ulceration is present; if one is seen, the visualized lesion is a visible vessel in an ulcer, not a Dieulafoy lesion. Endoscopic Doppler ultrasound can confirm the presence of a Dieulafoy lesion by visualizing a 2–3 mm diameter high-flow, pulsating submucosal artery. Lesions of the colon are similar in appearance to upper tract lesions.

Yamada's Handbook of Gastroenterology, Fourth Edition. John M. Inadomi, Renuka Bhattacharya, Joo Ha Hwang, and Cynthia Ko.

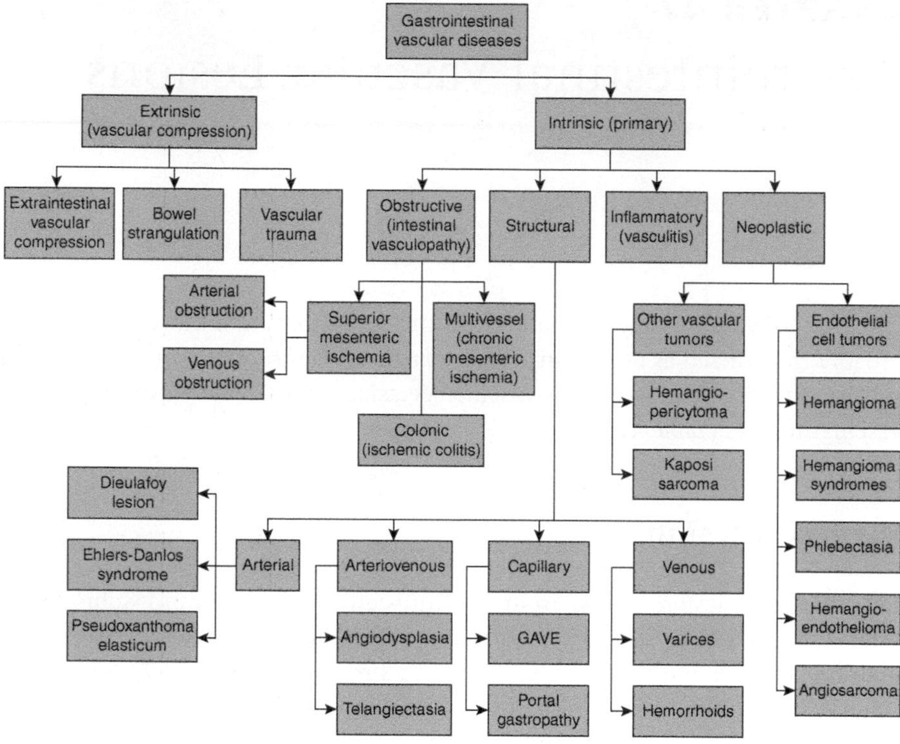

Figure 42.1 Classification of vascular gastrointestinal lesions. GAVE, gastric antral vascular ectasia. (Source: figure 127.1 from Podolsky et al. 2016.)

Table 42.1 Vascular lesions of the gastrointestinal tract

Vascular ectasia disorders
Angiodysplasia
Gastric antral vascular ectasia (GAVE) ("watermelon stomach")
Telangiectasia associated with multisystem disease (e.g. hereditary hemorrhagic telangiectasia [HHT], CREST syndrome, Turner syndrome)
Vascular tumors
Hemangiomas
Multiple hemangioma syndromes (e.g. intestinal hemangiomatosis, universal hemangiomatosis, blue rubber bleb nevus syndrome, Klippel–Trénaunay syndrome, Parkes–Weber syndrome)
Malignant vascular tumors (e.g. angiosarcoma, hemangiopericytoma, Kaposi sarcoma)
Other vascular lesions
Dieulafoy lesion
Miscellaneous (e.g. multiple phlebectasia, pseudoxanthoma elasticum, Ehlers–Danlos syndrome)

CREST, syndrome of calcinosis, Raynaud phenomenon, esophageal dysmotility, sclerodactyly, and telangiectasia.

Active bleeding may obscure endoscopic visualization, in which case angiography may be used to identify the bleeding vessel.

Management

Initial management consists of fluid resuscitation and replacement of blood loss. Endoscopic therapy is used to treat the Dieulafoy lesion: injection therapy with epinephrine (1 : 10,000 dilution) is commonly used initially to achieve initial hemostasis, followed by either bipolar electrocoagulation, thermal coagulation, or hemoclip placement. Band ligation has also been used successfully, but it can be associated with perforation or recurrent bleeding from the banding ulcer. It is important to tattoo the mucosa surrounding the lesion so that the location can be inspected in the case of recurrent hemorrhage. Angiography with selective left gastric artery embolization has been used with limited success to treat gastric Dieulafoy lesions. If nonsurgical attempts to control bleeding fail, surgical vessel ligation, wedge resection, or proximal partial gastrectomy may be necessary. Colonic lesions unresponsive to endoscopic therapy should be managed surgically.

Key practice points: Dieulafoy lesions

- A Dieulafoy lesion is identified endoscopically as a pigmented protuberance, possibly an adherent clot with little surrounding edema or ulceration.
- Endoscopic management includes injection of epinephrine for initial hemostasis followed by either hemostatic clipping, electrocautery, or band ligation.

Angiodysplasia

Angiodysplasia consist of dilated, tortuous, thin-walled blood vessels lined by endothelium with little or no smooth muscle. Vascular ectasias that occur in association with lesions of the skin or other organs are termed *telangiectasias*.

Clinical presentation

Angiodysplasia clinically manifests with painless gastrointestinal hemorrhage (melena or hematochezia). Most colonic lesions are located in the right colon and are associated with low-grade chronic bleeding or iron deficiency anemia, but 10% of patients present with acute massive hemorrhage. Up to 60% of patients have multiple angiodysplasias within the same portion of the intestinal tract. Traditionally, there has been an association between aortic stenosis and angiodysplasia (Heyde syndrome) that is clinically relevant because of case reports illustrating cessation of bleeding after aortic valve replacement; however, more recent evidence does not confirm this association and depletion of von Willebrand factor due to shear force across a stenotic aortic valve may account for the observed increase in hemorrhage.

Diagnostic investigation

Upper gastrointestinal endoscopy, small bowel enteroscopy, capsule endoscopy, and colonoscopy are the primary methods for identifying angiodysplasia in the gastrointestinal tract. The lesions appear as a dense reticular network of vessels ranging in diameter from 2 to 8 mm and are bright red due to the arterial source of blood without intervening capillaries. Angiography may identify colonic angiodysplasia overlooked on colonoscopy or angiodysplasia lesions in the small intestine not visualized by enteroscopy plus capsule endoscopy. The characteristic angiographic findings include a vascular tuft during the arterial phase of the study, rapid filling of the dilated vein, and slowly emptying veins. Because angiodysplasias bleed only intermittently, angiography demonstrates active bleeding in only 10–20% of patients. ^{99m}Tc-labeled erythrocyte scintigraphy is more sensitive in detecting acute hemorrhage but it can identify only the general region of bleeding. Patients with acute lower tract bleeding should undergo emergency colonoscopy or erythrocyte scintigraphy as the initial imaging procedure. Positive erythrocyte scans should be followed by angiography or colonoscopy.

Management and course

Many angiodysplasias are asymptomatic and are incidentally noted by endoscopy for nonbleeding indications. About one-quarter of patients who bleed from angiodysplasias experience recurrent hemorrhage within one year, and one half rebleed over a three-year period. Patients with mild, chronic blood loss who do not require transfusion are best managed conservatively with oral iron supplements. Octreotide (50–100 mcg subcutaneously twice per day, or once monthly intramuscularly using the long-acting form) has demonstrated efficacy in reducing transfusion requirements in patients who experienced recurrent bleeding from gastrointestinal vascular malformations. Thalidomide (25 mg four times daily) was shown to reduce bleeding episodes from vascular malformations; however, side effects include fatigue, constipation, dizziness, edema, abdominal distension. Other major adverse events with thalidomide include liver toxicity, venous thrombosis, peripheral neuropathy and severe birth defects. Estrogen and progesterone have been used to treat angiodysplasia; however, newer data fail to support their effectiveness.

Patients with acute bleeding or chronic bleeding who require transfusion should undergo more invasive therapy. Successful outcomes have been reported using multiple endoscopic methods, including argon plasma coagulation (APC), thermocoagulation (heater probe), electrocoagulation (multipolar electrocautery probe), or photocoagulation (laser). Balloon-assisted enteroscopy may be needed to reach the bleeding lesions. Local expertise and availability dictate the preference for instruments to control hemorrhage.

Angiography may be used to provide selective intra-arterial infusion of vasopressin to control acute bleeding, which is successful in 50–90% of cases. One-third of patients rebleed after infusion; thus angiographic embolization is often required to prevent recurrent hemorrhage. Complications of embolization include abdominal pain, fever, and occasionally bowel infarction, which necessitates emergency colectomy.

If medical and endoscopic therapies fail to control bleeding, surgical resection should be considered. Preoperative angiography can often define the extent of angiodysplasia in the small intestine and the colon. Recurrent hemorrhage after surgery occurs in one-quarter to one-third of patients and is generally from unresected lesions in the remaining intestine.

Key practice points: Angiodysplasia

- The majority of patients with angiodysplasias possess multiple lesions within the same portion of the intestinal tract.
- Recurrent bleeding from angiodysplasias is common.
- Medical therapy with octreotide or thalidomide may be effective in reducing recurrent bleeding.
- Endoscopic therapy with a noncontact method of electrocautery (APC) or laser can be effective, but multiple sessions are often required.
- If medical and endoscopic therapies fail, angiographic or surgical resection should be considered.

Gastric antral vascular ectasia

Gastric antral vascular ectasia (GAVE), or "watermelon stomach," is a distinctive syndrome of ectatic and sacculated mucosal vessels are visualized along longitudinal folds of the gastric antrum.

Clinical presentation and diagnosis

GAVE generally presents with iron deficiency anemia from chronic occult gastrointestinal bleeding. Overt upper gastrointestinal hemorrhage with melena or hematemesis is less common, and the lesion is painless.

Upper gastrointestinal endoscopy is the definitive means to diagnose GAVE. There is a characteristic appearance of erythematous longitudinal antral folds that converge toward the pylorus in a pattern reminiscent of a watermelon. Distinguishing GAVE from other gastropathies is based on the endoscopic pattern of dilated vessels or by demonstrating that the lesions blanch when compressed with biopsy forceps. Biopsy is not needed to establish the diagnosis, but histologically GAVE appears as hypertrophied mucosa with dilated and tortuous mucosal capillaries occluded by fibrin thrombi, and dilated or tortuous submucosal veins. Angiography and barium radiography are generally of limited diagnostic value for this condition.

Management

Patients may require iron supplementation and blood transfusion. Drugs that cause gastric mucosal injury (nonsteroidal anti-inflammatory drugs [NSAIDs]), antiplatelet agents and anticoagulants should be avoided if possible. Endoscopic therapy with APC is the preferred treatment modality, although alternatives include heater probe coagulation, endoscopic band ligation, radiofrequency ablation or laser therapy. Endoscopic therapy is generally well tolerated, but multiple sessions may be required and treatment is associated with complications such as perforation, stenosis, ulceration, and recurrent hemorrhage. Estrogen-progesterone therapy and other medical therapies have been largely anecdotal and are of uncertain clinical benefit. If patients do not respond to endoscopic therapy, antrectomy is essentially curative. Transjugular intrahepatic portosystemic shunt (TIPS) is not effective for treating GAVE in patients with cirrhosis.

Systemic telangiectasia syndromes

When angiodysplasia occurs in conjunction with vascular lesions of the skin and other organs, they are termed *telangiectasias*. Hereditary hemorrhagic telangiectasia (HHT), also known as *Osler–Weber–Rendu syndrome*, is an autosomal dominant disorder associated with vascular ectasia of the skin, mucous membranes, and internal organs. The disease prevalence is about 10 per 100,000 population, with equal sex distribution.

Clinical presentation, diagnosis, and management

Manifestations of HHT include orocutaneous telangiectasias (face, lips, tongue, oral mucosa, and hands), mucosal telangiectasias of the nasal and gastrointestinal tract, pulmonary telangiectasias, and cerebral telangiectasias. Patients usually present in childhood with recurrent and severe epistaxis. Bleeding from a posterior nasal or pharyngeal source presents similarly and should be considered in the differential diagnosis. Upper intestinal tract bleeding is more common than lower tract bleeding and may present as either iron deficiency anemia from chronic blood loss or hypovolemia and hypotension due to acute hemorrhage. Gastrointestinal lesions are identified by endoscopic examination, and most are located in the stomach and duodenum. Endoscopic APC, thermocoagulation, electrocoagulation, or photocoagulation are effective in controlling bleeding. Estrogen-progesterone therapy improves epistaxis and may reduce the rate of gastrointestinal bleeding. Data from studies using octreotide or thalidomide is sparse. The role of surgery is limited because of the diffuse nature of the disorder.

Bleeding gastrointestinal telangiectasias also occur in the CREST (calcinosis, Raynaud phenomenon, esophageal dysmotility, sclerodactyly, and telangiectasia) variant of progressive systemic sclerosis. These patients have vascular lesions on the hands, lips, face, and tongue as well as other signs of systemic sclerosis. Gastrointestinal hemorrhage is not a dominant feature of this disorder but has been reported from telangiectasias in the colon, stomach, and small intestine. The therapeutic approach is similar to that for sporadic angiodysplasia.

Hemangiomas

Intestinal hemangiomas are classified as capillary (small, closely packed vessels), cavernous (large, dilated vessels) or mixed.

Clinical presentation

Many hemangiomas are asymptomatic, but the most common clinical presentation is gastrointestinal hemorrhage. Capillary hemangiomas tend to cause low-grade chronic bleeding with iron deficiency anemia while cavernous lesions may produce massive bleeding. Most cavernous lesions are located in the rectosigmoid region, so painless hematochezia is a common presenting symptom. Large hemangiomas may cause nausea, vomiting, and abdominal pain as a result of obstruction or intussusception. Multiple hemangiomas throughout the digestive tract, a condition termed *intestinal hemangiomatosis,* affect 10% of patients. In the rare neonatal syndrome of universal hemangiomatosis, cavernous lesions are disseminated to other organs, including the brain and skin.

Rare disorders associated with diffuse cutaneous and gastrointestinal hemangiomas are the blue rubber bleb nevus syndrome, Klippel– Trénaunay syndrome and Parkes–Weber syndrome. Blue rubber bleb nevus syndrome consists of cutaneous lesions affect the limbs, trunk, and face. Their blue color and rubbery consistency are the source of the syndrome's descriptive name. Lesions also occur throughout the gastrointestinal tract and may produce occult bleeding. Patients with Klippel– Trénaunay syndrome have cavernous hemangiomas of the distal colon, port-wine cutaneous hemangiomas, bony and soft tissue hypertrophy, superficial varicose veins and atretic, hypoplastic or occluded deep veins that usually affect one lower extremity. Parkes-Weber syndrome has similar characteristics plus arteriovenous fistulae.

Diagnostic investigation

Upper and lower gastrointestinal endoscopy can diagnose hemangiomas. Capillary lesions appear as punctate red nodules, whereas cavernous lesions are violet-blue, sessile, polypoid lesions. The color, submucosal location, and compressibility distinguish the latter from colonic adenomas. Larger lesions can be mistaken for adenomatous polyps or carcinoma. Angiography and capsule endoscopy are useful for detecting hemangiomas in the small intestine. The characteristic pooling of contrast in the venous phase is a typical finding in angiographic images of large cavernous lesions but may be absent in images of small lesions.

Management

In disorders with multiple gastrointestinal hemangiomas, conservative therapy with iron supplementation is recommended initially. Blood transfusions may be necessary to treat chronic gastrointestinal bleeding. Small capillary hemangiomas may be amenable to endoscopic obliteration by coagulation, band ligation, sclerotherapy or polypectomy. Persistent hemorrhage or obstruction at a defined site requires surgical resection.

Key practice points: Hemangiomas

- Small capillary hemangiomas may be treated endoscopically with electrocautery such as APC or band ligation.
- Large cavernous venous lesions have high rates of hemorrhage or perforation with endoscopic therapy and may require surgical intervention.

Miscellaneous vascular lesions

Angiosarcomas, epithelioid hemangioendotheliomas, and hemangiopericytomas are malignant neoplasms that originate from the cellular components of blood vessels. All may be complicated by gastrointestinal hemorrhage or obstruction. Kaposi sarcoma is another vascular neoplasm that frequently disseminates to the gastrointestinal tract. This represents one of the most common causes of gastrointestinal bleeding in patients with acquired immunodeficiency syndrome. Gastrointestinal bleeding also occurs in patients with pseudoxanthoma elasticum, as a result of an abnormal vascular structure. This disorder of elastin synthesis typically presents with bleeding from arterioles in the gastric fundus. Gastrectomy is the definitive therapy.

Ehlers–Danlos syndrome is a heterogeneous group of genetic disorders of collagen metabolism. Patients characteristically have skin hyperextensibility, articular hypermobility and tissue fragility. Diagnosis is by clinical presentation, family pedigree analysis, and identifying genetic or biochemical defects. Patients with type IV Ehlers–Danlos syndrome can present with gastrointestinal hemorrhage from spontaneous arterial rupture due to vascular and perivascular connective tissue fragility. There is an increased risk of intramural intestinal hematomas, colonic diverticular hemorrhage, and intestinal perforation.

Case studies

Case 1

A 62-year-old man presents with melena, hematemesis, and hypotension. He has no prior history of bleeding and has no risk factors for liver disease or portal hypertension. His only medication is occasional use of NSAIDs for musculoskeletal pain. After resuscitation with saline and blood products, an upper endoscopy is performed that reveals large clots in the stomach but no evidence of varices, ulcers, or masses. He is transferred from the intensive care unit to the medical ward, where his vital signs and hemoglobin remain stable for two days; however, he has recurrence of hypotension and melena that require additional blood products and fluid. His endoscopy is repeated and after thorough lavage of his gastric contents, an actively spurting vessel is noted in the gastric fundus without surrounding ulceration. Epinephrine is injected around the bleeding site, which slows the rate of hemorrhage, allowing placement of three hemoclips that successfully stop the bleeding. The surrounding tissue is tattooed and the patient has no further episodes of rebleeding during the hospitalization.

Discussion

The diagnosis of a Dieulafoy lesion can be evasive because in the absence of active bleeding or a visible vessel indicating a fibrin clot, there is no endoscopic evidence of the source of hemorrhage. For this reason, after successful endoscopic treatment using injection of epinephrine for initial hemostasis followed by either hemostatic clipping, electrocautery, or band ligation, it is important to tattoo the area surrounding the lesion so that endoscopic therapy may be targeted to a specific location in the case of recurrent hemorrhage.

Case 2

A 53-year-old man presents to your clinic with iron deficiency anemia and intermittent melena. He has never been hospitalized but has received multiple blood transfusions and is on iron supplementation for anemia of at least three years duration. He has a history of chronic hepatitis C for which he has undergone successful eradication. He has undergone an upper endoscopy that did not reveal ulcerations, masses, or varices, and the endoscopist did not specify a bleeding lesion. His vital signs and physical examination are normal, and he has no stigmata of chronic liver disease. His laboratory tests are notable for a hemoglobin of 7.2 mg/dl, mean corpuscular volume (MCV) 68, ferritin 3, and normal liver enzymes. You decide to perform a colonoscopy and repeat the upper endoscopy. The colonoscopy is normal to the terminal ileum; however, the upper endoscopy is notable for erythematous longitudinal antral folds that converge toward the pylorus. You perform APC to the lesions, and after three endoscopic sessions the antrum appears normal. Three months later you see him in clinic follow-up and his hemoglobin and ferritin are normal and he denies further episodes of melena.

Discussion

GAVE is often misdiagnosed despite the characteristic appearance on endoscopy. The most common presentation is iron deficiency anemia, but occasional patients will have overt bleeding. The term *watermelon stomach* describes the erythematous linear streaks that line the gastric body and antrum. Biopsies are safe but not necessary to make the diagnosis. APC is the preferred endoscopic approach because the lesions are diffuse and superficial. Liver disease is common among patients with bleeding from GAVE, but portal hypertension is not causative so TIPS is not effective to treat bleeding.

Further reading

Podolsky, D.K., Camilleri, M., Fitz, J.G. et al. (eds.) (2016). *Yamada's Textbook of Gastroenterology*, 6e. Oxford: Blackwell.

CHAPTER 43

Medical, Surgical, and Endoscopic Treatment of Obesity

Obesity is a disease that is increasing in prevalence globally and has significant consequences in regards to increased risk of heart disease, diabetes, hypertension and hyperlipidemia. Obesity is defined as the presence of excessive body fat due to excess caloric intake relative to energy expenditure.

Clinical presentation

Evaluation of an obese patient should include a family history of obesity and obesity related diseases (heart disease, diabetes, hypertension, and hyperlipidemia) and a review of the patient's lifestyle (eating habits and physical activity). The possibility of an eating disorder should be investigated because patients with eating disorders should have interventions directed at treatment of the eating disorder before any treatment for obesity is considered. Medications should be reviewed for any that may promote weight gain. Evaluation for secondary causes of weight gain such has hypothyroidism, Cushing's syndrome, and polycystic ovarian syndrome should be investigated.

Physical examination

Measurement of the patient's weight and height are essential in order to calculate the patient's BMI. Body mass index (BMI) is a measure that correlates closely with the mass of adipose tissue and is used clinically to determine if a patient is underweight, normal, overweight, or obese (Table 43.1). BMI is calculated as follows: weight (kg)/[height (m)]^2. Waist circumference should also be measured because it is associated with risk of medical complications. Blood pressure should be measured with the appropriate-sized cuff to obtain an

Yamada's Handbook of Gastroenterology, Fourth Edition. John M. Inadomi, Renuka Bhattacharya, Joo Ha Hwang, and Cynthia Ko.

Table 43.1 Classification of weight by body mass index (BMI), waist circumference, and associated risk

BMI (kg/m^2)	Classification	Disease risk[a]	
		Waist circumference Men ≤40 in. (≤102 cm) Women ≤35 in. (≤88 cm)	**Waist circumference >40 in. (>102 cm) >35 in. (>88 cm)**
<18.5	Underweight	—	—
18.5–24.9	Normal	—	—
25.0–29.9	Overweight	Increased	High
30.0–34.9	Obese class I	High	Very high
35.0–39.9	Obese class II	Very high	Very high
≥40	Obese class III	Extremely high	Extremely high

[a] Disease risk for type 2 diabetes, hypertension, and cardiovascular disease, relative to normal weight and waist circumference.
Source: table 115.1 from Podolsky et al. 2016.

accurate measurement. The physical exam should also include investigating for any signs of hypothyroidism or Cushing's syndrome.

Diagnostic investigation

Laboratory studies

Laboratory studies include evaluation to screen for known complications of obesity including a fasting lipid panel, comprehensive metabolic panel, fasting glucose, hemoglobin A1C, and liver function tests. In addition, a thyroid-stimulating hormone level should also be measured.

Management

Obesity has been demonstrated to be associated with progressive excess mortality. Patients with a BMI of 30–35 kg/m^2 have a median survival that is reduced by 2–4 years and patients with a BMI of 40–45 kg/m^2 have a median survival that is reduced by 8–10 years.

Complications

The primary complication from obesity is the metabolic syndrome, which is the constellation of insulin resistance, visceral adiposity, hypertension, and dyslipidemia. This subsequently results in a two to three times increased risk of cardiovascular disease. In addition, obesity leads to significant osteoarthritis and increased the risk of developing obstructive sleep apnea. Other complications from obesity include nonalcoholic fatty liver disease (NAFLD), gastroesophageal reflux disease (GERD), and related complications such as Barrett's esophagus, gallstone disease, increased risk of pancreatitis, and increased risk of colon cancer.

Therapy

Lifestyle modifications

Patients with a BMI >25 kg/m^2 should be considered for weight loss interventions. Initial treatment should begin with diet, exercise, and behavioral therapy, with the goal of achieving a 10% weight reduction over a 6 months period. Combination of decreased caloric intake with increased energy expenditure with the goal of a loss of 500 kcal/day should result in a loss of 1 pound/week.

Pharmacotherapy

Anti-obesity drugs are indicated for patients with BMI ≥30 or patients with BMI ≥27 with comorbidities such as diabetes, hypertension, and/or hyperlipidemia, who have not achieved weight loss goals after lifestyle interventions. Pharmacologic agents that are currently approved for the treatment of obesity in the United States include orlistat, lorcaserin, phentermine, and phentermine/topiramate (Table 43.2).

Surgical therapy

Bariatric surgery should be considered for patients with a BMI ≥40 or BMI 35–39.9 with a serious comorbidity who have not met weight loss goals with lifestyle modifications and drug therapy. The goal of bariatric surgery is to obtain a sustained excess weight loss of >50% and resolution of comorbid conditions from obesity. Studies have demonstrated reduction in both morbidity and mortality with bariatric surgery. Bariatric surgeries have two potential mechanisms of action: restrictive and malabsorptive. The types of bariatric surgeries include: laparoscopic adjustable gastric band, sleeve gastrectomy, Roux-en-Y gastric bypass (RYGB), and biliopancreatic diversion with duodenal switch (BPD-DS) (Figure 43.1).

Laparoscopic adjustable gastric banding is a purely restrictive procedure that limits the volume of food that a patient can eat (Figure 43.1a). Weight loss is reported to be 40–55% of excess weight over 2–3 years with a slower resolution and improvement in comorbidities compared to the other procedures. Sleeve gastrectomy is also a restrictive procedure (Figure 43.1b); however, it also produces a metabolic effect by reducing ghrelin-producing cells from the greater curvature of the stomach, which becomes 65% of excess weight with resolution

Table 43.2 Weight loss agents currently approved by the US Food and Drug Administration (FDA)

Agent	Mechanism of action	Dose	Side effects	Notes
Orlistat	Lipase inhibitor	120 mg tid (prescription dose) 60 mg tid (over-the-counter dose)	Fat-soluble vitamin deficiency, fecal discharge, oily stool, flatulence, steatorrhea	Measure Vitamin D level periodically Take vitamin supplement 2 hours before or after medication
Lorcaserin	Selective serotonin 5 H2C agonist, appetite reduction	10 mg bid	Nausea, headache, fatigue, upper respiratory infections	Caution with serotonergic drugs
Phentermine/ Topiramate	Adrenergic agent (phentermine/ appetite suppression (topiramate)	Start 3.75/23 mg daily for 14 days then increase to 7.5/46 mg daily. Maximal dose: 15/92 mg daily	Tachycardia, hypertension, paresthesias, altered taste, dizziness, birth defects	Contraindicated in pregnant women or women trying to become pregnant
Phentermine	Adrenergic agent	15–37.5 mg/day	Tachycardia, hypertension, dry mouth	Monitor blood pressure and pulse

tid, three times daily.
Source: table 115.4 from Podolsky et al. 2016.

or improvement in diabetes, hypertension, and obstructive sleep apnea. RYGB combines a restrictive procedure (gastric pouch) with a malabsorptive procedure (gastric bypass) where a significant portion of the small bowel is bypassed, resulting in malabsorption (Figure 43.1c). BPD-DS involves the creation of a sleeve gastrectomy followed by a duodenoileostomy anastomosis to create the alimentary limb, and an ileoileostomy to connect the pancreaticobiliary limb to the ileum approximately 100 cm proximal to the ileocecal valve to create a common channel (Figure 43.1d). The primary mechanism for a biliopancreatic diversion is malabsorption. This surgery results in the greatest excess weight loss with the lowest rate of weight regain and results in resolution of comorbidities. Compared to RYGB, BPD-DS results in superior weight loss for extremely morbidly obese patients; however, it has higher associated morbidity and mortality from surgery, which are dependent on surgeon experience.

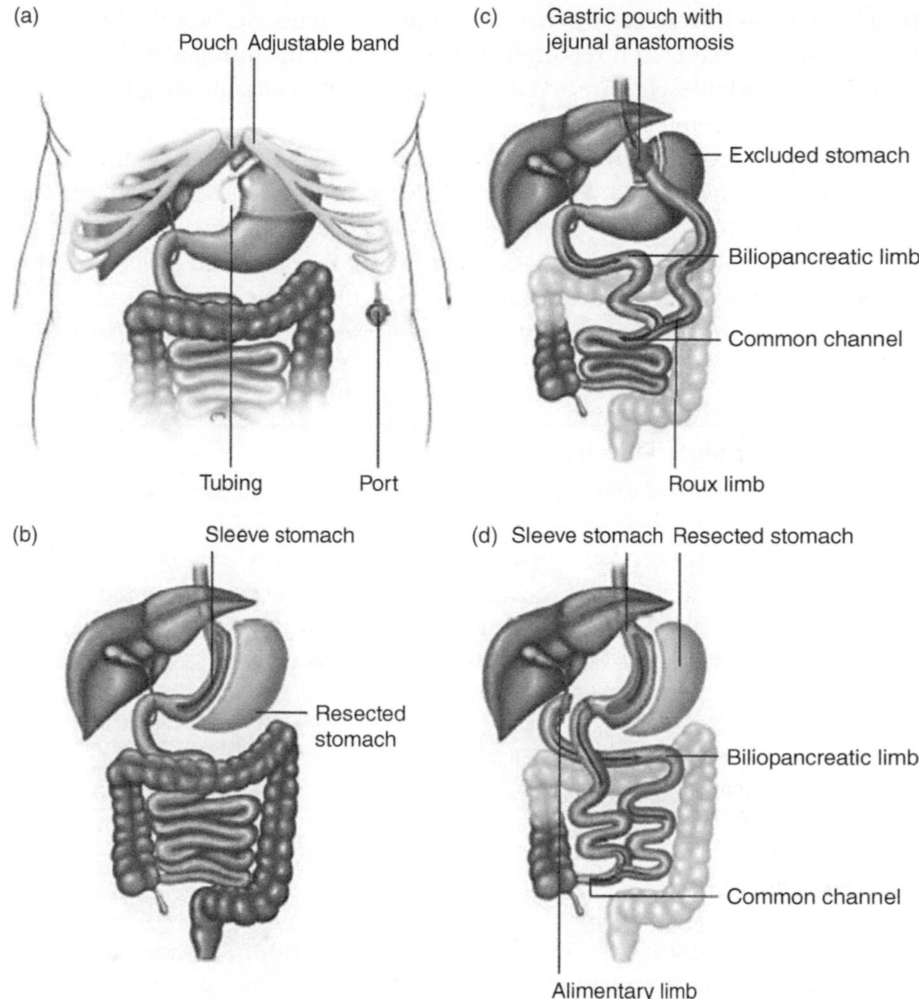

Figure 43.1 Types of bariatric surgical procedures. (a) Laparoscopic adjustable gastric band. (b) Sleeve gastrectomy. (c) Roux-en-Y gastric bypass (RYGB). (d) Biliopancreatic diversion with duodenal switch (BPD-DS). (Source: figure 116.3 from Podolsky et al. 2016.)

Endoscopic therapy

Endoscopic therapy for the treatment of obesity is an area of active investigation. Intragastric balloons have been developed and are currently available for placement in the United States. Intragastric balloons are endoscopically delivered devices that can be filled with saline to occupy the intragastric space. These devices are intended only for temporary placement (up to six months) and result in weight loss by decreasing food intake and reducing gastric emptying. Intragastric balloons have been demonstrated to be effective in achieving

10–15% weight loss. Adverse events including ulcer bleeding, bowel obstruction, and perforation have been reported. Treatment with the intragastric balloon in conjunction with lifestyle directed therapy can result in durable weight loss with improvement in comorbidities.

Endoscopic sleeve gastroplasty is another method that is currently being developed and investigated. Endoscopic sleeve gastroplasty is a procedure that is in evolution with the ongoing development of new endoscopic suturing devices. Preliminary studies of endoscopic sleeve gastroplasty compared to laparoscopic sleeve gastrectomy have demonstrated less weight loss for patients undergoing endoscopic sleeve gastroplasty; however, endoscopic sleeve gastroplasty had fewer adverse events.

Key practice points: Obesity

- BMI is an index relating the weight and height of a patient. BMI calculations are important in the diagnosis and management of obesity. BMI ≥30 is considered to be obese.
- Obesity has been demonstrated to be associated with progressive excess mortality
- Comorbidities of obesity include type 2 diabetes, cardiovascular disease, NAFLD, and sleep apnea.
- Bariatric surgery should be considered for patients with a BMI ≥40 or BMI 35–39.9 with a serious comorbidity who have not met weight loss goals with lifestyle modifications and drug therapy.
- The goal of bariatric surgery is to obtain a sustained excess weight loss of >50% and resolution of comorbid conditions from obesity.

Further reading

Podolsky, D.K., Camilleri, M., Fitz, J.G. et al. (eds.) (2016). *Yamada's Textbook of Gastroenterology*, 6e. Oxford: Blackwell.

CHAPTER 44
Questions and Answers

Questions

Chapter 1 – The Patient with Dysphagia or Odynophagia

1.1 A 65-year-old man presents with symptoms of dysphagia, coughing, and nasal regurgitation of solids and liquids with eating. What is the best initial test?

a. Barium esophagram
b. Video-fluoroscopic swallowing study
c. Upper endoscopy
d. Chest CT
e. Esophageal manometry

1.2 Which of the following is an etiology of odynophagia?

a. Gastroesophageal reflux disease
b. Schatzki's ring
c. Bacterial infection
d. Pill-associated ulceration

1.3 A 26-year-old man presents to the emergency department with symptoms of food stuck in his esophagus. On further questioning, he notes episodes of food "sticking" that have occurred one to two times per year for the past three to four years. He has never required medical attention for these episodes. He undergoes endoscopy with removal of the food impaction. Endoscopic findings are notable for multiple esophageal rings and longitudinal furrows. What histologic findings would be expected on biopsies taken from the proximal and distal esophagus?

a. Normal biopsies
b. Lymphocytic infiltration of the proximal and distal esophagus
c. Lymphocytic infiltration of the distal esophagus only

Yamada's Handbook of Gastroenterology, Fourth Edition. John M. Inadomi, Renuka Bhattacharya, Joo Ha Hwang, and Cynthia Ko.

d. Eosinophilic infiltration of the distal esophagus only
e. Eosinophilic infiltration of both the proximal and distal esophagus.

1.4 All of the following medications have been associated with pill-induced esophagitis except:
a. Bisphosphonates
b. Lisinopril
c. Doxycycline
d. Potassium supplements
e. Nonsteroidal anti-inflammatory drugs

Chapter 2 – The Patient with Heartburn or Chest Pain

2.1 True or false: A normal upper endoscopy excludes gastroesophageal reflux disease as a cause of heartburn or noncardiac chest pain.
a. True
b. False

2.2 Potential lifestyle modifications for patients with heartburn do *not* include:
a. Avoidance of spicy foods
b. Avoidance of fatty foods
c. Weight loss if patient is overweight or obese
d. Eating smaller meals
e. Eating a bedtime snack

2.3 All the following are consistent with an esophageal source of chest pain *except*:
a. Symptoms exacerbated by ingesting cold or hot liquids
b. Symptoms awaken the patient from sleep
c. Symptoms associated with exertion and relieved by rest
d. Symptom relief with antacids
e. Pain radiating to the neck

2.4 A 40-year-old man presents with persistent heartburn symptoms despite taking a PPI twice daily. He is otherwise healthy and takes no medications. He reports following antireflux lifestyle modifications. His body mass index is 25 kg/m^2. Upper endoscopy shows a 3 cm hiatal hernia but no esophagitis or Barrett esophagus. Esophageal manometry demonstrates normal esophageal motility. Twenty-four-hour ambulatory esophageal pH monitoring off PPIs shows abnormal esophageal acid exposure with good symptom correlation. Which of the following is a potential next step in his management?
a. Trial of an alternative PPI
b. Taper off PPI, with trial of high-dose H2-receptor antagonist

c. Trial of tricyclic antidepressant
d. Trial of selective serotonin reuptake inhibitor
e. Referral to consider Nissen fundoplication

2.5 According to recent guidelines, screening for Barrett esophagus would be appropriate in which of the following patients?
a. A 30-year-old African-American woman with two years of GERD symptoms
b. A 45-year-old Asian-American man with five years of GERD symptoms
c. A 60-year-old Caucasian man with 15 years of GERD symptoms
d. A 40-year-old Caucasian woman with seven years of GERD symptoms

Chapter 3 – The Patient with Gastrointestinal Bleeding

3.1 A 49-year-old healthy woman presents with small volume hematemesis. She does not have a history of liver disease and denies intake of nonsteroidal anti-inflammatory agents or aspirin. Her blood pressure is 100/70 and heart rate is 100. Physical examination is otherwise normal. Which of the following is *not* an appropriate up-front step in her evaluation and management?
a. Placement of two large-bore intravenous catheters
b. Resuscitation with intravenous crystalloid solution
c. Urgent upper endoscopy
d. Initiation of intravenous PPIs
e. Type and cross for potential transfusion of red blood cells

3.2 Endoscopic therapy is indicated for which of the following lesions in patients with acute upper GI bleeding?
a. Gastric ulcer with clean base
b. Duodenal ulcer with flat pigmented spot
c. Gastric ulcer with visible vessel in the base
d. Nonbleeding Mallory–Weiss tear
e. Gastric varices without bleeding stigmata

3.3 Which of the following is not recommended for the treatment of esophageal variceal hemorrhage?
a. Endoscopic sclerotherapy
b. Endoscopic variceal band ligation
c. Transjugular intrahepatic portosystemic shunt
d. Balloon tamponade
e. Argon plasma coagulation

3.4 A 75-year-old man presents with diffuse abdominal pain followed by rectal bleeding. He has a history of hypertension and diabetes. His initial blood pressure in 120/85 with a pulse of 76. On exam, he has diffuse abdominal tenderness without guarding or rebound. Rectal examination shows small amounts of rectal bleeding. What is the most likely diagnosis?

- **a.** Ischemic colitis
- **b.** Diverticulosis
- **c.** Internal hemorrhoids
- **d.** Colorectal cancer
- **e.** Colonic angiodysplasia

3.5 Which of the following is not indicated in the evaluation and management of patients with unexplained iron deficiency anemia after a negative upper endoscopy and colonoscopy?

- **a.** Video capsule endoscopy
- **b.** CT enterography
- **c.** CT of abdomen and pelvis with and without contrast
- **d.** MR enterography
- **e.** Oral iron supplementation

Chapter 4 – The Patient with Unexplained Weight Loss

4.1 Which of the following suggests malabsorption as a cause of unexplained weight loss?

- **a.** Normal fecal fat level
- **b.** Low fecal elastase level
- **c.** High serum carotene level
- **d.** Normal anti-tissue transglutaminase IgA level
- **e.** High serum vitamin D level

4.2 A 65-year-old man presents with postprandial abdominal pain, fear of eating, and a 20-pound unintentional weight loss. He denies any other gastrointestinal symptoms and has no shortness of breath. He has a history of well-controlled hypertension and a 30 pack-year history of smoking. He appears as a thin older man with normal affect and without localizing signs on physical exam. Laboratory studies are notable for mild anemia, albumin 3.2 g/dl, normal creatinine, and normal liver chemistries. Chest x-ray, upper endoscopy and colonoscopy are normal. Abdominal CT shows mild calcifications of the abdominal aorta but no other abnormalities. Which diagnosis is consistent with this presentation?

- **a.** Chronic pancreatitis
- **b.** Depression
- **c.** Adult rumination syndrome
- **d.** Chronic mesenteric ischemia
- **e.** Congestive heart failure

4.3 A 35-year-old man presents with an unintentional weight loss of 30 pounds. He reports poor appetite, loss of interest in daily activities, and insomnia. He denies gastrointestinal symptoms and does not take any current medications. Physical exam and laboratory investigation are unremarkable. What is the appropriate next step for evaluation and management?

a. Abdominal and pelvic imaging
b. Upper endoscopy
c. Colonoscopy
d. Initiation of appetite stimulant
e. Initiation of antidepressant medication

4.4 Unintentional weight loss can be caused by all of the following infections *except*:

a. Human immunodeficiency virus
b. Hepatitis C
c. Tuberculosis
d. Subacute bacterial endocarditis
e. Ascaris lumbricoides

4.5 A 35-year-old woman presents with 25-pound unintentional weight loss. She also reports symptoms of nausea, vomiting, abdominal distension, and constipation. Laboratory testing is notable for an albumin of 3.2 g/dl and normal thyroid tests, blood counts, and liver chemistries. HIV and tuberculosis testing are negative. Upper endoscopy and colonoscopy are normal. Abdominal CT scan shows a dilated stomach and dilated loops of small and large bowel without a transition point to normal caliber bowel. What is a possible diagnosis?

a. Anorexia nervosa
b. Bulimia nervosa
c. Adult rumination syndrome
d. Chronic intestinal pseudo-obstruction
e. Gastroparesis

Chapter 5 – The Patient with Nausea and Vomiting

5.1 Which of the following is most appropriate for a 17-year-old man with no significant past medical history, on no medications, who calls the nurse helpline reporting a one-day history of nausea and vomiting with myalgias and diarrhea?

a. Stool studies for ova and parasites
b. Colonoscopy
c. Barium upper GI study
d. No workup at this time
e. Gastric emptying study

5.2 Which of the following conditions would be most likely to have an associated succussion splash?
a. Diabetic gastroparesis
b. Viral gastroenteritis
c. Psychogenic vomiting
d. Erythromycin-associated vomiting
e. Intracranial hemorrhage

5.3 Which of the following would be most consistent with cannabinoid hyperemesis syndrome?
a. Small bowel distension on imaging
b. Relief of symptoms by hot bath or shower
c. Feculent emesis
d. Delayed gastric emptying on scintigraphy
e. Tachygastria on electrogastrography

5.4 Which of the following infections can cause nausea and vomiting?
a. *E. coli* O157:H7
b. *Bacillus cereus*
c. Adenovirus
d. *Clostridium difficile*
e. *Campylobacter jejuni*

5.5 Which of the following nongastrointestinal illnesses can cause nausea and vomiting?
a. Cushing's disease
b. Multiple sclerosis
c. Acute hepatitis B
d. Chronic obstructive pulmonary disease
e. Subacute bacterial endocarditis

Chapter 6 – The Patient with Abdominal Pain

6.1 In a patient with a suspected perforation, what test should be performed as quickly as possible?
a. Abdominal ultrasound
b. Abdominal series radiography (supine and upright or decubitus)
c. Upper endoscopy
d. Upper GI with barium

6.2 A patient presents with abdominal pain and has a positive Carnett sign on physical examination. What is the likely etiology of the patient's pain?
a. IBS
b. Cholecystitis

c. Rectus sheath hematoma
d. Appendicitis

6.3 A patient is evaluated in the emergency department for worsening RUQ abdominal pain. The patient has a positive Murphy sign on physical exam and has a fever to 39 °C. Labs demonstrate a leukocytosis but no liver function test (LFT) abnormalities. What is the next appropriate step in management?
a. Surgery
b. Request interventional radiology to place a percutaneous cholecystostomy tube
c. ERCP
d. IV hydration, pain management, and IV antibiotics

Chapter 7 – The Patient with Gas and Bloating

7.1 A 26-year-old woman complains of increased gas and flatulence. She denies weight loss, melena, hematochezia, or other alarm features, and she has no family history of inflammatory bowel disease or celiac disease. Her laboratory tests including hemoglobin, iron, albumin, B_{12}, folate, and fat-soluble vitamin concentrations are normal. Breath hydrogen and methane testing is normal. Of the following, which is the most reasonable recommendation?
a. Pancreatic enzyme supplementation
b. Rifaximin 550 mg three times daily for 14 days
c. Ciprofloxacin and metronidazole
d. Low FODMAP diet

7.2 Which of the following sources of complex carbohydrate is completely absorbed in healthy individuals?
a. Oat
b. Potato
c. Corn
d. Rice

Chapter 8 – The Patient with Ileus or Obstruction

8.1 What is the best initial management for a patient with acute colonic pseudo-obstruction?
a. Nasogastric tube suctioning, discontinuation of narcotics and other potential exacerbating drugs, and correction of potential electrolyte disturbances
b. Neostigmine
c. Interventional radiology placement of a cecostomy tube
d. Surgery

8.2 What is the best management of a patient who presents with acute small intestinal obstruction and does not respond to conservative measures (NPO, nasogastric tube suction, correction of electrolyte disturbances, frequent change of body position)?

a. Neostigmine
b. Water-soluble contrast enema
c. Colonic decompression by colonoscopy
d. Surgery

8.3 A patient with acute colonic pseudo-obstruction and a cecal diameter of 10 cm is initially treated with nasogastric tube insertion with suctioning, intravenous hydration, frequent position changes, and correction of electrolyte disturbances. The next day repeated plain abdominal radiographs reveal a cecum diameter of 13 cm. The patient describes abdominal distension and mild discomfort but has no peritoneal findings on examination. What is the best management option?

a. Neostigmine
b. Decompression of colon by colonoscopy
c. Cecostomy tube placement by interventional radiology
d. Surgery

Chapter 9 – The Patient with Constipation

9.1 A patient with chronic constipation responds to polyethylene glycol with increased bowel movements from one per week to once every third day; however, she reports her quality of life has not improved because she has persistent symptoms of "incomplete evacuation" with each movement. What is the next best test to identify the cause of symptoms?

a. Colonic transit test
b. Colonoscopy with biopsies
c. Anorectal manometry
d. CT abdomen and pelvis

9.2 What is the best initial therapy for dyssynergic defecation?

a. Sphincter myotomy
b. Botulinum toxin sphincter injection
c. Biofeedback
d. Nitroglycerin topical ointment

Chapter 10 – The Patient with Diarrhea

10.1 A 21-year-old woman with systemic lupus erythematosus (SLE) is sent to you in consultation for a three month history of nonbloody loose to watery stools five to six times per day. She has lost 17 pounds during this period. Her physical examination is notable for pitting edema of her lower extremities, but no abdominal masses or tenderness. Laboratory tests are notable for a normal complete blood count and electrolytes, but a low albumin (2.1 mg/dl). Stool tests are negative for red and white blood cells, and an enteric pathogen panel is negative. Fecal electrolytes include a sodium of 80 and potassium of 30. You perform a colonoscopy that is normal to the terminal ileum including random biopsies that reveal normal small intestinal and colonic biopsies. What is the next best test for her evaluation?

a. CT scan of the chest, abdomen, and pelvis
b. Fecal α1-antitrypsin clearance
c. Octreotide scan
d. SeHCAT testing

10.2 A 34-year-old woman presents with watery diarrhea. Her stool tests include the absence of red or white cells, negative bacterial culture and *C. difficile*, and concentrations of sodium of 65 and potassium 15. What is the most likely cause of her diarrhea?

a. Magnesium-containing laxative
b. IBS
c. VIP-secreting tumor
d. Senna-containing laxative

10.3 A 19-year-old college student complains of nausea, vomiting, and diarrhea since yesterday evening. She and several friends ate at an Asian restaurant in the afternoon, and within six hours, two of the five diners had acute onset of nausea and vomiting, followed by watery diarrhea. Minor abdominal cramping is also noted, but no blood is seen in stool. No travel history is noted. What is the most likely cause of symptoms?

a. Enterotoxigenic *E. coli*
b. *Bacillus cereus*
c. *Campylobacter jejuni*
d. *Shigella*

Chapter 11 – The Patient with an Abdominal Mass

11.1 On CT scan, a 45-year-old man was incidentally found to have a well-circumscribed, round, 3 cm mass that appears to arise from the wall of the stomach. What is the next appropriate step in evaluation?

a. Esophagogastroduodenoscopy
b. Upper GI series with barium
c. Follow-up CT scan in six months to assess for interval growth
d. EUS FNA

11.2 A 64-year-old woman presents to her physician with complaints of new-onset jaundice and a 15-pound unintentional weight loss over the past three months. LFTs demonstrate elevated bilirubin, alkaline phosphatase, AST, and ALT. CA 19-9 is also elevated. True or false: Given the elevated CA 19-9, a diagnosis of pancreatic cancer can be made.

a. True
b. False

Chapter 12 – The Patient with Jaundice or Abnormal Liver Biochemical Tests

12.1 A patient with prolonged jaundice due to primary biliary cholangitis would be expected to have all of the following except:

a. Vitamin D deficiency
b. Diminished bone density
c. Low cholesterol levels
d. Severe pruritus

12.2 Jaundice in the newborn may be due to physiological neonatal jaundice, breast milk jaundice, or Lucey–Driscoll syndrome. The pathophysiology of these conditions relates to:

a. Impaired hepatocyte secretion of bilirubin
b. Reduced activity of UGT
c. Increased destruction of red blood cells
d. Inadequate caloric intake

12.3 A patient has been hospitalized in the intensive care unit for postoperative sepsis and has been critically ill. Fortunately, he is responding to antibiotics and clinically improving. Of the following, the *least* likely etiology for persistent hyperbilirubinemia is:

a. Renal failure
b. Covalent binding of bilirubin to albumin
c. Development of gallstones
d. Ongoing use of TPN

12.4 Which of the following is true?

a. Antimitochondrial antibody is positive in approximately 50% of patients with primary biliary cholangitis
b. Anti-LKM antibody is associated with older patients with autoimmune hepatitis
c. Anti-LKM antibodies are associated with a more benign course of autoimmune hepatitis
d. Anti-smooth muscle antibodies may be present in up to 50% of PBC patients

12.5 Which of the following is *false* regarding the diagnosis of Wilson disease?
- **a.** Ceruloplasmin is a copper storage protein
- **b.** Free serum copper is low in Wilson disease
- **c.** Urinary copper can be markedly elevated in chronic cholestatic liver disease
- **d.** Ceruloplasmin can be low in advanced liver disease of any etiology

12.6 Which of the following diseases is typically characterized by a low serum alkaline phosphatase level?
- **a.** PBC
- **b.** PSC
- **c.** Wilson disease
- **d.** Cholangiocarcinoma

Chapter 13 – The Patient with Ascites

13.1 Routine analysis of ascites fluid should include all of the following with the *exception* of:
- **a.** Total protein
- **b.** White blood cell count with differential
- **c.** Albumin
- **d.** Glucose

13.2 All the following are associated with high SAAG, low protein ascites, *except*:
- **a.** Alcoholic hepatitis
- **b.** Hepatitis C cirrhosis
- **c.** Congestive heart failure
- **d.** Nodular regenerative hyperplasia

13.3 In a patient with tense ascites who develops hepatorenal syndrome (HRS), all the following should be part of management, *except*:
- **a.** Intravenous albumin
- **b.** Discontinue nephrotoxic medications
- **c.** Increase diuretic doses
- **d.** Consider use of octreotide and midodrine

Chapter 14 – The Patient Requiring Nutritional Support

14.1 Which of the following findings is not typically seen with hypocalcemia?
- **a.** Trousseau sign
- **b.** Hyporeflexia
- **c.** Heart block
- **d.** Seizures
- **e.** Paresthesias

14.2 What is the daily caloric requirement of a 70 kg person who is postoperative?

a. 1400–1750 kcal
b. 1750–2100 kcal
c. 2100–2800 kcal
d. 3000–4000 kcal

14.3 In a patient with an active Crohn's flare who is unable to tolerate any oral intake, how soon should TPN be initiated?

a. In 14–21 days
b. In 10–14 days
c. In one to seven days
d. TPN is contraindicated during a Crohn's flare

Chapter 15 – The Patient Requiring Endoscopic Procedures

15.1 Which of the following is not an accepted indication for performing endoscopy?

a. Surveillance of Barrett esophagus
b. Evaluation of suspected upper GI bleeding
c. Evaluation of suspected perforated duodenal ulcer
d. Evaluation of dysphagia

15.2 A 67-year-old man is scheduled for upper endoscopy for evaluation and management of solid food dysphagia. He is on coumadin for a mechanical heart valve in the mitral position. What is the appropriate management of his anticoagulation therapy?

a. Coumadin should be held for two days, and low molecular weight heparin should be administered until the night before the scheduled procedure
b. Coumadin should be held for five to seven days prior to the procedure, and low molecular weight heparin should be administered until the night before the scheduled procedure
c. Coumadin should be held for five to seven days. No bridge therapy is needed
d. Coumadin should not be held for the procedure

Chapter 16 – Motor Disorders of the Esophagus

16.1 What is the most common cause of noncardiac chest pain?

a. High-amplitude contractions of the esophageal body
b. Simultaneous contractions of the esophageal body
c. Gastroesophageal acid reflux
d. Hypertensive LES

16.2 The defining characteristic of type I (classic) achalasia includes an IRP $\geq$ 15 mmHg plus which of the following esophageal motility findings?
- **a.** Premature contractions
- **b.** Pan-esophageal pressurization
- **c.** Absent contractility
- **d.** Increased contractility

16.3 What is the most common cause of oropharyngeal dysphagia?
- **a.** Cerebrovascular accident
- **b.** Parkinson disease
- **c.** Myasthenia gravis
- **d.** Polymyositis

Chapter 17 – Gastroesophageal Reflux Disease and Eosinophilic Esophagitis

17.1 What is the most common adverse event associated with PPIs?
- **a.** *C. difficile*-associated diarrhea
- **b.** Nosocomial pneumonia
- **c.** Bone fracture
- **d.** Renal failure
- **e.** Increased heartburn upon discontinuation of drug

17.2 What is the most common cause of heartburn symptoms that persist despite PPI therapy?
- **a.** Excessive gastric acid production
- **b.** Functional heartburn
- **c.** Nonacid reflux
- **d.** Alkaline reflux

17.3 What is the most common endoscopic finding in patients with documented gastroesophageal reflux disease?
- **a.** Normal
- **b.** Barrett esophagus
- **c.** Erosive esophagitis
- **d.** Esophageal stricture

17.4 Which of the following food groups should you advise a patient to avoid when prescribing dietary management of eosinophilic esophagitis?
- **a.** Specific carbohydrates
- **b.** Fructans, galactans, fructose, and polyols
- **c.** Inulins, oligofructose, lactulose, and galacto-oligosaccharides
- **d.** Dairy, soy, wheat, egg, nuts, shellfish

Chapter 18 – Esophageal Neoplasia

18.1 Which of the following is the strongest risk factor for esophageal adenocarcinoma?
- **a.** Alcohol
- **b.** Smoking
- **c.** White race
- **d.** Intestinal metaplasia of the esophagus

18.2 What is the recommended management of Barrett esophagus with high-grade dysplasia?
- **a.** Chemoprevention with aspirin and high-dose PPI
- **b.** Endoscopic surveillance every three months
- **c.** Endoscopic radiofrequency ablation alone
- **d.** Endoscopic resection of visible lesions followed by ablation of flat Barrett mucosa
- **e.** Esophagectomy

18.3 Which of the following is associated with esophageal squamous cell carcinoma (ESCC)?
- **a.** White race
- **b.** Heartburn
- **c.** Alcohol
- **d.** Intestinal metaplasia

Chapter 19 – Disorders of Gastric Emptying

19.1 Which of the following scintigraphic-based gastric emptying protocols is most accurate for diagnosing gastroparesis?
- **a.** Two-hours liquid
- **b.** Two-hours solid
- **c.** Four-hours liquid
- **d.** Four-hours solid

19.2 For patients with established diabetic gastroparesis, which therapy should be pursued if medical therapy fails to alleviate symptoms?
- **a.** Gastric pacing
- **b.** Venting gastrostomy and feeding jejunostomy
- **c.** Total parenteral nutrition
- **d.** Total gastrectomy

19.3 In patients with early dumping syndrome, what is the best therapy in addition to dietary modifications?
- **a.** Omeprazole 40 mg daily
- **b.** Rifaximin 550 mg three times daily

c. Octreotide 50 mcg three times daily
d. Insulin, regularly titrated to maintain glucose below 130

Chapter 20 – Acid Peptic Disorders

20.1 What is the most common cause of hypergastrinemia in a 24-year-old patient presenting with recurrent duodenal ulcer disease?
a. Gastrinoma (Zollinger–Ellison syndrome)
b. Acid suppression therapy
c. Pernicious anemia
d. Laboratory error

20.2 What is the most clinically expeditious method to differentiate hypergastrinemia due to gastrinoma from gastrin elevation due to PPI therapy?
a. Basal and maximal acid output
b. Secretin stimulation
c. Gastric fluid pH
d. Serum chromogranin A

20.3 Which of the following is the most effective eradication therapy for patients who have persistent *H. pylori* after a 14-day course of clarithromycin, amoxicillin, and PPI?
a. Clarithromycin and metronidazole plus PPI
b. Bismuth, metronidazole, and tetracycline plus PPI
c. PPI plus amoxicillin for five days followed by clarithromycin and nitroimidazole for five days

20.4 A 58-year-old man is admitted to the hospital for symptoms of melena and epigastric pain for two days. His physical exam is notable for orthostatic hypotension, reduced bowel sounds, and epigastric tenderness with guarding. His rectal examination reveals melena, but his nasogastric lavage consists of bile-stained nonbloody fluid. His laboratory tests are notable for an Hb of 7.1 mg/dl, an HCT of 22, and a white blood count of 18.3 with a predominance of neutrophils. An intravenous PPI infusion is initiated, and he is resuscitated with normal saline and transfused two units of packed red blood cells. He is no longer orthostatic and repeated Hb is 9.7 mg/dl. What is the next best step in management?
a. Upper gastrointestinal endoscopy
b. Colonoscopy
c. CT scan of the abdomen
d. Interventional radiology embolization

Chapter 21 – Functional Dyspepsia

21.1 A 28-year-old woman is referred to your office for symptoms of epigastric discomfort, early satiety, nausea, and bloating. The symptoms have been constant for the past several months. She denies weight loss, nausea, and gastrointestinal bleeding. She does not take any prescription or over-the-counter medications. Her physical examination is normal and her laboratory testing shows a normal complete blood count and liver tests. What is the next best step in management?

a. Initiation of metoclopramide
b. *H. pylori* testing and eradication if positive
c. Upper endoscopy
d. CT scan of the abdomen

21.2 The patient in question 21.1 has negative *H. pylori* testing and is placed on a daily PPI. Her symptoms only respond partially, and an upper endoscopy is performed. What is the most likely finding?

a. Normal
b. Duodenal ulcer
c. Erosive esophagitis
d. Gastric malignancy

21.3 The patient in questions 21.1 and 21.2 remains symptomatic on PPI therapy despite providing reassurance and education about her symptoms. What is the next best step in management?

a. Abdominal CT scan
b. Gallbladder scintigraphy with ejection fraction
c. Magnetic resonance angiography
d. Trial of a tricyclic antidepressant

21.4 A 65-year-old Korean-American man presents with two months of dull epigastric discomfort. He reports a five-pound unintentional weight loss but denies symptoms of gastrointestinal bleeding. He has no family history of gastrointestinal illnesses or malignancies. What is the appropriate first step in management?

a. Abdominal CT scan
b. Test for *H. pylori* and treatment if positive
c. Trial of PPI
d. Abdominal ultrasound
e. Upper endoscopy

21.5 A potential mechanism of action for buspirone in patients with functional dyspepsia is:

a. Relaxation of the gastric fundus
b. Accelerating gastric emptying
c. Modulating visceral hypersensitivity
d. Inhibiting gastric acid secretion

Chapter 22 – Gastric Neoplasia

22.1 Which of the following is not a high-risk feature in evaluation of a gastrointestinal stromal tumor?
a. >10 mitosis/50 HPF
b. Tumor diameter >10 cm
c. Tumor with mucosal ulceration and GI bleeding
d. Tumor diameter >5 cm with >5 mitosis/50 HPF

22.2 A patient underwent EGD to evaluate epigastric pain and was found to have evidence of a 3 cm malignant-appearing ulcer with biopsies demonstrating intestinal-type gastric adenocarcinoma. Which is the next most appropriate test?
a. EUS
b. PET
c. CT
d. Upper GI series

Chapter 23 – Celiac Disease

23.1 Which of the following grains is tolerated by most patients with celiac disease?
a. Wheat
b. Barley
c. Buckwheat
d. Rye
e. Malt

23.2 Which of the following tests is no longer recommended as part of the diagnostic evaluation of suspected celiac disease?
a. Anti-tissue transglutaminase IgA antibody
b. Anti-endomysial antibody
c. Total IgA level
d. Anti-gliadin antibody
e. Small intestinal biopsy

23.3 All the following are true statements about celiac disease *except*:
a. The mainstay of treatment is a gluten-free diet
b. Celiac disease is associated with Down syndrome

- **c.** A gluten-free diet will result in gradual reversal of histologic findings
- **d.** Serologic tests will remain positive even with a gluten-free diet
- **e.** Histological findings on small bowel biopsy may be milder than expected due to gluten restriction in the diet at the time of diagnostic evaluation

23.4 Duodenal villous atrophy is *not* seen in which of the following entities?
- **a.** Crohn's disease
- **b.** Small intestinal bacterial overgrowth
- **c.** Intestinal lymphoma
- **d.** *Campylobacter jejuni* infection
- **e.** Eosinophilic enteritis

23.5 What is the most common cause of persistent gastrointestinal symptoms in a patient with established celiac disease?
- **a.** Inadvertent or ongoing gluten ingestion
- **b.** Type II refractory sprue
- **c.** Crohn's disease
- **d.** Pancreatic insufficiency
- **e.** Type I refractory sprue

Chapter 24 – Short Bowel Syndrome

24.1 A patient with Crohn's disease involving the small intestine becomes refractory to medical therapy and undergoes a segmental resection of the distal 80 cm of ileum. Two months after surgery, she describes persistent six to eight nonbloody watery bowel movements daily. Her CRP and fecal calprotectin are normal. Magnetic resonance enterography reveals an intact anastomosis and no inflammatory changes in the remaining small and large intestine. Stool testing includes a sodium of 90 and potassium of 35, negative qualitative fat, negative enteric pathogen panel, and absence of *C. difficile* toxin. Which of the following is the best therapeutic option:
- **a.** Prednisone
- **b.** Vedolizumab
- **c.** Oral vancomycin
- **d.** Cholestyramine
- **e.** Teduglutide

24.2 What is the most likely composition of nephrolithiasis in a patient with short bowel syndrome?
- **a.** Calcium oxalate
- **b.** Calcium phosphate
- **c.** Sodium hydroxyapatite
- **d.** Calcium urate

24.3 A patient with short bowel syndrome suddenly becomes obtunded after attending an annual cookie exchange event. A significant metabolic acidosis with respiratory alkalosis is revealed. What is the most likely etiology of this presentation?

a. Diabetic ketoacidosis
b. Alcoholic ketoacidosis
c. Salicylate overdose
d. D-lactic acidemia

24.4 What type of fat source is best absorbed in a patient with short bowel syndrome?

a. Short-chain triglycerides
b. Medium-chain triglycerides
c. Long-chain triglycerides

Chapter 25 – Small Intestinal Neoplasia

25.1 Patients with FAP syndrome should have which of the following performed every one to two years for surveillance purposes?

a. Double balloon enteroscopy
b. CT scan
c. Side-viewing upper endoscopy
d. Standard upper endoscopy

25.2 Which lab test should be ordered if carcinoid syndrome is suspected?

a. CA 19-9
b. CEA
c. Urinary 5-HIAA
d. Liver function panel

Chapter 26 – Diverticular Disease of the Colon

26.1 Which of the following statements about diverticular disease is *true*?

a. Diverticular hemorrhage more commonly originates from the left colon
b. Diverticulitis more commonly originates in the proximal colon (i.e. cecum, ascending and transverse colon) than in the sigmoid colon
c. Diverticulitis is precipitated by seeds, corn, or nuts
d. Most patients with diverticulosis will not develop complications (i.e. diverticulitis or bleeding) in their lifetime
e. Barium enema is recommended during an acute attack of diverticulitis to delineate the severity of strictures and determine if fistulization is present

26.2 Which of the following is *always* an indication for surgery for diverticulitis?
- **a.** Persistent symptoms after initial uncomplicated episode of diverticulitis
- **b.** Peritonitis
- **c.** Abscess formation
- **d.** Partial obstruction during acute episode of diverticulitis
- **e.** Recurrent uncomplicated diverticulitis

26.3 True or false: Diverticulosis commonly causes symptoms.
- **a.** True
- **b.** False

26.4 Which of the following is *not* an indication for inpatient treatment of diverticulitis?
- **a.** 2 cm pelvic abscess
- **b.** Immunosuppressive therapy
- **c.** Failure to improve with outpatient therapy
- **d.** Temperature of 38.0° C
- **e.** Colovesicular fistula

26.5 Which of the following is a risk factor for symptomatic diverticular disease?
- **a.** High levels of physical activity
- **b.** Low levels of red meat consumption
- **c.** Obesity
- **d.** Calcium channel blocker medications
- **e.** Excess alcohol consumption

Chapter 27 – Irritable Bowel Syndrome

27.1 Which of the following is effective for treating constipation-predominant IBS?
- **a.** Lubiprostone
- **b.** Dicyclomine
- **c.** Alosetron
- **d.** Tricyclic antidepressants
- **e.** Atropine with diphenoxylate

27.2 Which of the following is recommended for initial evaluation of a patient with suspected IBS?
- **a.** Fecal fat quantification
- **b.** Colonoscopy
- **c.** Complete blood count
- **d.** Abdominal CT imaging
- **e.** Colonic transit testing

27.3 Which of the following is an appropriate therapy for a patient with diarrhea-predominant IBS?

a. Linaclotide
b. Tegaserod
c. Lubiprostone
d. Tricyclic antidepressant

27.4 Which of the following is true about the medication eluxadoline?

a. It is indicated for treatment of constipation-predominant IBS
b. It has mu-opioid receptor agonist activity
c. It has delta-opioid receptor agonist activity
d. It has been associated with risk of ischemic colitis

27.5 Behavior and complementary therapies for IBS include all of the following *except*:

a. Massage therapy
b. Cognitive-behavioral therapy
c. Mindfulness-based stress reduction
d. Biofeedback and relaxation training
e. Hypnotherapy

Chapter 28 – Inflammatory Bowel Disease

28.1 A 34-year-old patient with ulcerative proctitis presents with worsened diarrhea, abdominal pain, and tenesmus. What is the best initial evaluation?

a. CT scan of the abdomen
b. Colonoscopy
c. Stool examination for *C. difficile* toxin
d. Stool electrolytes

28.2 A 38-year-old man with 20 years of pan-ulcerative colitis that has been previously in remission on infliximab and methotrexate presents with a three-day history of rapidly increasing abdominal pain, distension, and diarrhea. On examination, he is febrile (39.5 °C) and his abdomen is notable for absent bowel sounds, distension, and diffuse tenderness with rebound and guarding. WBC is 21,000 and stool testing is negative for *C. difficile* toxin and enteric pathogens. CT scan of the abdomen reveals dilation of the cecum to 10 cm with bowel wall edema but no free peritoneal air. What is the best step in management?

a. Intravenous steroids
b. Ustekinumab
c. Cyclosporine
d. Tofacitinib
e. Surgical intervention

28.3 A 29-year-old woman with ileal Crohn's disease presents with renal colic. What is the most likely composition of her stones?

a. Calcium phosphate
b. Calcium urate
c. Sodium hydroxyapatite
d. Calcium oxalate

Chapter 29 – Colonic Neoplasia

29.1 A 57-year-old patient presents with a positive result on a screening fecal immunochemical test. He is otherwise asymptomatic and has no family history of colorectal cancer. What is the best next step?

a. Repeat fecal immunochemical test
b. CT scan of the abdomen and pelvis
c. EGD
d. CT colonography
e. Colonoscopy

29.2 A 42-year-old man presents for his annual check-up. His review of systems is completely negative. He tells you that his sister was recently diagnosed with colorectal cancer at age 49. His mother was diagnosed with endometrial cancer in her 50s and his maternal uncle with colorectal cancer at age 63. What do you recommend?

a. Colonoscopy every 10 years beginning now
b. Colonoscopy every 10 years beginning at age 50
c. CT colonography every five years
d. Colonoscopy now, in addition to referral for genetics counseling
e. Annual fecal immunochemical test beginning at age 50

29.3 A 77-year-old woman with a history of a negative colonoscopy 10 years ago, diabetes mellitus, and oxygen-dependent COPD asks what colorectal cancer screening she should undergo. What do you recommend?

a. Annual FIT screening
b. CT colonography every five years
c. Flexible sigmoidoscopy with fecal immunochemical testing
d. Colonoscopy
e. None of the above

29.4 Which of the following is an extraintestinal manifestation of familial adenomatous polyposis syndrome?

a. Pancreatic adenocarcinoma
b. Desmoid tumors
c. Orocutaneous melanin pigmentation
d. Facial trichilemmomas
e. None of the above

29.5 Which of the following types of polyps has malignant potential?
- **a.** Sporadic juvenile polyp
- **b.** Sessile serrated adenoma
- **c.** Hyperplastic polyp
- **d.** Inflammatory polyp
- **e.** Sporadic Peutz–Jeghers polyp

Chapter 30 – Anorectal Diseases

30.1 Which of the following statements about hemorrhoids is *not* true?
- **a.** Hemorrhoids occur in up to 50% of adults in the United States
- **b.** Third-degree hemorrhoids prolapse and require digital reduction
- **c.** Surgical hemorrhoidectomy is the treatment of choice for most second-degree hemorrhoids
- **d.** Most first-degree hemorrhoids can be managed with high-fiber diet, adequate fluid intake, sitz baths, and good anal hygiene
- **e.** Thrombosis of an external hemorrhoid can produce severe pain and bleeding

30.2 Severe anal pain with scant red bleeding is a classic presentation of:
- **a.** Solitary rectal ulcer
- **b.** Anal fissure
- **c.** Pruritus ani
- **d.** Internal hemorrhoids
- **e.** Rectal prolapse

30.3 Fecal incontinence can be caused by all of the following *except*:
- **a.** Obstetric trauma
- **b.** Solitary rectal ulcer
- **c.** Rectal prolapse
- **d.** Ulcerative proctitis
- **e.** Multiple sclerosis

30.4 Which of the following is characteristic of levator ani syndrome?
- **a.** Tenderness and spasm of levator ani muscle on digital rectal exam
- **b.** Intense stabbing or aching pain lasting seconds to minutes
- **c.** Improvement with defecation
- **d.** Prolonged pain-free periods
- **e.** Exacerbation with intake of coffee

30.5 Which is true about anal fissures?
- **a.** Most fissures are located in the anterior or posterior midline
- **b.** Fissures due to Crohn's disease are always located in the midline
- **c.** Initial therapy should include botulinum toxin injection to the anal sphincter
- **d.** Anoscopy is necessary to confirm the diagnosis
- **e.** Topical steroids are necessary to assist healing

Chapter 31 – Pancreatitis

31.1 Which of the following is true regarding pancreatic enzymes therapy?

a. Immediate-release enzymes (nonenteric coated) have been shown to be effective in the treatment of chronic pancreatitis pain in a randomized controlled trial

b. Delayed-release enzymes (enteric coated) have been shown to be effective in the treatment of chronic pancreatitis pain in a randomized controlled trial

c. The mechanism of action of pancreatic enzyme replacement therapy is to increase pancreatic exocrine output in response to a meal

d. They are inexpensive

31.2 When should enteral nutrition with nasojejunal feeding be started in a patient diagnosed with severe acute pancreatitis?

a. On the seventh hospital day

b. Once the prediction of severe acute pancreatitis is made

c. Enteral nutrition should be avoided because it may exacerbate the patient's pancreatitis. Instead start TPN

d. Once the lipase is below five times the upper limit of normal

31.3 What is the theoretical advantage of placing a feeding tube past the ligament of Treitz?

a. Less likely that the tube will be displaced

b. Avoids the risk of tube tip trauma to the major papilla

c. Higher concentration of CCK and secretin-secreting cells in the duodenum

d. Lower concentration of CCK and secretin-secreting cells in the duodenum

31.4 In the setting of acute biliary pancreatitis, when should cholecystectomy be performed?

a. Always shortly after presentation

b. Shortly after presentation for mild acute pancreatitis, delayed days to weeks after presentation for severe acute pancreatitis

c. Shortly after presentation for severe acute pancreatitis, delayed days to weeks after presentation for mild acute pancreatitis

d. Always delayed days to weeks after presentation

e. Cholecystectomy is not necessary after acute biliary pancreatitis

31.5 Which of the following is not an indication for pseudo-cyst drainage?

a. Pseudo-cyst size greater than 6 cm

b. Vomiting due to gastric outlet obstruction

c. Infection of the pseudo-cyst

d. Obstructive jaundice with pruritus
e. Abdominal pain with anorexia and weight loss

Chapter 32 – Pancreatic Neoplasia

32.1 What is the best method for establishing the diagnosis of pancreatic cancer?
a. CA 19-9
b. CEA
c. CT scan
d. EUS FNA
e. PET/CT

32.2 What is the approximate risk of malignancy in a patient with main duct IPMN?
a. <20%
b. 25%
c. 50%
d. 70%

32.3 An EUS FNA is performed in a 40-year-old woman to evaluate a 2 cm pancreatic cyst in the body of the pancreas that was incidentally identified on CT scan. There are no pancreatic duct abnormalities identified, and no masses are appreciated. Cyst fluid aspiration is performed and demonstrates a CEA of 560 ng/dl and an amylase of 30 U/l. What is the most likely diagnosis?
a. Serous cystadenoma
b. Mucinous cystadenoma
c. Side branch IPMN
d. Main duct IPMN

Chapter 33 – Biliary Tract Stones and Cysts

33.1 Cholangiocarcinoma involving the hilum at the confluence of the left and right hepatic ducts is called a:
a. Bismuth tumor
b. Klatskin tumor
c. Krukenberg tumor
d. Caroli tumor

33.2 Which of the disorders listed below is *not* associated with primary sclerosing cholangitis?
a. Ulcerative colitis
b. Sjögren's syndrome
c. Osteopenia
d. Hypertriglyceridemia

33.3 Which type of biliary cyst is characterized by one or more cystic dilations of the intrahepatic ducts without extrahepatic duct disease?

a. Type I
b. Type II
c. Type III
d. Type IV
e. Type V

33.4 Which of the following symptoms is not part of the Charcot triad?

a. RUQ abdominal pain
b. Fever
c. Hypotension
d. Jaundice

33.5 A patient with a history of cholecystectomy presents with recurrent episodes of severe biliary-type pain. Evaluation of the patient during episodes of pain shows no laboratory or imaging abnormalities. If the patient has sphincter of Oddi dysfunction (SOD), with which type would it be most consistent?

a. Type I
b. Type V
c. Type IV
d. None of the above

Chapter 34 – Viral Hepatitis

34.1 True or false: A vigorous immune response to acute hepatitis B infection leads to greater clinical illness and a greater chance of chronic infection.

34.2 Hepatitis B is considered chronic if:

a. HBcAb IgG is present beyond six months
b. HBcAb IgM is present beyond three months
c. HBsAg is present beyond six months

34.3 Which of the following viruses is associated with acute (fulminant) liver failure in pregnant women?

a. Hepatitis D
b. Hepatitis C
c. Hepatitis E

Chapter 35 – Genetic and Metabolic Diseases of the Liver

35.1 Which of the following is true?

a. It is estimated that 50% of NASH patients will progress to cirrhosis
b. An HII of 2.0 is suggestive of hereditary hemochromatosis

c. The peak time of onset of Wilson disease is the fourth decade of life
d. Kayser–Fleischer rings are always present in patients with Wilson disease

35.2 Each of the following can be used in the pharmacotherapy of Wilson disease, except:
a. Penicillamine
b. Trientine
c. Zinc
d. Ursodiol

35.3 Each of the following is a typical histological feature of nonalcoholic steatohepatitis, except:
a. Hepatocyte ballooning
b. Steatosis
c. Pericellular fibrosis
d. Bile ductular proliferation

Chapter 36 – Cholestatic Liver Disease

36.1 Which of the following are potential causes of alkaline phosphatase elevation during the third trimester of pregnancy?
a. Placental release of alkaline phosphatase
b. HELLP syndrome
c. Cholestasis of pregnancy
d. All of the above

36.2 Typical diagnostic findings in PBC include all of the following except:
a. Positive AMA
b. Elevated serum IgM level
c. Dilated bile ducts on ultrasound
d. Granulomas on liver biopsy

36.3 Appropriate medications to prescribe for a patient with PBC include all the following *except*:
a. Ursodiol 15 mg/kg
b. Ursodiol 5 mg/kg
c. Calcium supplementation
d. Vitamin D supplementation

Chapter 37 – Alcoholic Liver Disease

37.1 Which of the following statements about alcoholic hepatitis is *false*?
a. Portal hypertension can exist without cirrhosis
b. Most patients admitted to hospital with alcoholic hepatitis have cirrhosis

c. Alcoholic hepatitis typically results in AST >300 IU/l
d. Continued use of alcohol is associated with a high mortality rate

37.2 Which of the following is *not* typical of liver biopsy findings in alcoholic hepatitis?
a. Pericentral steatosis
b. Lymphocytic inflammation
c. Pericellular fibrosis
d. Mallory hyaline

37.3 Which of the following statements is false among alcoholic hepatitis patients with a Maddrey discriminant function >32:
a. Have a 30-day mortality >50%
b. Will likely derive survival benefit from a course of corticosteroids
c. Are too ill to benefit from alcohol abstinence
d. Benefit from nutritional supplementation

Chapter 38 – Autoimmune Hepatitis

38.1 Which of the following is *false*?
a. Liver biopsy does not play a significant role in the diagnosis of AIH
b. AIH patients with a positive anti-LKM antibody (type 2) are unlikely to have a positive ANA
c. The diagnostic scoring systems for AIH account for the results of viral serologies
d. High levels of serum IgG support the diagnosis of AIH

38.2 Which of the following is *false* regarding liver biopsy findings in AIH?
a. Viral hepatitis and drug-induced hepatitis may have similar histological findings to AIH
b. Bridging necrosis can be seen on biopsies of patients with a severe presentation
c. Moderate (2–3+) iron staining is commonly seen on liver biopsy in AIH patients
d. The inflammation seen in AIH typically consists of lymphoplasmacytic inflammatory cells

Chapter 39 – Complications of Cirrhosis

39.1 Which of the following is *true*?
a. A patient with a HVPG of 15 is more likely to experience variceal bleeding than a patient with an HVPG of 12
b. Hepatopulmonary syndrome is due to pulmonary vascular vasoconstriction
c. Type 1 HRS is more severe than type 2 HRS
d. Type 1 HRS is associated with severe intrarenal vasodilation

39.2 Which of the following is not an appropriate choice for the purposes of variceal prophylaxis?

a. Propranolol
b. Carvedilol
c. Atenolol
d. Nadolol

Chapter 40 – Primary Hepatic Neoplasms

40.1 Which of the following statements about HCC is *false*?

a. 90% of patients with HCC have underlying cirrhosis
b. HCC affects men and women equally
c. HCC is the third leading cause of cancer deaths worldwide
d. HCC can occur in hepatitis B patients who do not have cirrhosis

40.2 Radiographic features of HCC include all of the following *except*:

a. HCC typically has arterial enhancement
b. HCC remains enhancing in portal and delayed phases of multiphase CT or MRI
c. CT and MRI can assess for portal venous invasion
d. Liver masses that meet radiographic criteria for HCC do not require biopsy for diagnosis confirmation

40.3 Which of the following statements about HCC treatment is *true*?

a. The majority of tumors are resectable
b. The recurrence rates after resection are approximately 5% at five years
c. A patient with a 3 cm HCC can receive priority for liver transplantation
d. TACE can be used safely in patients with bilirubin >5

Chapter 41 – Infections of the Gastrointestinal Tract

41.1 All the following are helpful in making the diagnosis of *C. difficile* colitis, except:

a. Tissue culture assay
b. Stool culture
c. Enzyme-linked immunosorbent assay for toxins A and B
d. Colonoscopic findings

41.2 Which of the following is *false* regarding EHEC infection?

a. The disease is caused by the O157:H7 strain
b. It is most prevalent in children <5 years of age
c. EHEC is associated with the development of hemolytic uremic syndrome
d. Treatment includes hydration and antibiotics

41.3 Which of the following is *false* regarding *Campylobacter jejuni* infection?
- **a.** *C. jejuni* is the most common cause of bacterial enterocolitis in the United States
- **b.** *C. jejuni* cannot be isolated from stool culture
- **c.** Infected individuals may present with right lower quadrant abdominal pain and bloody diarrhea
- **d.** Infection is associated with the development of Reiter syndrome and Guillain–Barré syndrome

Chapter 42 – Gastrointestinal Vascular Lesions

42.1 Which of the following is *not* consistent with the diagnosis of a Dieulafoy lesion?
- **a.** Ulcerated lesion with a pigmented protuberance
- **b.** Pigmented protuberance without an associated ulcer
- **c.** Adherent clot without an associated ulcer
- **d.** Large clot in the stomach without any obvious mucosal abnormality

42.2 Which of the following is *not* appropriate in the management of GAVE?
- **a.** Argon plasma coagulation
- **b.** Bipolar electrocautery
- **c.** TIPS
- **d.** Nd:YAG laser therapy

Chapter 43 – Medical, Surgical, and Endoscopic Treatment of Obesity

43.1 Which patients should be considered for bariatric surgery?
- **a.** Patient with a BMI of 36.0 with metabolic syndrome
- **b.** Patient with a BMI of 39.9 with no medical comorbidities
- **c.** Patient with a BMI of 45.0 and no medical comorbidities
- **d.** Both a and c

43.2 Which of the following has been demonstrated to result in the greatest excess weight loss with the lowest rate of weight regain and results in resolution of comorbidities?
- **a.** Laparoscopic adjustable gastric band
- **b.** Sleeve gastrectomy
- **c.** Biliopancreatic diversion with duodenal switch
- **d.** Roux-en-Y gastric bypass

Answers

1.1 (b) Videofluoroscopic swallowing study. The patient's symptoms of coughing and nasal regurgitation are suggestive of oropharyngeal dysphagia. This is best evaluated by videofluoroscopy, which can evaluate coordination of the oropharyngeal swallowing mechanisms.

1.2 (d) Pill-associated ulceration. Common causes of odynophagia include fungal or viral (but not bacterial) infection, caustic ingestions, foreign bodies, and pill-induced ulcerations. Gastroesophageal reflux disease and Schatzki's rings do not characteristically cause odynophagia.

1.3 (e) The history and endoscopic findings are consistent with eosinophilic esophagitis. Histologically, this is characterized by eosinophilic infiltration of both the proximal and distal esophagus. Eosinophilic infiltration of the distal esophagus is more consistent with gastroesophageal reflux disease than eosinophilic esophagitis. Lymphocytic infiltration is not seen in this condition.

1.4 (b) Lisinopril has not been associated with pill-induced esophagitis. Bisphosphonates, slow-release potassium supplements, nonsteroidal anti-inflammatory drugs, and doxycycline have all been implicated as causing pill-induced esophageal injury.

2.1 (b) False. Patients with nonerosive gastroesophageal reflux disease may not have demonstrated esophagitis or anatomic abnormalities on upper endoscopy.

2.2 (e) Commonly recommended lifestyle modifications for managing GERD include avoiding spicy, fatty, or acidic foods, weight loss (if appropriate), and eating smaller meals to avoid gastric overdistension. Eating meals or snacks close to bedtime may predispose to nocturnal reflux.

2.3 (c) Noncardiac chest pain from esophageal sources is often indistinguishable from angina, including radiation in a pattern similar to angina. However, esophageal pain is rarely brought on by exertion.

2.4 (e) The patient has persistent heartburn and regurgitation symptoms with objective documentation of reflux on esophageal pH monitoring. Because he has not responded to high-dose PPIs, referral to consider an antireflux procedure is reasonable. In most patients, switching to an alternative PPI does not provide much clinical benefit. Tapering off a PPI to an H2-receptor antagonist is usually not clinically effective. Because he has documented acid reflux and not reflux hypersensitivity or functional heartburn, trials of tricyclic antidepressants or selective serotonin reuptake inhibitors are not indicated.

2.5 (c) Recent guidelines from the American College of Gastroenterology recommend screening for Barrett esophagus in men with chronic (>5 years) and/or frequent (weekly or more) symptoms of GERD and two or more risk factors for Barrett esophagus or esophageal adenocarcinoma. Risk factors include age over 50 years. Caucasian race, central obesity, current or past smoking, and a confirmed family history of Barrett esophagus or esophageal adenocarcinoma. Only patient (c) meets these criteria.

3.1 (c) The initial management of patients with acute gastrointestinal bleeding should include hemodynamic stabilization and assessment of severity of blood loss. Sending a type and cross in case red blood cell transfusion is needed should be done with initial laboratory assessment. Endoscopy should be pursued only after hemodynamic stabilization unless the bleeding rate is too brisk. It may be pursued after hemodynamic stabilization in patients with less severe bleeding.

3.2 (c) Endoscopic therapy is indicated for patients with acute upper GI bleeding with certain high-risk lesions. These include peptic ulcers with active bleeding, a visible vessel, or an adherent clot with visible vessel or active bleeding. Peptic ulcers with clean bases or flat pigmented spots do not need endoscopic therapy. Esophageal varices with stigmata of bleeding such as red wale signs should also be treated endoscopically. Endoscopic therapy of gastric varices is generally less successful, and other interventional radiology techniques such as TIPS, BATO, or BRTO should be considered instead.

3.3 (e) Argon plasma coagulation. Endoscopic therapy for variceal hemorrhage includes sclerotherapy or band ligation. TIPS and surgical portocaval shunts can reduce the pressure gradient within the liver to reduce the risk of variceal hemorrhage. In the setting of massive variceal hemorrhage, balloon tamponade can help stabilize the patient prior to endoscopic or radiologic therapy. There is no role for argon plasma coagulation in the treatment of variceal hemorrhage.

3.4 (a) Ischemic colitis. Ischemic colitis typically presents with abdominal pain followed by hematochezia. It is more common in elderly patients with cardiovascular risk factors. Diverticulosis, internal hemorrhoids, angiodysplasias, and colorectal cancer typically do not present with abdominal pain.

3.5 (c) CT of the abdomen and pelvis with and without contrast. With unexplained iron deficiency anemia after an upper endoscopy and a colonoscopy, iron repletion and a small bowel evaluation are indicated. A CT of the abdomen and pelvis with and without contrast is relatively insensitive for small bowel lesions that might cause iron deficiency anemia. Video capsule endoscopy, CT enterography, and MR enterography will all provide more accurate small bowel evaluation than a standard CT of the abdomen and pelvis.

4.1 (b) A low fecal elastase level is seen with pancreatic insufficiency, which may lead to malabsorption of nutrients and unintentional weight loss. Normal fecal fat levels argue against malabsorption, whereas vitamin D and carotene levels are low with malabsorption. A normal anti-tissue transglutaminase IgA level suggests that celiac disease with resulting malabsorption is unlikely.

4.2 (d) Chronic mesenteric ischemia can be seen in patients with risk factors for cardiovascular disease. It presents with postprandial abdominal pain due to restricted mesenteric blood flow, resulting in fear of eating, poor oral intake, and unintentional weight loss. This diagnosis is suggested in this patient by the presence of cardiovascular risk factors and calcifications in the abdominal aorta, indicating atherosclerotic disease. Chronic pancreatitis is less likely with normal abdominal imaging and congestive heart failure with a normal chest x-ray. He does not present with symptoms of vomiting or regurgitation and has normal affect, making adult rumination syndrome and depression less likely.

4.3 (e) The patient's age and lack of localizing symptoms makes malignancy less likely, and he does not need age-appropriate cancer screening. The absence of gastrointestinal symptoms make upper endoscopy and colonoscopy less fruitful. His underlying symptoms are consistent with depression, which would respond best to behavioral therapy and initiation of an antidepressant. Initiation of an appetite stimulant would not address the underlying mood disorder.

4.4 (b) Hepatitis C. Chronic hepatitis C infection is not associated with unintentional weight loss. Weight loss can be a symptom of tuberculosis, human immunodeficiency virus, or Ascaris lumbricoides infections. Subacute bacterial endocarditis can also be associated with weight loss.

4.5 (d) Chronic intestinal pseudo-obstruction. The presence of a dilated stomach, small intestine, and large intestine on abdominal imaging suggests either a bowel obstruction or a motility disorder. The lack of transition to normal caliber distal bowel is inconsistent with a bowel obstruction, so chronic intestinal pseudo-obstruction is a possible diagnosis. A dilated stomach can be seen with gastroparesis but not dilated small or large bowel. Anorexia, bulimia nervosa, and adult rumination syndrome are not consistent with these imaging findings.

5.1 (d) No workup at this time. Acute onset of vomiting in association with myalgias and diarrhea suggests an infectious etiology. Diagnostic evaluation is reserved for patients with chronic symptoms or in the setting of comorbidity, such as in a person with diabetes in whom diabetic ketoacidosis must be excluded.

5.2 (a) A succussion splash, heard through a stethoscope placed on the abdomen during side-to-side movement of the abdomen, is classically found in gastric obstruction and gastroparesis.

5.3 (b) Relief of symptoms by hot bath or shower is typically reported by patients with cannabinoid hyperemesis syndrome. Small bowel distension suggests a motility disorder or obstruction. Delayed gastric emptying on scintigraphy suggests gastroparesis, whereas tachygastria on electrogastrography suggests gastric dysmotility. Feculent emesis suggests a distal bowel obstruction, gastrocolic fistulae, or bacterial overgrowth.

5.4 (b) *Bacillus cereus* infection is a common food-borne illness. The organism produces toxins that can cause nausea and vomiting or diarrhea. *E. coli* O157:H7, *Clostridium difficile*, and *Campylobacter jejuni* typically cause diarrhea but not nausea and vomiting. Adenovirus is a common respiratory virus but occasionally can cause diarrheal symptoms.

5.5 (c) Acute hepatitis B can cause nausea and vomiting. Adrenal insufficiency is another etiology of nausea and vomiting, but not Cushing's syndrome. Although neurologic disorders such as malignancy or intracranial hemorrhage can cause nausea and vomiting, multiple sclerosis is not a common cause. Nausea and vomiting are not typical symptoms of subacute bacterial endocarditis or chronic obstructive pulmonary disease.

6.1 (b) Abdominal series radiography (supine and upright or decubitus). Rapid diagnosis of a perforated viscus is essential, because these patients typically require surgical management. Abdominal radiography will demonstrate evidence of free air within the abdomen, rapidly confirming the diagnosis of a perforated viscus.

6.2 (c) Rectus sheath hematoma. The Carnett test can distinguish intra-abdominal discomfort from abdominal wall pain. Increased tenderness upon raising the head and tensing the abdomen suggests a superficial abdominal wall source.

6.3 (d) IV hydration, pain management, and IV antibiotics. This patient has evidence of acute cholecystitis. Initial management involves supportive care with IV hydration, pain management, and IV antibiotics. The patient should have a surgical consult; however, the timing of surgery will depend on the severity of symptoms and the patient's overall risk of undergoing surgery.

7.1 (d) Low FODMAP diet. Exclusion of small intestinal bacterial overgrowth by hydrogen and methane breath testing reduces the likelihood of response to antibiotic therapy such as ciprofloxacin and metronidazole. Rifaximin is also effective for small intestinal bacterial overgrowth as well as diarrhea-predominant IBS. Fat (including fat-soluble vitamins) malabsorption would also be evident if pancreatic insufficiency were present.

7.2 (d) Rice. Only rice and gluten-free wheat are 100% absorbed in healthy individuals.

8.1 (a) Nasogastric tube suctioning, discontinuation of narcotics and other potential exacerbating drugs, and correction of potential electrolyte disturbances. Neostigmine has been shown in controlled clinical trials to relieve symptoms and reduce colonic distension but should be reserved for patients in whom conservative measures have failed to improve symptoms.

8.2 (d) Surgery. Complete small intestinal obstruction should be treated surgically. Water-soluble contrast enemas are useful to rule out distal colonic obstruction and may be able to induce catharsis in patients with pseudo-obstruction but are not useful for small intestinal obstructive disease. Colonic decompression will not alleviate acute obstruction and neostigmine is contraindicated in acute small intestinal obstruction.

8.3 (a) Neostigmine. Although colonoscopic decompression is a viable alternative, the use of neostigmine in a patient without cardiovascular or other contraindications is less invasive and has proven of benefit in reducing distension and other symptoms.

9.1 (c) Anorectal manometry. Anorectal manometry, especially when coupled with a balloon expulsion test, can identify pelvic floor dyssynergia, which is the likely etiology of this patient's symptoms of "incomplete evacuation."

Colonic transit tests may be abnormal in defecatory disorders as well as slow colonic transit (colonic inertia). For this reason, assessment of colonic transit is recommended only after excluding a defecatory disorder. In this age group, malignancy and other structural lesions are unlikely; therefore, CT scans are rarely useful. Colonoscopy is likewise unlikely to identify the source of constipation, and biopsies would need to be full thickness in order to rule out Hirshsprung disease.

9.2 (c) Biofeedback has been demonstrated to reduce symptoms and improve physiology of patients with dyssynergic defecation. The principal focus is improved relaxation of the anal sphincter during defecation and improved pushing forces. Neither myotomy or botulinum injections to the sphincter lead to improvement in the majority of patients.

10.1 (b) Fecal α1-antitrypsin clearance. This patient has SLE and a protein-losing enteropathy. Protein-losing enteropathies may be primary, due to ulcerative (inflammatory bowel disease, *H. pylori* gastritis, gastrointestinal malignancy) or nonulcerative (Menetrier disease, parasitic infection, cystic fibrosis, eosinophilic gastroenteritis, celiac disease, SLE) enteropathies, or secondary to increased lymphatic hydrostatic pressure (mesenteric lymphatic obstruction, tuberculosis, sarcoidosis, lymphoma, intestinal lymphangiectasia, right heart failure). SLE is a well-documented etiology of protein-losing enteropathy resulting from epithelial leakage and lymphatic rupture. Treatment of protein-losing enteropathy in the setting of SLE includes steroids, cyclosporine, azathioprine for immunosuppression, plus octreotide to reduce diarrhea. Cross-sectional imaging (CT or MRI) and octreotide scans are useful to identify tumors that cause secretory diarrhea. SeHCAT testing is used to detect bile acid diarrhea, which is also a secretory diarrhea that is not consistent with this patient's fecal electrolytes.

10.2 (a) Magnesium-containing laxatives. The stool electrolytes indicate the presence of unmeasured osmotically active molecules. 290 mOsm (plasma) – 2 × ([Na] + [K]) = 130 mOsm. VIP-secreting tumors cause secretory diarrhea, as does senna ingestion. IBS does not cause osmotic diarrhea.

10.3 (b) *Bacillus cereus*. *Campylobacter* and *Shigella* would not present within hours of ingestion of the infected food. Enterotoxigenic *E. coli* is typically found in undercooked meat, whereas *B. cereus* most often occurs in the setting of cooked rice that is reheated (as is commonly used for fried rice).

11.1 (d) EUS FNA. The mass described in the CT scan is likely to represent a subepithelial mass that will require EUS to image and also to perform EUS-guided FNA of the lesion for a tissue diagnosis. EGD and upper GI series are unlikely to provide any additional information, and endoscopic imaging of the lesion can be performed at the time of EUS.

11.2 (b) False. Although the clinical presentation is consistent with pancreatic cancer, an elevated CA 19-9 can be seen in benign lesions in the presence of biliary obstruction as well as cholangiocarcinoma, which can present similarly. Furthermore, CA 19-9 should not be used to establish the diagnosis of pancreatic cancer; however, it can be a useful marker to monitor patients following surgery or response to chemotherapy. The baseline CA 19-9 should be established after the biliary system has been decompressed.

12.1 (c) Low cholesterol levels. Patients with prolonged cholestasis typically develop hypercholesterolemia, in addition to fat-soluble vitamin deficiency, bone density loss, and pruritus.

12.2 (b) Reduced activity of UGT. UGT is the hepatic enzyme responsible for bilirubin conjugation. Breast milk jaundice is due to the presence of a UGT inhibitor in breast milk. Lucey–Driscoll syndrome is due to a UGT inhibitor in the mother's blood. Physiological neonatal jaundice reflects inadequate UGT activity in many newborns, which typically improves by day 14 of life.

12.3 (c) Development of gallstones. In critically ill patients, hyperbilirubinemia can persist despite improvement of the underlying illness. With prolonged jaundice, circulating bilirubin may bind covalently to albumin, which prevents its elimination until the albumin is degraded. Conjugated bilirubin is cleared by renal glomeruli, and bilirubin levels may increase in renal failure. Total parenteral nutrition causes hyperbilirubinemia as a result of intrahepatic cholestasis. Although gallstones are a common cause of extrahepatic jaundice in the United States and can be caused by TPN use, they are less likely to be a cause of persistent jaundice in an ICU patient.

12.4 (d) Anti-smooth muscle antibodies may be present in up to 50% of PBC patients. Anti-LKM antibodies are associated with aggressive autoimmune hepatitis in young women. Antimitochondrial antibody is positive in approximately 90% of patients with primary biliary cholangitis.

12.5 (b) Although a disease of copper overload, the total serum copper (which includes the copper incorporated in ceruloplasmin) in Wilson disease is usually decreased in proportion to the decreased ceruloplasmin in the circulation. In patients with severe liver injury, total serum copper may be within the normal range, regardless of whether serum ceruloplasmin levels are elevated or not. In acute liver failure due to Wilson disease, levels of total serum copper are very elevated due to sudden release of copper from liver tissue. Normal or elevated serum copper, with decreased ceruloplasmin, indicates an increase in copper that is not bound to ceruloplasmin (nonceruloplasmin-bound copper, or "free copper"). Although assessment of nonceruloplasmin-bound copper may have utility for monitoring response to treatment in Wilson disease, its use as a diagnostic test for Wilson disease is dubious, particularly because the validity of the assessment is highly dependent upon the adequacy of the laboratory methods for measuring serum copper and ceruloplasmin.

12.6 (c) Wilson disease is typically associated with a low alkaline phosphatase level, with an elevated bilirubin to alkaline phosphatase ratio. PBC is a cholestatic liver disorder, with impaired bilirubin excretion and alkaline phosphatase elevation. PSC and cholangiocarcinoma can result in bile duct obstruction, with alkaline phosphatase elevation.

13.1 (d) Glucose. Routine analysis of ascites fluid should include total protein, albumin, and total cell count with differential. Ascites fluid may also be sent for culture (the highest yield occurring when the ascites fluid is inoculated into blood culture bottles at the bedside), if infection is suspected. Glucose should not be routinely checked in an initial evaluation of ascitic fluid, although it may be used when evaluating for secondary peritonitis.

13.2 (c) Congestive heart failure. Congestive heart failure is typically associated with high SAAG, high protein ascites.

13.3 (c) Increase diuretic doses. The development of HRS is a severe complication that can develop in patients with ascites. Management includes holding diuretics, providing intravenous albumin, potential use of octreotide and midodrine, and consideration of TIPS and/or liver transplantation. Increasing the dose of diuretics may only worsen renal function and impair renal perfusion further.

14.1 (b) Hyporeflexia. Hyperreflexia, as opposed to hyporeflexia, is typically seen in patients with hypocalcemia.

14.2 (c) 2100–2800 kcal. Healthy adults require 20–25 kcal/kg of body weight to satisfy daily caloric requirements. With the stress of disease or surgery, this need increases to 30–40 kcal/kg/day.

14.3 (c) In one to seven days. TPN should be initiated in one to seven days in patients requiring TPN who are catabolic and/or malnourished.

15.1 (c) Evaluation of suspected perforated duodenal ulcer. Endoscopy is contraindicated in the setting of any gastrointestinal perforation.

15.2 (b) Coumadin should be held for five to seven days prior to the procedure, and low molecular weight heparin should be administered until the night prior to the scheduled procedure. The patient is undergoing endoscopy for evaluation and management of solid food dysphagia with the potential of having a dilation performed. A dilation is considered a high-risk procedure for potential bleeding; therefore, anticoagulation with coumadin should be held five to seven days prior to the scheduled procedure. Bridge therapy with low molecular weight heparin should be administered while the coumadin is being held because a mechanical valve in the mitral position is considered a high-risk condition for a thromboembolic event.

16.1 (c) Gastroesophageal acid reflux. High-amplitude contractions (>180 mmHg) were proposed as a common etiology of noncardiac chest pain; however, this finding is common among asymptomatic persons and poorly correlated with symptoms of chest pain. Diffuse esophageal spasm and achalasia, which are characterized by aperistalsis of the esophageal body, can be associated with pain but more commonly present with dysphagia. Gastroesophageal reflux disease is the most common etiology of noncardiac chest pain and should be empirically treated or evaluated.

16.2 (c) Absent contractility. The Chicago Classification using high-resolution esophageal pressure topography defines classic (type I) achalasia as an IRP ≥ 15 mmHg and absent contractility. Type II achalasia with esophageal compression is associated with an IRP ≥15 mmHg and at least 20% of swallows with pan-esophageal pressurization to >30 mmHg. Type III (spastic) achalasia has an IRP ≥15 mmHg and premature esophageal contractions in ≥20% of swallows, with latency between upper esophageal sphincter relaxation and distal esophageal contraction <4.5 seconds. Increased contractions is not a feature of achalasia.

16.3 (a) Oropharyngeal dysphagia is most often the result of cerebrovascular accidents. The other etiologies can cause oropharyngeal dysphagia but are much less common.

17.1 (e) Increased heartburn upon discontinuation of PPI. Heartburn has been shown to occur after discontinuation of PPIs, presumably due to gastrin-induced hypertrophy of parietal cells. Whereas associations have been noted between PPI use and *C. difficile* infection, pneumonia, bone fracture, and hypomagnesemia, these associations, if true, are very rare.

17.2 (b) Functional heartburn. Excessive acid production is extremely rare and is associated with gastrin-producing tumors (gastrinoma). Nonacid reflux is the etiology of symptoms in a minority of patients nonresponsive to PPIs. Alkaline reflux occurs after surgery that allows reflux of duodenal contents into the stomach and esophagus but is a less frequent cause of refractory heartburn than functional disease.

17.3 (a) Normal. This is the most common endoscopic finding, even among patients with documented GERD. A minority of symptomatic patients have erosive disease, and 5–15% of patients with heartburn have Barrett esophagus. Strictures occur but in a small minority of patients.

17.4 (d) Dairy, soy, wheat, egg, nuts, shellfish. These six food groups are most often implicated in the genesis of eosinophilic esophagitis, and elimination of these from the diet of patients with eosinophilic esophagitis has been shown to normalize the esophageal inflammation and reduce dysphagia. A low FODMAP diet reduces fructans, galactans, fructose, and polyols and has been shown to reduce symptoms of IBS. Prebiotics including inulins, oligofructose, lactulose, and galacto-oligosaccharides have been suggested to improve a variety of diseases including inflammatory bowel disease; however, their use is not advocated until appropriately designed and powered studies prove their efficacy.

18.1 (d) Intestinal metaplasia of the esophagus. Esophageal adenocarcinoma is significantly more common among individuals with the following characteristics: white race, male sex, advanced age, GERD, and Barrett esophagus (intestinal metaplasia of the esophagus). Alcohol is not a risk factor, and although smoking is associated with cancer, it is not as strong a predictor as the other variables. Caucasians are more likely than non-Caucasians to develop Barrett esophagus and esophageal adenocarcinoma; however, intestinal metaplasia is a stronger risk factor and the only known precursor to esophageal adenocarcinoma

18.2 (d) Endoscopic resection of visible lesions followed by ablation of flat Barrett mucosa. Current guidelines for management of Barrett esophagus with high-grade dysplasia recommend endoscopic eradication therapy consisting of removal of any visible lesions (nodules, masses, ulceration) using mucosal resection or submucosal dissection followed by radiofrequency ablation or photodynamic therapy of the remaining Barrett esophagus. Patients refusing endoscopic therapy may undergo surveillance. Esophagectomy is reserved for patients with cancer. A recent randomized clinical trial demonstrated that chemoprevention with high-dose PPI (esomeprazole 80 mg daily) plus aspirin among individuals with Barrett esophagus without dysplasia reduced progression to high-grade dysplasia or cancer; however, this intervention has not been studied as treatment for high-grade dysplasia.

18.3 (c) Alcohol. The primary risk factors for ESCC include African-American race, alcohol, smoking, and male sex. These factors are different from those associated with esophageal adenocarcinoma (see question 18.1).

19.1 (d) The four-hours assessment of gastric emptying after ingestion of a solid radiolabeled meal is most accurate for diagnosing gastroparesis.

19.2 (b) Venting gastrostomy and feeding jejunostomy. This intervention has been illustrated to provide adequate symptom relief for patients with gastroparesis refractory to medical therapy. Although gastric electrical stimulation using high-frequency, low-energy pulses may reduce symptoms in patients with gastroparesis, gastric pacing (low-frequency, high energy pulses) is rarely effective in improving gastric emptying or symptoms. Total parenteral nutrition is an option but should be reserved for patients in whom all other alternatives have been examined due to the severe adverse events associated with this intervention. Total gastrectomy and other surgical options have had generally disappointing results.

19.3 (c) Octreotide delays gastric emptying and prevents the accelerated emptying seen in dumping syndrome. In addition, octreotide inhibits release of many of the enteric hormones and insulin secretion that play a role in symptom development. Rifaximin is approved for treatment of diarrhea-predominant IBS but has not been demonstrated to benefit patients with dumping syndrome. Omeprazole and glucose control with insulin have also not been established as effective treatment.

20.1 (b) Acid suppression. The most common etiology of elevated gastrin among patients presenting with recurrent peptic ulcer disease is acid suppression, usually due to PPI therapy. Acid is the most potent suppressor of gastrin production, and in the face of PPI therapy, gastrin elevations are common. Gastrinoma produces hypergastrinemia, but this is a rare tumor. Gastric atrophy associated with pernicious anemia is also associated with gastrin elevations, but this is not common in young patients.

20.2 (c) Gastric fluid pH. pH testing of gastric secretions is the most expeditious method of ruling out gastrinoma. Gastric pH will be acid (low) if hypergastrinemia is due to gastrinoma; however, causes of elevated gastrin due to hypochlorhydria (PPI use, atrophic gastritis) will reveal a relatively neutral pH. Secretin stimulation and acid output testing are useful to confirm the diagnosis of gastrinoma but require specialized equipment not as readily available as pH paper. Serum chromogranin A is a diagnostic test for gastrinoma but is not as expeditious as simply checking the gastric acidity.

20.3 (b) Bismuth, metronidazole, and tetracycline. The issue is antibiotic resistance, especially with the clarithromycin regimens. Although sequential therapy has excellent results, these are somewhat geographically disparate, and US trials have not observed the same rates of eradication as non-US studies. A regimen of clarithromycin and metronidazole plus PPI has excellent eradication results, but in treatment failures it is recommended to change clarithromycin to another agent. Quadruple therapy consisting of four times daily bismuth, metronidazole, and tetracycline (or doxycycline) with twice-daily PPI is an effective salvage regimen after failure of triple therapy.

20.4 (c) CT scan of the abdomen. The most likely diagnosis is perforated upper intestinal viscus due to peptic ulcer. Although the patient presented with evidence of hemodynamically significant upper gastrointestinal bleeding, there is no evidence of continued gastrointestinal hemorrhage; therefore, endoscopy is not emergent. The abdominal rebound tenderness with elevated WBC is worrisome for perforation, which can be detected by CT scan and would be a contraindication for endoscopy. Colonoscopy is useful to identify and treat colonic bleeding from vascular ectasias or diverticular disease, which can present as melena; however, the more urgent evaluation is to rule out perforation.

21.1 (b) *Helicobacter pylori* testing with eradication if positive. The patient is young and has no alarm features, making malignancy extremely unlikely. Testing and treatment, if needed, for *H. pylori* infection is a reasonable first step in her management. If the background prevalence of *H. pylori* infection is low, empiric acid suppression with PPIs would also be a reasonable first step. Upper endoscopy is not necessary in this case due to the low risk of malignancy or other serious organic disease. CT scans are rarely diagnostic in patients with dyspepsia without alarm features, especially with normal laboratory testing.

21.2 (a) Normal. The most likely diagnosis is functional dyspepsia, with which a normal examination is likely. Duodenal and gastric ulcers are generally associated with *H. pylori* infection and/or NSAIDs; therefore, they are of low probability in this patient. Erosive esophagitis is possible but unlikely if PPIs fail to alleviate symptoms. Gastric malignancy is unlikely in this age group and without alarm features.

21.3 (d) Trial of a tricyclic antidepressant. Reassurance and a supportive therapeutic relationship are important steps, and further investigation is unlikely to identify a structural cause of her symptoms. Tricyclic antidepressants can be effective at relieving symptoms in a patients with functional dyspepsia. Therapy should be initiated at a low dose with gradual dose titration as needed for management of symptoms and avoidance of side effects.

21.4 (e) Upper endoscopy. The patient is at an age where upper gastrointestinal malignancy is a concern. He also presents with alarm symptoms (i.e. unintentional weight loss) and has a high-risk ethnic background for gastric cancer. Therefore, upper endoscopy should be performed to exclude malignancy. Testing and treating for *H. pylori* or empiric PPI therapy is not appropriate due to his age and high-risk features. Abdominal CT or ultrasound have lower sensitivity for gastric malignancy than upper endoscopy.

21.5 (a) Relaxation of the gastric fundus. Buspirone may cause relaxation of the gastric fundus, and limited data suggest it may be helpful in patients with symptoms of early satiety and postprandial fullness. Buspirone does not modulate visceral hypersensitivity, accelerate gastric emptying, or affect gastric acid secretion.

22.1 (c) Tumor with mucosal ulceration and GI bleeding. GISTs often present clinically with GI bleeding and are found to have an overlying ulcer on EGD. The presence of an ulcer is generally associated with a larger tumor; however, the presence of an ulcer with GI bleeding is not necessarily a high-risk feature. Biopsy of the ulcer base should be performed if active bleeding is not present as it often will result in sufficient diagnostic tissue.

22.2 (c) CT. A CT scan should be performed once the diagnosis of gastric cancer is made to evaluate for metastatic disease. If metastatic disease is identified on CT scan, an EUS is not necessary because local/regional staging will not have an impact on overall stage of the disease (stage IV disease). If there is no evidence of metastatic disease on CT scan, then an EUS should be performed for local/regional staging.

23.1 (c) Buckwheat does not contain gluten and can be eaten in a gluten-free diet. Other safe grains include amaranth, corn, millet, quinoa, and sorghum. Oats appear to be safe for most patients with celiac disease. Grains that should be avoided include wheat, rye, and barley (including malt).

23.2 (d) Anti-gliadin antibodies. Anti-gliadin antibodies have lower specificity and sensitivity for celiac disease than newer tests including anti-tissue transglutaminase, anti-endomysial, and anti-deamidated gliadin peptide antibodies (a different test than anti-gliadin antibodies). Therefore, they are no longer recommended in the diagnostic evaluation. Total IgA may be assessed because up to 5% of celiac disease patients may be IgA deficient, leading to a false-negative IgA test. Positive serologic tests should be confirmed by small bowel biopsy showing characteristic histology with intraepithelial lymphocytosis and villous blunting.

23.3 (d) Levels of celiac-specific antibodies will gradually return to normal with a strict gluten-free diet, and histology will gradually normalize. However, some patients will continue to have intraepithelial lymphocytosis (Marsh 1) despite a gluten-free diet. The mainstay of treatment is a gluten-free diet, and histologic findings may be milder than expected if gluten is restricted at the time of initial diagnostic evaluation. The prevalence of celiac disease is higher in patients with Down syndrome than in the general population.

23.4 (d) *Campylobacter jejuni* infection. Duodenal villous flattening can be seen with some intestinal infections such as *Giardia lamblia* or norovirus but not with *C. jejuni*, which more typically causes an acute self-limited colitis. Crohn's disease, small intestinal bacterial overgrowth, intestinal lymphoma, and eosinophilic enteritis can all produce villous flattening and must be differentiated from celiac disease.

23.5 (a) Inadvertent or ongoing gluten ingestion. Inadvertent gluten ingestion is common due to the ubiquitous presence in foods and should be excluded in patients with persistent gastrointestinal symptoms. Other causes of diarrhea such as Crohn's disease or pancreatic insufficiency are much less common. Type I and type II refractory sprue also cause persistent gastrointestinal symptoms but are much less common than ongoing gluten intake.

24.1 **(d)** Cholestyramine. The most likely diagnosis is bile-salt-associated diarrhea. The amount of terminal ileum resected reduces the reabsorption of bile leading to excess bile exposure to the colon, causing a secretory diarrhea that may be treated using a bile sequestrate such as cholestyramine. Laboratory testing (CRP and fecal calprotectin) and imaging are not consistent with active Crohn's disease that would be amenable to treatment with prednisone or vedolizumab. Oral vancomycin would be appropriate for *C. difficile* infection. Teduglutide, a recombinant GLP-2 analogue, is indicated for short bowel syndrome; however, the absence of steatorrhea makes this diagnosis less likely than bile-associated diarrhea.

24.2 (a) Calcium oxalate. Hyperoxaluria is due to increased absorption of dietary oxalate, particularly in the colon. Steatorrhea causes an increase in luminal fatty acids, which preferentially bind to calcium, leaving oxalate that is readily absorbed in the colon. Note that oxalate stones would not be increased if this patient also had a colectomy.

24.3 (d) D-lactic acidemia. D-lactic acid is derived from malabsorbed fermentable carbohydrates that are metabolized by colonic lactobacilli to D-lactic acid. The clinical syndrome consists of encephalopathy and lactic acidosis with compensatory hyperventilation. It is acknowledged that if the cookie exchange also included an open bar, answer (b) could also be correct.

24.4 (b) Medium-chain triglycerides. Medium-chain triglycerides are absorbed in the absence of bile salts and do not require resynthesis in the enterocyte. Both short- and long-chain triglycerides require micelle formation that is facilitated by bile salts, which are deficient in short bowel syndrome.

25.1 (c) Side-viewing upper endoscopy. Patients with FAP are at increased risk for developing ampullary adenomas/adenocarcinomas. Therefore, side-viewing upper endoscopy should be performed every one to two years to examine the major papilla and duodenum for the development of adenomas. Double balloon enteroscopy and CT scans are not recommended for surveillance purposes. Standard upper endoscopy may also be performed for careful evaluation of the stomach; however, adequate visualization of the major papilla can be difficult with a forward-viewing endoscope.

25.2 (c) Urinary 5-HIAA. Carcinoid tumors produce and release serotonin, which is then metabolized to 5-HIAA. Carcinoid syndrome typically occurs in patients who have metastatic disease to the liver; therefore, a liver function panel (AST, ALT, alkaline phosphatase, bilirubin) should be ordered. However, abnormal liver enzymes alone will not support the diagnosis of carcinoid syndrome.

26.1 (d) The majority of patients with diverticulosis do not develop complications such as diverticulitis or diverticular bleeding. Although diverticula are more common in the sigmoid colon, diverticular bleeding more commonly originates from the proximal colon. However, diverticulitis is more common in the sigmoid colon. Barium enema is not indicated during an acute attack of diverticulitis, and consumption of seeds, nuts, or corn is not associated with development of diverticulitis.

26.2 (b) Peritonitis. Most diverticular abscesses can be managed by percutaneous drainage, but surgery may be indicated if percutaneous drainage is not possible or fails. Recurrent uncomplicated diverticulitis is not an indication for surgery. Although patients often have persistent low-grade symptoms after an initial attack of diverticulitis, surgery is not needed unless symptoms are severe and intractable. Partial obstruction during acute episodes of diverticulitis will often resolve with treatment and is not an indication for surgery.

26.3 (b) False. Most patients with diverticulosis are asymptomatic. There is some controversy as to whether or not uncomplicated diverticulosis can cause symptoms, which is termed *symptomatic uncomplicated diverticular disease*.

26.4 (d) Fever (temperature of 38 °C). Patients with complicated diverticulitis (e.g. abscess, fistula) or those with risk factors for treatment failure (e.g. immunosuppression, severe comorbidity) should be treated as inpatients. Patients with low-grade fevers but uncomplicated disease and no risk factors for treatment failure can be treated as outpatients with close follow-up. Inpatient admission is indicated for patients who fail to improve after three to four days of adequate outpatient therapy.

26.5 (c) Obesity. Obesity, particularly central obesity, is a risk factor for development of diverticulitis. Other risk factors include low levels of physical activity, high red meat consumption, use of aspirin or nonsteroidal anti-inflammatory agents, and smoking. Use of calcium channel blockers or alcohol have not been associated with diverticulitis.

27.1 (a) Lubiprostone. Lubiprostone is a chloride channel activator that increases intestinal fluid secretion and facilitates intestinal transit. Dicyclomine is an antispasmodic with anticholinergic properties that can cause constipation. Alosetron is a 5-HT3 receptor antagonist and is indicated for women with diarrhea-predominant IBS. Tricyclic antidepressants can modulate pain perception and may be most beneficial in patients with diarrhea but can worsen constipation through their anticholinergic effects. Atropine with diphenoxylate is an antidiarrheal.

27.2 (c) Complete blood count. Initial evaluation of a patient with suspected IBS should focus on screening for organic disorders. This can usually be done with a complete blood count and C-reactive protein or sedimentation rate. Fecal fat quantification is not needed in most patients with IBS, and colonoscopy or abdominal CT imaging is not required in patients with symptoms consistent with IBS without alarm features. Colonic transit testing can be used in patients with refractory constipation but is not indicated in the initial evaluation.

27.3 (d) Tricyclic antidepressant. Tricyclic antidepressants at low doses can improve stool form and relieve abdominal pain in patients with diarrhea-predominant IBS. Linaclotide, tegaserod, and lubiprostone can be used to treat constipation-predominant IBS. However, tegaserod was withdrawn from the US market due to risk of ischemic colitis.

27.4 (b) Eluxadoline has combined mu-opioid receptor agonist activity with delta-opioid receptor *antagonist* (not agonist) activity. It is indicated for treatment of diarrhea-predominant IBS, where it improves stool consistency and relieves abdominal pain. It has been associated with risk for acute pancreatitis, particularly in patients with prior cholecystectomy. Therefore, prior cholecystectomy is a contraindication for its use.

27.5 (a) Massage therapy. There are not evidence-based studies supporting massage therapy for IBS. Mindfulness-based stress reduction, cognitive-behavioral therapy, biofeedback with relaxation training, and hypnotherapy have all been successfully used for this patient population.

28.1 (c) Stool examination for *C. difficile*. The incidence of *C. difficile*-associated disease is elevated in IBD compared to non-IBD controls and can manifest in the absence of antibiotic use. Evaluation to rule out this infection is mandatory prior to initiation of immunosuppressive therapy.

28.2 (e) Surgical intervention. Steroids, biologics, cyclosporine, and tofacitinib are effective in inducing remission for moderate to severe ulcerative colitis; however, this patient meets criteria for toxic megacolon with peritoneal signs and warrants immediate surgical evaluation.

28.3 (d) Calcium oxalate. Small intestinal malabsorption of fat increases fatty acid binding to calcium, which in turn increases colonic absorption of oxalate leading to hyperoxaluria. Malabsorption in the small intestine also increases bile salt exposure to the colon, increasing permeability to oxalate.

29.1 (e) Colonoscopy. Positive results on screening fecal immunochemical tests should be followed-up by diagnostic colonoscopy. Repeating the fecal immunochemical test is inappropriate. Abdominal/pelvic CT will not be able to detect smaller or flat polyps. CT colonography will not allow biopsy or removal of colonic neoplasia and is also less sensitive than colonoscopy for small or flat polyps. EGD is not recommended to follow-up an abnormal colorectal cancer screening test.

29.2 (d) Colonoscopy now with referral for genetics counseling. This patient's family history meets the Amsterdam II criteria for the diagnosis of hereditary nonpolyposis colorectal cancer (HNPCC) because he has three relatives with HNPCC-associated cancers (colorectal and endometrial), involving at least two successive generations, and at least one cancer was diagnosed before age 50. Ideally, genetic testing of his affected relatives could be done to identify which mismatch repair gene is affected. If the patient does carry a Lynch syndrome-associated mutation, then he would require annual colonoscopy. Annual FOBT and colonoscopy every 10 years are appropriate for average-risk individuals but not for patients with Lynch syndrome or a family history of colorectal cancer diagnosed at age less than 50 years. CT colonography every five years is also recommended by some for average-risk individuals but is not appropriate for high-risk individuals.

29.3 (e) None of the above. The US Preventive Services Task Force recommends against routine screening in individuals aged 76–85. If this patient was in good overall health, particularly if she had not been previously screened, then screening may be appropriate. However, given her negative colonoscopy 10 years ago, her risk for colorectal cancer is below average. In addition, she has significant comorbidity that limits the relative benefits of screening.

29.4 (b) Desmoid tumors are found in patients with Gardner's syndrome, a sub-type of familial adenomatous polyposis. Pancreatic adenocarcinoma can be seen in Lynch syndrome, whereas orocutaneous pigmentation is a feature of Peutz–Jeghers syndrome. Facial trichilemmomas can be seen in Cowden's syndrome.

29.5 (b) Sessile serrated polyps are premalignant. Sporadic juvenile or Peutz–Jeghers polyps do not have malignant potential. Hyperplastic polyps are extremely common and also lack premalignant potential. Inflammatory polyps that arise in the setting of chronic inflammation do not develop into malignancy.

30.1 (c) Most first- and second-degree hemorrhoids can be treated with conservative measures such as high-fiber diet, fluid intake, and good anal hygiene. Surgical hemorrhoidectomy is not required for most second-degree hemorrhoids. Third-degree hemorrhoids prolapse but can be digitally reduced. Thrombosed hemorrhoids can cause severe pain and bleeding.

30.2 (b) Anal fissure. Thrombosed external hemorrhoids can also present with severe pain and scant bleeding but are easily differentiated from an anal fissure on rectal exam. Internal hemorrhoids typically are not painful. Solitary rectal ulcer can cause rectal bleeding but is less likely to cause pain. Rectal prolapse can present with the sensation of prolapse and bleeding but is also less likely to cause pain.

30.3 (b) Solitary rectal ulcer. Common causes of fecal incontinence include obstetric trauma and rectal prolapse. Additionally, proctitis from any etiology (e.g. inflammatory bowel disease, radiation, infection) can lead to fecal incontinence, as can central or peripheral nervous system disorders.

30.4 (a) Levator ani syndrome is characterized by chronic, aching, pressure-like pain, with tenderness of the levator ani muscle on digital rectal exam. Pain may worsen with defecation or prolonged sitting. In contrast, the pain with proctalgia fugax tends to be more fleeting but intense. Patients with proctalgia fugax have prolonged asymptomatic periods between episodes. Coffee intake is not associated with exacerbations of levator ani syndrome but has been associated with pruritus ani.

30.5 (a) Most fissures are located in the posterior or anterior midline. Fissures that are not in the midline require further evaluation to exclude Crohn's disease, malignancy, or infection. The diagnosis can be confirmed by physical examination. Anoscopy is not needed and is often poorly tolerated due to pain. Initial therapy should include high-fiber diet, topical anesthetics, and warm sitz baths. Topical corticosteroids play a limited role in therapy. Botulinum toxin injection can be used if conservative therapy or topical vasodilators such as nifedipine or nitroglycerin are not effective.

31.1 (a) Immediate-release enzymes (nonenteric coated) have been shown to be effective in the treatment of chronic pancreatitis pain in a randomized controlled trial. However, immediate-release enzymes were recently taken off the market by the FDA and are currently not available in the United States.

31.2 (b) Once the prediction of severe acute pancreatitis is made. Early initiation of enteral feeding in patients with severe acute pancreatitis has been demonstrated to decrease the risk of infection and decrease hospital stay, with a trend toward improving mortality.

31.3 (c) Higher concentration of CCK and secretin-secreting cells in the duodenum. Because there is a higher concentration of CCK and secretin-secreting cells in the duodenum, there is a theoretical advantage of bypassing this segment of bowel for enteral nutrition because feeding into the duodenum would stimulate release of CCK and secretin, resulting in increased stimulation of the pancreas.

31.4 (b) Shortly after presentation for mild acute pancreatitis, delayed days to weeks after presentation for severe acute pancreatitis. The guidelines for performing surgery in patients with acute biliary pancreatitis depend on the severity. For mild gallstone pancreatitis, laparoscopic cholecystectomy should be performed as soon as the patient has recovered and during the same hospital admission. In patients with severe gallstone pancreatitis, cholecystectomy should be delayed until there is a sufficient resolution of the inflammatory response and clinical recovery.

31.5 (a) Pseudo-cyst size greater than 6 cm. Size alone is not a sufficient reason to perform pseudo-cyst drainage. The decision to perform pseudo-cyst drainage should be based on symptoms or evidence of infection.

32.1 (d) EUS FNA. EUS FNA is the best method for obtaining tissue for diagnosis of pancreatic cancer. CA 19-9 can be useful for following response to therapy if elevated at the time of diagnosis; however, it should not be used to establish the diagnosis.

32.2 (d) 70%.

32.3 (b) Mucinous cystadenoma. The findings of an elevated CEA >200 ng/dl, low amylase, and no duct abnormalities on EUS examination suggest the diagnosis of mucinous cystadenoma. Theses lesions do have potential for malignant transformation and should either be resected or monitored closely. Mucinous cystadenomas almost exclusively occur in females.

33.1 (b) Klatskin tumor.

33.2 (d) Hypertriglyceridemia. Ulcerative colitis, Sjögren's syndrome, and osteopenia are associated with primary sclerosing cholangitis.

33.3 (e) Type V. Type V cysts are characterized by one or more cystic dilations of the intrahepatic ducts, without extrahepatic duct dilation. If multiple cystic dilations are present, then the disease is known as *Caroli disease*.

33.4 (c) Hypotension. The Charcot triad consists of RUQ abdominal pain, fever, and jaundice and is suggestive for cholangitis. The presence of hypotension and confusion added to the Charcot triad yields the Reynolds pentad, which is suggestive of a more fulminant course.

33.5 (d) None of the above. Despite the history of a proposed classification system for SOD as Types I, II, and III, data have shown that the patients previously categorized as Type III SOD (pain with normal liver enzymes and normal biliary imaging) do not respond to sphincterotomy, and the Type III classification of SOD does not actually exist.

34.1 False. A vigorous immune response is responsible for an aggressive clinical hepatitis but also is more likely to result in clearance of the virus.

34.2 (c) HBsAg is present beyond six months. Hepatitis B core antibody, regardless of class, may be present with acute, chronic, and resolved hepatitis B. The persistence of HBsAg beyond six months is considered an indication of chronic infection.

34.3 (c) Hepatitis E virus, which typically causes a self-limited infection after fecal–oral exposure, is associated with a high rate (15–25%) of fulminant hepatitis in women during the third trimester of pregnancy.

35.1 (b) An HII of 2.0 is suggestive of hemochromatosis. It is important to note, however, that although HII was used in the past to support a diagnosis of hereditary hemochromatosis (when HII was >1.9), the availability of genetic testing (HFE gene testing) has demonstrated that phenotypic expression of homozygosity can occur at a much lower HII, and thus, the HII should no longer be routinely used for a diagnosis of hereditary hemochromatosis. It is estimated that 15–20% of NASH patients may progress to advanced fibrosis/cirrhosis. The peak onset of Wilson disease is in the second decade of life. Kayser–Fleischer rings are not always present in Wilson disease, although they are commonly present in the setting of neurological involvement.

35.2 (d) Ursodiol. Penicillamine and trientine are chelators of copper. Zinc inhibits copper absorption from the gut, and therefore is not used to manage pre-existing copper overload but rather for maintenance after copper depletion. There is no role for ursodiol in the treatment of Wilson disease.

35.3 (d) Bile ductular proliferation. The characteristic histological features of NASH are steatosis, hepatocyte ballooning degeneration, lobular inflammation, pericellular fibrosis, and Mallory hyaline, with unremarkable bile ducts.

36.1 (d) All of the above. HELLP syndrome and acute fatty liver of pregnancy are two severe illnesses that can present with cholestasis during the third trimester. Cholestasis of pregnancy and placental release of alkaline phosphatase follow a benign course.

36.2 (c) Dilated bile ducts on ultrasound. Positive AMA and elevated IgM levels are the classic serological findings in PBC. The classic histological findings of PBC are small bile duct destruction with florid duct lesions, often with noncaseating granulomas. Imaging studies are not expected to show biliary dilation in PBC.

36.3 (b) The appropriate dose of ursodiol in PBC is approximately 15 mg/kg, not 5 mg/kg. PBC patients are likely to be deficient in fat-soluble vitamins and to have reduced bone density, so the routine use of calcium and vitamin D supplementation is appropriate.

37.1 (c) The typical pattern in alcoholic hepatitis is AST>ALT, with values under 300 IU/l. Although most patients admitted to the hospital with alcoholic hepatitis have disease that has progressed to cirrhosis, portal hypertension can exist without cirrhosis. Continued alcohol use is associated with a higher mortality.

37.2 (b) Lymphocytic inflammation. The inflammation on liver biopsy in alcoholic hepatitis is predominantly neutrophilic.

37.3 (c) Patients with alcoholic hepatitis benefit from alcohol cessation, regardless of disease severity.

38.1 (a) Liver biopsy plays a very important role in confirming the diagnosis of AIH. Patients with type 2 AIH are unlikely (<5%) to have a positive ANA. The absence of viral hepatitis and the presence of IgG elevation increase the likelihood of the diagnosis of AIH, with additional points provided in the diagnostic scoring systems.

38.2 (c) Moderate (2–3+) iron staining is commonly seen on liver biopsy in AIH patients. The histological findings of AIH are not specific and can overlap with those seen in viral and drug-induced liver disease. Bridging necrosis is not uncommon in those with severe hepatitis on presentation. The inflammatory cells typically seen on biopsy in AIH are lymphocytes and plasma cells.

39.1 (c) Type 1 HRS is more severe than type 2 HRS. Type 1 HRS is the more severe form of HRS and is typically irreversible without liver transplantation. It is associated with intrarenal vasoconstriction. Above an HVPG of 12, higher values do not correlate well with additional bleeding risk. Portopulmonary hypertension is due to pulmonary vascular vasoconstriction, whereas hepatopulmonary syndrome is related to intrapulmonary shunting.

39.2 (c) Atenolol. Nonselective β-blockers, such as propranolol, carvedilol, or nadolol, are recommended for variceal prophylaxis against bleeding.

40.1 (b) HCC affects men more than women, with a ratio of greater than 2:1. HCC can occur in patients with chronic hepatitis B without cirrhosis. 90% of patients with HCC do have underlying cirrhosis. HCC is the third leading cause of cancer mortality worldwide.

40.2 (b) HCC remains enhancing in portal and delayed phases of multiphase CT or MRI. HCCs typically show "washout" of contrast on portal and delayed images, resulting in a hypodense appearance.

40.3 (c) A patient with a 3 cm HCC can receive priority for liver transplantation. Patients with HCC within "Milan Criteria" (up to three lesions <3 cm or single lesion <5 cm) receive priority for liver transplant with MELD exception points. Only a minority of HCCs are resectable (5–20%), and the 5-year recurrence rates are approximately 50%. TACE can precipitate worsening liver function in patients with advanced liver disease, including those with high bilirubin.

41.1 (b) Stool culture is not able to distinguish between toxigenic and nonpathogenic strains of *C. difficile*, and therefore cannot differentiate asymptomatic carriers from patients with colitis. Although endoscopic evaluation is usually not necessary in the diagnosis and evaluation of *C. difficile* infection, findings of pseudo-membranes are suggestive of the infection.

41.2 (d) Antibiotics are not recommended for this infection because they do not diminish the duration of symptoms or prevent complications, and they may increase the risk of developing hemolytic uremic syndrome.

41.3 (b) Although it can be challenging to do so, *C. jejuni* can be isolated from stool culture.

42.1 (a) Ulcerated lesion with a pigmented protuberance. This is consistent with an ulcer and not a Dieulafoy lesion.

42.2 (c) TIPS. Although GAVE can be seen in the setting of portal hypertension, TIPS is generally not effective in managing bleeding due to GAVE. APC is the preferred method of treatment due to the noncontact electrocoagulation and ease of use, although bipolar electrocautery and laser therapy are effective alternatives.

43.1 (d) Both a and c. Bariatric surgery should be considered for patients with a BMI ≥40 or BMI 35–39.9 with a serious comorbidity who have not met weight loss goals with lifestyle modifications and drug therapy.

43.2 (c) Biliopancreatic diversion with duodenal switch.

Index

Yamada's Handbook of Gastroenterology, Fourth Edition. John M. Inadomi, Renuka Bhattacharya, Joo Ha Hwang, and Cynthia Ko.

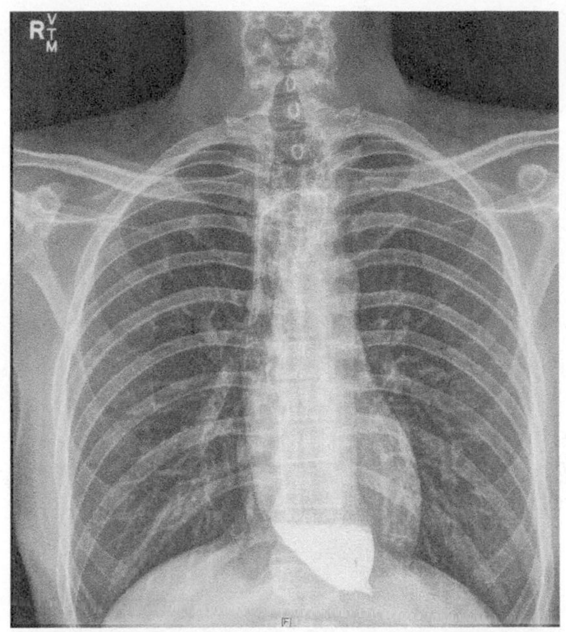

Chapter 16 Achalasia: barium esophagram demonstrating "bird's beak" at esophagogastric junction characteristic of achalasia.

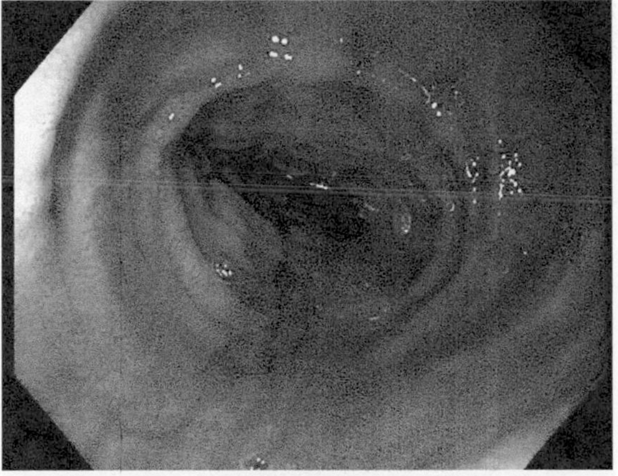

Chapter 17 Eosinophilic esophagitis: concentric rings and linear furrows.

Yamada's Handbook of Gastroenterology, Fourth Edition. John M. Inadomi, Renuka Bhattacharya, Joo Ha Hwang, and Cynthia Ko.

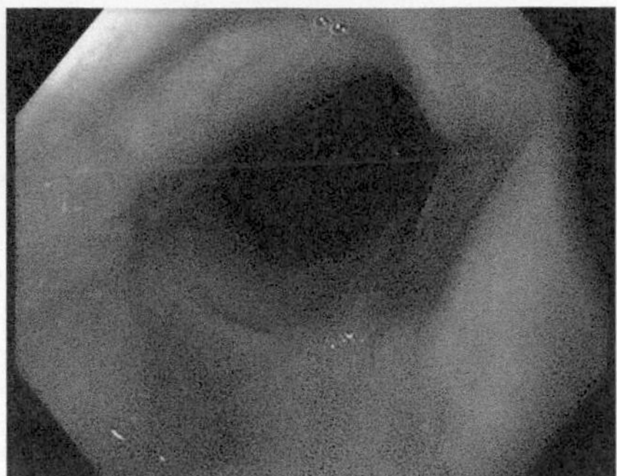

Chapter 17 Esophagitis: erythema of the distal esophagus due to gastroesophageal reflux.

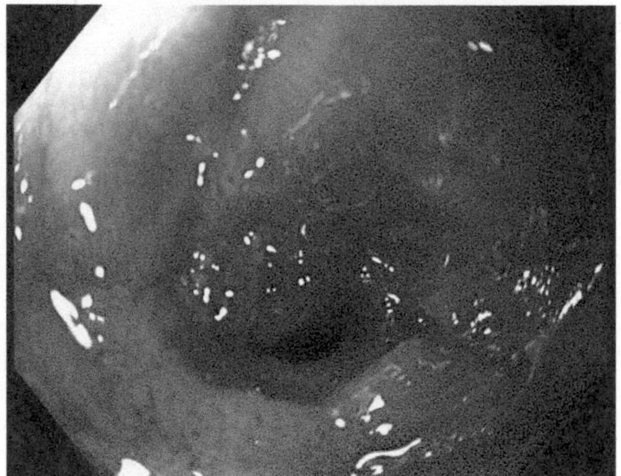

Chapter 17 Esophageal stricture: fibrous narrowing of the distal esophagus due to gastroesophageal reflux.

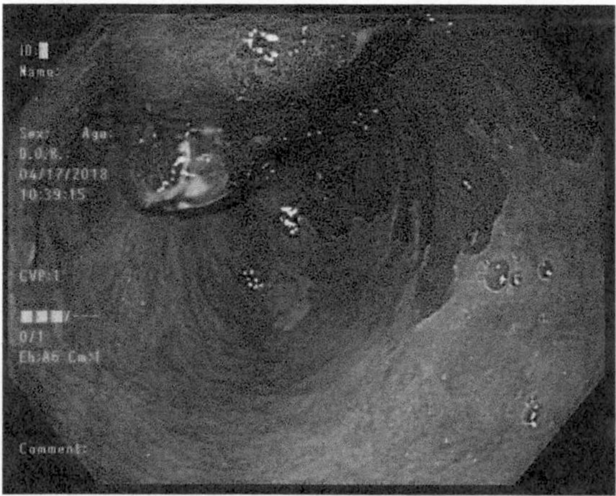

Chapter 18 Esophageal cancer: endoscopic view of esophageal adenocarcinoma.